ESSENTIALS OF

# Clinical Examination

## HANDBOOK
### Eighth Edition

**Editors-in-Chief:**

Yuhao Shi, BSc

Zahra Sohani, MSc, PhD

Brandon Tang, BSc

Florentina Teoderascu, MD, HBHSc

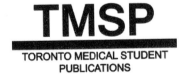

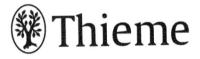

Toronto Medical Student Publications
Toronto, Ontario, Canada

Thieme
New York · Stuttgart · Delhi · Rio de Janeiro

*Essentials of Clinical Examination Handbook, Eighth Edition*, Copyright © 2017 Toronto Medical Student Publications

Editors:
Yuhao Shi
Zahra Sohani
Brandon Tang
Florentina Teoderascu

Cover Design: Wendy Gu

Thieme Publishers (www.thieme.com) is the exclusive worldwide distributor of Essentials of Clinical *Examination Handbook, Eighth Edition*.

In the Americas:
Thieme Publishers New York
333 Seventh Avenue
New York, NY 10001
United States of America
Email: customerservice@thieme.com
Tel: +1 800-782-3488 (Toll-free in US only)
Tel: +1-212-760-0888
Fax: +1-21 2-947-01 08

In Europe, Asia, Africa, and Australia:
Thieme Publishers Stuttgart
P.O. Box 30 11 20
70469 Stuttgart, Germany
Email: customerservice@thieme.de
Tel: +49 711-8931-421
Fax: +49 711-8931-410

In India, Bangladesh, Pakistan, Nepal, Sri Lanka, and Bhutan:
Thieme Medical and Scientific Publishers Private Limited A-12, Second Floor
Sector 2
NOIDA-201301
Uttar Pradesh, India
Email: customerservice@thieme.in
Tel: +91 120 427 4461 to 4464
Fax: +91 120 427 4465

Essentials of Clinical Examination Handbook, Eighth Edition, is provided for the sole use of the purchaser. This book, including all parts thereof, is legally protected by copyright. Any use, exploitation, or commercialization outside the narrow limits set by copyright legislation, without the publisher's consent, is illegal and liable to prosecution.

Notice: The editors of this edition have taken every effort to ensure that the information contained herein is accurate and conforms to the standards accepted at the time of publication. However, due to the constantly changing nature of the medical sciences and the possibility of human error, the reader is encouraged to exercise individual clinical judgment and consult with other sources of information that may become available with continuing research. The authors, editors, and publisher are not responsible for errors or omissions or for any consequences from application of the information in this book and make no warranty, expressed or implied, with respect to the currency, completeness, or accuracy of the contents of the publication. In particular, the reader is advised to check the manufacturer's insert of all pharmacologic products before administration.

*Seventh Edition* copyright © 2013   Editors: Justin Hall, Katrina Piggott, Miliana Vojvodic, and Kirill Zaslavsky

*Sixth Edition* copyright © 2010   Editors: Matthew Lincoln, Christopher Tran, Gordon McSheffrey, Denise Wong

*Fifth Edition* copyright © 2005   Editors: Woganee Filate, Dawn Ng, Rico Leung, Mark Sinyor

*Fourth Edition* copyright © 2002   Editors: Sonial Butalia, Catherine Lam, Hin Hin Ko, Jensen Tan

*Third Edition* copyright © 2000   Editors: Tyler Rouse, Cory Torgerson, Gilbert Tang, Hariette Van Spall

*Second Edition* copyright © 1999   Editors: Ashis Chawla, Rizwan Somani

*First Edition* copyright © 1997   Editors: Shane Burch, Derek Plausinis

Library and Archives Canada Cataloguing in Publication Information is available from the publisher.

ISBN 978-1-62623-944-9
eISBN 978-1-62623-945-6

Printed in the United States
5 4 3 2 1

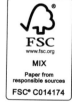

FSC
www.fsc.org
MIX
Paper from
responsible sources
FSC® C014174

# Table of Contents

# Preface and Acknowledgements

The *Essentials of Clinical Examination Handbook* is a publication made by students, for students. The *Handbook* was first published in 1997 to fill a need for a concise, portable, and affordable guide to clinical examination. This edition marks our 20th anniversary in aiding medical students and trainees of allied health professions around the world.

The *Eighth Edition* was written, illustrated, and edited by over 70 students and 60 faculty members at the University of Toronto. It has been revised to reflect evidence-based advances in clinical examination through incorporation of the *JAMA Rational Clinical Exam*, inclusion of succinct summary tables for differential diagnoses and clinical presentations, as well as new graphics to improve usability for students. Furthermore, we are proud to feature a companion mobile application (app) featuring clinical examination checklists which users can use to practice and test themselves on the go.

With the *Essentials of Clinical Examination Handbook*, students, residents, fellows, and staff physicians have come together to create a resource aimed at improving education for future doctors, nurses, and allied health professionals. The *Handbook* reflects a long tradition of excellence in medical education and research innovation at the University of Toronto, dating back to its inception as a medical school in 1843. Part of this tradition is to give back to our community and encourage social justice among healthcare students; as such, all revenue generated from the sales of this book are donated to support student charities and community health initiatives in Toronto and Mississauga, Ontario, Canada.

We would like to express our utmost appreciation to our team who made this edition into reality – including chapter editors, illustrators, layout editors, copy editors, resident reviewers, and faculty advisors. Their dedication, passion, and hard work have been invaluable. We would also like to acknowledge the University of Toronto Medical Society for their guidance in the production of this text. We extend our gratitude to our predecessors for their strong foundation on which we have built our new edition. Finally, we thank our international distributor *Thieme* for bringing this book to the desks of students worldwide.

To our readers, we hope that you enjoy learning from this book as much as we have enjoyed creating it.

Sincerely,

Editors in Chief, *Essentials of Clinical Examination Handbook Eighth Edition*
Yuhao Shi, Zahra Sohani, Brandon Tang, and Florentina Teoderascu

# Contributors

## Editors in Chief
Yuhao Shi
Zahra Sohani

Brandon Tang
Florentina Teoderascu

## Chief Layout Editors
Wendy Gu
Angela Han

Susan Le

## Art Editors
Erina He

Marina Spyridis

## Chapter Editors
Arnav Agarwal
Waleed S. Ahmed
Devon Alton
Gillian Bedard
Joshua Bernick
Andrea Copeland
Adrian Cozma
Matthew Da Silva
Maya Deeb
Ayan K. Dey
Ahmed Faress
Mohammed Firdouse
Claudia Frankfurter
Elise Fryml
Rushi Gandhi
Aaron Gazendam
Mena Gewarges
Lauren Glick
Joel Gupta
Sheliza Halani
Angela Han
Saurabh Kalra
Eli Kisilevsky
Reha Kumar
Sangwoo Leem
Marina Abdel Malak

Danny Mansour
Graham Mazereeuw
Yasmin Nasirzadeh
Erica Pascoal
Priyanka Patel
Armin Rahmani
Mark Shafarenko
Omid Shearkhani
Yuhao Shi
Qazi Zain Sohail
Zahra Sohani
Rebecca Stepita
Kota Talla
Brandon Tang
Florentina Teoderascu
Taraneh Tofighi
Gary Tran
Brian Tsang
Tiffanie Tse
Jane Wang
Marie Yan
Thomas Ying
Daniel Tae Oh Yoo
Ahmed Zaki
Stephanie Zhou
Jeremy Zung

## Resident Reviewers
Manreet Alangh, MD, FRCSC
Zenita Alidina, MD
Benny Dua. MD, PhD
Anjali Kulkarni, MD, MSc
Jenny Li, MD, BMSc
Fahim Merali, MD, MSc, CCFP

Emily Moon, MD, CCFP
Andrew Prine, MD
Shohinee Sarma, MD, MPH
Shixin Shen, MD, MSc
Amy Rebecca Zipursky, BA, MD
Tristan Juvet, MD, BSc

## Faculty Reviewers
Hosanna Au, MD, DipMEd, FRCPC
David N. Adam, MD, FRCPC
Anne Agur, PhD, MSc, BSc(OT)
Meyer Balter MD, FRCPC
Adrian Brown, MD, FRCSC
Esther Bui, MD, FRCPC
Kathy Cao, MD, FRCSC
Grant Chen, MD, FRCPC
Tulin Cil, MD, MEd, FRCSC

Maria Cino, MD, FRCPC
Natalie Clavel, MD, FRCPC
Scott Fung, MD, FRCPC
Jeannette Goguen, MD, FRCPC
David Hall, MD, PhD, FRCPC
Nathan Herrmann, MD, FRCPC
Kevin M. Higgins, MD, FRCSC
Douglas Ing, MD, FRCPC, FACC
Shinya Ito, MD, FRCPC

## Faculty Reviewers (continued)

Nasir Jaffer, MD, FRCPC
Jacqueline James, MD, FRCPC
Raymond Jang, MD, FRCPC
Michael Jewett, MD, FRCSC
David Juurlink, BPhm, MD, PhD, FRCPC
Yoo-Joung Ko, MD, MMSc, SM, FRCPC
Edward Kucharski, MD, CCFP
Shoba Sujana Kumar, MD, MSc, FRCPC
Paul Kuzyk, MD, MASc, FRCSC
Prateek Lala, MD, MSc
Jacques S. Lee, MD, MSc, FRCPC
Elyse Levinsky, MD, MHSc, FRCSC
Catherine Maurice, MD, FRCPC
Lawrence Mbuagbaw, MD, MPH, PhD, FRSPH
Andrew Morris, MD, SM, FRCPC
George Oreopoulos, MD, MSc, FRCSC
Richard Pittini, MD, MEd, FACOG, FRCSC
Susan M. Poutanen, MD, MPH, FRCPC
Angela Punnett, MD, FRCPC
Sudhashree Rajagopal, MD, FRCPC

Fahad Razak, MD, MSc, FRCPC
Evelyn Rubin, MD, CCFP
Ayal Schaffer, MD, FRCPC
Martin Schreiber, MD, MEd, FRCSC
Samir Sinha, MD, DPhil, FRCPC
Peter Stotland, MD, MSc, FRCSC
Gemini Tanna, MD, FRCPC
Richard Tsang, MD, FRCPC
Catherine Varner, MD, MSc, CCFP(EM)
Allan D. Vescan, MD, FRCSC
Kyle Wanzel, MD, MEd, FRCSC
Daniel Weisbrod, MD, FRCSC
Rory Windrim, MD, FRCSC
Camilla Wong, MD, FRCPC
Albert H.C. Wong, MD, PhD, FRCPC
Frances Wright, MD, MEd, FRCPSC
Doreen Yee, MD, FRCPC
Jensen Yeung, MD, FRCPC
Eugene Yu, MD, FRCPC, ABR
Eric Yu, MD, MEd, FRCPC, FACC

## Editorial Support

*Pediatrics*
Patrina Cheung
Rageen Rajendram
Taraneh Tofighi

*The Head, Neck, and Throat*
Terence Fu
Alvin Yang

*Sex and Gender Content*
Brian H. Kim
Edward Kucharski, MD, CCFP

## Artists

Ruth Chang
Ursula Florjanczyk
Wendy Gu
Angela Han
Susan Le

Melissa Lee
Alison McFadden
Sonia Seto
Marina Spyridis

## Cover Artist

Wendy Gu

## Copy Editors

Alexandre Coutin
Sarah Park
Arunima Sivanand
Alon Coret
Jae Eun Ryu
Eric Yung

Talha Maqbool
Irene Harmsen
Cecilia Alvarez
Tyler Hauer
Ananth Lionel
Sukhmani Sodhi

## Special Acknowledgements

We extend our gratitude to the following faculty members who provided us with direction for our unique vision of the Essentials of Clinical Examination Handbook, Eighth Edition:

Martin Schreiber, MD, MMedEd, FRCPC
Katina Tzanetos, MD, MSc, FRCPC

David Wong, MD, CCFP, FCFP, MScCH

We are also grateful for the work, creativity, and commitment of the app development team:

Ahmad Alhashemi
Zubair Baig
Arjun Balachandar
Matan Berson

Adrian Cozma
Sonia Seto
Kota Talla

# Common Abbreviations

| | |
|---|---|
| ACE | Angiotensin converting enzyme |
| ACTH | Adrenocorticotropic hormone |
| ALP | Alkaline phosphatase |
| ALT | Alanine transaminase |
| AP | Anterior-Posterior |
| aPTT | Activated partial thromboplastin time |
| ASA | Acetylsalicylic acid |
| AST | Aspartate aminotransferase |
| β-hCG | β-human chorionic gonadotropin |
| BMI | Body mass index |
| BP | Blood pressure |
| BPM | Beats per minute |
| BUN | Blood urea nitrogen |
| C&S | Culture and sensitivity |
| CAD | Coronary artery disease |
| CBC | Complete blood count |
| CC | Chief complaint |
| CHF | Congestive heart failure |
| CN | Cranial nerve |
| CNS | Central nervous system |
| COPD | Chronic obstructive pulmonary disease |
| Cr | Creatinine |
| CRP | C-reactive protein |
| CSF | Cerebrospinal fluid |
| CT | Computerized tomography |
| CVS | Cardiovascular system |
| CXR | Chest X-ray |
| DDx | Differential diagnosis |
| DHEAS | Dehydroepiandrosterone |
| DIP | Distal interphalangeal |
| DM | Diabetes mellitus |
| DOB | Date of birth |
| DRE | Digital rectal exam |
| DVT | Deep vein thrombosis |
| ECG | Electrocardiogram |

| | |
|---|---|
| EEG | Electroencephalography |
| ESR | Erythrocyte sedimentation rate |
| FHx | Family history |
| FI | Functional inquiry |
| FNAB | Fine needle aspiration biopsy |
| FSH | Follicle-stimulating hormone |
| GCS | Glasgow coma scale |
| GERD | Gastroesophageal reflux disease |
| GI | Gastrointestinal |
| GU | Genitourinary |
| Hb | Hemoglobin |
| HIV | Human immunodeficiency virus |
| HPI | History of present illness |
| HPV | Human papilloma virus |
| HR | Heart rate |
| HSV | Herpes simplex virus |
| HTN | Hypertension |
| Hx | History |
| IBD | Inflammatory bowel disease |
| ICU | Intensive care unit |
| ID | Identifying data |
| INR | International normalized ratio |
| IV | Intravenous |
| JVP | Jugular venous pressure |
| LFT | Liver function test |
| LOC | Level of consciousness |
| LR | Likelihood ratio |
| MAOI | Monoamine oxidase inhibitor |
| MI | Myocardial infarct |
| MMSE | Mini mental status exam |
| MRI | Magnetic resonance imaging |
| MS | Multiple sclerosis |
| MSK | Musculoskeletal |
| N/V | Nausea, vomiting |
| NSAID | Non-steroidal anti-inflammatory drug |
| OPQRST | Onset, palliating/provoking factors, quality, radiation, severity, temporal (progression) |
| OTC | Over-the-counter |
| PA | Posterior-Anterior |
| PE | Pulmonary embolism |
| PIP | Proximal interphalangeal |
| PMHx | Past medical history |
| PRN | Pro Re Nata, as needed |

| | |
|---|---|
| PSA | Prostate specific antigen |
| PT | Prothrombin time |
| PTH | Parathyroid hormone |
| PTT | Partial thromboplastin time |
| RBC | Red blood cells |
| ROM | Range of motion |
| ROS | Review of systems |
| RR | Respiratory rate |
| SHx | Social history |
| SLE | Systemic lupus erythematosus |
| SSRI | Selective serotonin reuptake inhibitors |
| STI | Sexually transmitted infections |
| TB | Tuberculosis |
| TCA | Tricyclic antidepressant |
| TIA | Transient ischemic attack |
| TSH | Thyroid stimulating hormone |
| U/S | Ultrasound |
| URTI | Upper respiratory tract infection |
| UTI | Urinary tract infection |
| WBC | White blood cells |

CHAPTER 1:

# The General History & Physical Exam

**Editors:**
Joshua Bernick, BEng, MASc
Adrian Cozma, MSc
Marina Abdel Malak, RN, BScN

**Faculty Reviewers:**
Shoba Sujana Kumar, MD, MSc, FRCPC
Evelyn Rubin, MD, CCFP

## TABLE OF CONTENTS

# 1. PREPARATION FOR THE INTERVIEW

GENERAL H&P

- Introduce yourself and explain your role
- If a third party is present, explain his/her role in the interview (e.g. evaluator, tutor, colleague)
- Explain to the patient that the contents of the interview will be kept confidential
- Recognize, however, that certain cases (e.g. child abuse, gunshot wounds, certain infectious diseases) may require mandatory reporting depending on government policies
- Posture and Positioning: sit at the same or at a lower level than the patient, in a position that permits but does not force eye contact. It is preferable to be on the patient's right side, at a comfortable distance that facilitates conversation but does not invade the patient's personal space
- Maintain eye contact and show interest
- Ask the patient how he/she would like to be addressed; clarify pronouns if necessary
- If the patient is accompanied by someone, suggest that he/she wait outside while you conduct the interview and physical exam

**Clinical Pearl: Perspective on Greetings in Medical Encounters[1]**
Physicians are encouraged to shake hands with patients but should remain sensitive to nonverbal cues that might indicate whether patients are open to this behavior or not. As a general rule for the initial interview, physicians should use both first and last names when introducing themselves and addressing patients.

# 2. GENERAL HISTORY

The general history is organized into the following sections:
- Identifying Data (ID)
- Chief Complaint (CC)
- History of the Present Illness (HPI)
    - Risk Factors
    - Associated Symptoms
- Past Medical History (PMHx)
- Family History (FHx)
- Medications (MEDS) and Allergies (ALL)
- Social History (SHx)
- Review of Systems or Functional Inquiry (ROS/FI)

## Identifying Data
- Record date of interview
- Patient's name, age, gender, occupation, ethnicity, relationship status, dependents, living status, as relevant
- If applicable, document translators and family members who are present during the interview

## Chief Complaint
- Brief statement in the patient's words
- Include duration of symptoms

## History of Present Illness
- A comprehensive and chronological account of the presenting chief complaint
- Symptom characterization:
    - **O** = **O**nset (when, what the patient was doing at the time) and duration
    - **P** = **P**alliating and **P**rovoking factors
    - **Q** = **Q**uality of pain (e.g. sharp, dull, throbbing)
    - **R** = does the pain **R**adiate?
    - **S** = **S**everity of pain ("on a scale from 1 to 10, with 1 being the least severe and 10 being the most severe")
    - **T** = **T**iming and progression ("is the pain constant or intermittent? worse in the morning or at nighttime?")

- ◆ **U** = "how does it affect '**U**' in your daily life?" - consider impact on self, work, family, friends, others
- ◆ **V** = Déjà **V**u ("Has this happened before?")
- ◆ **W** = "**W**hat do you think it is?" "**W**hat are you most worried about?"
- Also, explore:
  - ◆ Relevant risk factors
  - ◆ Associated symptoms, including pertinent positive and negative symptoms
  - ◆ Relevant past medical and family history
  - ◆ Patient's thoughts and feelings regarding their presenting problem; consider applying the FIFE framework (below)

---

 **Clinical Pearl: Taking a Focused History**

When collecting a "focused history", relevant content from the categories listed above (risk factors, associated symptoms, relevant past personal and family history, and FIFE framework) should be inquired about and reported as part of the HPI. Only relevant questions should be asked as they relate to the chief complaint – the goal is to remain focused as an attempt is made to confirm or refute possible items on the differential.

---

## Past Medical History
- Inquire about childhood illnesses, past medical illnesses, injuries, hospitalizations (age, reason, duration), operations (year, complications, hospital), gynecological and obstetrical history for women, immunizations, and screening procedures (e.g. Pap smear, mammogram, colonoscopy)
- Record dates

## Family History
- Inquire about all serious illnesses within immediate family (first-degree relatives); if relevant, include grandparents, aunts, and uncles
  - ◆ In the North American context, it's particularly important to ask about family history of cardiovascular disease, cancer (specifically breast and colon) and endocrine disorders
- Pay attention to illnesses/disorders that are familial or genetically transmitted
- Construct a genogram (also called a family tree or pedigree); record ages of family members, illnesses, and causes of death if applicable
  - ◆ e.g. Mrs. Jill Hill, the consultant, and Mr. Jack Hill are consanguineous in that their mothers are sisters. They have a healthy son and a healthy daughter who is 16 weeks pregnant. Jack has a healthy older sister and an older brother who died of an autosomal recessive (AR) disease. Jill has a healthy younger brother. Jill's uncle (mother's youngest brother) had a son who passed away of the same AR disease and two other healthy boys (see **Figure 1**)

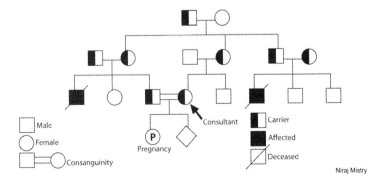

**Figure 1.** Family Tree

GENERAL H&P

## Medications
- Record prescription drugs (name, dosage, frequency, and route of administration), over-the-counter medications, all nutritional supplements and herbal remedies

## Allergies
- Record all environmental, ingestible, and drug-related allergies
- Include the response (rash, anaphylaxis) and timing (immediate or delayed), if it has been formally diagnosed, and how the patient manages symptoms (if applicable)

## Social History
- Living arrangements
  - Type of home (e.g. apartment, basement, house), location, occupants, privacy
- Education (highest level obtained)
- Occupation (current and past)
  - **WHACS**[2]: **W**hat do you do? **H**ow do you do it? **A**re you concerned about any of your exposures or experiences? **C**oworkers or others exposed? **S**atisfied with your job?
- Hobbies and leisure activities (e.g. sports, reading, traveling)
- Marital/relationship status, social support, finances, and living conditions; primary caregiver if applicable
- Sexual history "are you sexually active? with whom?" (see **Table 2**)
- Spirituality ("do you have any religious beliefs concerning your health or medical treatment?")
- Smoking ("have you ever smoked?" to determine pack years)
  - 1 pack year = (1 pack or 20 cigarettes a day) x (1 year)
- Alcohol (type, how much, how often)
  - Use **CAGE** to assess alcoholism: have you ever felt the need to **C**ut down on your drinking? have people **A**nnoyed you by criticizing your drinking? have you ever felt bad or **G**uilty about your drinking? have you ever had a drink first thing in the morning to steady your nerves or to get rid of a hangover – an **E**ye opener?
- Recreational drugs (type, how much, how often)
- Diet and stress

## Review of Systems/Functional Inquiry
- A head-to-toe review of the patient's current state of health ("at this time is there anything new?" or "has anything changed recently?")
- Primarily yes/no questions; positive answers should be explored in greater detail and can be asked with the rest of the HPI
- It is important to keep the history focused; questions asked from the review of symptoms should be guided by the CC and HPI

**Table 1.** Review of Systems

| Organ System | Symptoms to Ask About |
| --- | --- |
| **General** | Energy, appetite, weight or temperature changes, night sweats |
| **Dermatological (Derm)** | Rashes, lumps, sores, pruritus, changes in skin, nails, or hair |
| **Neuropsychiatric (Neuro/Psych)** | Weakness, seizures, problems with gait, memory and/or mood changes |
| **Head and Neck** | Headaches, dizziness, light-headedness<br>Swollen glands, lumps, goiter |
| **Eyes** | Visual changes, red eyes, pain |
| **Ears, Nose and Throat** | Tinnitus, vertigo, hearing loss, ear pain, discharge, nosebleeds, nasal congestion, sinus pain, dental disease, hoarseness, throat pain, difficulty swallowing |
| **Breast** | Lumps, pain, nipple discharge, skin changes |
| **Cardiovascular (CV)** | Chest pain, dyspnea, edema, palpitations, syncope, intermittent claudication, varicose veins |

| Organ System | Symptoms to Ask About |
|---|---|
| **Respiratory (RESP)** | Cough, dyspnea, sputum, hemoptysis, wheezing, chest pain |
| **Gastrointestinal (GI)** | Dysphagia, heartburn, abdominal pain, nausea, vomiting, diarrhea, constipation, hemorrhoids, changes in frequency of bowel movements or stool appearance |
| **Urinary (GU)** | Dysuria, frequency, urgency, polyuria, nocturia, hematuria, and in males: hesitancy, dribbling or decrease in caliber of urinary stream |
| **Sexual** | If relevant and warranted, inquire about the 5P's (see **Table 2**) Female: age of menarche, frequency and duration of periods, amount of bleeding, last period, dysmenorrhea, age of menopause, vaginal discharge or lesions, pregnancies (number, type of delivery, complications), abortions, dyspareunia Male: penile discharge, genital sores, testicular pain or masses |
| **Endocrine** | Polydipsia, polyuria, skin or hair changes, heat or cold intolerance |
| **Musculoskeletal (MSK)** | Joint pain, swelling, redness, stiffness |
| **Hematologic** | Anemia, easy bruising or bleeding, blood transfusions |

## 3. INTERVIEW SKILLS

- Progress from open-ended questions ("can you describe the pain?") to directed questions ("is the pain sharp, dull, or burning?", "does the pain radiate to your left arm?")
- Encourage the patient to continue ("uh-huh", "yes", "I understand, please continue") and do not interrupt the patient
- Redirect the patient when necessary ("it seems this is important to you and maybe we can discuss it further, but right now I would like to focus on...")
- Ask the patient to define vague terms (suddenly, a little, tired, dizzy, hurts, sick, weak), or any other terms you do not understand
- Ensure you are actively listening to the patient and maintain appropriate eye contact throughout the assessment
- Use the language, terms, and pronouns used by the patient
- Ask one question at a time
- Avoid leading questions ("you don't smoke, right?")
- Avoid medical jargon

At the end of the interview, summarize what you have discussed and what the plan moving forward will be. It is also important to ask the patient if they have any other questions, or if there is anything else that they wish to add to ensure all of their concerns have been addressed.

**Clinical Pearl: Nonverbal Behaviors Associated with Positive Health Outcomes[3]**
Nonverbal behaviors between a physician and his or her patient have been shown to be associated with variety of patient specific positive health outcomes. Outcomes can be divided into short term (patient satisfaction, trust in the physician), intermediate (compliance with medication and recommendations), and long term (quality of life, mortality). Positive non-verbal behaviours include forward leaning, head nodding, uncrossed arms and legs, arm symmetry, and less mutual gaze.

In addition, other nonverbal cues are critical to a complete assessment of the patient, for example, is the patient drinking ample water (could indicate diabetes, dehydration); is the patient fidgeting (could indicating a behavioral problem or underlying discomfort); is there a noticeable tremor (could suggest withdrawal or any underlying neurological problem).

## Helpful Acronyms in Clinical Situations:

*Emotion Handling Skills: NURSE[4]*
- **N**: **N**ame the emotion
- **U**: show **U**nderstanding
- **R**: handle the issue with **R**espect
- **S**: **S**how **S**upport
- **E**: ask the patient to **E**laborate on the emotion

*Understanding the Patient's Perspective: FIFE*
- **F**: **F**eelings and **F**ears ("what concerns you the most?")
- **I**: **I**deas ("what do you think is going on?")
- **F**: **F**unction ("how has your illness affected you day-to-day?")
- **E**: **E**xpectations ("how do you expect this treatment to help?" "What do you think will happen with your illness?")

*Breaking Bad News: SPIKES[5]*
- **S**: **S**etting up the interview
  - Deliver the news while sitting
  - Ensure privacy
  - Involve significant others (if appropriate)
  - Inform the patient about time constraints or interruptions
- **P**: **P**erception of the patient
  - Use open-ended questions to assess the patient's understanding of his/her situation
- **I**: **I**nvitation to disclose information
  - Ask the patient what he/she would like to know
- **K**: **K**nowledge giving
  - Warn the patient ("unfortunately I have some bad news…")
  - Deliver information in small chunks using non-technical words
  - Avoid being too blunt; be careful and considerate in your choice of words and phrasing
- **E**: **E**mpathizing with the patient's emotions
  - Allow the patient to express his/her emotions, identify the reason behind his/her emotions, and validate his/her emotions
- **S**: **S**trategize and **S**ummarize
  - Ask the patient to summarize his/her understanding of what was discussed
  - Elicit treatment goals and discuss suitable treatment plans

## 4. DIFFICULT INTERVIEWS

### Sexual & Gender History
- A sexual history should be part of every patient's comprehensive health assessment
- It is especially important to take a sexual history if the patient presents with:
  - Genitourinary symptoms:
    - Genital discharge, sores, ulcers, warts, or pruritis
    - Anorectal symptoms
    - Abdominal pain, pain with urination (dysuria), or intercourse (dyspareunia)
    - Blood in urine (hematuria)
    - Other signs suggestive of an STI
  - Express interest in becoming pregnant or undergoing STI or HIV testing
  - As part of an adolescent history (HEEADSS template)
- The presence of others in the room while taking a sexual history may compromise truthfulness, completeness, and validity of responses. Create a safe, non-judgmental, and comfortable space to ensure patient-centeredness
- Preface the interview by explaining why the sexual history is necessary, affirm confidentiality, and ask the patient for consent
  - An example of an opening statement could be: "now I am going to ask you a few very important questions about your sexual health and practices that will help me understand your overall health. These are personal questions, but I want you to know that I ask them of all my adult patients regardless of age, gender, sexual

orientation, or relationship status and the answers are kept in strict confidence. Do you have any questions before we get started?"
- Ask about the 5 P's (Partners, Practices, Protection, Past History, Pregnancy) of the Sexual History (see **Table 2**)
- It is very important to avoid making assumptions about a patient's sexual orientation, practices, relationship structure, or gender identity
- Do not make assumptions about your patient's anatomy (e.g. a transgender man may have a vagina)
- Do mirror your patient's language when referring to their anatomy (e.g., if your patient says 'chest' as opposed to their 'breasts,' refer to that part of their body as their 'chest')
- Ask about the patient's preferred name & pronoun(s) (e.g., he/him, she/her, they/their, ze, hir, and others)
- Ask about the patient's gender identity, gender expression, and assigned sex at birth

## Sexual and Contraceptive History (5 P's)

**Table 2**. 5 P's of Sexual and Contraceptive History

| Component of Hx Taking | Questions to Consider |
|---|---|
| **Partners** | • Current sexual activity, number and gender of partners (men, women, both, other), duration of marriage(s) or significant sexual or romantic relationship(s)<br>• Structure of current relationship(s) (monogamous, open, polyamorous, etc.)<br>• Inquire about sexual and/or romantic partners outside of the relationship(s) |
| **Practices** | • Type(s) of sexual practices (vaginal, oral, anal sex, digital, use of toys, other), high risk behaviours: exchange of fluids, genital piercings, sex work, survival sex<br>• Role in each sexual act (e.g., insertive and/or receptive partner for anal sex)<br>• Satisfaction (desire, arousal, orgasm, safety, comfortability) |
| **Protection** | • Type and frequency of protection against sexually transmitted infections (STIs)<br>• History or current use of pre- or post-exposure prophylaxis (PrEP or PEP, respectively) |
| **Past History** | • Age of onset of sexual activity<br>• Past STIs (type and duration) and treatment<br>• History of sexual assault or abuse |
| **Pregnancy**<br><br>This section applies to anyone with a uterus (i.e., includes transmen who have a uterus) | • GTPAL: gravida (# of gestations), term (pregnancies carried to ≥37 weeks of gestational age), preterm births (pregnancies carried for 20-37 weeks gestational age), abortions/terminations/miscarriages, live births<br>• Plans for pregnancy (if any); if not, type and duration of contraceptive methods<br>• Adherence, side effects, contraceptive failure, reasons for any discontinuation<br>• Menstrual history, past infertility issues and treatment, past extrauterine pregnancies |

## Cross-Cultural History Taking
- To improve communication it is important to be familiar with diverse cultures and beliefs
- Avoid using stereotypes
- If language is a barrier, use an interpreter who is not a relative of the patient
- Introduce the interpreter to the patient and ask the interpreter to translate in the patient's own words

- Maintain eye contact with and direct questions toward the patient
- Keep your sentences short and simple
- Ensure the patient's understanding of the content of the interview

## Spousal/Partner Abuse
- Types of Abuse
  - Physical: pushing, choking
  - Sexual: forced sexual contact, pregnancy, abortion
  - Emotional: name-calling
  - Psychological: social isolation, controlling behavior
  - Financial control
- Common Signs of Spousal Abuse[6]
  - Unexplained traumatic injuries inconsistent with history
  - Certain types of head or neck injuries taken with clinical suspicion: facial lacerations, fractures, burns, perforated eardrums, fractured teeth, retinal detachment, orbital blow-out fracture, retinal hemorrhages, skull fractures, subdural and epidural hematomas, multiple bruises at different stages of healing
  - Multiple visits for nonspecific and often stress-related complaints
  - Somatic symptoms, including headaches, insomnia, anxiety and depression
  - Suicidal ideation, suicide attempts
  - Substance abuse or eating disorders
  - Extra caution should be taken when a patient presents with physical injuries during pregnancy
- Approach to History and Physical Exam
  - Interview the patient alone (document if this is impossible)
  - Ensure confidentiality
  - Ask direct and specific questions:
    - "What happens when your partner loses his/her temper?"
    - "Do you feel safe at home?"
    - "Does your partner ever hit or abuse your children?" (inform the patient that suspected child abuse must be reported to Children's Aid Society)
  - Remind the patient he/she is not to blame
  - Assess his/her risk
    - Has the severity/frequency of assaults increased?
    - Have threats of homicide or suicide been made? Have these threats increased?
    - Have threats to any children been made?
    - Does your partner have access to a firearm?
    - Do you know where to call for help in an emergency?
  - Help the patient develop a safety plan that includes emergency numbers, key documents, a packed suitcase and money
  - Provide information on available community resources
  - Document the patient's history, physical exam, and medical treatment in detail, including any suspicions of ongoing abuse
  - If the patient provides consent, taking measurements or photographs of physical injuries may be helpful
  - Do not be frustrated if abuse is denied or help is declined; remain empathic and supportive
  - Arrange appropriate follow-up (if abuse is suspected, but the patient declines, one way to have the patient follow up would be to only renew prescriptions for a limited period of time, as this forces the patient to return to the office for prescription renewal, and gives the physician another opportunity to discuss the suspicions of abuse

## 5. PREPARATION FOR THE PHYSICAL EXAM

- Prepare the patient by explaining what you are going to do before proceeding
- Ensure patient comfort, and proper draping, positioning and lighting
- By convention, examine patients from the right side
- Avoid showing extreme reactions during the examination

## Principles of Infection Control
- Hand Hygiene
  - If hands are not heavily soiled, use alcohol-based hand cleanser before and after seeing each patient; if hands are soiled (i.e. with dirt, blood, etc.) use soap and warm water for 20 s
- Barrier Protection
  - Body substances include blood, oral secretions, sputum, emesis, urine, feces, wound drainage, and any additional moist body substances (excluding tears or sweat)
  - Assume that all patients are potentially infected with pathogens and all body substances are potential sources of transmission
  - Use barriers (gloves, gown, mask, eyewear) when appropriate (e.g. gloves when in contact with any bodily substances, masks when dealing with respiratory infections)

*Note:* additional precautions may apply when working with specific airborne pathogens and antibiotic-resistant organisms

## 6. GENERAL INSPECTION

### General Appearance
- Apparent state of health: any signs of distress (cardiac, respiratory, pain, anxiety, depression)? Any lines or tubes present (e.g. Foley catheter, IV line)? Quickly scan the room (e.g. bedside items, number of pillows for orthopnea, etc.) for clues. Does the patient appear unwell?
- Physical appearance: level of consciousness (alert, non-responsive, etc.), diagnostic facies (e.g. grimacing, fleeting eye contact), skin (color and obvious lesions), age and whether appears stated age, appropriate dress, grooming and personal hygiene (see **Table 3** and **Table 4**)
- Body structure: height, habitus, sexual development, fat distribution, symmetry, body posture and position, bony abnormalities (see **Figure 2**)
- Mobility: gait (normally shoulder-width base, with smooth, even strides), range of motion, involuntary movements (see **Geriatrics** and **Nervous System** Chapters)
- Behavior: facial expression, mood, affect, speech (articulation, fluency, hoarseness)
- Any odors of the breath or body

### Head
- Look for diagnostic facies, color abnormalities, swelling, scalp lesions, and abnormal hair distribution (alopecia, hirsutism)

**Table 3.** Color Abnormalities and Possible Causes

| Color Abnormality | Where to Look | Possible Causes |
|---|---|---|
| Blue | Tongue and mouth | Central cyanosis (pulmonary and/or cardiac disease) |
| | Lips, hands, and feet | Peripheral cyanosis |
| Blue-gray | General appearance | Hemochromatosis |
| Pale | Conjunctiva and oral mucosa | Anemia |
| Red | Can be generalized to whole body or localized to a specific part | Polycythemia, infections or drug reactions |
| Yellow | Sclera (jaundice) | Cholestasis, hepatic failure, hemolysis |

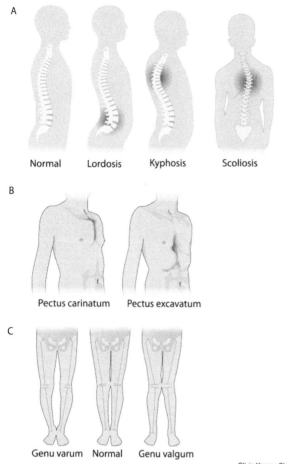

A

Normal     Lordosis     Kyphosis     Scoliosis

B

Pectus carinatum     Pectus excavatum

C

Genu varum    Normal    Genu valgum

Olivia Yonsoo Shim

**Figure 2.** Common Bony Abnormalities

**Table 4.** Common Diagnostic Facies and Possible Causes

| Signs and Symptoms | Possible Causes |
| --- | --- |
| Thick dry skin, loss of hair on head and lateral eyebrows | Hypothyroidism |
| Lid retraction, exophthalmos, sweating | Hyperthyroidism |
| Moon facies, acne, hirsutism, thinning of skin, and erythema | Cushing's syndrome |
| Large protruding jaw, wide spacing of teeth, protruding tongue, thick skin, prominent supraorbital ridges | Acromegaly |
| Periorbital edema (puffy eyes) | Nephrotic syndrome or thyroid disorder |
| Sunken eyes, temporal wasting | Malignancy, AIDS, advanced peritonitis |
| Dry sunken eyes, dry mucous membranes, reduced skin turgor | Dehydration |
| Malar flush with facial telangiectasias | Alcoholism |

| Signs and Symptoms | Possible Causes |
|---|---|
| Expressionless face, depressed affect, infrequent blinking | Parkinson's disease |
| Flat occiput and forehead, down-slanting palpebral fissures, low nasal bridge, large tongue | Down syndrome |

## Hands and Nails
- Inspect the hand for abnormal color or morphology
- Inspect shape, size, color, and consistency of nails

## 7. VITAL SIGNS

### Temperature
- Body temperature is influenced by age, the diurnal cycle, the menstrual cycle, and exercise (see **Table 5**)

**Table 5.** Normal Body Temperatures for Adult Men and Women

| Location | Mean Temperature (°C) | Temperature Range (°C) |
|---|---|---|
| Oral | 36.4 | 33.2-38.2 |
| Rectal | 36.9 | 34.4-37.8 |
| Tympanic | 36.5 | 35.4-37.8 |
| Axillary | 36.3 | 35.5-37.0 |

### Pulse Measurement
- Use the radial or carotid artery to determine:
  - Rhythm: regular, regularly irregular, irregularly irregular
  - Rate:
    - Regular rhythm: count for 30 s
    - Regularly irregular: count for 1 min
    - Irregularly irregular: count for 1 min using apex beat
  - Magnitude: weak (1+), normal (2+), or increased (3+) (see **Table 6**)
  - Symmetry: left vs. right
- Before palpating the carotid artery, auscultate for carotid bruits
- Never palpate both carotid arteries at the same time
- Normal adult pulse rate is 60-100 bpm
  - **Bradycardia**: an abnormally slow heart rate (<60 bpm)
  - **Tachycardia**: an abnormally fast heart rate (>100 bpm)

**Table 6.** Pulse Grading Scale

| Grade | Pulse |
|---|---|
| 4+ | Bounding |
| 3+ | Increased |
| 2+ | Normal |
| 1+ | Weak |
| 0 | Absent or Non Palpable |

### Respiratory Assessment
- Look for signs of respiratory distress (the use of accessory muscles, intercostal indrawing, pursed lip breathing, tripod positioning, heaving or audible wheezing)
- RR most reliably measured when patient is distracted from their own conscious breathing (e.g. while measuring their pulse)
- Count for 30 s if breathing is normal and for 1 min if you suspect abnormality
- Normal adult RR is 14-20 breaths/min[8]

GENERAL H&P

- ◆ **Bradypnea**: an abnormal decrease in RR (<14 breaths/min)
- ◆ **Tachypnea**: an abnormal increase in RR (>20 breaths/min)
- ◆ **Apnea**: absence of breathing, either periodic or sustained (i.e. cardiac arrest, CNS lesion)

## Blood Pressure Measurement
- Terminology
  - ◆ Systolic blood pressure (SBP): maximum arterial pressure during left ventricular contraction (see **Table 7**)
  - ◆ Diastolic blood pressure (DBP): resting arterial pressure between ventricular contractions (see **Table 7**)
  - ◆ Pulse pressure = SBP – DBP
  - ◆ Korotkoff sounds: arterial sounds heard during blood pressure measurement by auscultation
  - ◆ Auscultatory gap: transient loss of Korotkoff sounds during measurement of SBP
- Preparation (see **Figure 3**)
  - ◆ Patient should be relaxed, sitting with his/her back supported and feet flat on the floor
  - ◆ Wrap cuff around upper arm, 2-3 cm above antecubital fossa, with brachial marker over brachial artery
  - ◆ Ask the following questions:
    - ▪ "In the last 30 min, have you smoked, had caffeine, or exercised?" (note that this is context specific, since if you have been observing the patient for the last 30 minutes then this question does not apply)
    - ▪ "Is there any reason that you should not have your blood pressure taken on either of your arms?"
    - ▪ Unless advised otherwise, use the right arm

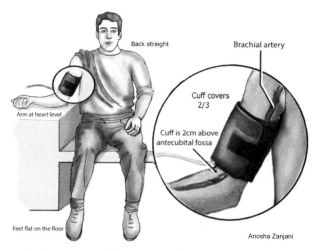

Back straight · Brachial artery · Cuff covers 2/3 · Arm at heart level · Cuff is 2cm above antecubital fossa · Feet flat on the floor · Anosha Zanjani

**Figure 3.** Blood Pressure Measurement Setup

- Systolic Pressure by Palpation
  - ◆ Is a particularly useful component of the blood pressure assessment. By first determining the pressure by palpation, the examiner is less likely to be confused by the auscultatory gap found between the 1st and 2nd Korotkoff Sounds, which could otherwise result in under-estimation of SBP and/or an over-estimation of DBP, if interpreted incorrectly
  - ◆ Palpate radial artery on arm
  - ◆ Inflate blood pressure cuff until radial pulse disappears
  - ◆ Slowly deflate approximately 2 mmHg/s
  - ◆ SBP is estimated when radial pulse can be felt again
- Systolic and Diastolic Pressure by Auscultation (see **Figure 4**)
  - ◆ Note in which arm BP is being measured

- Support upper arm at heart level
- Place stethoscope over brachial artery
- Inflate cuff to 20-30 mmHg above estimated SBP
- Slowly deflate approximately 2 mmHg/s
- SBP is read at the first Korotkoff sound
- DBP is read when the Korotkoff sounds disappear
- Repeat using other arm to assess symmetry
- Orthostatic Hypotension Measurement
  - Measure BP with the patient supine, then standing
  - Positive test: ≥20 mmHg fall in SBP or ≥10 mmHg fall in DBP upon standing[9]
  - Patients may also experience symptoms of cerebral hypoperfusion upon standing: dizziness, weakness, lightheadedness, visual blurring, darkening of visual fields, syncope (due to abrupt peripheral vasodilation without compensatory increase in cardiac output

**Table 7.** Blood Pressure Levels for Adults[10]

| Classification* | Systolic Pressure (mmHg) | Diastolic Pressure (mmHg) |
|---|---|---|
| Normal | <120 | <80 |
| Prehypertension | 120-139 | 80-89 |
| Stage 1 Hypertension | 140-159 | 90-99 |
| Stage 2 Hypertension | >160 | >100 |

*If the patient's SBP and DBP categories are not the same, classify them according to the more severe category

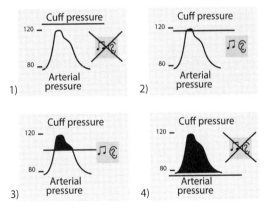

Prerna Patel

**Figure 4.** Korotkoff Sounds During BP Measurement
1. When cuff pressure is above SBP, blood flow is stopped; no Korotkoff sounds are heard.
2. When cuff pressure falls below SBP, turbulent blood flow causes Korotkoff sounds; a clear tapping sound is initially heard. This marks the SBP.
3. As cuff pressure continues to fall, the quality of the Korotkoff sounds changes.
4. When cuff pressure falls below DBP, laminar blood flow is restored and Korotkoff sounds disappear. This marks the DBP.

## Factors Influencing Blood Pressure
- Age (gradually rises throughout childhood until adulthood)
- Sex (generally lower in females until menopause, after which point females have higher blood pressure)
- Diurnal rhythm (lower in morning and higher in afternoon)
- Weight (higher in obese individuals)
- Exercise (lower in physically active individuals)
- Stress
- Ethnicity

## Body Mass Index (BMI)

- BMI is a simple, indirect measure of body fat and general health. It is derived from an individual's height and weight and is used internationally to classify patients as being underweight, healthy weight, overweight or obese (see **Table 8**)
  - Important disadvantage: does not accurately account for differences in body composition (proportion of fat, muscle and fluid) and so it is most reliable in adults of average proportions while decreasing in reliability in athletic or pregnant adults and children
- BMI = weight/height$^2$ (kg/m$^2$ or lbs/inches$^2$ x 703)

**Table 8.** BMI Classifications for Adults (Male and Female)

| Classification | Body Mass Index (kg/m$^2$) |
|---|---|
| Underweight | <18.5 |
| Healthy Weight | 18.5-24.9 |
| Overweight | 25.0-29.9 |
| Obese (Class I) | 30.0-34.9 |
| Obese (Class II) | 35.0-39.9 |
| Obese (Class III) | ≥40.0 |

## Waist Circumference (WC) Measurement

- Measure WC when the patient is standing, with abdominal muscles relaxed at the end of normal expiration (see **Table 9**)
- Position the measuring tape in a horizontal plane, level with the top of the iliac crest
- The circumference should be measured to the nearest 0.5 cm

**Table 9.** Ethnic-Specific Values for Waist Circumference

| Ethnicity/Country | Waist Circumference in cm (as a measure of central obesity) | |
|---|---|---|
| | Male | Female |
| European | ≤94 | ≤80 |
| Asian (East Asian, Chinese, South Asian) | ≤85 | ≤80 |
| African American, Hispanic or Middle Eastern | Use European-based cutoffs | |
| Aboriginal, African, Pacific Islanders, or South American | Unable to recommend | |

# 8. OVERVIEW OF THE PHYSICAL EXAM

*Four Principles of the Physical Exam for Each Body System*
\* Note: most physical exams follow this general structure (with some variation) and thus it is an excellent framework to help you stay organized throughout the process
- Inspection
- Palpation
- Percussion
- Auscultation

The following is a guideline for a general screening exam:

**Table 10.** General Screening Exam

| Organ System | What to Look for on Physical Exam |
| --- | --- |
| **General** | Note if the patient appears to be in any distress, their apparent state of health, presence of any tubes, IV lines or other objects |
| **Vitals** | Blood pressure, pulse, respiration, temperature |
| **Skin, Hair and Nails** | Skin: color, integrity, texture, temperature, hydration, excessive perspiration, unusual odors, presence of lesions<br><br>Hair: texture, distribution<br><br>Nail: morphology, texture, color, condition |
| **Head and Neck** | Lymph nodes: preauricular, postauricular, occipital, tonsillar, submandibular, submental, cervical (superficial, deep, posterior), supra- and infra-clavicular, epitrochlear, axillary, inguinal nodes; note size, shape, mobility, tenderness<br><br>Head: bruising, masses; check fontanelles in infants/young children<br><br>Neck: tracheal position, thyroid enlargement/nodules, lymphadenopathy, masses, carotid or thyroid bruits<br><br>(see **The Head, Neck and Throat** Chapter and **The Lymphatic System** Chapter) |
| **Eyes** | Ptosis, pupils (equal, round, pupillary light and accommodation reflexes), extraocular movements, visual fields and acuity, fundoscopy (red reflex, optic disc, retinal vessels), scleral icterus<br><br>(see **Ophthalmology** Chapter) |
| **Ears, Nose and Throat** | Ears: external ear, otoscopic findings in canals (cerumen, discharge, foreign body) and tympanic membranes (integrity, color, landmarks, and mobility), tenderness. Hearing: Weber and Rinne tests<br><br>Nose and Throat: nasal discharge, sense of smell, mucous membrane color and moisture, oral lesions, dentition, pharynx, tonsils, tongue, palate, uvula<br><br>(see **The Head, Neck and Throat** Chapter) |
| **Cardiovascular** | JVP, hepatojugular reflux; heart rate, rhythm, grade; apex beat, normal (S1, S2) and adventitious (thrills, heaves, S3, S4, murmurs) heart sounds,<br><br>(see **The Precordial Exam** Chapter) |
| **Respiratory** | Clubbing, central and/or peripheral cyanosis, bony abnormalities, chest expansion, tactile fremitus, percussion, diaphragmatic excursion, auscultation for adventitious sounds, egophony, whispered pectoriloquy<br><br>(see **The Respiratory System** Chapter) |

| Organ System | What to Look for on Physical Exam |
|---|---|
| **Peripheral Vascular** | Temporal, carotid, abdominal aortic, renal, iliac and/or femoral bruits; temperature, edema, pulses, capillary refill, pallor on elevation and rubor on dependency |
| | (see **The Peripheral Vascular Exam** Chapter) |
| **Breast** | Dimpling, tenderness, lumps, nipple discharge, axillary masses |
| | (see The **Gynecological Exam** Chapter) |
| **Abdomen** | Contour (e.g. flat, obese, distended), scars, dilated veins, visible peristalsis, ascites, ecchymoses, bowel sounds, bruits, tenderness, guarding, masses, liver and spleen size, costovertebral angle tenderness |
| | (see **The Gastrointestinal System** Chapter) |
| **Urological** | Inguinal masses or hernias, scrotal swelling, anal sphincter tone, rectal masses, prostate gland (nodules, tenderness, size), discharge, lesions, varicoceles |
| | (see **The Urological Exam** Chapter) |
| **Gynecological** | External genitalia, vaginal mucosa, cervical discharge and color, ovaries, uterine size and shape, masses (including adnexal), lesions |
| | (see **The Gynecological Exam** Chapter) |
| **Musculoskeletal** | Symmetry, deformities, muscle atrophy, erythema, temperature, tenderness, joint swelling, edema, ROM, crepitus, joint stability |
| | (see **The Musculoskeletal System** Chapter) |
| **Neuropsychiatric** | LOC, cranial nerves, mental status, speech, mood and affect |
| | Sensory: 1° sensory modalities (pain, temperature, fine touch, vibration, proprioception), 2° sensory modalities (stereognosis, graphesthesia, two point discrimination) |
| | Motor: tone, power (0-5), reflexes (0-4+), gait and coordination tests |
| | (see **The Nervous System** and **Psychiatry** Chapters) |

# REFERENCES

5. Laird JE, Tolentino JC, Gray C. Patient greeting preferences for themselves and their providers in a military family medicine clinic. *Mil Med.* 2013; 178(10): 1111-1114.
6. Schuman SH, Simpson WM. WHACS your patients. *J Occup Environ Med.* 1999; 41(10): 829.
7. Beck RS, Daughtridge R, Sloane PD. Physician-patient communication in the primary care office: A systematic review. *JABFP.* 2002; 15(1): 25-38.
8. Pollak KI, Arnold RM, Jeffreys AS, et al. Oncologist communication about emotion during visits with patients with advanced cancer. *J Clin Oncol.* 2007; 25(36): 5748-5752.
9. Baile WF, Buckman R, Lenzi R, et al. SPIKES—A six-step protocol for delivering bad news: Application to the patient with cancer. *Oncologist.* 2000; 5(4): 302-311.
10. Statistics Canada. *Family violence in Canada: A statistical profile.* Ottawa: Canadian Centre for Justice Statistics; 2004.
11. Sund-Levander M, Forsberg C, Wahren LK. *Scand J Caring Sci.* 2002; 16(2): 122-128.
12. Bickley LS, Szilagyi PG. Bates' guide to physical examination and history taking (9th Edition). Lippincott Williams & Wilkins; 2005.
13. Lanier JB, Mote MB, Clay EC. Evaluation and management of orthostatic hypotension. *Am Fam Physician.* 2011; 84(5): 527-536.
14. Chobanian AV, Bakris GL, Black HR, et al. The seventh report of the joint national committee on prevention, detection, evaluation, and treatment of high blood pressure: The JNC 7 report. *JAMA.* 2003; 289(19): 2560-2572.
15. Katzmarzyk PT, Mason C. Prevalence of class I, II and III obesity in Canada. *CMAJ.* 2006; 174(2): 156-157.
16. Lau DC, Douketis JD, Morrison KM, et al. 2006 Canadian clinical practice guidelines on the management and prevention of obesity in adults and children [summary]. *CMAJ.* 2007; 176(8): S1-S13.
17. Lear SA, James PT, Ko GT, Kumanyika S. Appropriateness of waist circumference and waist-to-hip ratio cutoffs for different ethnic groups. *Eur J Clin Nutr.* 2010; 64(1): 42-61.

CHAPTER 2A:

# The Precordial Exam

**Editors:**
Claudia Frankfurter, BHSc
Mena Gewarges, MD, MA, HBSc

**Resident Reviewers:**
Benny Dua, MD, PhD

**Faculty Reviewers:**
Eric Yu, MD, MEd, FRCPC, FACC
Douglas Ing, MD, FRCPC, FACC

## TABLE OF CONTENTS

# 1. ESSENTIAL ANATOMY AND PHYSIOLOGY

**Chambers of the Heart**

**Path of Electrical Impulses**

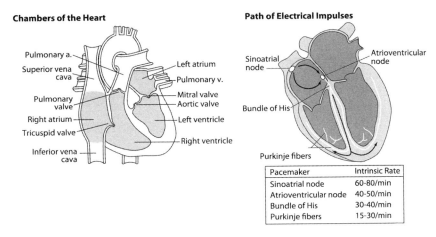

Pina Kingman 2010

**Figure 1.** Anatomy of the Heart

**Anterior**

**Posterior**

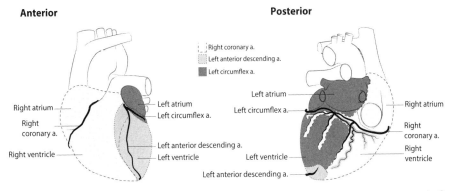

Joy Qu

**Figure 2.** Coronary Vessels and Vascular Territories (shaded)

## Abbreviations

RV=Right ventricle | LV=Left ventricle | RA=Right atrium | LA=Left atrium | RCA=Right coronary artery | LCA=Left coronary artery | LMA=Left main artery | LAD=Left anterior descending artery | CFX=Circumflex artery | PDA=Posterior descending artery | PLA=Posterior lateral artery | SA=Sinoatrial | SVC=Superior vena cava | AV=Atrioventricular | RBB=Right bundle branch | LBB=Left bundle branch | SNS=Sympathetic nervous system | PSNS=Parasympathetic nervous system | HR = heart rate | MAP = mean arterial pressure

## Review of Physiology

- Circulatory pathway has two components:
    - ◆ Pulmonary (low pressure) system:
        RV → pulmonary arteries → lungs for oxygenation → pulmonary veins → LA
    - ◆ Systemic (high pressure) system:
        LV→ aorta → body tissues for oxygen delivery → caval system → RA
- **Blood supply** to the heart is provided by the RCA and LCA, which are the first branches of the aorta
    - ◆ Left coronary system is comprised of a short LCA, which bifurcates into the LAD and left CFX
    - ◆ RCA gives off several branches, notably the right marginal artery and the PDA
    - ◆ Heart is perfused during diastole

- The venous drainage of the heart occurs through the coronary sinus, which empties into the RA and enters the pulmonary circulation
  - Anatomic variants of the coronary system are common
  - The dominant vessel is the one that supplies the posterior descending artery
  - Right-dominant circulation occurs 85% of the time (left-dominant 8% and co-dominant 7%)
- **Electrical conduction system** begins at the SA node located between the SVC and right atrial appendage → depolarizes both atria (LA via Bachmann's bundle) → internodal branches → AV node located between the coronary sinus and septal leaflet of tricuspid valve → His bundle → His-Purkinje system → RBB and LBB → Purkinje fibers (see **Figure 1**)
- Neural innervation of heart from both SNS and PSNS
  - SNS causes ↑ HR and ↑ AV node conduction rate
  - PSNS causes ↓ HR and ↓ AV node conduction rate
- Preload is the ventricular volume at the end of diastole, dependent on venous tone and blood volume
  - Decreased with standing up, increased with rapid squatting
- Afterload is the force against which the ventricle contracts, approximated by the MAP
  - Increased with hand gripping and rapid squatting

## 2. COMMON CHIEF COMPLAINTS AND DIFFERENTIALS

**Table 1.** Common Chief Complaints & Differentials

| CC | DDx (major-life threatening & most common) | Distinguishing features |
|---|---|---|
| Chest pain or discomfort | | **CARDIAC** |
| | Angina | • Retrosternal chest pain, tightness or discomfort radiating to left (± right) shoulder/arm/neck/jaw, associated with diaphoresis, nausea, anxiety<br>• Precipitated by exertion, emotions, eating<br>• Lasts <10-15 minutes, typically relieved by rest and nitrates<br>• Stress testing (pharmacologic or treadmill) may reproduce symptoms |
| | Acute coronary syndrome (ACS) | • Includes the spectrum of Unstable Angina (UA), ST-Segment Elevation Myocardial Infarction (STEMI), Non-ST-Segment Elevation Myocardial Infarction (NSTEMI)<br>• **UA**: accelerating pattern of pain; increased frequency, duration, decreased threshold of exertion, decreased response to treatment; angina at rest; new-onset angina; angina post-MI or post-procedure (i.e. PCI, CABG)<br>• **MI** = myocardial necrosis, diagnosed by rise of serum markers (i.e. high sensitivity troponin), plus one of: symptoms of ischemia (i.e. chest/upper extremity/mandibular/epigastric discomfort, dyspnea); ECG changes (i.e. ST-T changes, new BBB, pathological Q waves); evidence on imaging (i.e. loss of viability of the myocardium, wall motion abnormality, or intracoronary thrombus)<br>• **STEMI**: meets criteria for MI characterized by ST elevation or new LBBB<br>• **NSTEMI**: meets criteria for MI without ST elevation or new BBB |

| CC | DDx (major-life threatening & most common) | Distinguishing features |
|---|---|---|
| **Chest pain (cont'd)** | Aortic dissection | • Acute, severe chest pain, maximal at onset; sometimes tearing, radiating to the back, sometimes complicated by acute aortic regurgitation or tamponade<br>• Differential bilateral arm SBP >20mmHg<br>• Widened mediastinum on CXR<br>• CT chest can confirm dissection |
| | Pericarditis | • Chest pain with deep inspiration, worse supine and with cough, frequently following a viral prodrome<br>• Evanescent pericardial rub on physical exam<br>• In 5-10% of patients, ECG shows diffuse concave upwards ST elevation, PR depression, T wave abnormalities, and possible arrhythmia<br>• Echo may show pericardial fluid |

### PULMONARY

| | | |
|---|---|---|
| | Pulmonary embolism (PE) | • Pleuritic pain, dyspnea, tachypnea, cough, hemoptysis, diaphoresis, syncope<br>• High Wells-PE score (see **The Respiratory System chapter**)<br>• CT-pulmonary angiogram demonstrating PE<br>• Rule out using PERC Rule<br>• ECG: may have tachycardia, non-specific abnormalities, right axis deviation, RBBB, S1Q3T3, inverted T waves in anterior leads |
| | Pneumonia | • Malaise, chills, rigor, fever, cough (typically productive), dyspnea, chest pain (pleuritic, adjacent to infected area)<br>• Fever, tachypnea, tachycardia, crackles, bronchial breath sounds, egophony, dullness to percussion.<br>• Infiltrative process on CXR: air bronchogram(s), silhouette sign, spine sign. |
| | Pneumothorax | • Dyspnea, pleuritic chest pain<br>• Absent tactile fremitus, hyperresonance to percussion, decreased breath sounds on the affected side<br>• CXR shows radiolucent air, absence of lung markings juxtaposed between shrunken lobe or lung and the parietal pleura; tracheal deviation and mediastinal shift occur with large pneumothoraces |

| CC | DDx (major-life threatening & most common) | Distinguishing features |
|---|---|---|
| Chest pain (cont'd) | **GI** | |
| | Boerhaave's syndrome (full thickness perforation of the esophagus following a sudden rise in intra-esophageal pressure) | • Chest and abdominal pain, vomiting, hematemesis<br>• CXR shows mediastinal air, pleural effusion, or mediastinal widening |
| | Pneumomediastinum | • Substernal chest pain – can be severe<br>• Caused by alveolar rupture with dissection of air into mediastinum, esophageal perforation, or esophageal/bowel rupture with dissection of air from the neck or abdomen into mediastinum<br>• CXR shows air in the mediastinum |
| | Gasteroesophageal Reflux Disease (GERD) | • Heartburn, with or without regurgitation of gastric contents into the mouth<br>• Relieved with antacids, proton pump inhibitors, or H2 blockers |
| Dyspnea (shortness of breath) | **CARDIAC** | |
| | Congestive heart failure (CHF) | • Dyspnea, orthopnea, PND, supine cough, ankle swelling, fatigue, nocturia<br>• Jugular venous distention, peripheral edema, ascites, diaphoresis<br>• Abnormal cardiac exam (S3 with reduced ejection fraction; S4 with LV hypertrophy/noncompliance) displaced apex, parasternal lift, murmurs (pansystolic murmur of mitral regurgitation at the apex)<br>• Pulmonary findings may include early inspiratory basilar crackles that do not clear with coughing, and, if pleural effusion present, dullness to percussion and diminished breath sounds at the lung bases<br>• CXR may include enlarged cardiac silhouette, pleural effusion, fluid in major fissure, horizontal lines in periphery (Kerley B lines)<br>• ECHO can evaluate chamber dimensions, valve function, EF, wall motion abnormalities, LV hypertrophy, pericardial effusion<br>• ECG findings can include previous MI, LV hypertrophy, LBBB, or tachyarrhythmia (i.e., atrial fibrillation)<br>• Bedside U/S may reveal pleural effusion.<br>• Serum BNP is high (may help when clinical findings are unclear or other diagnoses such as COPD need to be excluded) |

| CC | DDx (major-life threatening & most common) | Distinguishing features |
|---|---|---|
| **Dyspnea (cont'd)** | Cardiac tamponade | • Beck's Triad – hypotension, jugular venous distention, muffled heart sounds<br>• Elevated venous pressure with preserved x descent, absent y descent, pulsus paradoxus<br>• ECG: low voltage, non-specific ST changes, electrical alternans<br>• Bedside ECHO shows diastolic right atrial and ventricular collapse and variation of tricuspid and mitral inflow velocities |
| | Acute coronary syndrome (ACS) | *Refer to previous entry* |
| | Arrhythmia | • Based on ECG interpretation |
| | Valvular dysfunction | • Physical exam findings (refer to page 29)<br>• ECHO demonstrating valvular abnormalities |

### PULMONARY

| | | |
|---|---|---|
| | Pulmonary embolism (PE) | *Refer to previous entry* |
| | Anaphylaxis | • Angioedema after exposure to known/unknown allergen |
| | Pneumonia | *Refer to previous entry* |
| | Chronic Obstructive Pulmonary Disease (COPD) | • Significant smoking history (with most patients having smoked ≥ 20 cigarettes/day for > 20 years)<br>• Previous PFTs indicating COPD<br>• Productive cough, progressive dyspnea, sputum production<br>• Wheezing, increased expiratory phase of breathing, lung hyperinflation with decreased heart and lung sounds, increased anteroposterior diameter of thorax (barrel chest)<br>• CXR shows lung hyperinflation, bullae, increased retrosternal airspace, and/or bronchial wall thickening |
| | Pleural effusion | • May be asymptomatic, or may cause dyspnea, pleuritic chest pain<br>• Absent tactile fremitus, dullness to percussion, and decreased breath sounds on the side of the effusion<br>• Pleural effusion visible on AP CXR with > 170-200mL of pleural fluid (or >50 mL on lateral CXR) |
| | Pneumothorax | *Refer to previous entry* |

| CC | DDx (major-life threatening & most common) | Distinguishing features |
|---|---|---|
| **Tachycardia (palpitations)** | | **CARDIAC** |
| | Regular tachyarrhythmia | *Narrow QRS (SVTs)*<br>• Sinus tachycardia<br>• Atrial tachycardia<br>• Junctional tachycardia<br>• Arial flutter<br>• AVNRT<br><br>*Wide QRS*<br>• Ventricular tachycardia<br>• SVT with BBB |
| | Irregular tachyarrhythmia | *Narrow QRS (SVTs)*<br>• Atrial fibrillation<br>• Multifocal atrial tachycardia<br><br>*Wide QRS*<br>• Polymorphic VT<br>• Premature ventricular contraction |
| | Valvular dysfunction | *Refer to previous entry* |
| | Hypertrophic cardiomyopathy (HOCM) | • Symptoms appear between ages 20-40 and are usually exertional; include dyspnea, chest pain (usually resembling angina), palpitations<br>• History of unexplained syncope (especially in young athletes), family history of unexplained sudden cardiac death<br>• Septal hypertrophy produces systolic ejection-type murmur that does not radiate to the neck, and may be heard at left sternal edge in 3rd or 4th intercostal space; mitral regurgitation murmur due to distortion of mitral apparatus may be heard at apex<br>• ECHO confirms diagnosis |
| | | **ENDOCRINE** |
| | Hyperthyroidism | • Anxiety, palpitations, hyperactivity, increased sweating, heat hypersensitivity, fatigue, increased appetite, weight loss, insomnia<br>• Presence of goiter, ophthalmologic changes (stare, eyelid lag, retraction)<br>• Diagnosis made by TSH, free T4 plus either free T3 or total T3, sometimes radioactive iodine uptake |
| | Hypoglycemia | • Sweating, nausea, warmth, anxiety, tremulousness, palpitations, hunger<br>• Diagnosed by blood glucose level correlated with physical findings, response to dextrose (or other sugar) administration |

| CC | DDx (major-life threatening & most common) | Distinguishing features |
|---|---|---|
| **Tachycardia (cont'd)** | | **SYSTEMIC** |
| | Fever | • Elevated body temperature (> 37.8°C orally, or > 38.0°C rectally) <br> • Evaluate surgical history, drug history, known conditions that predispose to infection (i.e., HIV, diabetes, cancer, organ transplantation, sickle cell disease, valvular heart disorders – especially if artificial valve present, rheumatologic disorders, SLE, gout, sarcoidosis, hyperthyroidism) <br> • Evaluate localizing symptoms (i.e., headache, cough) to guide evaluation <br> • Review vital signs for tachypnea, tachycardia, hypotension |
| | Anemia | • History of melena stools, epistaxis, hematochezia, hematemesis, or menorrhagia; vegan diet predisposes to B12 deficiency; alcoholism increases risk of folate deficiency <br> • Hemorrhagic shock (hypotension, tachycardia, pallor, tachypnea diaphoresis, confusion) <br> • Orthostatic hypotension in large GI loss; petechiae in thrombocytopenia or platelet dysfunction |
| | Medication induced | • Thorough medication history (with attention to stimulants and anticholinergic agents) |
| | | **PSYCHIATRIC** |
| | Anxiety | • Fear, uneasiness, worry <br> • May coexist with panic disorder, major depression, alcohol misuse |
| **Edema** | | **CARDIAC** |
| | Congestive heart failure | *Refer to previous entry* |
| | | **PERIPHERAL VASCULAR** |
| | Deep Vein Thrombosis (DVT) | • Acute pitting edema in a single limb, usually in lower extremity and accompanied with pain <br> • Redness, warmth, and tenderness; possibly less marked than in soft-tissue infection <br> • Sometimes a predisposing factor (e.g., recent surgery, trauma, immobilization, hormone replacement, cancer) <br> • High Well's DVT score  (see **The Respiratory System** chapter) <br> • U/S confirms diagnosis |
| | Chronic venous insufficiency | • Chronic edema in one or both lower extremities, with brownish discoloration, discomfort but not marked pain, and sometimes skin ulcers <br> • Often associated with varicose veins |

| CC | DDx (major-life threatening & most common) | Distinguishing features |
|---|---|---|
| Edema (cont'd) | **RENAL** | |
| | Nephrotic syndrome | • Diffuse edema, often significant ascites, and sometimes periorbital edema<br>• 24h urine collection to check for protein loss |
| | **GI** | |
| | Cirrhosis | • If chronic, look for stigmata of liver disease (clubbing, Terry's nails, asterixis, ascites, jaundice, spider angiomata, gynecomastia, palmar erythema, and testicular atrophy)<br>• Liver enzyme derangements, portal hypertension |
| | **INFECTIOUS** | |
| | Soft-tissue infection (i.e., cellulitis, necrotizing fasciitis, myonecrosis) | • If due to cellulitis, usually more erythematous, painful, and tender than that due to chronic venous insufficiency, and more circumscribed than that due to DVT.<br>• With necrotizing infections: severe pain (out of proportion to physical findings), constitutional symptoms, tachycardia, tachypnea, low grade fever. Hemorrhagic bullae, blistering, ulceration may develop. Necrotic areas can become insensate.<br>• U/S to rule out DVT, blood cultures to identify infection. |
| | Sepsis | • Life-threatening organ dysfunction due to a dysregulated host response to infection<br>• qSOFA score: patients with suspected infection and 2 of low blood pressure (SBP ≤ 100 mmHg), high respiratory rate (≥ 22 bpm), or altered mentation (GCS <15) are likely to have poor outcomes |
| | **DRUG INDUCED** | |
| | Medication induced | • Symmetric, dependent, painless, usually mild pitting edema<br>• Thorough medication history (with attention to minoxidil, NSAIDs, estrogens, fludrocortisone, dihydropyridine calcium channel blockers) |
| Syncope | **CARDIAC** | |
| | **Cardiac Conduction:** Bradycardia Long QT syndrome Wolff-Parkinson-White Heart block (Mobitz II, 3rd degree) Intermittent VT | • Based on ECG interpretation |

| CC | DDx (major-life threatening & most common) | Distinguishing features |
|---|---|---|
| **Syncope (cont'd)** | **Cardiac pump:** Aortic stenosis Hypertrophic Obstructive Cardiomyopathy (HOCM) Acute Coronary Syndrome (ACS) | • Based on physical exam and echo |

| | | |
|---|---|---|
| | **PULMONARY** | |
| Hyperventilation | | • Often tingling around mouth or on fingers prior to syncope<br>• Usually in context of a distressing situation<br>• Requires thorough clinical evaluation |
| Pulmonary embolism | | *Refer to previous entry* |
| Pneumothorax | | *Refer to previous entry* |
| | **VASCULAR** | |
| Severe carotid stenosis | | • Cerebral angiogram demonstrating changes in the carotid arteries, vertebrobasilar system |
| Ruptured abdominal aortic aneurysm (AAA) | | • Patients who do not die immediately present with abdominal or back pain, hypotension, tachycardia<br>• Diagnosed with U/S or CT angiography or MRI angiography<br>• Requires immediate open surgery or endovascular stent grafting |
| Orthostatic hypotension | | • Etiologies: Primary and secondary autonomic disorders, volume depletion, medication-induced<br>• BP supine and standing; BP and HR are measured after 5 min supine, and at 1 and 3 min after standing; patients unable to stand may be assessed while sitting upright<br>• Positive test: decrease in at least 20 mmHg systolic, 10mmHg diastolic, or increase in heart rate by at least 30 bpm) |
| | **METABOLIC** | |
| Hypoglycemia | | *Refer to previous entry* |
| Anemia | | *Refer to previous entry* |
| | **NEUROLOGICAL** | |
| Intracranial hemorrhage | | • Sudden onset headache, focal neurological deficits, impaired consciousness in patients with risk factors (i.e. chronic arterial hypertension, cigarette smoking, obesity, cocaine and other sympathomimetic drugs)<br>• Immediate CT or MRI to diagnose |

| CC | DDx (major-life threatening & most common) | Distinguishing features |
|---|---|---|
| Syncope (cont'd) | **REFLEX-MEDIATED** | |
| | Vasovagal | • Precipitated by noxious stimuli, stress, fear<br>• Warning/prodromal symptoms (i.e. dizziness, nausea, sweating)<br>• Recovery is prompt, but not immediate (5-15 min, sometimes up to hours) |
| | Situational | • Precipitated by cough, micturition, post-exercise |
| | Carotid sinus hypersensitivity | • Precipitated by pressure on carotid sinus (i.e. tight collar, shaving) |

## 3. FOCUSED HISTORY

### Risk Factors for Cardiac Disease
- Nonmodifiable risk factors:
    - Age (M >45 yr, F>55 yr)
    - Sex (M 10 yrs earlier than F)
    - Family history (MI <55 yr in M relatives, <65 yr in F relatives; or <60 yr in first-degree relatives)
    - Ethnic groups (South Asians and African-Americans are at higher risk than the general population)
- Modifiable risk factors:
    - HTN (BP >140/90 mmHg or taking antihypertensive medications)
    - Diabetes mellitus
    - Hypercholesterolemia
    - Smoking (or recent ex-smoker)
    - Postmenopausal
    - Obesity
    - Sedentary lifestyle
    - Stress
    - High alcohol consumption
    - Depression
    - Hyperhomocysteinemia

### Chief Complaint and History of Present Illness
*Chest Pain (OPQRST)*
- Onset/duration: sudden vs. gradual, hours vs. days, previous similar symptoms, frequency, progression, course (constant vs. intermittent), pleuritic, after meals (postprandial)
- Precipitating and relieving factors: better or worse with exercise/rest/sleep/position
- Quality: crushing, pressing, squeezing, burning, stabbing, tightening, aching, general uncharacteristic chest discomfort; for women in particular, general uneasiness with aching, generalized chest discomfort
- Location: epigastric, periumbilical, flank, back
- Radiation: to neck, jaw, axilla, back, arm (either or both arms can be involved)
- Associated symptoms: fatigue, palpitations, diaphoresis, peripheral edema, nausea/vomiting, dyspnea
- Stable vs. unstable angina:
    - **Stable angina** is intermittent chest pain during exertion or emotional stress, relieved by rest
    - **Unstable angina** is characterized by:
        - New onset (<2 mo) that is severe (CCS III or IV) and/or frequent
        - Progression of symptoms (crescendo pattern)
        - At rest or nocturnal
        - Post-MI

*Note:* always assess functional class of angina (see **Table 2** and **Table 3**)
- Risk factors for cardiovascular disease
- Medications: prescribed vs. OTC, antiplatelets, antithrombin therapies, β-blockers, ACE inhibitors, angiotensin receptor blockers (ARBs), calcium channel blockers (CCBs), diuretics, antiarrhythmics, lipid-modifying agents
- See **Table 1** for differential diagnosis of chest pain

**Table 2.** Canadian Cardiovascular Society (CCS) Functional Classification of Angina

| Class | Activity Evoking Angina | Limits to Physical Activity |
|---|---|---|
| 0 | Asymptomatic | None |
| I | Prolonged exertion | None |
| II | Walking >2 blocks or >1 flight of stairs | Slight |
| III | Walking <2 blocks or <1 flight of stairs | Marked |
| IV | Minimal activity or at rest | Severe |

**Table 3.** New York Heart Association (NYHA) Functional Classification of Congestive Heart Failure

| Class | Activity evoking angina | Limits to physical activity |
|---|---|---|
| I | None | None |
| II | Ordinary physical activity | Slight |
| III | Walking <2 blocks or <1 flight of stairs | Marked |
| IV | Minimal or at rest | Severe |

*Dyspnea*
- See **Table 1** and **The Respiratory System Chapter**

*Peripheral Vascular Disease*
- Peripheral edema
- See **Peripheral Vascular Exam**

## 4. FOCUSED PHYSICAL EXAM

**General**
- Patient's level of comfort or distress
- Skin color (pale vs. pink)
- Cyanosis: central (blue mucous membranes) vs. peripheral (blue fingers/toes)
- Respiratory distress: tachypnea, accessory muscle use, intercostal indrawing, position
- Presence of edema in lower limbs
- Extracardiac features: xanthomata (lipid skin deposits), rash, petechiae, nail splinter hemorrhages

**Vitals**
- HR: rate, rhythm (regular vs. regularly irregular vs. irregularly irregular), amplitude (strong vs. soft)
- BP: both arms
- RR, $O_2$ saturation
- Temperature
- Orthostatic vitals (HR, BP)

**JVP**
- Direct assessment of the pressure in the right atrium (i.e. central venous pressure) via visualization of the internal jugular vein
- Assessment includes four parameters: height, waveform, Kussmaul's sign, hepatojugular/abdominojugular reflux
- Differentiate internal jugular pulse from carotid pulse (see **Table 4**)
- Bedside U/S of intrahepatic IVC is a more reliable measure of volume status

**Table 4.** Characteristics of Internal Jugular vs. Carotid Pulse

| Feature | Internal Jugular Pulse | Carotid |
|---|---|---|
| Palpable | No | Yes |
| Number of Waveforms | Double | Single |
| Finger Pressure above Clavicle | Disappears | Persists |
| Inspiration/Elevation of the Head of the Bed* | Decreases | No change |
| Hepatojugular Reflux/ Lowering of the Head of the Bed* | Increases | No change |

*Change in bed position causes changes in jugular vein position in the neck

*JVP Height* (see **Figure 3**)
- Position the patient at 30° elevation and turn the patient's head slightly to the left, then adjust the angle of elevation until jugular pulsations are observed
- Look between the two heads of the sternocleidomastoid for pulsations: if difficult to observe, shine a light tangentially across the right side of the patient's neck, and look for shadows of pulsations
  - The JVP is more of an inward, double waveform movement and will cast a shadow with tangential light
- Determine JVP by measuring the vertical distance from the sternal angle to a horizontal line drawn from the top of the jugular pulsation
  - Normal JVP: ≤4 cm
- Elevated JVP suggests increased pressure in the right atrium due to:
  - Right heart failure (may be secondary to left heart failure)
  - Constrictive pericarditis or tamponade physiology
    - **Note:** Other causes of high JVP can occur irrespective of right atrium changes; e.g. superior vena cava (SVC) obstruction

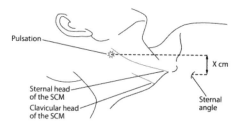

Pina Kingman

**Figure 3.** Measuring JVP Height

*Kussmaul's Sign*
- Rising of JVP with inspiration (paradoxical) suggests that the blood flow into the right heart is impaired. This could result from:
  - Constrictive pericarditis
  - Right heart failure
  - SVC obstruction
  - Tricuspid stenosis
  - Restrictive cardiomyopathy

CIRCULATORY

*Hepatojugular/Abdominojugular Reflux (HJR/AJR)*
- To assess high JVP and RV function:
  - Position the patient so that the top of the JVP is visible
  - Place the right hand over the liver in the right upper quadrant or anywhere in the abdomen
  - Apply moderate pressure (25-30 mmHg) and maintain compression for 10s
  - The JVP may rise or remain unchanged; a sustained elevation of the JVP height (>4 cm) after 2 spontaneous breaths (to ensure patient is not having a Valsalva maneuver) is pathological

*Waveforms*

The JVP is a multiple waveform entity (see **Figure 4**), and an understanding of each of the wave components is essential to conceptualizing how certain diseases are reflected by changes in the JVP:
- a-wave: Atrial contraction
- c-wave: Closing of the tricuspid valve increases atrial pressure during relaxation
- x-descent: Atrial relaxation following contraction
- v-wave: Increasing atrial pressure with venous return
- y-descent: Opening of the tricuspid valve decreases atrial pressure

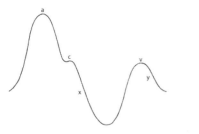

Alison McFadden

**Figure 4.** JVP Waveform

*Precordial Exam*
- Divide the precordium into 4 areas where sounds and murmurs from the heart valves are best auscultated. Please note that the classic area of auscultation is not representative of actual valvular location, but radiation of the murmur (see **Figure 5**)

*Inspection*
- Chest shape: normal vs. excavatum (hollow) vs. carinatum (pigeon-like)
- Apex beat (5th intercostal space, mid-clavicular line)
- Abnormal motions (pulsations)
- Scars

*Palpation*
- Palpate over the 4 auscultation areas and along the sternum
- Palpate for heaves (sustained outward motion), thrills (vibration over area of turbulent blood flow), and impulses (systolic vs. diastolic)
- Palpate over the apex beat and describe it in terms of location, amplitude, duration, size (LADS)

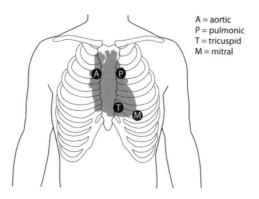

A = aortic
P = pulmonic
T = tricuspid
M = mitral

Pina Kingman 2010

**Figure 5.** Classic Auscultation Areas of Heart Sounds and Murmurs

**Table 5.** Palpable Findings in Precordial Exam

| Auscultation Area | Abnormal Findings | Possible Pathology |
|---|---|---|
| A | Systolic impulse | Systemic HTN<br>Dilated aortic aneurysm |
| P | Systolic impulse | Pulmonary HTN |
| T | Heave, thrill | RV enlargement (2° to pulmonary HTN or left-sided heart disease) |
| M | Thrill | Mitral regurgitation (MR) |

*Auscultation*
- Auscultate over the 4 auscultation areas for heart sounds and murmurs
- Focus on identifying S1 and S2 first, then listen during systole and during diastole
- Physiological splitting of S2 sound into the aortic and pulmonic components can occur upon inspiration due to delayed closure of pulmonic valve

**Table 6.** Heart Sounds

| | Auscultation | Physiologic Significance | Possible Pathologies |
|---|---|---|---|
| S1 | Diaphragm over left lower sternal border (T), apex (M) | Closing of mitral and tricuspid valves | **Loud S1:** mitral stenosis, increased contractility, short PR interval<br><br>**Soft S1:** first degree AV block, LV failure, LBBB<br><br>**Variable S1:** AF, AV dissociation, ventricular pacing, Mobitz I 2nd degree block<br><br>**Split S1:** RBBB |

| | Auscultation | Physiologic Significance | Possible Pathologies |
|---|---|---|---|
| S2 | Diaphragm over left 2nd intercostal space | Closing of aortic and pulmonic valves | **Loud S2**<br>Loud A2: systemic HTN, hyperdynamic circulation, dilated aorta<br>Loud P2: pulmonary HTN<br><br>**Soft S2:** AS or PS<br><br>**Split S2:**<br>Wide: RBBB, WPW, PS, pulmonary HTN, MR<br>Fixed: ASD<br>Paradoxical: LBBB, AS, WPW, HCM |
| **Mid-Systolic Click** | Diaphragm over apex and LLSB while asking patient to squat from standing | Not physiologic | Mitral valve prolapse |
| **Opening snap** | Diaphragm at apex and LLSB | Not physiologic | Mitral stenosis |
| S3 | Bell at apex with patient in left lateral decubitus | **Children and young adults:** physiologic<br><br>**Adults:** pathologic | CHF<br><br>**Left-sided:** MR, AI<br><br>**Right-sided:** TR, PI |
| S4 | Bell over apex | Not physiologic (atria contracting against stiffened ventricle) | **Left-sided:** LVH, AS, systemic HTN, CAD, cardiomyopathy<br><br>**Right-sided:** RVH, PS, pulmonary HTN |

AF = atrial fibrillation, AI = aortic insufficiency, AS = aortic stenosis, ASD = atrial septal defect, AV = atrioventricular, HCM = hypertrophic cardiomyopathy, LLSB = left lower sternal border, L/RBBB = left/right bundle branch block, L/RVH = left/right ventricular hypertrophy, LV = left ventricle, MR = mitral regurgitation, PI = pulmonary insufficiency, PS = pulmonic stenosis, TR = tricuspid regurgitation, WPW = Wolff-Parkinson-White

*Murmurs*
- Describe murmurs in terms of:
- Timing: systolic, diastolic, continuous
- Shape: crescendo, decrescendo, crescendo-decrescendo, plateau
- Location of maximal intensity
- Radiation: axilla, back, neck
- Duration
- Intensity
    - 6-point scale (see **Table 7**)
    - Intensity of murmur not necessarily related to clinical severity
    - Grade diastolic murmurs using 4-point scale (see **Table 8**)
- Pitch: high, medium, low
- Quality: blowing, harsh, rumbling, musical, machine-like, or scratchy
- Relationship to respiration

- Relationship to body position
- Effect of special maneuvers

**Table 7.** Murmur Intensity Scale

| Grade | Definition |
|---|---|
| I | Softer than S1 and S2 |
| II | Intensity of murmur same as S1 and S2 |
| III | Intensity of murmur louder than S1 and S2 but no palpable thrill |
| IV | Loud murmur with palpable thrill |
| V | Loud murmur with palpable thrill, audible with only one rim of stethoscope touching chest |
| VI | Loud murmur with palpable thrill and audible with stethoscope lifted off chest |

**Table 8.** Diastolic Murmur Grading Scale

| Grade | Description |
|---|---|
| I | Barely audible |
| II | Audible, but soft |
| III | Easily audible |
| IV | Loud |

- Murmur is likely nonpathological if:
  - ◆ Early systolic, short duration, and low intensity (usually grade 1-2/6)
  - ◆ Nonradiating, not associated with other CV abnormalities/murmurs
  - ◆ Found in otherwise healthy children, especially in states of hyperdynamic blood flow (e.g., exercise, fever, anxiety)
  - ◆ Decreases or disappears upon sitting
- Special maneuvers for auscultation (see **Table 9**)

**Table 9.** Special Positions and Maneuvers for Auscultation of Heart Sounds

| Position | Effect on Heart Sounds | |
|---|---|---|
| **Sitting upright, leaning forward, holding exhalation** | ↑ AS, AR, pericardial rubs | |
| **Left lateral decubitus (LLD) (use bell of stethoscope)** | S3, S4, MS | |
| **Maneuver** | **Physiological** | **Effect on Heart** |
| **Quiet inspiration, sustained abdominal pressure, leg elevation** | ↑ *venous return* | ↑ *right-sided murmurs, TR, PS* |
| **Fist-clenching (isometrics)** | ↑ *systemic arterial resistance* | ↑ *some left-sided murmurs (MS, AR, VSD)* <br> ↓ *AS* |
| **Standing (Valsalva strain)** | ↓ *venous return* <br> ↓ *vascular tone* | ↑ *MVP, HCM* <br> ↓ *AS* |
| **Squatting (Valsalva release)** | ↑ *venous return* <br> ↑ *vascular tone* | ↓ *MVP, HCM* <br> ↑ *AS* |

AR = aortic regurgitation, AS = aortic stenosis, HCM = hypertrophic cardiomyopathy, MR = mitral regurgitation, MS = mitral stenosis, MVP = mitral valve prolapse, PS = pulmonic stenosis, TR = tricuspid regurgitation, VSD = ventricular septal defect

## Common Murmurs and Heart Sounds

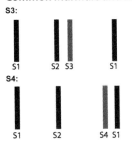

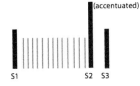
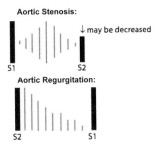
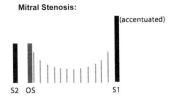

**Figure 6.** Common Murmurs and Heart Sounds

## Respiratory Exam
- See **Respiratory System**

## Peripheral Vascular Exam
- See **Peripheral Vascular Exam**

> **Clinical Pearl: Pediatrics Corner**
> - Benign heart murmurs are common, especially in the pediatric population, and can be exacerbated by high output states.
> - Characteristics of benign murmurs are often: harmonic/musical, systolic, and low grade.

## 5. COMMON INVESTIGATIONS

Table 10. Cardiac Investigations

| Study Type | Test | Description | Indication |
|---|---|---|---|
| **Stress Tests** | Exercise Stress Test | Echocardiogram or ECG monitoring while patient exercises on treadmill at increasing speed until chest discomfort, inordinate dyspnea, abnormal ECG changes or target HR is observed | Suspected CAD Post MI |
| | Pharmacologic stress | In patients who are unable to exercise maximally, medications such as dobutamine, dipyridamole, and adenosine can be used | |
| **Perfusion** | Cardiac Perfusion Test[1] | Radiographic visualization of coronary territory following introduction of contrast material | Assessment of CAD, heart failure |
| **Enyzmes** | Creatine phosphokinase MB isoenzyme (CK-MB), Troponins | Enzymes released into circulation following damage to cardiac muscle; used to diagnose myocardial injury/ infarctions | Suspected MI |

# 6. COMMON CLINICAL SCENARIOS

**Table 11.** Summary of Common Clinical Scenarios

| Key Symptoms | Physical Exam | Investigations | Management |
|---|---|---|---|
| **ST-Elevation Myocardial Infarction (STEMI)** | | | |
| • Deep, substernal, visceral pain described as aching or pressure, often radiating to one or more of the following areas: back, jaw, left arm, right arm, shoulders<br>• Dyspnea, diaphoresis, nausea, and vomiting<br>• Relieved little or only temporarily by rest or nitroglycerin<br>• Women & diabetics are more likely to present with atypical chest discomfort<br>• Elderly patients may report dyspnea as presenting complaint (angina equivalent)<br>• Patients may interpret their discomfort as indigestion<br>• Patients may be asymptomatic | • Skin may be pale, cool, and diaphoretic<br>• Peripheral or central cyanosis may be present<br>• Pulse may be thready, and BP is variable, although many patients initially have some degree of hypertension during pain<br>• Heart sounds are usually somewhat distant; an S4 may be present<br>• A soft systolic blowing apical murmur (reflecting papillary muscle dysfunction) may occur<br>• In right ventricular (RV) infarction, signs include elevated RV filling pressure, distended jugular veins (often with Kussmaul sign), clear lung fields, and hypotension | • Serial ECGs (ST-segment elevation ≥ 1 mm in 2 or more contiguous leads subtending the damaged area)<br>• ST depressions in V1-V2 could represent a posterior MI (RV infarct)<br>• Serial cardiac markers (high sensitivity troponin, CK) | • Pre-hospital care: $O_2$ (if arterial saturation < 90%), aspirin, nitrates and/or opioids for pain, and triage to an appropriate medical centre<br>• Drug treatment: Antiplatelet drugs, antianginal drugs, anticoagulants<br>• Reperfusion therapy: Fibrinolytics or angiography with percutaneous coronary intervention (PCI) or coronary artery bypass surgery<br>• Post-discharge rehabilitation and chronic medical management |
| **Non-ST Elevation Myocardial Infarction (NSTEMI)** | | | |
| *As above* | *As above* | • As above, with high sensitivity troponin elevation without acute ST-segment elevation<br>• ECG changes such as ST-segment depression, T-wave inversion, or both may be present | • Risk scores (i.e. TIMI and GRACE) stratify patients into high and low risk groups<br>• Uncomplicated NSTEMI requiring PCI within 24-48h after presentation, and complicated NSTEMI (i.e. hospital course was complicated by recurrent angina or infarction, heart failure, or sustained recurrent ventricular arrhythmias) requiring urgent PCI |

## Congestive Heart Failure (CHF)

- Dyspnea, orthopnea, PND, supine cough, nocturia, jugular venous distention, peripheral edema, ascites, fatigue, diaphoresis

- Abnormal cardiac exam (S3 with reduced ejection fraction; S4 with preserved ejection fraction) displaced apex, parasternal lift, murmurs (pansysytolic murmur of mitral regurgitation at the apex)
- Pulmonary findings may include early inspiratory basilar crackles that do not clear with coughing, and, if pleural effusion present, dullness to percussion and diminished breath sounds at the lung bases

- CXR may include enlarged cardiac silhouette, pleural effusion, fluid in major fissure, horizontal lines in periphery (Kerley B lines), cephalization/ vascular marking redistrictuion
- ECHO can evaluate chamber dimensions, valve function, EF, wall motion abnormalities, LV hypertrophy, pericardial effusion
- Serum BNP is high (may help when clinical findings are unclear or other diagnoses such as COPD need to be excluded)
- ECG findings can include previous MI, LV hypertrophy, LBBB, or tachyarrythmia (i.e. atrial fibrillation)

- Treatment of cause
- Supplemental $O_2$ (if arterial saturation < 90%)
- IV diuretic (furosemide)
- ± Nitrates
- ± IV inotropes
- ± Morphine
- +/- NIPPV (i.e. Airvo/ Optiflow, BiPAP)
- ± Ventilatory assistance

## Atrial Fibrillation (AFib)

- Often asymptomatic, but may have palpitations, vague chest discomfort, or symptoms of heart failure (e.g., weakness, light-headedness, dyspnea), particularly when the ventricular rate is very rapid (often 140-160 beats/min)
- May also present with symptoms and signs of acute stroke or of other organ damage due to systemic emboli

- Irregularly irregular pulse with loss of a waves in the jugular venous pulse
- A pulse deficit (the apical ventricular rate is faster than the rate palpated at the wrist) may be present (LV stroke volume is not always sufficient to produce a peripheral pressure wave at fast ventricular rates)

- ECG - absence of P waves, f (fibrillatory) waves between QRS complexes (irregular in timing, irregular in morphology; baseline undulations at rates >300/min not always apparent in all leads), and irregularly irregular R-R intervals
- ECHO
- Thyroid function tests, electrolytes

- Rate control with drugs (BB, CCB) or AV node radiofrequency ablation
- Sometimes rhythm control with cardioversion, drugs (Amiodaraone), or AF substrate ablation
- Prevention of thromboembolism (CHADS score ≥ 1 requires oral anticoagulation)

CIRCULATORY

**CIRCULATORY**

**Infective endocarditis**

| Key Symptoms | Physical Exam | Investigations | Management |
|---|---|---|---|
| • Low-grade fever (< 39° C), night sweats, fatigability, malaise, and weight loss, chills, arthralgias | • May be normal or include: pallor, fever, change in a pre-existing murmur or development of a new regurgitant murmur, tachycardia<br>• Petechiae<br>• Refer to Table 12 for further details | • CBC, electrolytes, extended electrolyte panel, creatinine, liver enzymes, coagulation panel<br>• Blood cultures x 3 (from separate sites)<br>• Transthoracic ECHO (TTE)<br>• Transesophageal ECHO (TEE): should be done when endocarditis is suspected in patients with prosthetic valves, when TTE is non-diagnostic, and when diagnosis of infective endocarditis has been established clinically | • IV antibiotics (based on the organism and its susceptibility)<br>• Sometimes valve debridement, repair, or replacement<br>• Surgical indications include refractory infection, new CHF, or recurrent major systemic emoblization |

## 6.1 Acute Myocardial Infarction (AMI)
### Symptoms
- **Pain:** classically retrosternal, heavy, squeezing or crushing pain, radiating to arm, abdomen, back, neck, jaw, prolonged (often lasting >30 min)
- **Atypical Pain:** "silent" AMI (more often in patients with DM, hypertension, increased age)
- **Associated Symptoms:** diaphoresis, N/V, weakness, pallor, dizziness, palpitations, cerebral symptoms, sense of impending doom

### Physical Exam
- **JVP:** normal, ↑ with RV infarct
- **Pulse:** variable, most commonly rapid and regular, may be normal, ↓ pulse volume, variable BP
- **Palpation:** ↓ point of maximum impulse (PMI), abnormal systolic pulsation 3rd-5th left intercostal space
- **Auscultation:** S3, S4, ↓ intensity of heart sounds, paradoxical split S2, transient apical systolic murmur, mitral regurgitation, pericardial rub
- **Extracardiac Findings:** ↑ Increased RR, pulmonary crackles, signs of arteriosclerosis

## 6.2 Congestive Heart Failure: Left and Right Heart
### Symptoms
- Dyspnea, orthopnea, PND, cough, Cheyne-Stokes respiration, fatigue, weakness, abdominal symptoms (anorexia, nausea, abdominal pain), cerebral symptoms, nocturia, peripheral edema, weight gain

### Physical Exam
- **JVP:** increased, positive hepatojugular reflux
- **Pulse:** ↓ pulse volume, ± pulsus alternans (alternating stronger and weaker beats), sinus tachycardia
- **Palpation:** PMI may be sustained, diffuse and displaced, S3 may be palpable, ± left parasternal lift
- **Auscultation:** S3, S4; S2 may be paradoxically split (often associated with LBBB), murmurs often associated with mitral regurgitation, and tricuspid regurgitation
- **Extracardiac:** systemic hypotension, diastolic pressure may be increased, pulmonary HTN, peripheral cyanosis, pulmonary crackles, hepatomegaly, ascites, edema, pleural effusion, cachexia

**EBM: Congestive Heart Failure**

Features most suggestive of diagnosis of congestive heart failure are the overall clinical judgment, history of heart failure, a third heart sound, jugular venous distension, radiographic pulmonary venous congestion or interstitial edema, and electrocardiographic atrial fibrillation.

The single finding that most decreases the likelihood of heart failure is a brain natriuretic peptide (BNP) <100 pg/mL.

Wang CS, et al. 2005. *JAMA* 294(15):1944-1956.

## 6.3 Mitral Stenosis
**Symptoms**
- Pulmonary edema, atrial arrhythmias, fatigue, abdominal discomfort, edema, hemoptysis, recurrent pulmonary emboli, pulmonary infection, systemic embolization

**Physical Exam**
- **JVP:** elevated if RHF, no "a" wave if atrial fibrillation (AF)
- **Pulse:** normal contour, normal volume, may be irregularly irregular as in AF
- **Palpation:** PMI normal, S1 may be palpable, loud S2 suggests pulmonary HTN
- **Auscultation:** loud S1, opening snap, mid-diastolic decrescendo murmur with presystolic accentuation (lost in AF), possible PR (Graham Steell's murmur)
- **Extracardiac:** ± evidence of pulmonary HTN

## 6.4 Aortic Stenosis
**Symptoms**
- Dyspnea, angina pectoris, exertional syncope, CHF signs and symptoms in later course

**Physical Exam**
- **JVP:** normal or prominent "a" wave (septal hypertrophy)
- **Pulse:** pulsus parvus et tardus (small volume and slow-rising pulse), apical-carotid delay, brachial-radial delay
- **Palpation:** sustained apical beat, systolic thrill may be palpable over aortic area
- **Auscultation:** soft S2, delayed A2, S2 splitting may be lost or paradoxical, systolic crescendo-decrescendo ejection murmur radiating to neck/sternal border, S4 (late peaking correlates with severe AS)

**EBM: Aortic Stenosis**

Effort syncope, slow rate of rise of the carotid artery pulsation, timing of peak murmur intensity in mid or late systole, and decreased intensity of S2 are all associated with an increased likelihood for aortic stenosis.

Absence of a systolic murmur or murmur radiating to the right common carotid artery is associated with a decreased likelihood of aortic stenosis.

Etchells E, Bell C, Robb K. 1997. *JAMA* 277(7):564-571.

## 6.5 Atrial Fibrillation (AF)
**Symptoms**
- Pulmonary congestion, angina pectoris, syncope, fatigue, anxiety, dyspnea, cardiomyopathy, signs of pulmonary emboli

**Physical Exam**
- **JVP:** absent "a" wave
- **Pulse:** irregularly irregular pulse, often tachycardic, variable pulse pressure in the carotid arterial pulse
- **Auscultation:** S1 usually varies in intensity

## Investigations

- **ECG:** P waves not discernable, undulating baseline or sharply inscribed atrial deflections with varying amplitude and frequency (350-600 bpm)
- **Echocardiogram:** LA size helps to determine the likelihood of successful cardioversion and maintenance of sinus rhythm thereafter; also helps to identify underlying cardiac cause of AF (valvular heart disease or cardiomyopathy)

## 6.6 Mitral Regurgitation (MR)

### Symptoms

- Fatigue, exertional dyspnea, orthopnea, symptoms of right-sided heart failure and LV failure

### Physical Exam

- **JVP:** abnormally prominent "a" waves in patients with sinus rhythm and marked pulmonary hypertension and prominent "v" waves in those with accompanying severe TR
- **Pulse:** usually normal, arterial pulse may show a sharp upstroke in patients with severe MR
- **Palpation:** systolic thrill often palpable at cardiac apex, brisk systolic impulse and a palpable rapid-filling wave, apex beat often displaced laterally, RV heave palpable in patients with marked pulmonary hypertension
- **Auscultation:** systolic murmur of at least grade 3/6 intensity, may be holosystolic or decrescendo, S1 generally absent, soft or buried in the systolic murmur, wide splitting of S2, a low-pitched S3 occurring 0.12 to 0.17 s after the aortic valve closure sound, S4 often audible[2]
- **Extracardiac:** pulmonary edema, hepatic congestion, ankle edema, distended neck veins, ascites

---

**EBM: Mitral Regurgitation**

Absence of a mitral area murmur or a late systolic/holosystolic murmur significantly reduces the likelihood of mitral regurgitation.

Etchells E, Bell C, Robb K. 1997. *JAMA* 277(7):564-571.

---

## 6.7 Infective Endocarditis (IE)

- Life-threatening infection of the endocardial surface of the heart, usually on the valves
  - Duke's criteria may be helpful in diagnosis

**Table 12.** Infectious Endocarditis

| History | Signs/Symptoms |
| --- | --- |
| • Rheumatic fever<br>• Prosthetic valves<br>• Previous IE<br>• IV drug users<br>• Intravascular devices (e.g. arterial lines)<br>• Most congenital heart malformations<br>• Valvular dysfunction<br>• Hypertrophic cardiomyopathy<br>• MVP with MR<br>• Recent surgeries<br>• Indwelling catheters or hemodialysis | • Constitutional: fever, chills, malaise, night sweats, anorexia, arthralgias<br>• Cardiac: murmur, palpitations, heart failure<br>• Pulmonary: septic pulmonary embolism<br>• Neurological: focal deficit, headache, meningitis<br>• Metastatic infection: organ infarction<br>• Embolic manifestations:<br>  • Petechiae: conjunctivae, buccal mucosa, palate<br>  • Splinter hemorrhages: linear dark red streaks under nails<br>  • Janeway lesions: nontender hemorrhagic macules on palm and soles<br>  • Osler's nodes: small painful nodules on fingers, toe pads, lasting hours to days<br>  • Roth spots: retinal hemorrhage with pale center near optic disc<br>• Immune-mediated phenomena: vasculitis, glomerulonephritis, splenomegaly, synovitis |

# 7.ECG INTERPRETATION

## ECG Leads
- Six limb leads record voltages from the heart directed onto the frontal plane of the body - 3 bipolar leads I, II, and III; 3 augmented unipolar leads (automated volt left, right, and foot [aVL, aVR, aVF])[3]
- The six chest leads (V1 to V6) record voltages from the heart directed onto the horizontal plane of the body (6 unipolar leads)
- A wave of depolarization moving toward an electrode will record a positive deflection on an ECG; a negative deflection represents a wave of depolarization moving away from an electrode
  - Direction of atrial depolarization: down and right to left
  - Direction of septal depolarization: down and left to right
  - Direction of ventricular depolarization: down and right for RV, down and left for LV, net effect down and left since LV mass >> RV mass

CIRCULATORY

Table 13. Anatomical Correspondence of the ECG Leads

| Leads | Anatomical View |
|---|---|
| V1-V2 | Right ventricle, posterior heart, septum |
| V3-V4 | Interventricular septum, anterior LV wall |
| V5-V6 | Anterior and lateral LV walls |
| V1-V2 | Posterior part of the heart |
| V1-V4 | Anterior part of the heart |
| R chest leads | Right side of the heart |
| I, aVL, V5-V6 | Lateral part of the heart |
| II, III, aVF | Inferior part of the heart |

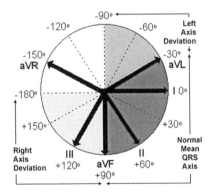

Gilbert Tang 2005

Figure 7. Axial ECG Leads and their Normal Ranges

## 8. APPROACH TO THE ECG
- Heart rate
- Rhythm
- Mean QRS axis
- Waves and segments
- Hypertrophy and chamber enlargement
- Ischemia/infarction

## 8.1 Heart Rate
- Each small box is 40 ms; each large box is 200 ms
- If HR is regular, divide 300 by the number of large squares between two consecutive R waves (e.g. HR is 60 if 5 large squares between consecutive R waves since 300/5 = 60)
- If a rough estimate of HR is required, simply count off the number of large boxes between two consecutive QRS complexes, using the sequence 300, 150, 100, 75, 60, 50: this corresponds to the HR in beats/min
- If HR is irregular, multiply the number of complexes in 6 s (30 large squares) by 10 to determine the average ventricular rate
- Normal sinus rhythm = 60-100 bpm; sinus bradycardia <60 bpm; sinus tachycardia >100 bpm

## 8.2 Rhythm
- Rhythm is considered regular if both RR and PP intervals are equal:
  - Sinus rhythm (i.e. every P wave followed by QRS, and every QRS preceded by P, P wave is positive in leads I or II, and aVF)
- QRS complex: wide or narrow
- Relationship between P waves and QRS complexes, prolonged PR intervals
- Ectopic beats
- Pattern: regular or irregular
- If irregular, note if regularly irregular or irregularly irregular

## 8.3 Mean QRS Axis
- Many methods are available for a fast approximation of the mean QRS axis
- Normal mean QRS axis falls between -30° and +90° (up to +105°)

### Lead Method (I, II)
1. Is the QRS complex of lead I positive or negative?
2. Is the QRS complex of lead II positive or negative?
3. Determine in which quadrant the mean QRS axis lies (e.g. if I is positive and II is positive, then the mean QRS lies between -30° and +90°, which is normal)
4. If lead I is positive and lead II is negative, a left axis deviation is suggested.

### Isoelectric Lead Method (more precise)
1. Look for the most isoelectric lead (i.e. the net area under the curve for the QRS complex is 0): between the baseline and the curve
2. Find the perpendicular lead: is it positive or negative?
3. If positive, the mean QRS complex lies in the positive direction of that lead
- **Left Axis Deviation:** mean axis between -30° and -90°
  - Common causes: left anterior hemiblock, inferior MI, LBBB, WPW
  - Associated causes: heart movement during respiration or an elevated left diaphragm associated with pregnancy, ascites or abdominal tumors
- **Right Axis Deviation:** mean axis between +90° and 180°
  1. Common causes: RVH, RBBB, dextrocardia, acute heart strain (e.g. massive pulmonary embolism), may also be seen in thin individuals, left posterior hemiblock (diagnosis of exclusion)

**Table 14.** Important ECG Characteristics

| | Significance | Parameters |
|---|---|---|
| **P Wave** | Represents atrial depolarization Rhythm is sinus if P wave is positive in leads I, II, and aVF | <2.5 mm in height and <120 ms |
| **PR Interval** | Represents time taken for impulse to travel from SA node to ventricles | Measured from beginning of P wave to beginning of QRS (120-200 ms) |
| **QRS Complex** | Represents ventricular depolarization | • Narrow QRS complex (<120 ms)<br>• Normal (120 ms)<br>• Wide QRS (>120 ms) represents abnormally slow ventricular activation |
| **QT Interval** | Represents time taken for ventricles to depolarize and then repolarize | • Measured from the beginning of QRS complex to end of T wave<br>• Normal is ½ of the preceding RR interval (HR between 60-90 bpm)<br>• QTc = QT Corrected:<br> • Male <450 ms<br> • Female <460 ms |
| **ST Segment** | Represents time interval between depolarization and repolarization | Shorter ST segment with higher heart rate |
| **T Wave** | Represents ventricular repolarization | • Usually positive in all leads except aVR<br>• An inverted T wave in leads V3-V6 is usually abnormal |

CIRCULATORY

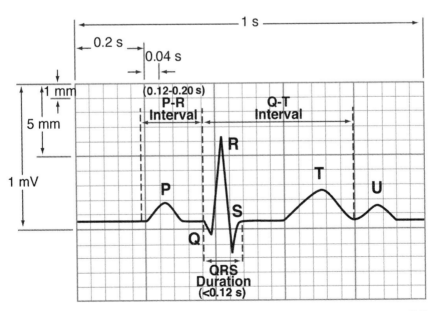

Pina Kingman 2010

**Figure 8.** ECG and Normal Values

**Table 15.** Common Arrhythmias (List not exhaustive)

| Location | Example | |
|---|---|---|
| **Atrium** | | |
| **Premature Atrial Contractions (PAC)** | | * |
| **Atrial Flutter** | | † |
| **Atrial Fibrillation (AF)** | | † |
| **Supraventricular Tachycardia (SVT)** | | † |
| **AV Node** | | |
| **Conduction Blocks:** <br> **1° Atrioventricular Block** <br> (↑ PR interval) | | * |
| **2° Atrioventricular Block** <br> (Wenckebach shown to the right) <br> – Mobitz Type 1 (Wenckebach) <br> – Mobitz Type 2 (Classic) | | * |
| **3° Atrioventricular Block** <br> (complete heart block) | | * |
| **Ventricle** | | |
| **Premature Ventricular Contractions (PVC)** | | * |
| **Ventricular Tachycardia (VTach)** | | † |
| **Torsades de Pointes** | | † |
| **Ventricular Fibrillation (VF)** | | † |

*GE Marquette, 2000
†Patient samples

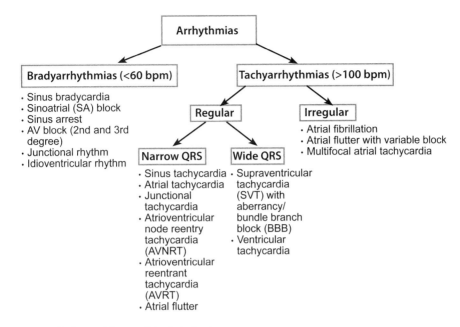

CIRCULATORY

**Figure 8.** General Approach to Arrhythmias

## 8.4 Waves and Segments (P Wave Abnormality)

- Left Atrial Enlargement
    - LA enlarges posteriorly (downward deflection in V1)
    - In V1 a deep terminal component that is ≥40 ms and ≥1 mm deep
    - P wave has double peaks and P wave >120 ms (P mitrale) in lead II
- Right Atrial Enlargement
    - RA enlarges vertically (tall P wave in inferior leads)
    - Large P wave >2.5 mm (height) in leads II, III or aVF
    - In V1 a large positive wave >1.5 mm may be seen

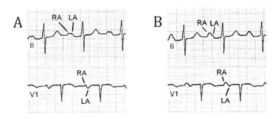

**Figure 9.** (A) Left and (B) Right Atrial Enlargement ECG (Tracing Dr. F. Yanowitz, 1999)

## 8.5 Hypertrophy and Chamber Enlargement

- Left Ventricular Hypertrophy (LVH):
    - Leads I, aVL, V5, and V6 show taller R waves
    - Leads V1 and V2 show deeper than normal S waves
    - Criteria for the diagnosis of LVH:
        - S in V1 + R in V5 or V6 >35 mm above 40 yr (>40 mm for age 31-40 yr, >45 mm for age 21-30 yr)
        - R in aVL>11 mm
        - R in I + S in III >25 mm
    - Additional criteria: left atrial enlargement, ventricular strain (asymmetric ST depression in leads I, aVL, V4-V6)
        - Associated features: delayed intrinsicoid deflection (longer QR interval, >0.05 s)

- Right Ventricular Hypertrophy (RVH):
  - ◆ Results in a large R wave in V1 and a large S wave in V6
  - ◆ Criteria for the diagnosis of RVH:
    - ◆ Right axis deviation
    - ◆ R/S ratio >1 or qR in lead V1
    - ◆ RV strain pattern: ST segment depression and T wave inversion in leads V1-V2
- Bundle Branch Blocks:
  - ◆ Left bundle branch block (LBBB)
    - ◆ Right ventricle depolarizes first due to LBBB
    - ◆ QRS >120 ms
    - ◆ Broad-notched R wave in V5, V6, I, aV
  - ◆ Right bundle branch block (RBBB)
    - ◆ QRS >120 ms
    - ◆ QRS positive in lead V1 (rSR')
    - ▪ Broad S wave in leads I, V5-V6 (>40 ms)
    - ▪ Use first 60 ms of the QRS complex to determine mean QRS axis

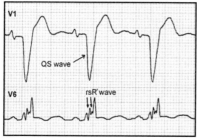

**Figure 10.** LBBB ECG Tracing (GE Marquette, 2000.)

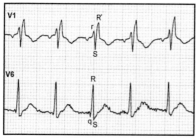

**Figure 11.** RBBB ECG Tracing (GE Marquette, 2000.)

## 8.6 Ischemia/Infarction
### Transmural MI
- Q waves are possible evidence of a prior transmural MI
- A significant Q wave must be either 40 ms wide (1 small box or greater) or one-third the height of the R wave
- For the Q waves to be suggestive of prior infarction, Q waves should be present in at least 2 leads in the same territory

**Table 16.** Localization of the Acute MI

| Anatomical Location | Leads with Abnormal ECG Complexes | Associated Coronary Artery |
|---|---|---|
| Posterior | V1, V2 (tall R, not Q) | RCA or CFX (distal) |
| Inferior | II, III, aVF | RCA |
| Anterior Septal | V1, V2 | LAD |
| Anterior Apical | V3, V4 | LAD (distal) |
| Lateral | I, aVL, V5, V6 | CFX |
| Anterior | V2-V5 | LAD (proximal) |
| Right Ventricle | R chest leads V3, V4 | RCA |

CFX = left circumflex artery, LAD = left anterior descending artery, RCA = right coronary artery

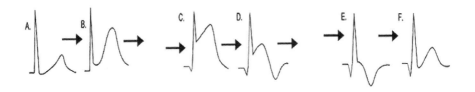

**Figure 12.** ECG Evolution during Acute Q-Wave MI (Dr. F. Yanowitz, 1999.)

**Table 17.** Legend Corresponding to Figure 12

| Time Frame | ECG Changes |
|---|---|
| A. Normal | None |
| B. Acute | ST elevation |
| C. Hours | ST elevation, depressed R wave, Q wave begins |
| D. 1-2 Days | T wave inversion, increased Q wave |
| E. Days | ST normalizes, T wave inverted |
| F. Weeks | ST and T normal, Q wave remains |

### 8.7 ST Segment and T Wave Abnormalities

- Non-Q wave MI involves only the subendocardial layers of the myocardium (not transmural)
- Results in ECG changes, such as T wave inversion and ST segment depression
- Causes of ST segment depression[4]:
  - Angina (ischemia)
  - Subendocardial infarction
  - Acute posterior wall MI (V1 and V2)
  - LVH strain
  - LBBB
- Causes of ST segment elevation[4]:
  - Acute MI
  - Post MI
  - Acute pericarditis
  - Ventricular aneurysm
  - Early repolarization

# REFERENCES

1. Braunwald E, Zipes DP, Libby P. *Heart Disease: A Textbook of Cardiovascular Medicine.* Philadelphia: Saunders; 2011.
2. Lilly LS (Editor). *Pathophysiology of Heart Disease: A Collaborative Project of Medical Students and Faculty,* 5th ed. Philadelphia: Wolters Kluwer/Lippincott Williams & Wilkins; 2011.
3. Casella L, Nader A. *ECG Made Simple.* http://www.ecgmadesimple.com. Accessed May 2016.
4. Wesley K. *Basic Dysrhythmias and Acute Coronary Syndromes: Interpretation and Management.* St. Louis: Mosby Jems; 2011.
5. Bickley LS, Szilagyi PG, Bates B. *Bates' Guide to Physical Examination and History Taking,* 10th ed. Philadelphia: Lippincott Williams & Wilkins; 2009.
6. Dugani S, Lam D (Editors). *The Toronto Notes 2009: Comprehensive Medical Reference.* Toronto: Toronto Notes for Medical Students, Inc; 2009.
7. Fauci AS. *Harrison's Principles of Internal Medicine.* New York: McGraw-Hill; 2008.
8. Swartz MH. *Textbook of Physical Diagnosis: History and Examination,* 6th ed. Philadelphia: Saunders Elsevier; 2010.
9. Arnold, M. Heart Failure. *Merck Manual Online.* http://www.merckmanuals.com/en-ca/professional. Accessed May 2016.
10. Dumitru I, et al. Heart Failure. *Medscape and TheHeart.Org.* http://emedicine.medscape.com/. Accessed May 2016.
11. Higginson, L. Symptoms of Cardiovascular Disorders. *Merck Manual Online.* http://www.merckmanuals.com/en-ca/professional. Accessed May 2016.
12. Huckell, V. Endocarditis. *Merck Manual Online.* http://www.merckmanuals.com/en-ca/professional. Accessed May 2016.
13. Tunkel, F. Fever. *Merck Manual Online.* http://www.merckmanuals.com/en-ca/professional. Accessed May 2016.
14. Warnica, J. Coronary Artery Disease. *Merck Manual Online.* http://www.merckmanuals.com/en-ca/professional. Accessed May 2016.
15. Wise, R. COPD. *Merck Manual Online.* http://www.merckmanuals.com/en-ca/professional. Accessed May 2016.

CIRCULATORY

CHAPTER 2B:

# The Peripheral Vascular Exam

**Editors:**
Mohammed Firdouse, BHSc
Qazi Zain Sohail, BSc
Yuhao Shi, BSc

**Resident Reviewer:**
Benny Dua, MD, PhD

**Faculty Reviewers:**
George Oreopoulos, MD, MSc, FRCSC

## TABLE OF CONTENTS

# 1. COMMON CHIEF COMPLAINTS

**Table 1.** Common presentations and differential diagnoses

| Chief Complaints | Differential Diagnosis | Distinguishing Features |
|---|---|---|
| **Intermittent leg pain** | Chronic limb ischemia (vascular claudication) | Highly reproducible exertional pain, relieved with rest; atherosclerosis risk factors |
| | Neurogenic claudication | Position dependent; hx of spinal disc issues |
| | MSK related | Hx of injury; reproducible pain with movement |
| **Acute onset non-traumatic leg pain** | Acute limb ischemia | Severe pain, sensory and motor deficits, pallor, absent distal pulses |
| | Infection (cellulitis, necrotizing fasciitis) | May have accompanying fever, increased WBC, rapidly spreading erythema |
| | Deep vein thrombosis (DVT) | Hx of immobility, surgery, hypercoagulable state, previous DVTs |
| **Constant leg pain** | Critical limb ischemia | Hx of claudication, ulcers, rest pain |
| | Osteosarcoma | Constitutional symptoms, pathological fractures |
| | MSK related | Hx of trauma |
| **Skin ulcerations** | Diabetic ulcer | Poorly controlled diabetes, decreased peripheral sensations, neuropathic pain |
| | Venous ulcer | Often medial malleolus, skin changes (lipodermatosclerosis), varicose veins |
| | Arterial ulcer | Distal regions of foot, well demarcated, absent distal pulses |
| | Malignant ulcer | Constitutional symptoms, atypical appearance |
| | Traumatic ulcer | Hx of trauma |
| **Acute abdominal/ back pain** | Symptomatic/ruptured Abdominal Aortic Aneurysm (AAA) | Pulsatile abdominal mass, hemodynamic instability; Retroperitoneal bruising if ruptured |
| | For full DDx for abdominal pain, see **The Gastrointestinal System** Chapter | |
| **Uncommon problems** | Aortic dissection | Hx of sudden onset tearing chest pain, BP difference in each arm |
| | Mesenteric ischemia | Hx of postprandial pain, weight loss, hematochezia |
| | Thoracic outlet syndrome | Pain or numbness in arm, swelling and bluish discoloration of arm after physical exertion. |

CIRCULATORY

**Other common presentations:**
· Varicose veins
· Incidental finding of asymptomatic abdominal aortic aneurysm on imaging
· Neurological events (TIAs/stroke) in the setting of carotid disease

## 2. FOCUSED HISTORY

### 2.1 Risk Factors
- Atherosclerosis
  - Smoking
  - HTN
  - DM
  - Family history
  - Lifestyle (e.g. exercise, diet)
  - Elevated cholesterol
- Thromboembolic event
  - Atrial fibrillation, post-myocardial infarction <3 mo, valvular disease, prosthetic valves, endocarditis, cardiomyopathy, myxoma

### 2.2 Previous Medical History
- History of heart disease:
  - Congestive heart failure (CHF) - peripheral edema, pulmonary congestion, exercise intolerance
- History of arterial disease:
  - Myocardial infarction (MI) or coronary artery disease (CAD)
  - Signs and symptoms of MI or CAD (see **The Precordial Exam** Chapter)
  - Peripheral vascular disease (PVD) often considered a "CAD equivalent"
- Stroke/TIA
  - Cerebrovascular occlusive disease
  - Signs and symptoms of stroke (see **The Nervous System** Chapter) including: unilateral or bilateral weakness/paralysis of limbs, sensory deficits, speech difficulties, diplopia or amaurosis fugax, and facial droop
  - Neurological symptoms (e.g. dizziness, presyncope, and syncope)
  - Hemispheric symptoms
- Vasculitis
  - Skin changes, mucosal ulcerations
  - Joint pain
  - Changes in vision and/or eye pain
- History of venous disease:
  - Varicose veins
  - Venous ulcers, skin discolorations
  - Previous deep vein thrombosis (DVTs)
  - Risk factors for DVTs:
    - Recent prolonged immobilization
    - Postoperatively (especially orthopedic, thoracic, GI, GU)
    - Trauma (fractures of femur, pelvis, spine, tibia, etc.)
    - Post-MI, CHF
    - Long travel
    - Hormone-related: pregnancy, oral contraceptive pill use, hormone replacement therapy, selective estrogen receptor modulators (SERMs)
    - Inheritable hypercoagulability states:
    - APLA syndrome, Factor V Leiden, Prothrombin G20210A, etc.
    - Underlying malignancy or blood dyscrasias

### 2.3 History of presenting illness
### Symptoms of acute limb ischemia  (6 P's)
- **P**olar /poikilothermia (cold): typically first notable symptom
- **P**ain: absent in 20% of cases due to prompt onset of anesthesia and paralysis
- **P**allor: replaced by mottled (network-like appearance) cyanosis within a few hours
- **P**aresthesia*: light touch lost first (small fibers) followed by other sensory modalities

(larger fibers)
- **P**aralysis*/Power loss: further progression of ischemia, indicative of severity
- **P**ulselessness
- *Paresthesia and paralysis suggest critical ischemia
- Do NOT expect all of the **6 P**'s to be present and do NOT rely on pulses

### Critical Ischemia
- Acute
  - **6 P**'s
  - Neuromotor dysfunction
- Chronic
  - Night pain
  - Pain at rest (pain at all times and not relieved by dependency)
  - Tissue loss (ulceration/gangrene)

### Pain
- **OPQRSTUVW** with emphasis on:
  - Onset (e.g. exertional pain in legs and amount of exercise required)
  - Location (muscles, abdomen)
  - Reproducible pain with similar exertion (consistent pattern)

### Skin
- Changes in color, temperature, appearance
- Ulceration
  - Classification (traumatic, ischemic, neoplastic, venous, mixed, malignant)
  - Time and rate of development
  - If resulting from minor trauma (e.g. toes, heel), may indicate chronic ischemia
- Gangrene: wet (infectious) vs. dry (noninfectious)

## 3. FOCUSED PHYSICAL EXAM

### 3.1 General
- Ensure the patient is adequately exposed with draping in between the legs
- Remember to compare sides
- Vitals: bilateral and orthostatic blood pressures (see **General History and Physical Exam**)

### 3.2 Inspection
- Specific locations
  - Upper & Lower extremities
    - Inspect for SEADS: Swelling, Erythema, Atrophy, Deformity, Skin changes (shiny skin, hair loss, ulcers)
- Arterial insufficiency
  - Cyanosis: central (frenulum and buccal mucosa) and peripheral (nails)
  - Skin: cool, pale extremities, increased pigmentation, swelling, heaviness and aching in legs (usually medial lower third of legs)
  - Ulcers: ischemic ulceration due to trauma of the toes and heel, develops rapidly, painful, and has discretely visible edges
- Venous stasis
  - Skin: warm, thickening and erythema over the ankle and lower leg (dependent areas), thickened (woody) fibrosis/lipodermatosclerosis of subcutaneous tissues
  - Ulcers: stasis ulceration of ankle or above medial malleolus, develops slowly, painless, diffuses with no distinct borders, exudate
  - Veins: engorgement, varicosities
    - Prominent veins in edematous limb may be secondary to hereditary varicose veins or venous obstruction
    - Pemberton's sign: facial flushing, distension of neck veins, elevation of JVP, and stridor when patient raises arms above head (sign of vena cava obstruction)
  - Chronic venous insufficiency: warm, erythematous, thickened skin, increased pigmentation, ± brown ulcers around ankles
  - Superficial phlebitis: warm, painful, erythema secondary to inflammation around

vein, superficial changes, swelling of distal part of extremity

**Clinical Pearl: Deep Vein Thrombosis**
Painless swelling in the affected limb is a common symptom of DVT, which is a risk factor for PE.

- **Vasculitis**
  - Skin:
    - Livedo reticularis rash (bluish-red discoloration, network pattern)
    - Malar or discoid rash on face in SLE
    - Raynaud's phenomenon: episodes of sharply demarcated pallor and/or cyanosis, then erythema of the digits (see **Common Clinical Scenarios**, p. 57)
    - Purpura
  - Mucosa: oral or nasal ulcers (SLE, Wegener's, Behçet's)
  - Joints: look for "active" swollen joints
  - Eyes: episcleritis, scleritis, anterior uveitis (iritis)
  - Venous and arterial thrombosis/ulcers, gangrene as above

## 3.3 Palpation and Auscultation

### Arterial
- Skin temperature: feel with back of hand: warm vs. cool
- Capillary refill: compress nailbeds and determine the duration for return of circulation: normal = 2-3 s
- **Pulses**
  - Rate: tachycardia >100 bpm, bradycardia <60 bpm
  - Rhythm: regular, regularly irregular (consistent pattern), irregularly irregular
  - Amplitude:

| Amplitude of Pulses | |
|---|---|
| 0 | Absent |
| 1 | Diminished |
| 2 | Normal |
| 3 | Increased |
| 4 | Aneurysmal (often exaggerated, widened pulse) |

  - Always compare both sides for presence and symmetry

*Characteristic Pulse Patterns*
- **Hyperkinetic Pulse**
  - Strong, bounding pulse
  - Increased stroke volume in heart block
  - Hyperdynamic circulation and increased stoke volume in fever, anemia, exercise, anxiety
  - Reduced peripheral resistance in patent ductus arteriosus, AV fistula
- **Pulsus Tardus**
  - Small, slowly rising pulse that is delayed with respect to heart sounds
  - Seen in aortic stenosis
- **Pulsus Parvus (Hypokinetic)**
  - Small, weak pulse due to diminished left ventricular (LV) stroke volume
  - Seen in hypovolemia, LV failure, MI, restrictive pericardial disease, shock, arrythmia, and aortic stenosis

**Table 2.** Description of Characteristic Wave Forms

| Waveform | Description | Representative Diagram | Associated with/ Etiology |
|---|---|---|---|
| Pulsus Parvus et Tardus (anacrotic) | Small, slow rising pulse with drop or notch in ascending portion | | Aortic stenosis |
| Collapsing | Quick rise, quick fall | | Increased $CO_2$ |
| Water-Hammer | Sudden rapid pulse with full expansion followed by sudden collapse | | Aortic regurgitation or arterial obstruction |
| Bisferiens | Double-peaked pulse with mid-systolic dip | | Aortic regurgitation, ± aortic stenosis, hypertrophic cardiomyopathy |
| Alternans | Alternating amplitude of pulses | | CHF, more easily detected in conjunction with BP measurement |

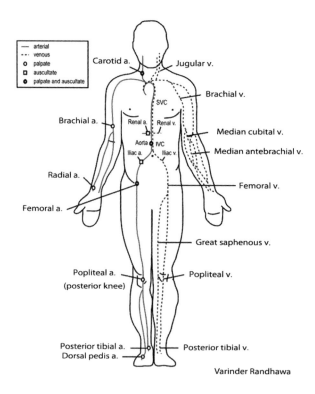

Varinder Randhawa

**Figure 1.** Location of Pulses

*Examine the following pulses (see Figure 1):*
- **Carotid**
  - ◆ Auscultate for bruits (absent, mild/soft, harsh/loud)
  - ◆ If no bruits, palpate one carotid artery at a time

- **Brachial**
  - May use thumb to palpate
- **Radial**
  - Use the pads/tips of three fingers
  - Significant delay of the radial pulse after the brachial pulse may suggest aortic stenosis
- **Abdominal Aorta**
  - Normal width of abdominal aorta is about 2 cm
  - Palpate deeply for pulsations (lay patient flat, ensure abdomen is relaxed)
  - Auscultate for abdominal bruits
  - Midline pulsatile abdominal mass may be an abdominal aortic aneurysm (AAA)
  - Midline abdominal bruit suggests atherosclerotic disease of the aorta or renal vessels
- **Renal Arteries**
  - Auscultate for bruits at positions 5 cm above the umbilicus and     3-5 cm to either side of the midline or from the back
- **Femoral**
  - Palpate at midpoint of the inguinal ligament
  - Auscultate for bruits
  - Compare timing of femoral pulse with radial pulse to rule out radio-femoral delay
  - Significant delay of the femoral pulse after the radial pulse suggests coarctation of the upstream aorta (most commonly thoracic, however abdominal coarctation is also possible)
- **Popliteal**
  - Flex the knee approximately 10-20°
  - Using two hands, place thumbs on the tibial tuberosity and palpate deeply in the popliteal fossa with 3-4 fingers from each hand (allow knee to relax/fall into both hands)
  - A decreased or absent pulse indicates partial or complete arterial occlusion proximally; all pulses distal to occlusion are typically affected
  - Prominent pulse may predict popliteal aneurysm
- **Posterior Tibial**
  - Palpate behind and slightly below the medial malleolus
  - Chronic arterial occlusion of the legs causes intermittent claudication, postural color changes and skin alterations
- **Dorsalis Pedis**
  - Palpate on dorsum of the foot, lateral to extensor hallicus longus tendon

---

**Clinical Pearl: Dorsalis Pedis**
Dorsalis pedis is absent in 15% of normal populations.

---

## Venous
*Edema*
- Check for pitting (venous) or nonpitting (lymphatic) edema
  - Press firmly with thumb over bony prominences for >5 s
    - Over the dorsum of each foot
    - Behind each medial malleolus
    - Over the shins
    - If nonambulatory, check for sacral edema
  - Pitting: depression caused by the pressure from your thumb
    - Pitting suggests orthostasis, chronic venous insufficiency or CHF
    - Firm, nonpitting edema (lymphedema) suggests lymphatic obstruction (see **The Lymphatic System** Chapter)
  - Note height of leg edema and if swelling is unilateral or bilateral
  - Unilateral edema may suggest DVT
  - When following patients with chronic edema (venous or lymphatic), it may be useful to document calf circumference at serial visits
    - A difference between the two sides suggests edema

- Muscular atrophy can also cause differences in leg circumference
  - ◆ Note unusually prominent veins
  - ◆ Chronic venous insufficiency can lead to dependent edema ('heaviness in the legs')
  - ◆ With DVT, extent of edema may suggest location of occlusion:
    - A calf DVT when the lower leg or ankle is swollen
    - An iliofemoral DVT when the entire leg is swollen

## Special Tests

*Arterial: Arterial Insufficiency*
- Allen Test
  - ◆ Purpose: test for good collateral flow through the ulnar artery before proceeding with puncture of the radial artery for arterial blood gases
  - ◆ Method
    - Using your thumbs, occlude the patient's radial and ulnar arteries at the wrist
    - Ask patient to open his/her hand with the palm up: palm should be blanched
    - Then release pressure on the ulnar artery only, watch palm for "blushing"
  - ◆ Normal Result: color returns to the hand in <5 s
  - ◆ **Abnormal Result**: if color does not return within 10 s, DO NOT perform arterial puncture at this site, as this may indicate incomplete palmar arch or insufficient collateral flow
- Straight Leg Raise Test (Pallor on Elevation)
  - ◆ Raise the leg 45-60° for 30 s, or until pallor of the feet develops
  - ◆ Normal Result: mild pallor on elevation
  - ◆ **Abnormal Result**: marked pallor on elevation may suggest arterial insufficiency
- Rubor on Dependency
  - ◆ After performing the straight leg raise test, ask the patient to sit up and dangle both legs over the side of the bed
  - ◆ Normal Result: return of color within 10 s, filling of the superficial veins of the foot within 15 s
  - ◆ **Abnormal Result**: persistent pallor of the feet for >10 s followed by rubor (marked redness) on dependency (after 1-2 min) may be seen in patients with critical ischemia; the marked redness is due to arterial dilation following the tissue hypoxia induced by elevation of a leg with arterial insufficiency

*Venous: Incompetent Saphenous Vein*
- Brodie-Trendelenburg Maneuver
  - ◆ Ask the patient to lie supine and raise his/her legs 90° for 15 s to empty the veins
  - ◆ Place a tourniquet around the patient's upper thigh after the veins have drained (do not occlude arterial pulse)
  - ◆ Instruct the patient to stand
  - ◆ Watch for venous filling with the tourniquet on for 60 s
  - ◆ Normal Result: superficial saphenous system should fill slowly from below the tourniquet within 35 s
  - ◆ **Abnormal Result**:
    - Fast filling: indicates incompetence of the deep and perforator veins
    - Slow filling: remove the tourniquet and observe the superficial venous system
    - Retrograde flow: suggests superficial venous incompetence
  - ◆ Tourniquet can be used above and below knee to differentiate between long and short saphenous incompetence

## 4. COMMON INVESTIGATIONS

## Blood Work
- Prior to CT angiogram: consider Cr for renal function
- Prior to catheter angiogram: CBC, PT, INR, PTT and Cr
- For risk factor assessment: HbA1C, total cholesterol, LDL, and HDL
- Hypercoagulability work-up:
  - ◆ aPTT, PT/INR, fibrinogen, factor assay

- ◆ Deficiency of antithrombin III, protein C or S
- ◆ Lupus anticoagulant, anticardiolipin antibody
- ◆ C-anti-neutrophil cytoplasmic antibody (C-ANCA), P-ANCA
- ◆ D-dimers: useful to rule out venous thromboembolism (VTE) if negative and low clinical suspicion

## Ankle-Brachial Index (ABI)

- ABI for each ankle = ankle systolic pressure / higher brachial systolic pressure of the two arms
- ABI diagnoses the presence (sensitivity = 95%, specificity = 100%) and severity of peripheral artery disease (PAD)
- ABI >0.90 is normal, ABI >1.3 suggests calcification, 0.5-0.8 is claudication range, <0.4 suggests possible critical ischemia[1]

## Duplex Ultrasonography

- Detects the direction, velocity, and turbulence of blood flow with an accurate anatomical view
- Can assess location and degree of stenosis as well as patency of bypass grafts; in detecting >50% stenosis in iliac arteries, generally has a sensitivity of 90% and a specificity of 95%
- Normal arteries produce biphasic or triphasic waveform signals, while monophasic signals are associated with an upstream stenosis; a significant increase in arterial flow velocity also suggests stenosis

## CT Angiogram (CTA)

- Very helpful in assessing underlying atherosclerosis, aneurysm, and dissection
- Requires IV contrast, but is associated with less radiation than conventional angiogram
- In detecting >50% stenosis in iliac arteries, has a sensitivity from 89-100%, and a specificity from 92-100%

## MR Angiogram (MRA)

- Gadolinium dye is used for delineating anatomy
- Useful in minimizing radiation exposure

## Conventional Cathether-Based Angiography

- Arterial or venous access followed by contrast injection and image using fluoroscopy; is often intraoperative to facilitate thrombolytic or endovascular therapy
- Detects narrowing of vessels and vessel anatomy
- Gold standard technique, but is invasive and uses high doses of radiation

# 5. COMMON CLINICAL SCENARIOS

**Table 3.** Summary of Common Disorders

| Signs/ Symptoms | On exam | Investigations | Management |
|---|---|---|---|
| **Acute Arterial Occlusion** | | | |
| Sudden pain, local neurological symptoms, +/- Hx of claudication +/- skin changes | Cool temperature, sluggish capillary refill and weak arterial pulses. 6P's (see above) | CBC, aPTT, PT/INR; ECG, Echo (embolus) CT angiography | Depends on thrombus vs embolus (see Table 4) Medical: heparinization Surgical: endovascular thrombolysis/embolectomy; bypass graft |

**CIRCULATORY**

### Chronic Arterial Occlusion

| Signs/ Symptoms | On exam | Investigations | Management |
|---|---|---|---|
| Atrophic changes of skin and muscle, intermittent claudication, rest pain, night pain | Hair loss, shiny skin, hypertrophic nails, pallor on elevation/rubor on dependency, Allen test | Routine blood work<br>ABI<br>Duplex ultrasonography<br>CT Angiography | Manage risk factors<br><br>Medical: aspirin, clopidogrel<br><br>Surgical: endovascular stenting, bypass graft |

### Aortic Dissection

| Signs/ Symptoms | On exam | Investigations | Management |
|---|---|---|---|
| Acute onset tearing chest/inter-scapular pain. Presentation varies according to aortic branches involves - Coronary (MI), carotids (Syncope, Horner's, neurological deficits), mesenteric, renal, iliac (ischemic limb) | Hypotension in Type A and hypertension in Type B. Asymmetric pulses or BP. | Routine blood work<br>ECG, CXR<br>CTA | Resuscitation<br><br>Medical: beta-blocker, analgesia (BP target 100-120 systolic)<br><br>Surgical:<br>Type A: open surgery<br><br>Type B: if complicated, endovascular or open repair |

### AAA

| Signs/ Symptoms | On exam | Investigations | Management |
|---|---|---|---|
| Generally asymptomatic until they rupture. Often misdiagnosed as renal colic. Surgical emergency | Flank ecchymosis, pulsatile abdominal mass, hypotension | Blood work<br>Abdominal U/S<br>CT abdomen (assess extent) | Ruptured: proximal aortic control endovascularly/ surgical<br><br>Asymptomatic: conservative management or surgical repair |

### Carotid Artery Disease

| Signs/ Symptoms | On exam | Investigations | Management |
|---|---|---|---|
| May be asymptomatic; TIA, Amaurosis fugax, Stroke | Hollenhorst plaques on fundoscopy, +/- carotid bruits | Blood work<br>Duplex ultrasonography<br>MRA<br>Catheter based angiography (Gold standard) | Risk factor management<br>Aspirin/ clopidogrel<br><br>Asymptomatic: surgery if >60% stenosis<br><br>Symptomatic: surgery if >50% stenosis |

### VTE

| Signs/ Symptoms | On exam | Investigations | Management |
|---|---|---|---|
| Sudden unilateral pain, swelling of limb, erythema and warmth that is relieved with elevation | Venous distention is exacerbated in upright position, collateral vein distentions, leg swelling (>3 cm difference), Homan's sign | Blood work<br>D-dimer if very low suspicion (sensitive)<br>ECG CXR<br>Doppler ultrasonography | Prophylaxis in moderate-high risk: LMWH or UFH<br><br>Long-term therapy: anticoagulation (warfarin, NOAC), IVC filter if anticoagulation contraindicated; massive PE may require aggressive thrombolysis |

| Signs/ Symptoms | On exam | Investigations | Management |
|---|---|---|---|
| **Vasculitis** | | | |
| Joint pain, vision changes, renal failure, neuropathy, Raynaud's phenomenon | Depends on underlying condition (see below for details) | Autoimmune work up: ESR, CRP, ANCA, RF, C3, C4, ANA, anti-phospholipid antibodies Urinalysis Consider biopsy | Treat underlying cause; commonly use immunosuppressants |
| **Superficial Venous Thrombosis** | | | |
| Tenderness, induration, redness | No swelling of limb, localized swelling along course of the vein | Clinical diagnosis | Conservative: warm compress, ambulate Medical: consider heparin/ anti-platelet Surgical if above fails |
| **Varicose Veins** | | | |
| Dull aching, burning or cramping provoked by prolonged standing or menstruation. Edema resolves over night. | Varicose veins, ulceration, Brodie-Trendelenburg maneuver | Duplex ultrasonography | Conservative: compression stockings Surgical: indicated if symptoms bad, prominent tissue changes Sclerotherapy Stripping Endovenous Laser Treatment (EVLT) |

## 5.1 Arterial

## Acute Arterial Occlusion/Insufficiency
- Patient has 6 h before irreversible muscle injury (in the setting of complete ischemia). This is a vascular emergency!

*Etiology*
- Important to differentiate embolism from thrombosis because the treatment for the two varies
- **Embolus**
  - Cardiogenic embolus: (80-90%)
  - Atrial fibrillation (most common)
    - MI <3 mo (anterior MI most common)
    - Valvular disease (e.g. endocarditis)
    - Cardiomyopathy with severe LV dysfunction
    - Atrial myxoma (very rare)
  - Arterial embolus:
    - Atheroembolism (e.g. ulcerated plaque)
    - Aneurysms (e.g. popliteal)
  - Paradoxical embolism
    - History of venous embolus passing through intracardiac shunt
    - May have history of oral contraceptive pill (OCP) use, VTE, PE, TIA, or stroke
- *In situ* **Thrombosis**
  - Atherosclerotic artery with underlying severe disease

- Bypass graft occlusion (most common example)
- Increased risk associated with hypercoagulable state (e.g. malignancy) and stasis (e.g. CHF)
- **Trauma**
  - Iatrogenic (e.g. arterial catheterization)
- **Idiopathic**

**Clinical Pearl: Acute Arterial Occlusion**
If there is neuromuscular compromise (i.e. paralysis and/or absent sensation) emergent revascularization is indicated.

**Table 4.** Embolus vs. *In situ* Thrombosis in Acute Arterial Occlusion

| Feature | Embolus | In situ Thrombus |
|---|---|---|
| Onset of Pain | Sudden | Acute-on-chronic or gradual |
| Neuromuscular Status | Severe loss of function | Less severe loss (due to collaterals) |
| History of Claudication | Unlikely | Maybe |
| Contralateral Pulses | Usually normal | Diminished or absent |
| Chronic Skin Changes | No | Maybe |
| Possible Associated Symptoms | Focal neurological deficits (stroke), abdominal pain (splenic, mesenteric, renal), shortness of breath, blue toe syndrome | Usually local process |

*Signs and Symptoms*
- Depend on the etiology (see **Table 4**)
- Compartment syndrome:
  - Characterized by elevated interstitial pressure due to reperfusion injury and edema in the rigid compartments of the lower limb
  - Treatment is fasciotomy
  - Note that pulse may be normal
  - Pain may be refractory to narcotics or passive stretch of muscles in the affected compartment.

*Physical Exam*
- Vitals
- Inspect limbs for pallor, chronic skin changes, and signs of critical ischemia (e.g. ulcerations, gangrene)
- Palpate limbs for cool temperature, sluggish capillary refill, and arterial pulses
- Assess neuromuscular status of limbs
- Neurological, cardiorespiratory, and abdominal exams

*Investigations*
- If physical exam findings are severe, may have to immediately treat without the delay of investigations
- CBC, aPTT, PT/INR, troponin (consider: Cr, LFTs, lactate)
- ECG (rule out atrial fibrillation or MI)
- Echocardiogram (identify valvular disease, intracardiac thrombus, or aortic dissection)
- Bedside ABI with Doppler (consider duplex ultrasonography)
- Computed tomography angiography (CTA)
- Conventional angiography (usually intraoperatively)

*Treatment*
- Medical: immediate heparinization, consider long-term antiplatelet and/or anticoagulation

depending on underlying etiology
- Surgical/endovascular: intraarterial thrombolysis, embolectomy, thrombectomy ± bypass graft ± endovascular therapy, primary amputation
- Treat underlying cause

## Chronic Arterial Occlusion/Insufficiency

*Etiology*
- Atherosclerosis (most common)
- Rare causes include (vasculitis, see p. 67): giant cell arteritis, Takayasu disease, Buerger's disease, polyarteritis nodosa

*Signs and Symptoms*
- Chronic atrophic changes of the skin and muscles
- Intermittent claudication: pain or discomfort in calves or thighs with exertion that is relieved rapidly with rest. Classically reproducible in the same location with the same amount of exertion
- Critical ischemia: rest pain, night pain, and/or tissue loss
- Leriche's syndrome: if male patient complains of buttock or thigh pain while walking, inquire about impotence (intermittent claudication and impotence are features caused by chronic aortoiliac obstruction)
- Chronic mesenteric ischemia: classically describe history of weight loss, and "food fear" due to postprandial pain

**Table 5.** Vascular Claudication vs. Neurogenic Claudication vs. Musculoskeletal Pain

| Feature | Vascular | Neurogenic | MSK |
|---|---|---|---|
| Onset of Pain | Dependent on discrete, reproducible amount of exercise | Sudden discomfort with locomotion or change in position | Sudden discomfort with locomotion or movement |
| Location of Pain | Can be unilateral - involves muscles of lower extremities (calf, thigh or buttock) | Usually bilateral - involves whole leg and can be associated with numbness and tingling | Localized to affected joints or muscles, somtimes improves with movement |
| Resolution of Pain | Rest (usually <5 min) | Rest (>5 min) | Rest (>5 min), often variable |
| Alleviating and Provoking Factors | No change with position | Flexion of spine relieves pain | Pain is often insidious and gradually progresses over years, with flare-ups and remissions |
| Pulses | Diminished or absent | Present | Present |
| Skin | Atrophic changes | No changes | No changes |

*Physical Exam*
- Inspect for signs of chronic poor perfusion: hair loss and/or shiny skin, pallor, arterial ulcers, hypertrophic nails, muscle atrophy
- Palpate for cool temperature and sluggish capillary refill
- Assess for decreased or absent pulses
- Auscultate for significant bruits, which may be heard if 50% occlusion (if severe stenosis present, bruits may be absent)
- Pallor on elevation/rubor on dependency
- Allen Test (upper extremity disease)

*Investigations*
- Routine blood work, fasting metabolic profile
- ABI
- Duplex ultrasonography

CIRCULATORY

*Treatment*
- Conservative:
  - Exercise rehabilitation, risk factor modification (smoking, HTN, dyslipidemia, type 2 DM)
- Medical:
  - Antiplatelet therapy (e.g. ASA, clopidogrel)
- Surgical/endovascular revascularization:
  - Endovascular angioplasty/stenting
  - Endarterectomy
  - Bypass graft
- Primary amputation (for unreconstructable critical limb ischemia or profound tissue loss +/- active infection)

## Aortic Dissection
- Disruption of aortic intima causing blood to flow into the media: considered acute if <14 d
- Classification (Stanford)[1]:
  - Type A: involves ascending aorta ± arch and/or descending aorta
  - Type B: does not involve ascending aorta (usually distal to left subclavian artery)
- Risk Factors: smoking, HTN, male, >70 yr, family history, history of vascular disease (CAD, cerebrovascular disease [CVD], PVD)

*Etiology*
- Atherosclerotic degeneration (most common)
- Other Factors: collagen vascular disease (Marfan's, Ehlers-Danlos), arteritis, bicuspid aortic valve, infection (e.g. syphilis), iatrogenic, trauma
- DDx: MI, massive PE, esophageal rupture, cardiac tamponade, aortic aneurysm

*Signs and Symptoms*
- Classically present with acute onset tearing chest/interscapular pain
- Dissection is painless in ~10% of cases[1]
- Signs and symptoms vary according to aortic branches involved: coronary (MI), carotids (syncope, Horner's, neurological deficits), mesenteric, renal, iliac (ischemic limb)
- Respiratory symptoms if dissection ruptures into pleura
- Heart failure if dissection ruptures into pericardium causing tamponade
- Hypovolemic shock if dissection ruptures into peritoneum

*Physical Exam*
- Vitals
  - Hypotension (Type A), HTN (Type B), asymmetrical pulse or BP (>20-30 mmHg suggests dissection)
- Abdominal exam
- Cardiorespiratory exam: aortic regurgitation (AR) murmur, heart failure, tamponade
- Peripheral vascular exam: limb ischemia, signs of heart failure
- Neurological exam: focal deficits

*Investigations*
- Blood work: CBC, creatinine, LFTs, troponin, lactate, type and cross
- ECG: may show LVH or ST changes
- CXR: may show widened mediastinum
- CTA (84-94% sensitive, 87-100% specific): allows rapid and accurate assessment of anatomy to diagnose and facilitate planning for surgical repair[1]
- Echocardiogram (transesophageal echocardiogram more sensitive and specific than transthoracic echocardiogram): can confirm dissection and assess aortic valve competence
- Conventional aortogram performed as part of any endovascular repair if indicated

*Treatment*
- Hemodynamically unstable: aggressive resuscitation
- Medical: β-blockers, analgesia, vasodilators (target systolic BP: 100-120 mmHg)
- Surgical/endovascular repair:
  - Type A: open surgery is only definitive therapy

- Type B:
  - Uncomplicated (i.e. no malperfusion syndrome or rupture): no surgery required
  - Complicated: open or endovascular repair (emerging technique)

## Abdominal Aortic Aneurysm (AAA)
- Localized dilatation of the abdominal aorta that is 2 times normal diameter
- Clinically significant aneurysms are > 5cm in diameter or greater
- True Aneurysm: wall is made of all 3 layers of the artery (intima, media, adventitia)
- False Aneurysm: wall is made of fibrous tissue or graft (e.g. complication postcatheterization)
- Classification: infrarenal (~90%), juxtarenal, suprarenal, thoraco-abdominal
- Risk Factors: smoking, HTN, >70 yr, family history, history of vascular disease (CAD, CVD, PVD)

*Etiology*
- Atherosclerotic degeneration
- Other Factors: collagen vascular disease (Marfan's, Ehlers-Danlos), arteritis, infection (e.g. syphilis), trauma

*Signs and Symptoms*
- Aneurysms are generally asymptomatic until they rupture, and are often incidentally found on physical exam or imaging
- Ruptured AAA
  - Other symptoms include syncope and shock (pale skin, hypotension, shallow, fast respirations, decreased LOC)
  - Surgical emergency
  - Classic presentation is most often misdiagnosed as renal colic

**Clinical Pearl: Ruptured AAA**
Classic triad: abdominal pain radiating to back, pulsatile mass, hypotension.

*Physical Exam*
- Do not delay treatment if highly suspicious history
- Vitals
- Inspect for flank ecchymosis (retroperitoneal hemorrhage)
- Abdominal exam: palpate for pulsatile mass
- Cardiorespiratory, peripheral vascular, and neurological exams
- Typical signs in classic triad may not be present
  - Expansile mass may be hard to feel if person is obese
  - Hypotension may be absent in person who is normally hypertensive

*Investigations*
- Screening with abdominal U/S is recommended among men aged >50 yr with risk factors, all men >65 yr, and women >65 yr with risk factors
- Blood work: CBC, electrolytes, creatinine, aPTT, PT/INR, ESR, blood culture, type and cross (10 units pRBCs)
- Abdominal U/S (nearly 100% sensitive and specific for diagnosis)
- CT abdomen
  - Done to assess extent of aneurysms
  - Usually abdomen and pelvis, however include chest if thorax involved
  - Also identifies anatomic abnormalities: retroaortic vein, left sided vena cava, dilatation of ureters, enhancing rim of aorta seen with inflammatory aneurysm
- Conventional aortography
  - Only done when using endovascular aneurysm repair (EVAR)
  - Risk of false aneurysm, hematoma, or atheroembolism is 1-2%

*Treatment*
- Ruptured AAA:
  - Proximal aortic control by surgical or endovascular means (small-volume resuscitation can reduce the risk of further bleeding)

- No investigations are necessary if patient is hemodynamically unstable
- Asymptomatic:
  - Conservative: exercise rehabilitation, risk factor modification, surveillance every 6 mo-3 yr with abdominal U/S
  - Surgical repair or EVAR

> **Clinical Pearl: AAA**
> Repair is recommended for aneurysms exceeding 5.5 cm in men and 5.0 cm in women.

## Carotid Artery Disease

- Stenosis of the internal carotid artery, usually near the bifurcation of the common carotid artery
- Stenosis can be origin of thrombemboli to distal sites, leading to symptoms (e.g. TIA, amaurosis fugax, stroke)
- Risk Factors: age, smoking, HTN, DM2, dyslipidemia, family history, history of CAD, PVD, and AAA

*Etiology*
- Atherosclerotic degeneration (~90%)
- Other: dissection, aneurysm, arteritis, fibromuscular dysplasia
- DDx: cardioembolic (e.g. atrial fibrillation), *in situ* thrombosis of intracranial artery, vertebral artery disease, idiopathic (~32%)[2]

*Signs and Symptoms*
- May be asymptomatic: incidental finding
- TIA: lateralizing neurologic deficit (usually middle cerebral artery [MCA] territory), lasting less than 24 h (usually 1 h), and that completely reverses (CT normal)
  - MCA territory: contralateral hemiplegia and hemianesthesia, aphasia
- Amaurosis fugax: transient blindness (total or sectorial) due to ipsilateral retinal insufficiency (Takayasu syndrome is associated with retinal findings)
- Stroke: similar to a TIA but lasting more than 24 h, and usually associated with CT findings (carotid stenosis is underlying etiology in 30% of ischemic strokes)[2]

*Physical Exam*
- Inspect retina by fundoscopy: look for "Hollenhorst plaques", emboli that are visible as small bright flecks at arterial bifurcations in the retina
- Auscultate for carotid bruits: bruits do not correlate with severity of stenosis, and absence of bruits does not rule out severe disease. They merely correlate with the presence of atherosclerosis at the carotid bifurcation.

> **Clinical Pearl: Carotid Artery Disease**
> If patient has known carotid artery atherosclerosis (especially symptomatic and/or bruits), do not palpate the carotid pulse due to theoretical risk of atheroembolism and ischemic stroke.

- Neurological exam: assess for lateralizing neurological deficits and cerebellar abnormalities
- Precordial and peripheral vascular exams: assess for arrhythmias, cardiomegaly, murmurs, extra heart sounds, and signs of arterial insufficiency in lower limbs

*Investigations*
- Blood work: CBC, creatinine, aPTT, PT/INR, metabolic profile
- Duplex ultrasonography: indicates presence of disease (for >50% stenosis, 98% sensitivity and 88% specificity) and severity of stenosis (mild/moderate/severe)[3]
- CT angiography (88% sensitivity, 100% specificity)[3]
- MRA (95% sensitivity, 90% specificity): can concurrently evaluate cerebral circulation[3]
- Catheter-based angiography (gold standard): usually performed with angioplasty and stenting (not diagnostic test), and carries a 1/200 risk of stroke

*Treatment*
- Risk factor modification (smoking, HTN, DM2, dyslipidemia)
- Antiplatelet therapy (e.g. ASA ± clopidogrel)
- Statin therapy
- Asymptomatic disease[4]
  - ◆ >60% stenosis benefit from carotid endarterectomy (CEA): controversial
  - ◆ <60% stenosis benefit from CEA: no benefit
- Symptomatic disease[5]
  - ◆ Patients with >50% stenosis benefit from CEA (70-99% stenosis see greater benefit than 50-69%)
- Carotid angioplasty/stenting can be considered in poor surgical candidates with severe disease: controversial[6]

## 5.2 Venous

### Venous Thromboembolism (VTE)
- Blood clot formation, and subsequent inflammation, in one of the major deep veins in the leg, thigh, or pelvis

*Etiology*
- Virchow's triad: hypercoagulability, stasis, endothelial damage (see **Table 6**)
- Increasing age and family history are risk factors

*Signs and Symptoms*
- Establish index of suspicion according to risk factors (see **Table 6**)
- Classically presents as sudden unilateral pain, swelling, erythema, and warmth that is relieved with elevation

**Table 6.** Virchow's Triad

| Hypercoagulability | Stasis | Endothelial Damage |
|---|---|---|
| Surgery/trauma | Obesity | Trauma |
| Neoplasms | Recent travel | Previous VTEs |
| Estrogen related (e.g. OCP, pregnancy, HRT) | Postoperative bed rest | Venulitis |
| Blood dyscrasias or hyperviscosity (e.g. polycythemia and sickle cell disease respectively) | Trauma and subsequent immobilization | |
| Antiphospholipid antibody syndrome | Right heart failure | |
| Nephrotic syndrome | | |
| Inherited thrombophilias (e.g. protein C & S deficiency, antithrombin deficiency) | | |

HRT = hormone replacement therapy, OCP = oral contraceptive pill, VTE = venous thromboembolism

*Physical Exam*
- Absence of physical findings does not rule out VTE
- Examine the patient both upright and supine, venous distension is exacerbated in the upright position
- Vitals
- Inspect for erythema, collateral vein distension, and leg swelling (>3 cm difference in calf circumference is significant)
- Palpate for temperature difference, pitting edema, and indurated tender venous cord
- Attempt to elicit calf pain on dorsiflexion (Homans' sign)
- Cardiorespiratory exam

> **Clinical Pearl: Pulmonary Embolism**
> About 10% of cases of VTE are associated with pulmonary embolism. Clinically significant symptoms and signs include: shortness of breath, tachypnea (RR >16), tachycardia (>100 bpm), cough, hemoptysis, chest pain, fever, and anxiety.

*Investigations*
- Blood work: CBC, aPTT, PT/INR, creatinine, LFTs
- D-dimer (if low index of suspicion: sensitive but nonspecific)[8,9]
- Consider hypercoagulability work-up
- ECG, CXR
- Doppler ultrasonography (highly sensitive and specific)
- CT abdomen/pelvis with contrast (if proximal veins suspected)
- Venography (definitive but rarely used)
- If suspicious of PE, consider: ventilation-perfusion (V/Q) scan or CT with PE protocol

*Treatment*
- Prophylaxis
  - Conservative: early ambulation, compression stockings
  - Moderate to high risk: consider unfractionated heparin (UFH) or low molecular weight heparin (LMWH)
- Initial Therapy
  - UFH, LMWH, or fondaparinux
  - In select patients, catheter-directed thrombolytics or thrombectomy may be considered
- Long-Term Therapy
  - Anticoagulation (e.g. warfarin, dabigatran)
  - If anticoagulation is contraindicated (e.g. active bleeding), consider IVC filter
  - Duration ranges from 3-12 mo or indefinite therapy depending on risk factors
- Pulmonary Embolism (PE)
  - Admission for observation
  - Treatment for mild-moderate PE is similar to VTE
  - Massive PE: aggressive resuscitation, thrombolysis (systemic or catheter-directed) or thrombectomy ± IVC filter (with contraindication to anticoagulation)

## Superficial Venous Thrombosis (SVT)

*Etiology*
- 20% associated with occult VTE
- SVTs may be caused by varicose veins, trauma (e.g. recent sclerotherapy), intravenous indwelling catheters, autoimmune disease (e.g. Buerger's), malignancy, or hypercoagulable state
- Most commonly in greater saphenous vein
- Migratory SVT often associated with malignancy (Trousseau's disease)
- Can be misdiagnosed as cellulitis

*Signs and Symptoms*
- Often history of previous SVTs
- Tenderness, warmth, induration, redness, and localized swelling along course of vein
- Typically no generalized swelling of the limb

*Physical Exam*
- Inspect the area for redness, swelling, and varicose veins
- Palpate the affected vein and determine if it is hard and cord-like

*Investigations*
- Tests are not necessary for diagnosis of SVT, but should be done to rule out VTE
- Doppler ultrasonography

*Treatment*
- Conservative: warm compress, ambulation, NSAIDs

- Medical: depending on risk factors, consider antiplatelet or heparinization
- Surgical excision if conservative and medical measures fail. Specifically reserved for septic thrombophlebitis.

## Varicose Veins
- Distended tortuous superficial veins due to venous insufficiency from incompetent valves in the lower extremities

*Etiology*
- Hereditary incompetence of venous valves i.e. varicose veins
- Increasing age, female gender
- Situation of increased pressure (pregnancy, prolonged standing, ascites, tricuspid regurgitation)
- Previous VTE

*Signs and Symptoms*
- Dull aching, burning, or cramping provoked by prolonged standing or menstruation
- Edema which resolves overnight
- In some cases, chronic venous insufficiency (CVI) leads to skin damage
    - Pruritus, hyperpigmentation (hemosiderin deposits), stasis dermatitis, lipodermatosclerosis, bleeding, or ulceration

*Physical Exam*
- Inspect for evidence of varicose veins, skin damage, swelling, or ulceration
- Palpate for tenderness or edema
- Test for incompetent saphenous vein with Brodie-Trendelenburg maneuver (see **Special Tests**, p. 56)
- Peripheral vascular exam

*Investigations*
- Duplex ultrasonography: assess for reversed flow

*Treatment*
- Usually a cosmetic problem
- Conservative
    - Elastic/compression stockings
    - Leg elevation
- Surgical: indicated with symptomatic varices, prominent tissue changes, or failure of conservative measures
    - Sclerotherapy: injection of sclerosant drug by U/S-guidance into vein to cause vein shrinkage
    - Stripping, removal of all or part of saphenous vein trunk
    - Endovenous laser therapy (EVLT), endovenous RFA, endovenous glue embolization

## 5.3 Vasculitis

*Etiology*
- Inflammation of any blood vessel
- Can involve any organ system, but some may present with symptoms of peripheral vascular disease

*Disease-specific Findings*
- Behçet's Disease
    - Multisystem leukocytoclastic vasculitis
    - Ocular involvement
    - Recurrent oral and vaginal ulcers
    - SVT
    - Skin and joint inflammation
- Buerger's Disease
    - Thromboangiitis obliterans (TAO)

- Inflammation secondary to clotting of small- and medium-sized vessels
- Most common in Asian males
- Strong association with cigarette smoking
- May lead to distal claudication and gangrene
- Giant Cell (Temporal) Arteritis
    - Inflammation of aorta and its branches
    - New headache, jaw claudication
    - Scalp tenderness, may have pulseless or "ropy"/thickened temporal artery
    - Female > Male, >50 yr
    - Elevated ESR
    - May present with sudden, painless loss of vision ± diplopia
    - Aortic arch syndrome: involvement of subclavian and brachial arteries
        - Pulseless disease, aortic aneurysm ± rupture
- Polyarteritis Nodosa
    - Necrotizing vasculitis of small- to medium-sized vessels
    - May lead to thrombosis, aneurysm or dilatation at any lesion site
    - Associated with hepatitis B surface antigen positivity
    - Livedo reticularis of the skin
    - Diastolic BP >90 mmHg
    - Renal failure
    - Neuropathy
- Takayasu's Arteritis
    - "Pulseless" disease
    - Chronic inflammation of aorta and its branches
    - Usually in young Asian females
    - Constitutional symptoms
- Raynaud's Phenomenon
    - Pain and tingling in the digits due to vasospasm
    - Episodes of sharply demarcated pallor and/or cyanosis followed by erythema
    - Normal pulses present
    - Triggered by cold or emotional stress
    - May be primary or secondary; associated with SLE, scleroderma, rheumatoid arthritis (RA), cryoglobulinemia
- Antiphospholipid Antibody Syndrome
    - Multisystem vasculopathy often associated with SLE
    - Recurrent thromboembolic events (arterial and venous)
    - Recurrent spontaneous abortions
    - Skin changes (e.g. livedo reticularis, purpura, leg ulcers, gangrene)

*Investigations*
- Routine blood work
- Autoimmune work-up: ESR, CRP, ANCA, RF, C3, C4, antinuclear antibody (ANA), ferritin, anticardiolipin, and lupus anticoagulant antibodies
- Urinalysis (active sediment, proteinuria), BUN, creatinine
- Consider synovial fluid analysis if joint involvement
- Fundoscopy ± slit lamp examination
- CT scan
- Angiography
- Biopsy of affected organ, skin, or suspected blood vessel

*Treatment*
- Often dependent on condition
- Mainstay of treatment is immunosuppressive agents, most often with corticosteroids and/or cyclophosphamide
- Consider anticoagulation if thromboembolism involved
- NSAIDs for pain control with joints, eye and/or skin involvement

## 5.4 Lymphatics
- See **The Lymphatic System** Chapter

# REFERENCES

1. Hagan PG, Nienaber CA, Isselbacher EM, Bruckman D, Karavite DJ, Russman PL, et al. 2000. The International Registry of Acute Aortic Dissection (IRAD): New insights into an old disease. *JAMA* 283(7):897-903.
2. Barnett HJ, Gunton RW, Eliasziw M, Fleming L, Sharpe B, Gates P, et al. 2000. Causes and severity of ischemic stroke in patients with internal carotid artery stenosis. *JAMA* 283(11):1429-1436.
3. Chappell FM, Wardlaw JM, Young GR, Gillard JH, Roditi GH, Yip B, et al. 2009. Carotid artery stenosis: Accuracy of noninvasive tests - Individual patient data meta-analysis. *Radiology* 251(2):493-502.
4. Halliday A, Mansfield A, Marro J, Peto C, Peto R, Potter J, et al. 2004. Prevention of disabling and fatal strokes by successful carotid endarterectomy in patients without recent neurological symptoms: Randomised controlled trial. *Lancet* 363(9420):1491-1502. Erratum in: *Lancet* 2004;364(9432):416.
5. North American Symptomatic Carotid Endarterectomy Trial Collaborators. 1991. Beneficial effect of carotid endarterectomy in symptomatic patients with high-grade carotid stenosis. *New Engl J Med* 325(7):445-453.
6. Brott TG, Hobson RW 2nd, Howard G, Roubin GS, Clark WM, Brooks W, et al. 2010. Stenting versus endarterectomy for treatment of carotid-artery stenosis. *New Engl J Med* 363(1):11-23. Erratum in: *New Engl J Med* 2010;363(5):498, and *New Engl J Med* 2010;363(2):198.
7. Wells PS, Owen C, Doucette S, Fergusson D, Tran H. 2006. Does this patient have deep vein thrombosis? *JAMA* 295(2):199-207.
8. Kearon C, Ginsberg JS, Douketis J, Crowther M, Brill-Edwards P, Weitz JI, et al. 2001. Management of suspected deep venous thrombosis in outpatients by using clinical assessment and D-dimer testing. *Ann Intern Med* 135(2):108-111.
9. Bickley LS, Szilagyi PG, Bates B. *Bates' Guide to Physical Examination and History Taking*, 10th ed. Philadelphia: Lippincott Williams & Wilkins; 2009.
10. Orient JM, Sapira JD. *Sapira's Art and Science of Bedside Diagnosis*, 4th ed. Philadelphia: Lippincott Williams & Wilkins; 2010.

CIRCULATORY

CHAPTER 3:

# The Endocrine System

**Editors:**
Ahmed Faress, MD
Lauren Glick, BSc

**Resident Reviewer:**
Andrew Prine, MD

**Faculty Reviewers:**
Jeannette Goguen, MD, FRCPC
Jacqueline James, MD, FRCPC

## TABLE OF CONTENTS

# 1. COMMON CHIEF COMPLAINTS

**Table 1.** Common Chief Complaints with Associated Differential Diagnoses

| Chief Complaint | Differential Diagnosis |
|---|---|
| Polydipsia | **Endocrine:** Diabetes Mellitus, Diabetes Insipidus (central or nephrogenic) |
| | **Metabolic:** excessive volume loss, dehydration (e.g. diarrhea, excessive sweating), hypernatremia, hypercalcemia (via nephrogenic DI) |
| | **Other:** psychogenic, drugs (anticholinergics, etc.) |
| Atraumatic/pathological fracture | **Endocrine:** osteoporosis, primary hyperparathyroidism |
| | **Bone disorders:** osteomalacia, osteogenesis imperfecta, Paget's disease |
| | **Neoplasia:** bone cancer/tumor, multiple myeloma, metastatic cancer |
| Thyroid mass/goiter | **Neoplasm:** thyroid adenoma (colloid, hyperplastic), thyroid cancer, lymphoma |
| | **Inflammatory (goiter):** thyroiditis (Hashimoto's, De Quervain's) |
| | **Other:** multinodular goiter, thyroglossal duct cyst |
| Gynecomastia | **Drugs:** anti-androgens, spironolactone, HAART, anabolic steroids, alcohol, atypical antipsychotics |
| | **Liver disease:** cirrhosis |
| | **Endocrine:** male hypogonadism, thyrotoxicosis, puberty, aging, obesity |
| | **Neoplasm:** testicular or adrenal |
| | **Other:** tea tree oil, lavender oil, malnutrition/starvation |
| Hirsutism | **Endocrine:** Metabolic Reproductive Syndrome (MRS previously called PCOS), Cushing's, classic CAH (21 alpha-hydroxylase deficiency), non-classic CAH, acromegaly, hyperprolactinemia, thyroid dysfunction |
| | **Neoplasm:** androgen-secreting tumor (adrenal or ovarian) |
| | **Drugs:** exogenous androgens, danazol, valproic acid |
| | **Other:** idiopathic, obesity and insulin resistance may be associated with MRS and exacerbate it |
| Fatigue | **Physiologic:** pregnancy |
| | **Endocrine:** hypothyroidism, thyrotoxicosis, adrenal insufficiency, Cushing's syndrome, hyperparathyroidism |
| | **Psychiatric:** depression |
| | **Organ failure:** liver, kidney, heart, respiratory |
| | **Other:** (many) chronic diseases, cancer, fibromyalgia, neurological disorders, anemia |

**Table 2.** Common Lab Abnormalities with Associated Differential Diagnoses

| Lab Abnormality | Differential Diagnosis |
|---|---|
| Hyperglycemia | T1DM, T2DM, Gestational diabetes |
| | **Other specific types:**<br>**Endocrinopathies:** Cushing's Syndrome, acromegaly, hyperthyroidism, pheochromocytoma |
| | **Diseases of Exocrine Pancreas:** pancreatic cancer, pancreatitis, pancreatectomy, cystic fibrosis, hemochromatosis |
| | **Genetic:** MODY |
| | **Other:** stress (critical illness), drugs (corticosteroids, antipsychotics, anti–retroviral, thiazides etc.) |
| Hypoglycemia | **Drugs:** insulin or insulin secretagogues, alcohol, pentamidine, salicylates, quinine |
| | **Endocrine Deficiencies:** cortisol, growth hormone, glucagon |
| | **Critical illness:** hepatic failure, renal failure, sepsis, starvation |
| | **Other:** insulinoma, non-beta-cell tumors (IGF2 production), insulin autoimmune syndrome, post-gastrectomy, disorders in infancy (diabetic mother, enzyme defects), factitious |
| Dyslipidemia | **Genetic:** familial hypercholesterolemia, familial hypertriglyceridemia, familial combined hyperlipidemia, polygenic hypercholesterolemia |
| | **Secondary causes:**<br>**Endocrine:** diabetes, hypothyroidism, obesity |
| | **Renal:** chronic kidney disease, nephrotic syndrome |
| | **Other:** sedentary lifestyle, primary biliary cirrhosis, drugs (thiazides, beta blockers, retinoic acid, atypical antipsychotics, antiretroviral agents, etc.), alcohol |

# 2. COMMON CLINICAL SCENARIOS

## 2.1 Disorders of Carbohydrate Metabolism

**Table 3.** Overview of Clinical Presentation and Management of Carbohydrate Metabolism Disorders

| | Key Symptoms | Physical Exam Findings | Investigations | Management |
|---|---|---|---|---|
| **Type 1 Diabetes** | • Polyuria and nocturia<br>• Enuresis<br>• Lethargy, fatigue<br>• Polyphagia, polydipsia<br>• Sudden weight loss | • Vitals: weight loss<br>• Signs of complications (retinopathy, peripheral arterial disease, peripheral neuropathy) | • High fasting plasma glucose, oral glucose tolerance test, HbA1c | • Insulin (basal and pre-meal bolus) |

ENDOCRINE

| | Key Symptoms | Physical Exam Findings | Investigations | Management |
|---|---|---|---|---|
| **Type 2 Diabetes** | · Often none and detected by routine labs<br>· Polyuria, polydipsia, polyphagia | · Vitals: overweight or obese, high BP common<br>· Signs of complications (retinopathy, peripheral arterial disease, peripheral neuropathy) | · High fasting plasma glucose, oral glucose tolerance test, HbA1c | · Lifestyle changes: diet and exercise<br>· Metformin<br>· Other oral antihypergly-cemic agents<br>· Insulin |
| **Hypoglycemia** | · Weakness<br>· Hunger<br>· Sweating, tremor, palpitations<br>· Blurred vision<br>· Confusion<br>· Loss of consciousness | · General: cool, diaphoretic skin<br>· Vitals: high HR and systolic BP<br>· Neuro: tremor, confusion, seizure, coma | · Low plasma glucose | · Administer simple carbohydrate (glucose tablets, sugary beverage/food, IV dextrose if necessary) |

## 2.1a Diabetes Mellitus (DM)

### Classification
· Types 1 and 2 DM

**Table 4.** Summary Table of Carbohydrate Metabolism Disorders

| | Type 1 DM (T1DM) | Type 2 DM (T2DM) |
|---|---|---|
| **Pathophysiology** | Lack of insulin due to autoimmune destruction of B-cell mass | Three-step pathophysiology: 1) insulin resistance 2) B-cell failure 3) increased hepatic glucose production |
| **Etiology** | Multifactorial: genetic predisposition, autoimmune, environment | Multifactorial: genetic predisposition, obesity is major environmental risk factor |
| **Age of Onset** | Usually childhood or young adulthood, but can be seen at any age | Usually during older adulthood, but depending on population and obesity rates, can been seen in younger adults or childhood |
| **Presentation** | Usually lean, and symp-tomatic of hyperglycemia at presentation, ketosis prone | Variable: May be asymptomatic, present with complication of diabetes, not ketosis prone |
| **Family History** | Usually none, but helpful if positive | Often present |
| **Lab Markers** | At onset, anti-GAD, anti-islet, anti-insulin antibodies may be present, C-peptide levels low. These tests are not typically ordered unless diagnosis is unclear | Antibodies usually negative but not typically ordered |
| **Treatment** | Requires exogenous insulin for survival | Requires diet modification and exercise, anti-hyperglycemic agents, anti-obesity agents and possibly insulin |

- **Other Specific Types of DM:** accounts for <10% of all DM;
  - ◆ Monogenic forms (MODY genes, e.g. HNFα)
  - ◆ Endocrinopathies (e.g. Cushing's disease, acromegaly, pheochromocytoma)
  - ◆ Disorders of exocrine pancreas (e.g. hemochromatosis)
  - ◆ Drug related (e.g. commonly glucocorticoids)
- **Gestational DM:** Diabetes first diagnosed in pregnancy. Usually in the early 3rd trimester in predisposed individuals and typically resolves postpartum

## Focused History

- **Past Medical History:** diabetes history (age at diagnosis, presenting signs and symptoms), history of other autoimmune disorders
- **Family History:** diabetes, other autoimmune disorders
- **Risk Factors:** family history, ethnicity, central obesity, weight changes, lifestyle (exercise, dietary habits)
- **Blood sugar control:** diet, exercise, use of insulin and/or anti-hyperglycemic agents, basal and bolus settings for insulin pump users, home blood glucose monitoring, episodes of hypoglycemia, diabetes education, presence of acute and chronic complications
- **Social History:** (which may impact self-management of diabetes) e.g., occupation, social supports, medication costs, health benefits, psychiatric disorders, addictions, driving. For women: birth control, family planning, pregnancy history

## Common Chief Complaints

- T1DM: hyperglycemic symptoms (e.g. polyuria, polydipsia, nocturia, hyperphagia, weight loss, blurred vision, fatigue)
- T2DM: same as T1DM, but often asymptomatic and identified on blood glucose screening[1]

## Acute Complications

- Hyperglycemic conditions include diabetic ketoacidosis (DKA) and hyperglycemic hyperosmolar syndrome (HHS; formerly HONKS)

**Table 5.** Differentiating DKA vs. HHS[2,3]

|  | DKA | HHS |
|---|---|---|
| **Presentation** | T1DM, younger patient, rapid onset | T2DM, older patient, onset over days-weeks |
| **Precipitants** | Inadequate insulin treatment or nonadherence, new onset of diabetes, acute illness/stress (infection, trauma, etc.) | Inadequate pharmacologic treatment or nonadherence, acute illness, drugs (e.g. glucocorticoids), previously undiagnosed diabetes |
| **Symptoms/signs** | Fatigue, abdominal pain, nausea, vomiting, Kussmaul respirations, altered mental status, acetone-odoured breath | Profound dehydration, shallow breathing, decreased level of consciousness, possible focal neurologic signs |

- Microvascular complications:
  1. Retinopathy: change in vision, last eye specialist visit
  2. Nephropathy: urinary albumin excretion, HTN
  3. Neuropathy
     - Autonomic: postural hypotension, gastroparesis, urinary retention, diarrhea/ constipation, erectile/sexual dysfunction
     - Peripheral: numbness, tingling or decreased sensation in hands and/or feet, foot ulcers
- Macrovascular complications:
  - ◆ Presence of chest pain/discomfort, shortness of breath, atypical cardiac symptoms ("silent" ischemia), claudication, symptoms of TIA/stroke
  - ◆ Cardiovascular risk factors: smoking, HTN, dyslipidemia, family history of premature CAD (e.g. angina, MI, stroke, TIA, peripheral vascular disease [PVD], gangrene, infection)

- Other complications: peripheral arterial disease, immune suppression

*Focused Physical Exam*
- **General:** height, weight, waist circumference (central obesity), BMI, BP (supine and standing), pulse
- **H&N:** eyes (fundoscopy), thyroid
- **CVS:** signs of CHF, peripheral pulses and bruits
- **GI:** hepatomegaly from fatty liver
- **MSK:** foot inspection, limited joint mobility, arthropathy, color/temperature of limbs
- **Neuro:** screen for peripheral neuropathy using vibration tuning fork and ankle reflexes or monofilament
- **Derm:** inspection for cutaneous infections, problems with injection/pump sites

*Focused Investigations*
Diagnostic Criteria for Diabetes Mellitus[4]

---

**Random plasma glucose (PG) ≥11.1 mM with symptoms of DM (polyuria, polydipsia, unexplained weight loss)**

## OR

**2+ Abnormalities from amongst the following:**

| Fasting PG ≥7.0 mM | 2 h post 75 g oral glucose tolerance test (OGTT) ≥11.1 mM | HbA1c ≥ 6.5% |

---

\*\*Screening for hyperglycemia should begin at age 40

*Important Laboratory Markers*
- Blood: HbA1c, glucose, lipids, creatinine, electrolytes, AST
- Urine: albumin/creatinine ratio

## 2.1b Hypoglycemia

*Classification*
- **Fasting:** resulting from an imbalance of hepatic glucose production (too little) and peripheral glucose utilization (too much)
  - **Iatrogenic:** insulin or insulin secretagogues
  - **Metabolic:** hormonal deficiencies (cortisol, GH, glucagon), renal or liver failure, sepsis, starvation
  - **Neoplastic:** insulinoma, non-β cell tumor
- **Postprandial** (within 4 h of food consumption): glucose levels fall more rapidly than insulin levels
  - **Iatrogenic:** alimentary hypoglycemia post gastric surgery
  - **Metabolic:** early T2DM
  - **Idiopathic**

*Focused History*
- **Neurogenic Signs and Symptoms:** sweating, pallor, tachycardia, palpitations, tremor, anxiety, tingling and paresthesias of mouth and fingers, hunger, N/V
- **Neuroglycopenic Signs and Symptoms:** weakness, headache, dizziness, blurred vision, mental dullness/confusion, abnormal behavior, amnesia, seizures, loss of consciousness, transient focal neurologic deficit

*Focused Physical Exam*
- **General:** cool, diaphoretic skin
- **Vitals:** elevated HR, systolic BP
- **Neuro:** tremor, confusion, which may escalate to seizures and coma

*Focused Investigations*

*Diagnostic Criteria for Hypoglycemia*
- Patients with diabetes: plasma glucose <4.0 mM
- Patients without diabetes: Whipple's Triad (low plasma glucose, symptoms of hypoglycemia, relief of symptoms with correction of plasma glucose). Typically plasma glucose <3.0mM

*Important Laboratory Markers*
- If spontaneous onset: measure plasma glucose, insulin, proinsulin, C-peptide, insulin antibodies, cortisol, urine sulfonylurea level while hypoglycemic
- If onset not spontaneous: perform 72 h fast until plasma glucose low (<2.5-3.0 mM). Measure insulin, C-peptide, proinsulin, B-hydroxybutyrate levels to diagnose suspected insulinoma

## 2.2 Pituitary Disorders

- The pituitary hormones are:
  - **Anterior pituitary:** growth hormone (GH), luteinizing hormone (LH), follicle-stimulating hormone (FSH), thyroid-stimulating hormone (TSH), adrenocorticotropic hormone (ACTH), prolactin (PRL)
  - **Posterior pituitary:** antidiuretic hormone (ADH), oxytocin
- Disorders of the pituitary can present with one or more of the following: mass effect, hyperfunction, or hypofunction

**Table 6.** Summary Table of Pituitary Disorders

| | Key Symptoms | Investigations | Management |
|---|---|---|---|
| **Mass Effect** | • Headache<br>• Neuro: CN II, III, IV, V1, V2, VI defect | • MRI sella<br>• Visual field testing | • Drugs, surgery, or radiation |
| **Hyperfunction** | | | |
| **PRL** | • Galactorrhea<br>• Amenorrhea<br>• Infertility<br>• Low libido, erectile dysfunction<br>• Hypogonadism | • High prolactin<br>• (No suppression testing) | • 1st line = dopamine agonists<br>• Surgery or radiation if unresponsive |
| **GH** | • Enlarged hands, feet, jaw, tongue<br>• High BP<br>• Carpal tunnel syndrome<br>• Sleep apnea | • High baseline GH and IGF-1<br>• Suppression test: GH not suppressed by oral glucose challenge | • 1st line = surgery<br>• Drugs or radiation |
| **ACTH** | • Central obesity, abnormal fat deposition<br>• High BP<br>• Muscle weakness<br>• Bruising, purple striae<br>• Psychiatric complaints | • High cortisol and ACTH<br>• Suppression test: Cortisol suppressed by high dose DXM, but not low dose | • 1st line = surgery<br>• Drugs or radiation |
| **Hypofunction** | | | |
| **GH** | • Short stature (children)<br>• Fatigue, bone mass depletion, high fat mass, low muscle mass (adult) | • Low IGF-1<br>• Little response of GH to hypoglycemia in insulin tolerance test | • Hormone therapy: GH |

| | Key Symptoms | Investigations | Management |
|---|---|---|---|
| **FSH/LH** | • Amenorrhea<br>• Infertility<br>• Erectile dysfunction, low libido<br>• Hypogonadism | • Low LH, FSH, estradiol (female) and testosterone (male) | • Hormone therapy: sex hormones |
| **TSH** | • Fatigue<br>• Weight gain<br>• Constipation<br>• Poor concentration<br>• Menorrhagia | • Low TSH and free T4 | • Hormone therapy: T4 |
| **ACTH** | • Weight loss<br>• Weakness, fatigue<br>• Dizziness<br>• Nausea and vomiting<br>• Low BP | • Low cortisol<br>• Little response of cortisol to hypoglycemia in insulin tolerance test | • Hormone therapy: cortisol |
| **PRL** | • Inability to lactate | • Low prolactin | • None |
| **ADH** | • Polyuria, polydipsia | • High [Na+] | • Hormone therapy: ADH |

## 2.2a Pituitary Mass Effect

- Classified as either micro (<1 cm) or macro (>1 cm)
- Any pituitary tumor can cause normal pituitary to underproduce GH, LH, FSH, TSH, ACTH and increase prolactin (via stalk compression)
- Pituitary tumors and can also cause compression of the optic nerve (CNII), compression of cranial nerves of the cavernous sinus (CN III, IV, V1, V2, VI), and can increase intracranial pressure

*Focused History and Physical Exam*
- Headache
- Cranial nerve II defect
    - Visual field defect (bitemporal hemianopsia most common)
    - Fundoscopy (pale optic disc)
    - RAPD
- Cranial nerve III, IV, VI defect: Abnormal extra-ocular movements (see the **Nervous System** Chapter)
- Cranial nerve V1, V2 defect: loss of facial sensation in V1, V2 distribution

*Diagnostic Criteria*
- History and physical
- Visual field assessment
- MRI sella

## 2.2b Pituitary Hyperfunction

*Etiology*
- Increased hormone secretion usually resulting from benign adenomas of the pituitary
- Most commonly overproduce PRL (prolactinoma) or GH (acromegaly) or ACTH (Cushing's syndrome), rarely TSH (see **Table 6**)
- PRLs account for 30% of all pituitary adenomas

**Clinical Pearl: Prolactin Overproduction**
Overproduction of PRL can be caused by pregnancy/breastfeeding/nipple stimulation, pituitary tumor (prolactinoma or nonsecretory with stalk effect), decreased clearance as in liver and renal failure, drugs (psychiatric, GI motility), and/or primary hypothyroidism (via thyrotropin releasing hormone [TRH]).

> **Clinical Pearl: Pituitary Hypofunction**
> **Go Look For The Adenoma Please** is a mnemonic for the order of hormone loss in pituitary hypofunction (GH, LH/FSH, TSH, ACTH, PRL).

**Table 7.** Summary of Laboratory Findings in Various Forms of Cushing's Syndrome[5]

| Type of Cushing's | Plasma ACTH | 24h Urine Cortisol | Low dose DXM Test | High Dose DXM Test |
|---|---|---|---|---|
| **Adrenal Cushing's** | | | | |
| **Adenoma, carcinoma, bilateral nodular adrenal hyperplasia** | ↓ACTH | ↑Cortisol | Cortisol not suppressed | Cortisol not suppressed |
| **Pituitary Cushing's** | | | | |
| **Pituitary ACTH-producing adenoma** | ↑ACTH | ↑Cortisol | Cortisol not suppressed | Cortisol suppressed |
| **Ectopic ACTH-Secreting Tumor** | | | | |
| **Small cell lung cancer, bronchial carcinoma** | ↑↑ACTH | ↑Cortisol | Cortisol not suppressed | Cortisol not suppressed |
| **Exogenous Corticosteroid** | | | | |
| **Exogenous corticosteroid use** | ↓ACTH | ↑Cortisol | Cortisol not suppressed | Cortisol not suppressed |

DXM = dexamethasone

> **Clinical Pearl: Cushing's Syndrome**
> The commonest cause of Cushing's syndrome is iatrogenic use of glucocorticoid therapy.

## 2.2c Pituitary Hypofunction

*Etiology*
- **Neoplasia:** pituitary adenoma, craniopharyngioma
- **Cystic lesions:** Rathke's cleft cyst, arachnoid cyst
- **Iatrogenic:** pituitary surgery or radiation
- **Necrosis:** (e.g. Sheehan's syndrome)
- **Infection/Infiltration:** TB, histiocytosis X, lymphocytic hypophysitis, sarcoidosis
- **Other:** empty sella syndrome, hemorrhage (pituitary apoplexy), trauma
- **Hypothalamic dysfunction**

For each individual pituitary hormone, there exists a factor that stimulates its release arising from the hypothalamus. Prolactin is only pituitary hormone that is controlled by tonic inhibition (by dopamine) (see **Figure 1** below)
- Therefore, hypothalamic lesions (tumors, aneurysms, genetic syndromes) can cause pituitary hormone deficiencies, which are referred to as "tertiary" deficiencies

*Focused History and Physical Exam*

**Table 8.** Focused History and Physical Exam for Pituitary Hypofunction

| Hormone Hypofunction | Focused History and Physical | Diagnostic Criteria |
|---|---|---|
| **Anterior Pituitary** | | |
| **ACTH** | Signs and symptoms of adrenal insufficiency (see section 2.3b) | ↓8 AM cortisol (↓cortisol with cortisol stimulation test) |
| **GH** | Low energy, osteoporosis, dyslipidemia, short stature (in children) | ↓IGF-1 |
| **PRL** | Inability to lactate | ↓Prolactin |
| **TSH** | Signs and symptoms of hypothyroidism (see section 2.4b) | ↓TSH and ↓free T4 |
| **FSH/LH** | Women: amenorrhea, infertility Men: erectile dysfunction, loss of libido, decreased secondary sexual characteristics (body hair, breast development) | ↓LH, ↓FSH ↓Estradiol ↓Bioavailable testosterone |
| **Posterior Pituitary** | | |
| **ADH** | Polyuria, polydipsia, confusion, coma | May have hypernatremia |

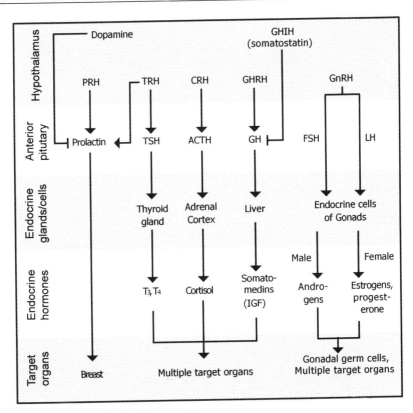

**Figure 1.** Hypothalamic-Pituitary Hormonal Axes

CRH = corticotropin-releasing hormone, GnRH = gonadotropin-releasing hormone
GHIH = growth hormone-inhibiting hormone, GHRH = growth hormone-releasing hormone,
PRH = prolactin-releasing hormone, TRH = thyrotropin-releasing hormone

## 2.3 Adrenal Disorders

- The adrenal gland cortex makes three classes of steroid hormones:
  - Glucocorticoids (regulate blood sugar, metabolism, and immunity)
  - Mineralocorticoids (absorbs Na+, excretes K+, regulates plasma [K+], ECFV and BP)
  - Sex hormones (affect 2° sex characteristics: axillary/pubic hair, libido)
- The adrenal medulla produces catecholamines (epinephrine and norepinephrine)
- Disorders of the adrenal gland cause problems related to disturbance in endocrine functions leading to overproduction or underproduction of adrenal hormones

**Table 9.** Summary Table of Adrenal Disorders

| | Key Signs and Symptoms | Investigations | Management |
|---|---|---|---|
| **Adrenal Cushing's Syndrome** | · Central obesity, abnormal fat deposition<br>· Metabolic syndrome<br>· Muscle weakness<br>· Bruising, purple striae<br>· Psychiatric complaints | · High cortisol<br>· Low ACTH<br>· Cortisol not suppressed by low or high dose DXM test | · Surgical removal with glucocorticoid taper |
| **Conn's Syndrome** | · High BP | · High aldosterone<br>· High aldosterone:renin<br>· Low potassium | · Surgical removal |
| **Pheochromocytoma** | · 3 Ps: Pain (headache), palpitations, perspiration<br>· High BP | · High urine and serum catecholamines or metanephrines | · Surgical removal |
| **Adrenal Insufficiency** | · Fatigue, weakness, dizziness<br>· Nausea, vomiting<br>· Postural hypotension<br>· Skin hyperpigmentation<br>· Salt craving | · Low baseline plasma cortisol<br>· High ACTH<br>· Low cortisol following stimulation test | · Hydrocortisone and fludrocortisone |

### 2.3a Adrenal Hyperfunction

*Cushing's Syndrome*
- See **Table 6** (ACTH) and **Table 7** (Cushing's)
- Adrenal Cushing's has overproduction of cortisol secondary to adrenal adenoma, hyperplasia, or rarely carcinoma
- Unlike ACTH-dependent Cushing's, no excess of androgens

*Conn's Syndrome*
- Overproduction of aldosterone secondary to adrenal adenoma, hyperplasia or rarely carcinoma
- *Focused History and Physical Exam*
  - Severe or resistant HTN, often with hypokalemia
- *Diagnostic Criteria*
  - ↑aldosterone and ↑aldosterone:renin ratio
  - Aldosterone does not suppress with salt load
  - Adrenal vein sampling used to localize overproducing adrenal gland(s)

*Pheochromocytoma*
- Overproduction of catecholamines and metanephrines by adrenal glands or extra-adrenal sympathetic nervous tissue
- *Focused History and Physical Exam*

- ◆ Spells with 3 Ps: Pain (headache), palpitations, perspiration
- ◆ Severe HTN
  - ▪ Associated genetic syndrome (MEN 2, MEN3 (previously MEN 2A and 2B), von Hippel Lindau, NF-1, familial paraganglioma syndromes
- • *Diagnostic Criteria*
  - ◆ Elevated catecholamines and/or metanephrines in 24 h urine collection and/or elevated plasma metanephrines (when available)

## 2.3b Adrenal Hypofunction

*Etiology of Adrenal Insufficiency*
1. **Primary** (adrenal hypofunction, ↓adrenal gland hormones, ↑ACTH):
   - ◆ Autoimmune destruction (may be associated with type 1 or 2 autoimmune polyglandular syndrome)
   - ◆ Infectious (TB, systemic fungal infection, opportunistic infection, e.g. in HIV)
   - ◆ Tumor (metastatic carcinoma, especially of breast, lung, kidney, or bilateral lymphoma)
   - ◆ Other (hemorrhage [e.g. Waterhouse-Friderichsen syndrome], necrosis, thrombosis, congenital)
2. **Secondary** (pituitary hypofunction, low ACTH, normal aldosterone):
   - ◆ See section 2.2c
3. **Tertiary** (low CRH secretion, low ACTH) (can't measure CRH):
   - ◆ Hypothalamic tumors
   - ◆ Long-term glucocorticoid therapy

*Focused History*
- • **Common Chief Complaints:**
  - ◆ Fatigue, weakness, loss of appetite, weight loss, dizziness, nausea, vomiting
- • **Associated Symptoms:**
  - ◆ Hyperpigmentation of skin (seen in 1° adrenal insufficiency), muscle and joint pain, amenorrhea, salt craving, more severe cases present with frank hypotension
  - ◆ Related to **cause of adrenal disease**:
    - ▪ Consider secondary adrenal insufficiency: pituitary tumor symptoms (headache, loss of peripheral vision, symptoms of low levels of other pituitary hormones)
  - ◆ Related to **consequences and complications**:
    - ▪ Adrenal crisis: hypotension with loss of consciousness; preceded by fever, N/V, abdominal pain, weakness and fatigue, and confusion (occurs in primary adrenal insufficiency often due to infection, trauma or stress)
    - ▪ Symptoms of hypoglycemia: more common in acute secondary/tertiary adrenal insufficiency

*Focused Physical Exam*
- • **H&N:** assess pituitary findings (headache [on history], visual symptoms)
- • **CVS:** postural hypotension
- • **GI:** tenderness on palpation of abdomen
- • **MSK:** diffuse, nonspecific weakness
- • **Derm:** vitiligo, hyperpigmentation (primary adrenal insufficiency) especially in areas exposed to light (face, neck, backs of hands) and areas exposed to chronic mild trauma (e.g. elbows, knees, spine, knuckles, waist, shoulders, buccal mucosa along dental occlusion and inner surface of lips)

*Diagnostic Criteria*
- • Low plasma cortisol (classically less than 100 nM at 8 AM), especially if still less than 500 nM after Cortrosyn® (cosyntropin) stimulation testing (ACTH) or following insulin-induced hypoglycemia for secondary deficiency

## 2.4 Thyroid Disorders

- The thyroid gland makes two forms of thyroid hormone: the main circulating hormone $T_4$ and smaller amounts of the active hormone $T_3$
- $T_4$ enters cells and is converted to $T_3$; $T_3$ has nuclear receptors that have different effects depending on the organ; in general, T3 increases metabolic rate, heart rate, and energy levels, and regulates bone health
- Disorders of the thyroid gland cause problems related to endocrine function (overproduction or underproduction of thyroid hormones) or mass effect (dysphagia, dysphonia, stridor or incidentally found)

**Table 10.** Summary Table of Thyroid Disorders

| | Key Symptoms | Physical Exam Findings | Investigations | Management |
|---|---|---|---|---|
| **Thyrotoxicosis** | · Weight loss despite increased appetite<br>· Palpitations<br>· Poor concentration<br>· Mood swings<br>· Heat intolerance<br>· Tremor<br>· Exophthalmos (Graves') | · High HR, high systolic BP<br>· Warm moist skin<br>· Eyes: lid retraction or lag, exophthalmos, periorbital edema<br>· Thyroid: palpable goiter or nodule<br>· Tremor, hyperreflexia | · High free $T_3$, free $T_4$<br>· Low TSH<br>· Positive TSI if Graves' Disease | · Beta blockers for symptoms<br>· Thiouracil (methimazole or PTU), radioactive iodine (RAI) or thyroidectomy for overproduction (not for thyroiditis) |
| **Hypothyroidism** | · Weight gain despite decreased appetite<br>· Constipation<br>· Apathy, psychomotor slowing<br>· Cold intolerance<br>· Dry skin and hair loss | · Low HR, high diastolic BP<br>· Dry, thick, cool skin<br>· Periorbital edema<br>· Thyroid: palpable goiter<br>· Non-pitting edema, carpal tunnel syndrome | · Low free $T_3$, free $T_4$<br>· High TSH<br>· Positive anti-TPO and anti-thyroglobulin if Hashimoto's | · Levothyroxine (Synthroid®, EltroxinTM) |

### 2.4a Thyrotoxicosis

*Etiology*
- **Excess Production** (Hyperthyroidism):
  - **Primary** ($\downarrow$TSH, $\uparrow T_4/T_3$): Graves' Disease (most common), toxic multinodular goiter, toxic adenoma, hyperemesis gravidarum, trophoblastic tumors, struma ovarii, drugs (e.g. amiodarone)[3]
  - **Secondary** ($\uparrow$TSH, $\uparrow T_4/T_3$): TSH-secreting anterior pituitary adenoma; pituitary resistance to $T_4/T_3$
- **Excess Hormone Release** (Thyroiditis, $\downarrow$TSH, $\uparrow T_4/T_3$): usually subacute, post-viral, postpartum, drug-induced (e.g. amiodarone), radiation-induced or idiopathic
- **Exogenous Thyroid Hormone** ($\downarrow$TSH, $\uparrow T_4/T_3$): thyroid medications (excess dosage or surreptitious use); hamburger thyrotoxicosis

> **Clinical Pearl: Thyrotoxicosis vs. Hyperthyroidism**
> Thyrotoxicosis is any condition that results in elevated levels of thyroid hormone, including hyperthyroidism. Hyperthyroidism is the excess <u>production</u> (and not just leak) of thyroid hormone by the thyroid gland itself.

ENDOCRINE

*Focused History*
- **History of presenting illness** (see **Table 11**)
  - ◆ **Symptoms associated with high thyroid hormone**
    - ▪ "Anxiety", weight loss with increased appetite, fatigue and weakness, frequent bowel movements, heat intolerance/sweating, palpitations, chest pain, shortness of breath, insomnia
  - ◆ **Symptoms associated with enlarged thyroid**
    - ▪ Enlarged thyroid/nodule, "mass effect": dysphagia, dyspnea, dysphonia (pressure on laryngeal nerve)
  - ◆ **Complications of elevated thyroid hormone**
    - ▪ Chest pain due to decompensated heart disease
    - ▪ Osteoporosis and bone fractures
    - ▪ Thyroid storm: a rare, life-threatening condition characterized by an exaggeration of the usual symptoms of thyrotoxicosis; can develop in cases of untreated thyrotoxicosis or may be precipitated by stress such as surgery, trauma or infection
- **Past Medical History**
  - ◆ Personal or family history of autoimmune, thyroid or endocrine disorders (e.g. T1DM), and management (drugs, surgery, head/neck irradiation)
  - ◆ Recent history of viral infection, pregnancy
  - ◆ Medication use (e.g. amiodarone, lithium, L-Thyroxine), goitrogen ingestion (e.g. seaweed, kelp, iodine)
  - ◆ Personal or family history of eye symptoms (e.g. Graves' exophthalmos, eye grittiness, discomfort, excess tearing)

*Focused Physical Exam*

**Table 11.** Physical Signs and Symptoms of Thyrotoxicosis[6]

| System | Symptoms | Signs |
|---|---|---|
| General | Weight loss with good appetite, heat intolerance | Fever, decreased LOC in thyroid storm |
| H&N | Bulging eyes (Graves') | Exophthalmos (Graves'); stare, lid lag |
| CVS | Palpitations | Tachycardia, wide pulse pressure, bounding pulse, aortic systolic murmur, atrial fibrillation, systolic hypertension, signs of congestive heart failure |
| GI | Increased bowel movements | None |
| GU | Women: menstrual irregularities | None |
| Neuro | Feeling shaky, difficulty climbing the stairs | Fine tremor, proximal muscle weakness, hyperreflexia |
| Derm | Warm, smooth and silky skin, increased perspiration, hair thinning | Warm, silky, diaphoretic, vitiligo, pretibial myxedema (Graves') |
| Psych | Anxiety, irritability | |

*Focused Investigations*

**Table 12.** Laboratory and Radiological Findings in Thyrotoxicosis[7]

| Disorder | TSH | Free T4/T3 | Thyroid Antibodies | Radioactive Iodine Uptake/Scan |
|---|---|---|---|---|
| Graves' Disease | ↓ | ↑ | TSI | Increased uptake (homogeneous) |
| Toxic Multinodular Goitre | ↓ | ↑ | None | Increased uptake, (heterogeneous), multiple "hot" nodules |

| Disorder | TSH | Free T4/T3 | Thyroid Antibodies | Radioactive Iodine Uptake/Scan |
|---|---|---|---|---|
| Toxic Adenoma | ↓ | ↑ | None | Increased uptake in hot nodule, low uptake in rest of the gland |
| Thyroiditis | ↓ | ↑ | None | Decreased uptake |
| Endogeneous thyroid hormone (struma ovariae, etc.) | ↓ | ↑ | None | Decreased uptake |
| Exogeneous thyroid hormone | ↓ | ↑ | None | Decreased uptake |

## 2.4b Hypothyroidism

*Etiology*
- **Primary (↑TSH, ↓T$_4$):**
  - ◆ Iatrogenic: post-thyroid surgery or radioactive iodine ablation (e.g. in treatment of thyroid cancer or Graves' disease)
  - ◆ Autoimmune: Hashimoto's thyroiditis, subacute thyroiditis
  - ◆ Drug-induced: goitrogens (iodine), thionamides (propylthiouracil, methimazole), lithium, amiodarone
  - ◆ Infiltrative disease: progressive systemic sclerosis, amyloid
  - ◆ Other: iodine deficiency, congenital, subacute granulomatous Thyroiditis (De Quervain's), subacute painless thyroiditis
- **Secondary (↓TSH, ↓T$_4$):**
  - ◆ Hypopituitarism: tumors, surgery, trauma, infiltrative disorders
    - ▪ Bexarotene treatment
- **Tertiary**: hypothalamic disease leading to TRH reduction

*Focused History*
- **History of presenting illness (see Table 13)**
  - ◆ **Symptoms associated with low thyroid hormone:**
    - ▪ Weight gain, fatigue, cold intolerance, constipation, dry skin, hair loss, difficulty concentrating
  - ◆ **Symptoms associated with complications of low thyroid hormone:**
    - ▪ Myxedema coma: a severe disease where the body cannot adapt to the hypothyroidic changes causing organ failure; may lead to coma, hypothermia, hypotension, bradycardia and respiratory failure; is usually precipitated by another illness

*Focused Physical Exam*

**Table 13.** Physical Signs and Symptoms of Hypothyroidism

| System | Symptoms | Signs |
|---|---|---|
| General | Weight gain, cold intolerance, fatigue, depression | Increased weight, hypothermia |
| H&N | Periorbital edema, hoarseness | Signs of goiter |
| CVS | None | Diastolic HTN, bradycardia, hyperlipidemia |
| GI | Constipation | None |
| GU | Women: menorrhagia | None |
| Neuro | Tingling, hand pain and weakness | Delirium, coma, proximal muscle weakness, carpal tunnel syndrome, delayed relaxation of reflexes |

| System | Symptoms | Signs |
|--------|----------|-------|
| Derm | Dry skin, hair loss | Dry skin, brittle hair and nails, yellow or pale skin |
| Psych | Difficulty concentrating | Decreased memory in elderly (pseudo-dementia) |

## 2.5 Metabolic Reproductive Syndrome (Formerly PCOS)

- Characterized by oligomenorrhea, hirsutism, obesity, and polycystic appearing ovaries due to large ovarian follicles
- **Prevalence**: 5-10% of reproductive age women, leading cause of infertility, may be underdiagnosed because condition is masked by oral contraceptive pills[4]. Age of onset is often around menarche, adolescence or young adulthood
- **Etiology**: causes are not well understood, both genetic and environmental influences

*Diagnostic Criteria*
- 2003 Rotterdam European Society of Human Reproduction and Embryology (ESHRE)/ American Society for Reproductive Medicine (ASRM) criteria require 2 of the following 3 criteria[8,9]:
    - Oligoovulation or anovulation
    - Clinical and/or biochemical signs of hyperandrogenism
    - Polycystic appearing ovaries on transvaginal ultrasound (ovary size >10 mL and/or >12 follicles 2-9 mm)
- Rule out disorders that can mimic metabolic reproductive syndrome (hyperandrogenism and/or ovulatory dysfunction) (see **Table 14**)

*Focused History*
- **Past medical history:**
    - **Reproductive history:** menstrual history, irregular vaginal bleeding, infertility, miscarriage, endometrial hyperplasia/cancer
    - **History of metabolic disorders:** weight gain, gestational diabetes, T2DM, HTN, dyslipidemia (increased TG, low HDL), cardiovascular disease, sleep apnea
    - **Dermatologic history:** male-pattern hair growth on face, back, chest, and abdomen, acne, hair loss
- **Family history:** infertility, insulin resistance, DM, and androgen excess

*Focused Physical Exam*
- **General:** height, weight, BMI, waist circumference (>80 cm in women)
- **H&N:** thyroid exam, androgenic alopecia (male pattern baldness)
- **CVS:** elevated blood pressure
- **GU:** adnexal size and masses
- **Derm:** acanthosis nigricans (hyperpigmented skin, usually in the posterior folds of the neck, axilla, groin, and umbilicus), hirsutism, acne, male pattern alopecia, skin tags

**Table 14.** Conditions to Exclude for the Diagnosis of Metabolic Reproductive Syndrome

| Differential Diagnosis | Clinical Features | Laboratory Features |
|------------------------|-------------------|---------------------|
| Pregnancy | Amenorrhea, breast tenderness | Positive BHCG |
| Androgen-Secreting Tumor (adrenal or ovarian) | Virilization, (clitoromegaly, severe hirsutism, increased muscle bulk, male pattern alopecia, deepening voice), rapid onset | ↑↑↑DHEAS and/or ↑↑↑testosterone |
| Hypothalamic Amenorrhea | Excessive exercise, Anorexia Nervosa, low body mass, lack signs of hyperandrogenism | ↓FSH and LH ↓Estradiol |

| Differential Diagnosis | Clinical Features | Laboratory Features |
|---|---|---|
| **Primary ovarian insufficiency** | Amenorrhea, symptoms of estrogen deficiency - hot flashes and urogenital symptoms, may have other autoimmune disorders | ↑FSH<br>↓Estradiol |
| **Acromegaly** | See GH Hyperfunction, Table 6 | ↑IGF-1 |
| **Congenital Adrenal Hyperplasia** | Family history of infertility and hirsutism | ↑17-OH progesterone |
| **Cushing's Syndrome** | Obesity, hirsutism, moon facies, HTN, purple striae (see Table 7) | ↑24 h urinary free cortisol |
| **Hyperprolactinemia** | Galactorrhea, amenorrhea | ↑Prolactin |
| **Thyroid Dysfunction** | Goiter, signs of hypothyroidism (see Table 13) | ↑TSH and ↓T4 |
| **HAIR-AN Syndrome** | Hyperandrogenism, insulin Resistance, acanthosis Nigricans | ↑↑↑Insulin following oral glucose challenge |
| **Idiopathic Hirsutism** | No menstrual irregularities | Normal serum androgen |
| **Exogenous Androgen Administration** | History of androgen therapy or Danazol use | |

## 2.6 Disorders of Calcium Metabolism

- Parathyroid hormone (PTH) production by the parathyroid gland is stimulated by hypocalcemia and hyperphosphatemia
- PTH is suppressed by hypercalcemia and hypophosphatemia
- PTH function[7]:

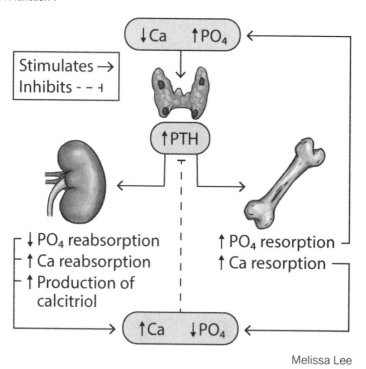

Melissa Lee

**Figure 2.** Parathyroid Hormone Regulation

**Table 15.** Summary Table of Calcium Disorders

| | Key Symptoms | Physical Exam Findings | Investigations | Management |
|---|---|---|---|---|
| **Hypercalcemia** | • Bone pain<br>• Nausea and vomiting<br>• Constipation, abdominal pain, anorexia, weight loss<br>• Flank pain, dysuria | • High BP<br>• Confusion, stupor or coma<br>• Muscle weakness, hypotonia | • High corrected or ionized calcium | • Fluid resuscitation<br>• Bisphosphonates<br>• Calcitonin<br>• Glucocorticoids if lymphoma or granulomatous disease<br>• Dialysis if severe |
| **Hypocalcemia** | • Muscle twitches or spasms<br>• Tingling around lips, fingers, toes | • Muscle spasm, tetany, Chvostek sign, Trousseau sign | • Low corrected or ionized calcium | • Oral or IV calcium<br>• Calcitriol |

## 2.6a Hypercalcemia

*Etiology:*
- PTH Dependent (↑serum calcium, ↑/normal PTH)[10]:
  - ◆ Primary Hyperparathyroidism
    - ▪ Elevated secretion of PTH, leading to hypercalcemia and hypophosphatemia
    - ▪ Can be caused by parathyroid adenoma (most common), primary hyperplasia of parathyroid glands, carcinoma
    - ▪ Familial forms are associated with multiple endocrine neoplasia (MEN) I, and MEN 2 (previously 2A) syndromes (autosomal dominant inheritance)
  - ◆ Familial Hypercalcemic Hypocalciuria
- PTH Independent (↑serum calcium, ↓PTH)[10]:
  - ◆ Malignancy: osteolytic metastases, humoral hypercalcemia (PTHrP), 1,25-dihydroxyvitamin D secreting tumor
  - ◆ Increased intake: milk alkali syndrome, hypervitaminosis A or D
  - ◆ Drugs: lithium, thiazide diuretics, theophylline
  - ◆ Granulomatous disease: sarcoid, TB, lymphoma
  - ◆ Other: thyrotoxicosis, adrenal insufficiency, pheochromocytoma, immobilization

*Focused History and Physical Exam*
- **Common Chief Complaints:**
  - ◆ Usually asymptomatic; otherwise fatigue, pain from kidney stones (if severe: constipation, polyuria, decreased level of consciousness, abdominal pain)
  - ◆ "Moans, bones, stones and groans" represents the presence of myalgias, bone pain, renal stones, abdominal pain respectively.

**Table 16.** Physical Signs and Symptoms of Hypercalcemia[10,11]

| System | Symptoms | Signs |
|---|---|---|
| **H&N** | Jaw pain or mass (osteitis fibrosa cystica: bone lesions due to increased osteoclast activity (very rare) | Eyes: band keratopathy (deposition of calcium across the cornea of the eye) |
| **CVS** | None | Diastolic HTN |
| **GI** | Constipation, abdominal pain | None |
| **GU** | Flank pain, dysuria | Renal stones |
| **MSK/ Neuro** | Muscle weakness, bone pain | Clinical evidence of osteoporosis/osteopenia |

**Table 17.** Laboratory Values in Hyperparathyroidism

|  | PTH | Calcium | PO4 |
|---|---|---|---|
| **Primary** | ↑ | ↑ | ↓ |
| **Secondary** | ↑ | ↓/N | ↑/N |
| **Tertiary** | ↑ | ↑ | ↑ |
| **Ectopic PTHrP** | ↓ | ↑ | ↓ |

## 2.6b Hypocalcemia

*Etiology:*
- Primary hypocalcemia (↓serum calcium, ↑ PTH)[10]:
  - Hypovitaminosis D due to chronic kidney disease
  - Malabsorption syndromes: Crohn's disease, celiac disease, Whipple's disease, post-bariatric surgery
  - Inadequate sun exposure/Vitamin D supplementation
- Hypoparathyroidism (↓serum calcium, ↓PTH)[10]:
  - Iatrogenic (most common): following thyroid or parathyroid surgery
  - Autoimmune, congenital DiGeorge syndrome
  - Infectious: HIV/AIDS
  - Impaired PTH secretion: hypomagnesemia, EtOH

*Focused History*
- **History of presenting illness:**
  - **Symptoms associated with hypocalcemia:** muscle twitches or spasms tingling around lips, fingers or toes, dysphagia, abdominal pain, biliary colic
- **Past medical history:** history of thyroid or parathyroid surgery, history of autoimmune disease (may be associated with Addison's disease and autoimmune polyglandular syndrome type I), history of malabsorption syndromes or malnutrition, HIV infection

*Focused Physical Exam*
- **H&N:** cataracts (chronic hypocalcemia)
- **MSK:** muscle twitches/spasms, tetany, Chvostek sign (tapping of facial nerve will cause twitching of facial muscles), Trousseau sign (inflating blood pressure cuff over brachial artery can cause flexion of the wrist and extension of the interphalangeal joints)
- **Resp:** bronchospasm, stridor
- **CVS:** arrhythmias (prolonged QT), CHF, hyper/hypotension
- **Neuro:** confusion, disorientation, numbness/paresthesias (perioral and in fingers/toes), seizures, basal ganglia calcification and movement disorder if chronic
- **Derm:** dry skin/hair, brittle nails

## 2.7 Dyslipidemia

- Elevated plasma cholesterol and/or triglyceride levels or a low plasma high density lipoprotein (HDL) level

*Etiology:*
- Primary (genetic):
  - Polygenic hypercholesterolemia, familial hypercholesterolemia, familial hypertriglyceridemia, familial combined hyperlipidemia, hypoalphalipoproteinemia, lipoprotein lipase deficiency, familial dysbetalipoproteinemia
- Secondary:
  - T2DM, sedentary lifestyle/obesity, hypothyroidism, nephrotic syndrome, chronic kidney disease, cholestatic liver disease, alcohol consumption, cigarette smoking, drugs (thiazides, beta blockers, retinoic acid derivatives, etc.)

*Focused History*
- **Common Chief Complaints:** usually asymptomatic but can lead to symptomatic vascular disease or xanthomas; elevated triglycerides can cause pancreatitis
- **Risk factors:** family history, diet, sedentary lifestyle, social history (alcohol, cigarettes), medication history, other secondary causes of dyslipidemia
- **Associated Symptoms**
  - ◆ **Complications:** coronary artery disease, peripheral artery disease, cerebrovascular disease

*Focused Physical Exam*
- **General:** height, weight, BMI
- **H&N:** High cholesterol: xanthelasma palpebrum (yellow plaque under eyelids), arcus cornealis (white/gray rings at edge of cornea); High triglycerides: lipemia retinalis ("tomato soap" appearance of blood in retinal vessels)
- **MSK:** High cholesterol: tuberous xanthoma (collections of cholesterol deposits over the palms, knees, heels or elbows), tendinous xanthoma (cholesterol deposits above the tendons)
- **Derm:** High triglycerides: eruptive xanthoma (small yellow-red papules)

## 3. COMMON PHARMACOLOGICAL THERAPIES

**Table 18.** Pharmacological Therapy for Common Clinical Scenarios in Endocrinology[4]

| | |
|---|---|
| **T1DM** | · Combination of basal insulin (glargine, detemir) and pre-meal bolus insulin (aspart, lispro, glulisine)<br>· Insulin pump with rapid insulin for basal and bolus needs |
| **T2DM** | · Lifestyle intervention: nutrition and physical activity<br>· Metformin<br>· Other oral antihyperglycemic agents, individualize for patient needs:<br>  • SGLT2 inhibitor: e.g. canagliflozin<br>  • Alpha-glucosidase inhibitor: eg. acarbose<br>  • DPP-4 inhibitors: e.g. sitagliptin<br>  • GLP-1 agonist: e.g. exenatide<br>  • Thiazolidinediones: e.g. pioglitazone<br>  • Meglitinides: e.g. nateglinide<br>  • Sulfonylureas: e.g. glyburide<br>  • Insulin can be added to oral agents (see T1DM above). Insulin pumps not routinely used for T2DM in Canada |
| **Diabetic Ketoacidosis** | · Fluid resuscitation with IV normal saline<br>· IV regular insulin to correct metabolic acidosis (add IV D5W if hypoglycaemia)<br>· Manage hyperosmolality: correct no faster than 3mmol/kg/hr<br>· IV K+<br>· Identify precipitating cause: insulin omission, new diagnosis, MI, infection, drugs, thyrotoxicosis |
| **Prolactinoma** | · 1st line: Dopamine Agonists<br>  • Cabergoline (often 1st choice agent)<br>  • Bromocriptine<br>  • Quinagolide<br>· Other options if unresponsive to medications:<br>  • Surgery<br>  • Radiation |
| **Thyrotoxicosis** | · Thiouracils (methimazole, propylthiouracil), radioactive iodine therapy, surgery<br>· For symptom management: beta-blockers, analgesics (painful thyroiditis)<br>· Glucocorticoids, for severe thyrotoxicosis, storm |
| **Hypothyroidism** | · Levothyroxine (Synthroid®, EltroxinTM); consider in symptomatic patients, or asymptomatic patients pregnant/trying to conceive or have TSH>10 |

| Hypercalcemia | · Start with fluid resuscitation with normal saline ± furosemide to prevent volume overload<br>· Bisphosphonates<br>· Calcitonin in patients with serum calcium >3.5 mM<br>· Glucocorticoid therapy (for hypercalcemia due to lymphoma, or granulomatous disease)<br>· Dialysis if severe |
| --- | --- |
| **Primary Adrenal Insufficiency** | · Hydrocortisone and fludrocortisone |
| **MRS (PCOS)** | · Weight reduction if obese, ± GLP1 Agonists<br>· Low-dose oral contraceptives<br>· Spironolactone for hyperandrogenism<br>· ± Metformin |

# REFERENCES

1. Laffel L, Svoren B. *Epidemiology, presentation, and diagnosis of type 2 diabetes mellitus in children and adolescents.* In: UpToDate. Waltham, MA: UpToDate; 2012.
2. Kitabchi AE, Umpierrez GE, Murphy MB, Kreisberg RA. *Hyperglycemic crises in adult patients with diabetes: A consensus statement from the American Diabetes Association.* Diabetes Care. 2006; 29(12): 2739-48.
3. Canadian diabetes association. *2013 clinical practice guidelines for the prevention and management of diabetes in Canada.* Can J Diabetes. 2013; 37: S1-S212.
4. Goldenberg R, Clement M, Hanna A, et al. *Pharmacologic management of type 2 diabetes: 2016 interim update.* Can J Diabetes. 2016; 193-195.
5. Goljan EF. Endocrine disorders. In: *Rapid Review: Pathology.* 3rd ed. Philadelphia: Mosby; 2010.
6. Reid JR, Wheeler SF. *Hyperthyroidism: Diagnosis and treatment.* Am Fam Physician. 2005; 72(4): 623-630.
7. Justice T, Makedonov I. Endocrinology. In: Merali Z, Woodfine J, eds. *Toronto Notes.* Toronto, ON: Toronto Medical Student Publications; 2016.
8. Franks S. *Controversy in clinical endocrinology: Diagnosis of polycystic ovarian syndrome: In defense of the Rotterdam criteria.* J Clin Endocrinol Metab. 2006; 91(3): 786-789.
9. Rotterdam ESHRE/ASRM-Sponsored PCOS consensus workshop group. *Revised 2003 consensus on diagnostic criteria and long-term health risks related to polycystic ovary syndrome (PCOS).* Hum Reprod. 2004; 19(1): 41-47.
10. Palazzo F. Primary hyperparathyroidism. *In: Epocrates Online Diseases.* San Mateo, CA: Epocrates Inc; 2012.
11. Stack, BC Jr, Chou FF, Schneider V. Secondary hyperparathyroidism. *In: Epocrates Online Diseases.* San Mateo, CA: Epocrates Inc; 2012.

ENDOCRINE

# CHAPTER 4:

# The Gastrointestinal System

GASTROINTESTINAL

**Editors:**
Sheliza Halani, BASc
Elise Fryml, MSc, BSc

**Resident Reviewer:**
Shohinee Sarma, MD, MPH

**Faculty Reviewers:**
Scott Fung, MD, FRCPC
Maria Cino, MD, FRCPC
Grant Chen, MD, FRCPC

---

## TABLE OF CONTENTS

# 1. ANATOMICAL REGIONS

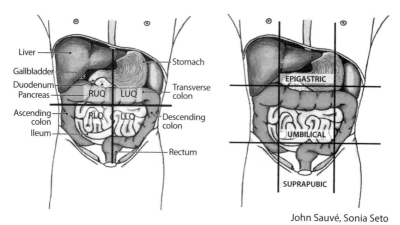

John Sauvé, Sonia Seto

**Figure 1.** Anatomical Regions of the Gastrointestinal Tract

**Table 1.** Structures of the abdomen by quadrant[17]

| Quadrant | Right | Left |
|---|---|---|
| **Upper** | Liver (right lobe), gallbladder, pylorus, duodenum, pancreas (head), right adrenal gland, right kidney (upper pole), hepatic flexure, ascending colon (portion), transverse colon (portion) | Liver (left lobe), spleen, stomach, pancreas (body), left adrenal gland, left kidney (upper pole), splenic flexure, transverse colon (portion), descending colon (portion) |
| **Lower** | Right kidney (lower pole), cecum, appendix, ascending colon (portion), right ovary, right fallopian tube, right ureter, right spermatic cord, uterus (if enlarged), bladder (if enlarged) | Left kidney (lower pole), sigmoid colon, descending colon (portion), left ovary, left fallopian tube, left ureter, left spermatic cord, uterus (if enlarged), bladder (if enlarged) |

RUQ = right upper quadrant, RLQ = right lower quadrant, LUQ = left upper quadrant, LLQ = left lower quadrant

## 2. OVERVIEW OF COMMON CLINICAL PRESENTATIONS AND DIFFERENTIAL DIAGNOSES

**Table 2.** Overview of Common Clinical Presentations and Differential Diagnoses

| Chief Complaint | Differential Diagnosis | Distinguishing Features |
|---|---|---|
| **Abdominal Pain** | Refer to Table 3 for DDx of abdominal pain by location | |

| Chief Complaint | Differential Diagnosis | Distinguishing Features |
|---|---|---|

**Dysphagia**  See algorithm below[22]

Refer to **The Head, Neck, and Throat** Chapter for details on oropharyngeal dysphagia

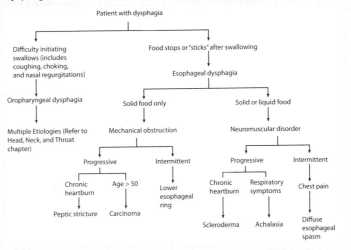

**Nausea and Vomiting[12]**

### 1. Neuropsychiatric

| | |
|---|---|
| CNS (brainstem lesion, increased ICP), migraine | Headache, stiff neck, vertigo, focal neurological deficits, ataxia |
| Vestibular causes (vestibular neuritis, Meniere's Disease, BPPV) | Tinnitus, hearing loss, vertigo, aural fullness, headache |
| Psychiatric (depression, conversion disorder), substance use disorder | Continuous; Major depression = irregular vomiting, not associated with food intake |

### 2. Gastrointestinal

| | |
|---|---|
| Motility Disorder | Insidious, 1 - 4 hours after a meal, with early satiety and postprandial bloating (gastroparesis), Diabetes Mellitus, reflux disease (GERD), Partially digested (gastric outlet obstruction, gastroparesis) |
| Inflammatory (cholecystitis, gastroenteritis, pancreatitis) | Abrupt pain, fever |
| Obstructions | Bile may be present<br>Feculent or odorous if obstruction with bacterial degradation of food contents<br>Abdominal distention with tenderness<br>Bowel sounds: decreased (ileus), increased (obstruction) |
| Malignancy | 1 – 4 hours after a meal, weight loss |

| Chief Complaint | Differential Diagnosis | Distinguishing Features |
|---|---|---|
| Nausea and Vomiting (continued) | **3. Systemic Disorders** | |
| | Pregnancy: morning sickness | Insidious, usually before breakfast but can occur at any time during the day |
| | Pregnancy: hyperemesis gravidarum | More severe than morning sickness and can result in dehydration and weight loss |
| | Infectious (viral/bacterial/parasitic) | Diarrhea, myalgias, malaise, headache, sick contacts, travel |
| | Endocrine (Cortisol deficiency, hypercalcemia, hyperthyroid, uremia, DKA) | Associated signs and laboratory abnormalities |
| | Medication side effects | Chemotherapy, analgesics, diuretics, cardiovascular medications, antibiotics, nicotine, sulfasalazine, azathioprine, narcotics, antiparkinsonian drugs, anticonvulsants, theophylline, radiation therapy |
| Diarrhea | Secretory Diarrhea (infection, inflammatory: IBD, microscopic colitis, malignancy, medications, motility disorder) | Watery stools, stool volume continues with fasting<br>If inflammatory and colonic: frequent, small-volume, bloody stools, may have tenesmus, fever, or severe abdominal pain, iatrogenic with hospital stay (C.difficile) |
| | Mucosal Diseases (ex. Celiac disease, cirrhosis, lactose intolerance) | Fatty stools, weight loss, greasy bulky stools, difficult to flush, oily film in toilet bowl |
| | Osmotic Diarrhea (laxatives, antacids, carbohydrate malabsorption) | Watery stools, stool volume decreases with fasting |
| | Drug-Induced Diarrhea | Caffeine, antibiotics, NSAID's, mycophenolate mofetil, Vitamin C, magnesium |
| | Endocrine (hyperthyroidism, pancreatic insufficiency) | |

**Table 3.** Differential for Abdominal Pain by Location

| Location of pain | Differential Diagnosis | Characteristics |
|---|---|---|
| **RUQ** | Liver | *Acute hepatitis*: Gradual onset, constant, fever, jaundice, fatigue, nausea, vomiting |
| | | *Abscess:* Acute onset, fever. May have jaundice, nausea, vomiting, hepatomegaly, sepsis & SIRS criteria |

| Location of pain | Differential Diagnosis | Characteristics |
| --- | --- | --- |
| **RUQ (cont.)** | Gallbladder/ biliary tract | *Biliary colic:* acute onset, intermittent duration, worse with inspiration, radiation to the right shoulder or back, may be related to fatty meals, nausea, vomiting. Resolves on its own. |
| | | *Cholecystitis:* Similar to biliary colic but more persistent and often associated with fever. |
| | | *Cholangitis:* Similar to cholecystitis with associated jaundice, fever, sepsis risk<br>• Charcot's triad: jaundice, fever, RUQ pain<br>• Reynold's pentad: Charcot's triad + hypotension (shock), altered mental status |
| | Renal colic/ pyelonephritis | Acute, severe pain, fever (with pyelonephritis) usually starting in the right flank and radiating down into the right groin. May have dysuria, hematuria and history of renal stones, costovertebral angle tenderness |
| | Pleural inflammation (pleuritis) | Infarct (pulmonary embolism), infection or malignancy. Acute onset, worse with inspiration, radiation to right shoulder Always keep chest pain on differential |
| **Epigastric pain** | Gastroesopha- geal | *Gastroesophageal reflux:* Intermittent, burning, radiation into chest/throat, related to eating and supine position |
| | | *Peptic ulcer disease:* Acute onset (severe if perforated), burning pain, better with food, history of H. Pylori |
| | | *Gastric cancer:* Early satiety, nausea, weight loss |
| | Pancreatitis | Acute onset, severe, radiates to the midback Penetrating pain accentuated by reclining, relieved by sitting up; Exacerbated by food, alcohol; Pain has a rapid onset Associated nausea and vomiting |
| | Cardiovascular | *Myocardial infarction:* Acute dull pain, radiates to the chest, shoulders, arms, related to exertion, associated dyspnea, relieved with rest or nitroglycerin |
| | | *Pericarditis:* Acute onset, sharp, worse with inspiration, may have associated fever, dyspnea |
| | | *Abdominal aortic aneurysm (AAA):* abrupt onset, severe tearing, diffuse (if ruptured) |
| | | *Aortic dissection:* Similar to ruptured AAA, tearing back pain, blood pressure difference in arms |
| **LUQ** | Splenic infarct/ rupture | Acute onset, radiation to left shoulder, fever, chills, associated history of trauma (if ruptured) |
| | Renal colic/ pyelonephritis | Acute, severe pain, fever (with pyelonephritis) usually starting in the left flank and radiating down into left groin. May have dysuria, hematuria and history of renal stones |
| | Pleural inflammation (pleuritis) | Infarct (pulmonary embolism), infection or malignancy. Acute onset, worse with inspiration, radiation to left shoulder |

**GASTROINTESTINAL**

| Location of pain | Differential Diagnosis | Characteristics |
|---|---|---|
| **RLQ** | Appendicitis | Acute onset, starts as vague and diffuse and progresses to severe pain in the RLQ. Worse with movement/walking. May have associated nausea, vomiting, and fever |
| | Ileitis (Crohn's Disease) | Gradual onset, colicky/crampy, maybe associated with diarrhea, fever, anorexia, weight loss |
| **LLQ** | Diverticulitis | Acute onset, may have constipation and fever, history of diverticulosis, distention, bleeding if perforation, hypotension (shock) |
| | Sigmoid volvulus | Acute onset, obstipation with abdominal distention |
| **Lower abdominal pain** | Colitis | Gradual onset, crampy with bloody diarrhea. May have fever, nausea, vomiting, distention, tenderness |
| | Irritable bowel syndrome | Intermittent, crampy pain relieved with a bowel motion, altered bowel habit (diarrhea, constipation or mixed) |
| | Gynecological | *Ectopic pregnancy:* must be ruled out in child-bearing aged females. Acute onset, sharp and constant. May have associated vaginal bleeding |
| | | *Pelvic inflammatory disease, endometriosis, ruptured ovarian cyst:* Acute onset, diffuse lower abdominal/pelvic pain, often related to menstrual cycle. Worse with intercourse (dyspareunia). PID (History of STI's) |
| **Diffuse** | Gastroenteritis | Gradual onset, crampy, anorexia, fever, history of travel or sick contacts |
| | Small bowel obstruction | Acute onset, crampy, colicky, distention, nausea and vomiting (feculent), history of abdominal surgery (adhesions), hernia, shock |
| | Peritonitis from any intra-abdominal cause | Severe, rigid abdomen, rebound tenderness with guarding, shock |
| **Other** | Sickle cell crisis | Associated with diffuse body pain |
| | Diabetic ketoacidosis | General abdominal pain, nausea, vomiting |

## 3. FOCUSED HISTORIES

- See General History and Physical Exam for a detailed approach to history taking
- OPQRSTUVW questions regarding each complaint
- Location and aggravating/alleviating factors are especially important

## Complaint-specific questions

### Abdominal Pain
- OPARST-AAA (aggravating/alleviating factors, associated symptoms, and attributions/adaptations)
- Location:
  - RUQ: cholecystitis, hepatitis, choledocolithiasis, cholangitis, pancreatic cancer
  - Epigastric: peptic ulcer disease, pancreatitis, thoracic (MI, pericarditis, aortic aneurysm), gallstones, reflux disease (GERD)
  - LUQ: ruptured spleen, gastric ulcer/cancer, splenic infarct
  - Flank: pyelonephritis, nephrolithiasis, retroperitoneal bleeding
  - Lower Abdomen: aortic aneurysm, appendicitis, diverticulitis, colorectal cancer, pelvic inflammatory disease, sigmoid volvulus, bowel perforation
- Association with meals (worse, better)
- Radiation of pain
- **Family History:**
  - Colorectal cancer, hepatocellular cancer, pancreatic cancer
  - Genetic syndrome: familial adenomatous polyposis, Lynch syndrome
  - Inflammatory bowel disease
  - Celiac disease, liver disease
- **Red Flags**
  - Constitutional symptoms: fever, night sweats, weight loss
  - Abrupt, excruciating pain: rule out myocardial infarction, ruptured aneurysm, ectopic pregnancy
  - Hypotension, tachycardia, tachypnea (signs of shock)

>
> **Clinical Pearl: Abnormal Etiology of Abdominal Pain**
> Diseases of the heart and lungs, such as coronary artery disease and pneumonia, can present with upper abdominal pain, especially in pediatric and geriatric populations.

### Dysphagia
- OPQRST
- Type: Solid, liquid or both
- Timing
  - Progressive or intermittent
  - Difficulty initiating swallowing or food "sticks"
- Associated symptoms: chronic heartburn, respiratory symptoms, chest pain, odynophagia, choking, aspiration, and history of stroke or other neurological disorders

### Nausea and Vomiting
- OPQRST
- Timing: During the meal, right after, within a few hours? Continuous or irregular? Does it occur at a particular time of day? With a particular consistency of food? Intentional? Bilious? Associated chest pain?
- **Medical History:** pregnancy, depression, conversion disorder, neuropathy, brainstem lesion
- Medications or illicit drugs
- Exposure history to infections, travel history
- **Complications:** Hypochloremic metabolic alkalosis, esophageal tear (Mallory-Weiss, Borhaave syndrome, undernutrition)

### Bowel Habits (Diarrhea, Constipation)
- OPQRST
- Chronic or acute change in bowel patterns: establish baseline bowel habits
- Change in number of stools per day
- Frequency and volume of stools, type of stool (Bristol stool chart)
- Constipation, diarrhea, tenesmus (straining, passing little or no feces, sense that all stool has not been passed)
- Character of stools: solid/loose, floating, malodorous, presence of blood (mixed with

stool/on the surface/separate), mucus (true mucus in irritable bowel syndrome vs pus in inflammatory bowel disease), color (red, black, or pale; other colors have no diagnostic significance)
- Associated symptoms (e.g. fever, abdominal pain, vomiting)
- Food history
- Exposure history (e.g. contact with ill persons, travel history, illicit drug use)
- If bowel obstruction suspected: absence of flatus (+/- obstipation) suggests obstruction is complete
- **Past Medical History:**
    - Ask about constipation (overflow diarrhea)
    - History of IBD (Crohn's, ulcerative colitis), celiac disease, and other GI disorders
- **Medications/Supplements:**
    - Detailed review of prescribed and non-prescribed medications including caffeine, antibiotics, NSAID's, mycophenolate mofetil, vitamin C, magnesium, artificial sweeteners (gum/candy), laxatives
- Associated symptoms (e.g. fever, abdominal pain, vomiting, other constitutional symptoms)

## Gastrointestinal Bleeding
- Ask about onset, timing, volume, brisk frank blood vs. drops of blood in toilet
    - Hematemesis: vomiting blood from gut (bright red or "coffee-grounds")
    - Melena: black, tarry, malodorous stools
    - Hematochezia: blood in stools (bright red/maroon)
- Previous history of GI bleeding, history of Aspirin or other anti-platelets, NSAID's, liver disease, anti-coagulants, previous endoscopy/colonscopy, peptic ulcer disease, alcohol use disorder

**Table 4.** Gastrointestinal Bleeding

|  | Upper GI Bleed | Lower GI Bleed |
|---|---|---|
| **Description** | Bleeding that originates proximal to the ligament of Treitz Hematemesis and/or melena Hematochezia if bleeding is brisk (other clues: hemodynamic instability, elevated BUN/Cr ratio) | Distal to ligament of Treitz (jejunum, ileum, colon) Often presents as hematochezia Can present as melena if originates from distal small bowel or right colon especially if slow rate of bleeding |
| **Potential Causes** | PUD, varices, esophagitis, Mallory-Weiss tear, tumors, angiodysplasia, Dieulafoy lesion, Zollinger-Ellison syndrome (gastrinomas) | *Painless:* diverticulosis, external haemorrhoids, angiodysplasia, colon cancer or large polyps, Meckel's diverticulum, post-polypectomy *Painful:* anal fissure, internal hemorrhoids *Bloody diarrhea*: ischemic colitis, infectious colitis, IBD |

## Jaundice and Scleral Icterus
- Onset, duration
- Ask about pale stools and dark urine -- suggest hepatobiliary disease (and less likely hemolysis) and can be an indicator of hepatobiliary disease before jaundice develops
- Associated symptoms: fever, pruritus (cholestatic liver disease)
- Alcohol intake: CAGE questionnaire* (see Social History in **General History and Physical** Chapter, pg. 4) *to be used for screening only and not for diagnosis
- Medications
    - All medications (especially new ones)
    - Consider statins, antibiotics, excessive acetaminophen use, anti-epileptics
    - Herbal products (complementary medicines), over-the-counter meds, supplements
    - If altered bowel habits, ask about narcotics as well as pro-motility agents
- Industrial chemical exposure
- Risk factors for hepatitis (see social history below)

- **Past Medical History**
  - Previous episodes of jaundice
  - History of acute hepatitis or liver disease
  - Past abdominal/GI/GU surgery
  - History of autoimmune diseases
  - Hemodialysis and prior hospitalization
- **Family History**
  - Hepatitis (HBV) and liver cancer in 1st degree relative
  - GI or liver disease (jaundice, viral hepatitis, cirrhosis)
  - Cirrhosis and liver failure/liver transplant
  - Cholangiocarcinoma and gallbladder cancer
  - Pancreatic cancer
  - Other GI cancers, ovarian/endometrial cancer
  - Gallstones
  - IBD: ulcerative colitis (UC) or Crohn's disease (CD)
  - Celiac disease or other autoimmune diseases
- **Social History**
  - Menstrual patterns as a clue to onset of a chronic disease
  - Sexual practices (e.g. anal intercourse, unprotected sex)
  - Smoking history
  - Recreational or intravenous drug use
  - Country of birth of parents and patient
  - History of incarceration, institutionalization
  - Tattoos, body piercings
  - Blood product exposure
  - Ask about travel (for infectious diseases causing jaundice)
  - Diet and exercise levels (nonalcoholic fatty liver disease)

**Clinical Pearl: Jaundice**

In a patient with jaundice, long-standing history of decreased libido and abnormal menstruation suggests chronic liver disease or cirrhosis.

## 4. FOCUSED PHYSICAL EXAM

In any of the following physical exams, the following elements would be included at the beginning:

- **Prepare the patient:** adequate lighting, warm room, comfortable environment, explain examination to patient
- **Always look at patient's facial expressions for pain/discomfort during abdominal exam**
- Adjust bed to flat position
- Patient lying supine, arms at his/her side
- Appropriate draping: exposure of abdomen from below nipple line to symphysis pubis
- Stand on the patient's right side
- **Vital Signs:** BP, HR, RR, SpO2 and temperature

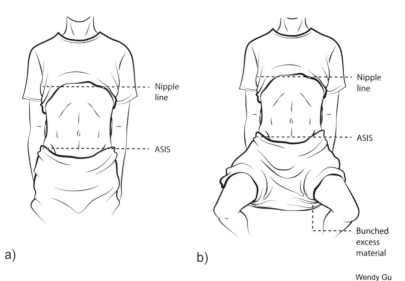

a)  b)

Wendy Gu

**Figure 2**. Abdominal Exam Draping
a) Standard draping b) Draping if leg maneuvers need to be performed

### 4.1 General Abdominal Exam

**Inspection:** look at the abdomen from the foot of the bed
- General appearance: distress, jaundice (scleral icterus), level of consciousness
- Contour
  - Normal: note symmetry
  - Scaphoid: normal, malnourished
  - Protuberant: **6 F's** (Fat, Fluid, Feces, Flatus, Fetus, Fatal growth)
  - Distended lower half: suggests pregnancy, leiomyoma (fibroid), ovarian tumor, hernias
  - Distended upper half: suggests gastric dilatation, enlarged lobe
- Umbilicus
  - Umbilical hernia: suggestive of increased abdominal pressure usually due to fluid or mass
  - Bluish discoloration due to intra or retroperitoneal hemorrhage (Cullen's sign, see **Table 4**)
  - Nodular (Sister Mary Joseph Node): metastatic abdominal or pelvic malignancy
- Hernias (see **The Urological Exam** Chapter)
- Flanks: bulging (suggests ascites), bluish discolouration (retroperitoneal hemorrhage: Grey-Turner's sign) and striae (stretch marks in the skin, associated with rapid weight gain/growth or endocrine causes (Cushing's syndrome)
- Superficial Veins
  - Visible in thin patients and in vena cava obstruction
  - Caput medusae (surrounding umbilicus)
  - Cephalad drainage pattern in IVC obstruction, caudad drainage in SVC obstruction, normal flow pattern (cephalad above umbilicus and caudad below umbilicus) in portal hypertension without caval obstruction

**Auscultation:**
- Bowel sounds
  - Listening to one quadrant is sufficient
  - Listen for 2 min before concluding absent
- Vascular bruits
  - Aortic (1-2 inches above umbilicus at midline)
  - Renal arteries (1 inch on either side off midline from aortic)
  - Bifurcation of the common iliac arteries (halfway between umbilicus and ASIS)
- Other

- If vomiting, assess for succussion splash: gently shake patient from side-to-side while auscultating in the epigastrium for the "whoosh" noise indicating gastric outlet obstruction

**Percussion:** Percuss all 4 quadrants (usually tympanic; note any dullness)

**Palpation:**
- Light palpation: Detects abdominal tenderness, areas of muscle spasm/rigidity
  - Lightly palpate entire abdomen using palmar surface of either hand
  - Lift hand entirely from the skin when moving from area to area
  - In the case of a ticklish patient try placing the patient's hand on top of your hand while palpating
- Ask patient to breathe through his/her mouth
- If areas of tenderness are identified, further palpation can be used to delineate the area
  - Start away from stated areas of tenderness first
  - If areas of tenderness identified, assess for guarding and rebound tenderness by comparing degree of tenderness on palpation vs. releasing (pain worse on release suggests peritonitis)
- If hernia suspected, examine inguinal hernial rings and male genitalia, ask patient to cough while palpating to elicit herniation
- Palpate costovertebral angle tenderness:
  - Place one hand flat on the costovertebral angle to assess for tenderness
  - If pain not elicited, attempt fist palpation (using the ulnar surface of your fist, strike the costovertebral angle and assess for pain)
  - For assessment of retroperitoneal abscess, and pyelonephritis
- Deep palpation: Detects presence of masses, appendiceal abscess, etc
  - Using both hands, rest one hand on the abdomen and apply gentle but steady pressure with the other over top
  - If abdominal wall is tense, it can be relaxed by maximally flexing knees (heels close to buttocks), by placing a pillow under patient's head and/ or knees or by placing the patient's hand onto your palpating hand (this may also help with "ticklish" patients, and children)

## 4.2 Liver and Gallbladder Exam

**Inspection**
- Skin abnormalities
  - Pallor, cyanosis, erythema, scleral icterus
  - Striae (recent = pink, blue; purple = Cushing's; silver = old, obese, postpartum)
  - Scars (surgical and hypertrophic/keloid)
  - Spider angiomas on chest and abdomen
- Gynecomastia, testicular atrophy, frontal balding, pectoral alopecia, decreased body hair in men
- Level of consciousness
- Abdominal distention, flank distention
- Fetor hepaticus (sulphur-smelling breath)
- Hands and Nails
  - Thenar wasting
  - Palmar erythema
  - Dupuytren's contracture
  - Interossei wasting
  - Clubbing
  - Leukonychia (white spots, streaks on nails)
- Other: JVP (see **The Precordial Exam** Chapter), pedal edema

---

**Clinical Pearl: Liver Disease and JVP**
In ascites, elevated JVP may be the only clinical clue to a cardiac cause of liver disease (tricuspid insufficiency, pericarditis), whereas in other causes of cirrhosis, JVP is low. Also be alert to a pulsatile liver.

---

**Auscultation (optional in Liver Exam)**
- Bruit: suggests hepatocellular carcinoma, alcoholic hepatitis
- Venous hum: suggests portal hypertension

**Percussion**
- Done in in mid-clavicular line from RLQ to right costal margin looking for tympany to dullness and from above right nipple down looking for resonance to dullness
- Measure the span
  - Normal: M: 8-12 cm, F: 6-10cm MCL
  - Falsely increased span (lung dullness, e.g. right pleural effusion)
  - Falsely decreased span (gas in the right upper quadrant, e.g. gas in the colon)

**Palpation**
- **Method 1: Standard Technique**
  - Start in the mid-clavicular line of the RLQ - Place the right hand on the abdomen with fingertips positioned superiorly parallel to the rectus abdominus muscle and push inwards and upward toward patient's head during each inspiration until the liver edge is felt
  - The hand inches forward/upward during expiration
  - To check for tenderness, the examiner's left hand is placed on the liver while the ulnar side of the right fist strikes the left hand
- **Method 2:** Hooking Technique (useful method if a patient is obese, optional technique)
  - Stand near the head of the patient with examiner facing patient's feet
  - Place both hands below the right costal margin to "hook" over the liver edge
  - The examiner pushes inward and toward the patient's head during inspiration
- ***Note:*** the edge of an enlarged liver may be missed by starting palpation too high on the abdomen
- When describing your examination of the liver, always include:
  - Length of liver below costal margin
  - Total liver span
  - Liver edge characteristics
    - Texture of liver edge (i.e. smooth or nodular)
    - Consistency of liver edge (i.e. firm or soft)
  - Presence of bruits

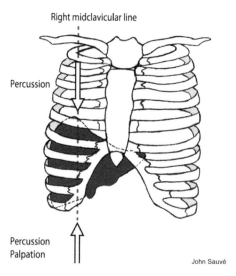

Right midclavicular line

Percussion

Percussion
Palpation

John Sauvé

**Figure 3.** Liver Percussion

## Palpation of Gallbladder
- To attempt palpation of gallbladder, the lower liver edge should be first identified
- Palpate the lower liver edge at the mid-clavicular line
- If the liver edge is not palpable, go to right costal margin
- Ask the patient to breathe in deeply
- A sudden stop in inspiration is a positive Murphy's sign and is suggestive of acute cholecystitis

**Clinical Pearl: Hepatomegaly**
A palpable liver is not necessarily enlarged, but increases the likelihood of hepatomegaly. A nonpalpable liver edge does not rule out hepatomegaly, but reduces its likelihood.

**Clinical Pearl: Biliary Neoplasm**
A palpable gallbladder with painless jaundice (Courvoisier sign) is likely pancreatic or biliary neoplasm until proven otherwise.

## 4.3 Ascites Exam
### Inspection
- Bulging flanks: suggests ascites but need to differentiate from obesity
- Increased abdominal girth
- Ankle edema

### Percussion
- **Shifting Dullness**
  - Determine the border of tympany and dullness by percussion in supine position, beginning at the umbilicus and moving laterally (mark this spot with a pen). Repeat percussion in the same direction with the patient rolled to that same side
  - In the presence of ascites, the tympany-dullness margin will move 'upward' (toward the umbilicus) as the ascitic fluid pools in the dependent side of the peritoneal cavity
  - In the absence of ascites, the margin does not move

### Palpation
- **Fluid Wave (sensitivity = 50-80%, specificity 82-92%)[24]**
  - Ask the patient to place the ulnar side of his/her hand in the midline of the abdomen (to avoid the patient's arm getting in the way and compressing the abdomen and patients are more relaxed when their wrists are flexed rather than extended)
  - Tap on lateral side of abdomen and assess the transmission of a wave to contralateral side using the other hand – if the fluid thrill can be palpated by this hand, the abdominal distension is likely due to ascites
    - **Note:** the tap must be below the level of tympany

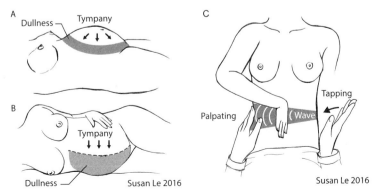

**Figure 4.** Ascites Tests. Part (a) and (b) Shifting Dullness (c) Fluid Wave

## 4.4 Spleen Exam

### Percussion
- **Traube's Space**
    - ◆ Have the patient lie supine and breathe normally
    - ◆ Percuss in the area bounded by the sixth rib superiorly, left anterior axillary line laterally, and the left costal margin inferiorly (Traube's space)
    - ◆ Normal or small spleen sounds resonant or tympanic
    - ◆ Enlarged spleen sounds dull[1]
- **Castell's Sign**
    - ◆ Have the patient lie supine and breathe in and out deeply in a continuous manner
    - ◆ While patient is breathing continuously, percuss the lowest intercostal space in the left anterior axillary line
    - ◆ Have the patient take a full inspiration, percuss in the same area and compare the percussion notes
    - ◆ Normal or small spleen sounds tympanic on inspiration
    - ◆ Enlarged spleen sounds dull on inspiration[2]

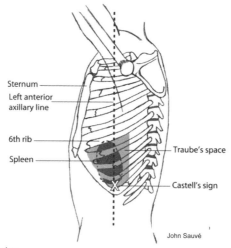

Sternum

Left anterior axillary line

6th rib

Spleen

Traube's space

Castell's sign

John Sauvé

**Figure 5.** Spleen Percussion

---

**Clinical Pearl: Splenomegaly**
Start with Percussion when testing the spleen. The clinical examination is more specific than sensitive and is useful for ruling in the disease when it is suspected. Percussion may indicate but does NOT confirm splenomegaly.

---

**Clinical Pearl: Percussing the Spleen Postprandially**
Since food in the stomach causes dullness in the left upper quadrant, interpret dullness cautiously if patient has eaten within the past four hours.

---

### Palpation
- Stand on the right side of the supine patient
- Place left hand behind the patient's left rib cage and right hand in the right lower quadrant (area of the appendix) angled toward the left anterior axillary line
- Use the right hand to push inwards and upwards toward patient's head during each inspiration
- Incrementally move the right hand diagonally upward to the left costal margin palpating for the spleen
- When the right hand reaches the left costal margin, gently dig deep under the left costal margin while the patient inspires deeply, searching for an enlarged spleen (i.e. palpate for the tip of the spleen coming forward against fingertips)

THE ESSENTIALS OF CLINICAL EXAMINATION HANDBOOK, 8TH ED.

## 4.5 Kidney Exam

**Palpation**
- The kidney is not usually palpable in an adult except in polycystic kidney disease
- Stand on the patient's right side
- Palpate deeply with the right hand below the right costal margin
- Left hand is placed on the patient's back between the right costal margin and the right iliac crest and is used to lift upward
- For the left kidney, stand on the left side of the patient and repeat the maneuvers switching hands
- To check for tenderness, ask patient to sit up; strike the two costovertebral angles with the ulnar side of your fist (lightly). Proceed in a downward vertical direction

**Table 5.** Differentiating Enlarged Spleen vs. Enlarged Kidney

| Enlarged Spleen | Enlarged Kidney |
| --- | --- |
| LUQ percussion is dull | LUQ percussion is tympanic |
| Can probe with fingers deep to the medial and lateral borders but not between the mass and the costal margin | Can probe with fingers between the mass and costal margin, but not deep to its medial and lower borders |
| Cannot ballot | Can ballot the kidney |
| Notch can be felt on the medial side | No notch |
| Moves with inspiration | |
| Edge may extend beyond the midline when it enlarges or during respiration (moves toward RLQ) | Edge does not extend beyond midline (enlarges down and forward) |

**Clinical Pearl: The Equivocal Patient**
To differentiate between involuntary or malingering pain try to distract patient by pretending to auscultate by pushing in the stethoscope.
**Note:** Do not do this routinely, only when pain is questionable!

## 4.6 Acute Abdomen Exam

**Inspection**
- State of the patient:
  - Completely still: may indicate peritonitis
  - Writhing: suggests colic
  - Curled up in fetal position: suggests visceral pain
  - One hip flexed: suggests splinting
  - Sitting up and leaning forward: suggests retroperitoneal irritation

**Special Tests**
- Elicit cough tenderness
  - Coughing often elicits localized pain in an inflamed area
- Shake tenderness: shake the bed
- Sudden movements can be used to elicit peritoneal signs

**Auscultation**
- Decreased or absent bowel sounds (ileus)
- Lightly push down on stethoscope to look for pain

## Palpation
- Always look at patients face (see 4.1 General Abdominal Exam section above)
- Voluntary Guarding: result of patients' fear commonly rather than actual pain itself. Distracting the patient or relaxation techniques may partially or fully eliminate the guarding
- Involuntary Guarding: Reflexive spasm of the abdominal muscles due to peritonitis (peritoneal inflammation) and as such it cannot be overcome
- Also check for other signs. See **Table 6** below

**Table 6.** Specific Signs and Their Possible Interpretation

| Sign/Special Test | Description | Possible Pathology |
|---|---|---|
| Rovsing's Sign | RLQ pain on LLQ palpation | Appendicitis |
| Obturator Test | Pain when thigh is flexed to a right angle (with the hip and knee at 90 degrees), gently rotate the hip, first internally then externally | Pelvic appendicitis<br>Diverticulitis<br>PID<br>Other causes of inflammation in region of obturator internus muscle |
| McBurney's Sign | Tenderness at McBurney's point (1/3 along line extending from the ASIS to the umbilicus) | Appendicitis |
| Rebound Tenderness | Pain on quick withdrawal of palpation Check for peritonitis before assessing rebound tenderness by asking patient to cough or by lightly jarring the bed; if this reproduces the abdominal pain, there is no need to maximize the pain by demonstrating rebound tenderness | Peritonitis |
| Murphy's Sign | Arrest of deep inspiration on RUQ palpation (hand contact with gallbladder elicits pain) | Cholecystitis |
| Courvoisier's Sign | Painless, palpable distended gallbladder | Biliary obstruction usually from malignancy (pancreatic or biliary tract) |
| Cullen's Sign | Blue discoloration of periumbilical area caused by retroperitoneal hemorrhage tracking around to anterior abdominal wall | Acute hemorrhagic pancreatitis<br>Ectopic pregnancy<br>Intra-peritoneal hemorrhage<br>Abdominal trauma |
| Grey-Turner's Sign | Blue discoloration of the flank area caused by retroperitoneal hemorrhage | Acute hemorrhagic pancreatitis<br>Ruptured abdominal aortic aneurysm |
| Kehr's Sign | Severe left shoulder pain exacerbated by elevating foot of bed (referred pain; diaphragmatic involvement) | Splenic rupture |
| Carnett's Sign | **Positive Carnett's Sign**<br>Abdominal pain/tenderness exacerbated when patient lifts feet above the bed without bending knees | Source of pain is abdominal wall (strain/sprain/abdominal wall hernia) because stretching of abdominal wall worsens any lesion within wall (positive Carnett's sign) |
| | **Negative Carnett's Sign**<br>Abdominal pain/tenderness alleviated when patient lifts feet above the bed without bending knees | Source of pain is inside abdominal cavity because stabilizing abdominal wall protects the organs within the abdominal cavity (negative Carnett's sign) |

ASIS = anterior superior iliac spine, PID = pelvic inflammatory disease, R/LLQ = right/ left lower quadrant, RUQ = right upper quadrant

THE ESSENTIALS OF CLINICAL EXAMINATION HANDBOOK, 8TH ED.

GASTROINTESTINAL

**Clinical Pearl: Appendicitis**
Appendicitis is often suspected with a positive psoas sign, pain migration, RLQ pain, and rigidity. In children, aside from abdominal pain, fever is the single most useful sign associated with appendicitis[15]

## Abdominal Aortic Aneurysm
- See **The Peripheral Vascular Exam** Chapter

## Digital Rectal Exam
- Male: see **The Urological Exam** Chapter
- Female: see **The Gynecological Exam** Chapter

# 5. COMMON INVESTIGATIONS

Table 7. Common Investigations

| Test | Description | Indication for Test |
| --- | --- | --- |
| **Stool Microbiology** | Detection of microbes in stool<br><br>C&S (Culture and Sensitivity): bacterial infection<br><br>O&P (Ova and Parasites): parasitic infection<br><br>C. Difficile toxin | To test for chronic diarrhea (C. difficile especially with history of antibiotic or hospital exposure) |
| **FOBT** (Fecal occult blood test)<br><br>**FIT** (Fecal Immuno-chemical test) | Detects small volumes of blood in the stool | ONLY for colon cancer screening in appropriate asymptomatic individuals |
| **Colonoscopy*** | Provides best direct view of colon mucosa and opportunities for biopsy | Used to rule out or establish diagnosis of multiple mucosal conditions (e.g. colorectal cancer, IBD) |
| **MRCP** | MRI evaluation of the bile duct, gallbladder, and pancreatic duct | To diagnose biliary obstruction as a cause of jaundice or elevated liver enzymes |
| **ERCP*** | Endoscopic procedure to examine the common bile duct and pancreatic duct | Used for suspected bile duct obstruction requiring intervention such as sphincterotomy, stent, biopsy |
| **Upper Endoscopy (OGD)** | Provides a direct view of the esophagus, stomach, and duodenum | Look for esophageal varices, esophagitis, peptic ulcer, small bowel biopsy to rule out intestinal disease, such as celiac disease, etc.<br><br>Evaluation of the upper GI tract with biopsies for inflammation (including H. pylori), ulcers, malignancy, varices and other mucosal disease such as celiac disease<br><br>Opportunity for intervention in upper GI bleeding |

| Test | Description | Indication for Test |
|------|-------------|---------------------|
| **Schilling Test*** | Measurement of urinary radioactive labeled vitamin B12 following oral ingestion | Evaluate vitamin B12 absorption to test for pernicious anemia, ileal disease, bacterial small bowel overgrowth, pancreatic insufficiency |
| **C-14 Urea Breath Test (UBT)**<br><br>**C-13 Non-Radioactive** | Detection of the enzyme urease, produced by Helicobacter pylori. If gastric urease present, then orally administered C-14 urea will be hydrolyzed into ammonia and $^{14}CO_2$. The $^{14}CO_2$ can be detected in the expired breath. Analogous test possible with non-radioactive $^{13}CO_2$, but is more expensive<br><br>C-13: Sensitivity 93% and specificity 92%<br><br>C-14 UBT: Sensitivity 88-95% and specificity 95-100% [21] | Presence of Helicobacter pylori infection of stomach<br>Confirmation of eradication of H. Pylori following antibiotic therapy |

*Gold standard in indicated pathology

FOBT = fecal occult blood test, ERCP = endoscopic retrograde cholangiopancreatography, MRCP = magnetic resonance cholangiopancreatography, OGD = oesophago-gastro-duodenoscopy

## 6. TEN COMMON CLINICAL SCENARIOS

**Table 8.** Ten Common Clinical Scenarios

| Key Symptoms | Physical Exam Findings | Investigations | Management |
|--------------|------------------------|----------------|------------|
| **Gastro-esophageal Reflux Disease** | | | |
| • Acid regurgitation, heartburn, retrosternal chest pain, worse with certain foods, nighttime, response to antacids, cough<br><br>• MUST distinguish from cardiac disease<br><br>• Red flags: GI bleed/anemia, odynophagia, dysphagia, anorexia, weight loss, pain with exertion | • GERDQ questionnaire | • Endoscopy if red flags<br><br>• Empiric PPI trial in those without red flags; Endoscopy if PPI fails | • Lifestyle (weight loss, avoidance of dietary triggers: caffeine, mint, smoking, alcohol, spicy foods, etc.)<br><br>• PPI |

**GASTROINTESTINAL**

### Peptic Ulcer Disease

| Key Symptoms | Physical Exam Findings | Investigations | Management |
| --- | --- | --- | --- |
| • Burning epigastric pain, may be post-prandial, often relieved w/ food, antacid<br><br>• Rule out red flags: weight loss, N/V, early satiety, GI bleed/anemia, new onset in advanced age<br><br>• MUST distinguish from cardiac disease (i.e. relation to exertion and other risk factors) | • May have epigastric tenderness on physical exam | • If no red flags, non-invasive testing with H. pylori serology or urea breath test<br><br>• If persistent symptoms despite treatment or H. pylori-negative testing, upper endoscopy (OGD) +/-abdominal ultrasound | • H. pylori eradication regimens<br><br>• Stop offending medications (including NSAID's)<br><br>• Acid suppression (PPI) |

### Cirrhosis

| Key Symptoms | Physical Exam Findings | Investigations | Management |
| --- | --- | --- | --- |
| • Spectrum from alcoholic fatty liver to alcoholic hepatitis to cirrhosis (end stage)<br><br>• Jaundice, abdominal distention, confusion (hepatic encephalopathy), may have RUQ abdominal pain, anorexia, fever | • Gynecomastia, spider nevi, altered pectoral alopecia, palmar erythema, testicular atrophy, caput medusae, hemorrhoids<br><br>• Splenomegaly<br><br>• Portal hypertension, ascites, encephalopathy, variceal bleeding, spontaneous bacterial peritonitis | • CBC, extended electrolytes, renal function, liver profile<br><br>• AST:ALT > 2:1 (alcoholic liver disease)<br><br>• Increased GGT<br><br>• Increased MCV<br><br>• Anemia, thrombocytopenia (from hyerpsplenism), may have impaired liver function ($\uparrow$ INR, $\downarrow$ albumin, $\uparrow$ bilirubin)<br><br>• Abdominal U/S (to assess liver morphology and signs of portal HTN: ascites, splenomegaly, portal and hepatic vein blood flow)<br><br>• Work up for etiology of liver disease, including viral hepatitis (HBV, HCV), metabolic disorders (ferritin, iron profile, ceruloplasmin, alpha-1 antitrypsin), autoimmune disorders i.e. primary biliary cirrhosis (ANA, anti-SM, anti-liver/kidney, anti-mitochondrial Abs, Ig) | • Treat underlying etiology and manage complications of liver disease (sodium-restriction/ diuretics for ascites, beta-blockade/banding for varcies, lactulose/ rifaximin for encephalopathy)<br><br>• Alcohol cessation: counseling, support groups<br><br>• MELD score <15: monitor for complications<br><br>• MELD score >15 or <15 with complications: referral for transplant if alcohol abstinent<br><br>• Child–Pugh Scoring System also used for prognosis |

**GASTROINTESTINAL**

### Gallstones

| Key Symptoms | Physical Exam Findings | Investigations | Management |
|---|---|---|---|
| • <u>Cholelithiasis</u>: Incidental/asymptomatic (seen incidentally on imaging)<br><br>• <u>Biliary colic</u>: intermittent RUQ pain associated with fatty foods with radiation to shoulder or back<br><br>• <u>Acute cholecystitis</u>: same pain as biliary but persistent, may be associated with N/V, fever<br><br>• <u>Ascending cholangitis</u>: fever, jaundice, RUQ pain, signs of sepsis | • <u>Biliary colic</u>: normal physical exam<br><br>• <u>Acute cholecystitis</u>: Murphy's sign<br><br>• <u>Ascending cholangitis</u>: fever, RUQ tenderness, signs of sepsis - tachycardia, hypotension, decreased LOC | • Ultrasound<br><br>• Hepatobiliary iminodiacetic acid scan<br><br>• CT scan<br><br>• MRCP<br><br>• CBC, liver enzymes (ALT, AST), total bilirubin, alkaline phosphatase, amylase, and lipase levels<br><br>• Mild leukocytosis<br><br>• Note: testing is only for acute cholecystitis<br><br>• ERCP/MRCP is only when there is a suspected concomitant choledocholithiasis (elevated liver profile, bilirubin)<br><br>• Blood cultures | • Cholelithiasis: no testing or surgery needed<br><br>• Biliary colic: elective laparoscopic cholecystectomy<br><br>• Acute cholecystitis: more urgent surgery |

### Acute Pancreatitis

| Key Symptoms | Physical Exam Findings | Investigations | Management |
|---|---|---|---|
| • Sudden onset LUQ, periumbilical, or epigastric pain; worse after eating/ drinking<br><br>• N&V<br><br>• Indigestion, fullness, distension<br><br>• Fever | • Hypotension, tachycardia, tachypnea, diaphoresis, jaundice<br><br>• Significant tenderness on palpation<br><br>• Decreased bowel sounds<br><br>• Cullen's; Grey Turner<br><br>• May have signs of peritonitis (rigidity, rebound tenderness)<br><br>• Signs of dehydration | • CBC, extended chemistry panel (electrolytes, creatinine, liver profile, amylase/ lipase, calcium, Mg/ phosphate, LDH, triglycerides)<br><br>• Urinalysis<br><br>• Blood cultures if signs of sepsis<br><br>• ABG, CRP may be helpful in severe cases | • Bowel rest (NPO or clear fluids to start), IV fluids, narcotic analgeisa<br><br>• If gallstones present, ERCP if presence of biliary obstruction |

**GASTROINTESTINAL**

## Pancreatic Cancer

| Key Symptoms | Physical Exam Findings | Investigations | Management |
|---|---|---|---|
| • Symptoms related to location<br><br>• Head of pancreas, symptoms usually present in late stage of disease, painless jaundice +/• anorexia and weight loss;<br><br>• Body/tail: often symptomatic and much larger | • Cachexia, scleral icterus, may have palpable supraclavicular node (Virchow's node), palpable abdominal mass | • CT scan for staging<br><br>• MRI<br><br>• Biopsy<br><br>• Endoscopy ultrasound (EUS)<br><br>• Liver profile | • Curable disease: surgical resection +/• neoadjuvant chemoradiation or palliative chemotherapy<br><br>• ERCP with stenting if biliary obstruction present (i.e. jaundice) |

## Appendicitis

| Key Symptoms | Physical Exam Findings | Investigations | Management |
|---|---|---|---|
| • Migration of pain from peribumbilical region to RLQ pain, anorexia, N&V<br><br>• Low grade fever | • Localized tenderness on percussion<br><br>• Psoas sign, obturator sign, Rovsing's sign, flank tenderness in RLQ, guarding | • Elevated WBC count<br><br>• Radiology: ultrasound, CT scan | • Surgical removal |

## Acute Diarrhea

| Key Symptoms | Physical Exam Findings | Investigations | Management |
|---|---|---|---|
| • May have fever, dehydration, bloody stool, anorexia, weight loss, myalgias, arthalgias | • Assess dehydration status (see **Fluids, Electrolytes, and Acid/Base Disturbances** Chapter)<br><br>• Assess full abdomen including rectal exam for pain, masses, abdominal distention, bleeding | • Not usually indicated<br><br>• Blood work (CBC, electrolyte panel, and renal function) with stool microbiology if symptoms are severe | • Oral rehydration<br><br>• Antimicrobial therapy only for specific pathogens and in severe cases<br><br>• Anti-diarrheals can be considered in mild cases |

GASTROINTESTINAL

## Inflammatory Bowel Disease

| Key Symptoms | Physical Exam Findings | Investigations | Management |
|---|---|---|---|
| • Diarrhea (+/• blood), lower abdo cramps, urgency<br><br>• Weight loss, low-grade fever, nausea, vomiting, anorexia<br><br>• Extra-intestinal manifestations: joint swelling, eye pain/redndess, skin findings (erythema nodosum, pyoderma gangrenosum) | • Full abdominal exam<br><br>• Palpable mass in RLQ (Crohn's disease)<br><br>• Distention may suggest bowel obstruction (due to stricture)<br><br>• DRE to look for perianal disease | • Standard blood work (CBC, extended electrolytes, renal function, liver profile, B12/ferritin, CRP),<br><br>• Stool microbiology<br><br>• Colonoscopy | • Lifestyle modifications (lower residue diet for flares, obstructive symptoms)<br><br>• Anti-diarrheal medications<br><br>• Immunosuppressive therapy, 5-ASA, corticosteroids, biologics, surgery |

## Colorectal Cancer

| Key Symptoms | Physical Exam Findings | Investigations | Management |
|---|---|---|---|
| • Hematochezia, melena, anemia<br><br>• Change in bowel habits (constipation and/or diarrhea)<br><br>• Iron deficiency anemia, change in caliber of stool<br><br>• Weight loss, anorexia if severe due to liver metastases | • May have palpable abdominal mass, or rectal mass on DRE | Screening:<br>• FOBT/FIT<br>• Flexible sigmoidoscopy<br>• Colonoscopy<br><br>Symptomatic patients:<br>• Colonoscopy and/or CT scan (for staging of confirmed colorectal cancer) | • Surgical removal after TNM staging |

# REFERENCES

1. Grover SA, Barkun AN, Sackett DL. 1993. The rational clinical examination. Does this patient have splenomegaly? JAMA 270(18):2218-2221.
2. Castell DO, Frank BB. 1977. Abdominal exam: Role of percussion and auscultation. Postgrad Med 62(6):131-134.
3. Feighery C. 1999. Fortnightly review: Coeliac disease. BMJ 319(7204):236-239.
4. Hobbs FD. 2000. ABC of colorectal cancer: The role of primary care. BMJ 321 (7268):1068- 1070.
5. Horwitz BJ, Fisher RS. 2001. The irritable bowel syndrome. N Engl J Med 344(24):1846-1850.
6. Longstreth GF, Thompson WG, Chey WD, Houghton LA, Mearin F, Spiller RC. 2006. Functional bowel disorders. Gastroenterology 130(5):1480-1491.
7. Moayyedi P, Talley NJ, Fennerty MB, Vakil N. 2006. Can the clinical history distinguish between organic and functional dyspepsia? JAMA 295(13):1566-1576.
8. O'Donohue J, Williams R. 1996. Primary biliary cirrhosis. QJM 89(1):5-13.
9. Bickley LS, Szilagyi PG, Bates B. Bates' Guide to Physical Examination and History Taking. Philadelphia: Lippincott Williams & Wilkins; 2007.
10. Canadian Hypertension Education Program. 2008. The 2008 Canadian Hypertension Education Program recommendations: The scientific summary – an annual update. Can J Cardiol 24(6):447-452.
11. Examination of the Spleen. http://stanfordmedicine25.stanford.edu/the25/spleen.html   Published by Standford Medicine 2016. Accessed December 27, 2016.
12. Scorza, K et al. 2007.  Evaluation of Nausea and Vomiting. American Family Physician.  76(1): 76 -  84.
13. Sweester, S. (2012).  Evaluating the Patient with Diarrhea: A Case-Based Approach.  87(6): 596-602.
14. Trowbridge, R. L., Rutkowski, N. K., and Shojania, K.G.  (2003).  Does This Patient Have Acute Cholecystitis?  JAMA.  289(1): 80-86.
15. Bundy, D.G. et al. (2007).  Does This Child Have Appendicitis? JAMA.  298(4): 438-451.
16. Abdominal Pain. http://www.slideshare.net/azanero33/acute-abdominal-pain-presentation Published 2008.  Accessed December 27, 2016.
17. University of Toronto Faculty of Medicine .  The Art and Science of Clinical Medicine Book 4.  University of Toronto Faculty of Medicine Retrieved from http://emodules.med.utoronto.ca/ASCM1/ASCM1_Book4.pdf
18. Smith, J.A. Refuerzo, J.S. & S. M. Ramin. (2016). Treatment and outcome of nausea and vomiting in pregnancy.  In: UpToDate, Post TW (Ed), UpToDate, Waltham, MA. (Accessed on December 27, 2016.)
19. Srygley, F. D. Gerardo, C. J. & T. Tran. (2012).  Does this patient have a severe upper gastrointestinal bleed? JAMA, 307(10): 1072 – 1079.
20. Merali, Z, Woodfine, J.D., Kim, J. & I. Mukovozov.  (2016).  The Toronto Notes 2016: Comprehensive medical reference and review for the Medical Council of Canada Qualifiying Exam Part 1 and the United States Medical Licensing Exam Step 2.  Toronto: Toronto Notes for Medical Students, Inc, 2016.
21. S. E. Crowe.  (2015).  Indications and diagnostic tests for Helicobacter pylori infection. In: UpToDate, Post TW (Ed), UpToDate, Waltham, MA. (Accessed on December 27, 2016).
22. M. R. Spieker. (2000).  Evaluating Dysphagia.  American Family Physician, 61(12): 3639 – 3648.
23. G.F. Longstreth. (2016).  Approach to the Adult with Nausea and Vomiting.  In: UpToDate, Post TW (Ed), Waltham, MA. (Accessed on December 27, 2016).
24. Physical Examination: Ascites or Fluid Wave Assessment.  http://www.ebmconsult.com/articles/physical-exam-fluid-wave-ascites Last Updated June 2015.  Accessed December 27, 2016.

**GASTROINTESTINAL**

CHAPTER 5:

# The Head, Neck, and Throat

**Editors:**
Yuhao Shi, BSc
Florentina Teoderascu, MD, HBHSc

**Faculty Reviewers:**
Kevin M. Higgins, MD, FRCSC
Allan D. Vescan, MD, FRCSC

## TABLE OF CONTENTS

HEAD, NECK & THROAT

# 1. EAR

## 1.1 Essential Anatomy

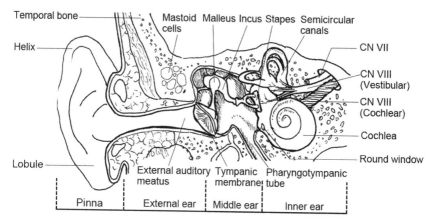

**Figure 1.** Overview of ear anatomy

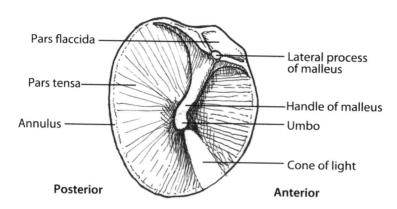

**Figure 2.** Tympanic membrane anatomy

HEAD, NECK & THROAT

**Table 1.** Differentials for Specific Otological Complaints

| Chief Complaint | Diffrential Diagnosis | Differentiating Features |
|---|---|---|
| Ear pain[1,2] | **External Ear Causes** Infections | May be accompanied by constitutional symptoms such as fever |
| | Otitis externa | Recent swim. White discharge. Swollen and red external auditory canal |
| | Cellulitis | Recent insect bite, scratch, or piercing. Rapid progression. Often earlobe involvement |
| | *Perichondritis | Recent insect bite, scratch, or piercing. Rapid progression. Persistent redness, swelling, pain that is more severe than cellulitis |
| | *Necrotizing otitis externa | Suspect in refractory otitis externa in patients who are immunocompromised or diabetic patients. |
| | Trauma (including frost bites) | History of trauma, or exposure to cold weather |
| | Foreign body | Presence of foreign object in external canal |
| | Cerumen impaction | Presence of cerumen on ear drum and in external canal |
| | **Middle Ear Causes** Infection | May be accompanied by constitutional symptoms such as fever |
| | Otitis media | Recent upper respiratory infection. Night restlessness in children. Red or cloudy tympanic membrane that is immobile on pneumatic otoscopy. |
| | Mastoiditis | Recent or concurrent otitis media. Retroauricular pain. Protrusion of auricle.Tender edematous mastoid. |
| | Myringitis | Presents in association with otitis media. May have more pain than otitis media alone. |
| | Trauma | History of barotrauma or other trauma. |
| | Referred pain | See Clinical Pearl below |

HEAD, NECK & THROAT

| Chief Complaint | Diffrential Diagnosis | Differentiating Features |
|---|---|---|
| **Conductive hearing loss**[3] | **External ear causes** Cerumen impaction | Canal occlusion with cerumen visualization. Often sudden, painless hearing loss |
| | Otitis externa | Narrow canal with debris. Evidence of inflammation. Sudden painful loss of hearing. |
| | Foreign object | Visualization of foreign body in external canal |
| | Growths/tumors(e.g. exostosis, osteoma, polyps, squamous cell carcinoma) | Visible on otoscopy. Slow, painless hearing loss. |
| | Middle ear causes Otitis media with effusion | Middle ear effusion seen on exam. |
| | Otosclerosis | Tympanic membrane often normal. Gradual painless loss of hearing. |
| | Tympanic membrane perforation | History of barotrauma, and other sources of trauma |
| | Cholesteatooma | Retracted or perforated tympanic membrane with chronic drainage. Gradual painless hearing loss. |
| | Tumors (e.g. glomus) | May be visualized on otoscopy behind the tympanic membrane. Gradual painless loss. |
| **Sensorineural hearing loss**[3] | Presbycusis | Bilateral, symmetric. Gradual loss. Tobacco use. Elderly patients. |
| | Noise-induced | Noise exposure. Gradual hearing loss. Tinnitus. Bilateral, symmetric loss centered at 4,000Hz. |
| | *Autoimmune | Rapid progressive, possibly fluctuating, bilateral loss. Poor speech discrimination on audiogram. |
| | *Medication induced | Associated with tinnitus and/or vertigo. High frequency loss. Bilateral. (see table 2 for ototoxic medications). |
| | Meniere's disease | Sudden, fluctuating, unilateral loss with tinnitus and vertigo. Low-frequency loss on audiogram. |
| | Acoustic neuroma | Gradual unilateral loss with tinnitus. Possible facial nerve weakness. |
| | Perilymph fistula | Sudden unilateral loss, tinnitus, vertigo. History of trauma, training. |

| Chief Complaint | Diffrential Diagnosis | Differentiating Features |
|---|---|---|
| **Vertigo (must be differentiated from dizziness)[4]** | Benign positional vertigo | Lasts seconds to minutes. Provoked by head movement. |
| | Meniere's disease | Lasting minutes to hours. Sensurineural hearing loss. Tinnitus and/or perception of aural fullness. |
| | Vestibular neuronitis | Acute phase: vertigo/nausea/vomiting and nystagmus<br>Convalescent phase:<br>Imbalance, motion sickness lasting weeks. |

\* Medical emergency

**Clinical Pearl: 10Ts + 2**
Ear pain may be referred pain from the sensory branches of cranial nerve V, VII, IV, X, and cervical roots C2 and C3. These can be remembered with the 10Ts + 2 mnemonic[5].
- Eus**t**achian Tube
- **T**MJ syndrome (pain in front of the ears)
- **T**rismus (spasm of masticator muscles, early symptom of tetanus)
- **T**eeth
- **T**ongue
- **T**onsils (tonsillitis, tonsillar cancer, post-tonsillectomy)
- **T**ic (glossopharyngeal neuralgia)
- **T**hroat (cancer of larynx)
- **T**rachea (foreign body, tracheitis)
- **T**hyroiditis
- Geniculate herpes and Ramsay Hunt syndrome type 2

**Table 2.** Ototoxic compounds

| Class | Examples |
|---|---|
| **Aminoglycosides[6]** | Gentamicin, tobramycin, amikacin, neomycin |
| **NSAIDs[7]** | Aspirin, acetaminophen |
| **Antimalarials[8]** | Quinine, chloroquine |
| **Heavy metals[9]** | Lead, mercury, cadmium, arsenic |
| **Loop diuretics[8]** | Furosemide, ethacrynic acid |
| **Chemotherapy agents[10]** | Cisplatin, 5-fluorouracil, bleomycin |
| **Other antibiotics[8]** | Erythromycin, tetracycline |
| **Phosphodiesterase-5 inhibitors[11]** | Sildenafil, tadalafil, vardenafil |

## 1.3 Focused Histories

- See **General History and Physical Exam** for a detailed approach to history taking
- HPI:
  - **OPQRSTUVW** questions regarding each complaint
  - Unilateral vs. bilateral (**Note:** be cautious of unilateral concerns)
  - Onset, duration, progression, frequency
  - Ask about concurrent ear symptoms:
    - Hearing loss
    - Otalgia
    - Otorrhea (discharge)
    - Tinnitus
    - Vestibular symptoms, such as vertigo and imbalance
  - Recent or past head/ear trauma

- ◆ Noise exposure
- ◆ Risk factors for tumor (>50yo, tobacco, alcohol use)
- PMH:
  - ◆ Previous surgery
  - ◆ Concurrent systemic disease (e.g. MS, SLE, DM)
  - ◆ Recent infections (local, systemic)
- Family history
- Medications (especially ototoxic meds, see **Table 2**)

## Key questions in complaint-specific history

### Otalgia[1]
- Location, duration, severity. Constant vs intermittent
- Does pain occur with swallowing or jaw movement?
- Age – young children (more likely middle ear disease) vs older children/adults (more likely otitis externa, throat infections, TMJ issues)
- Concurrent symptoms:
  - ◆ hearing loss, tinnitus, otorrhea, vertigo suggest primary cause
  - ◆ Issues with teeth, temporomandibular joint, cervical spine may cause secondary ear pain (See Clinical Pearl)
- History of trauma
- Presence of constitutional symptoms: fever, weight loss

### Otorrhea[12]
- Quality (bloody vs clear vs purulent, color, odor, quantity, consistency)
- Duration, frequency, onset
- Associated symptoms: ear pain, headaches, fever, hearing loss
- History of swimming, insertion of objects, use of ear drops – can be source of trauma or infection
- Recent or recurrent ear infections
- History of head trauma – can cause CSF leakage in the ear
- Presence of ystemic disease: elderly, diabetes, immunocompromised – predisposition to necrotizing otitis externa

### Tinnitus[13]
- Subjective (heard by patient) vs. objective (can be heard by others, e.g. with stethoscope) ear ringing
  - ◆ Subjective tinnitus suggests otologic disorders
  - ◆ Objective tinnitus is usually due to vascular abnormalities, Eustachian tube dysfunction, or neurologic disease
- Unilateral vs bilateral
  - ◆ Unilateral causes include cerumen impaction, otitis external, otitis media
  - ◆ Unilateral + sensorineural hearing loss hallmark of acoustic neuroma
- Characteristic of ear sound (ringing, buzzing, or hissing)
  - ◆ Low-pitch rumble – Meniere's disease
  - ◆ High-pitched – sensorineural hearing loss
- Pattern
  - ◆ Continuous – associated with sensorineural hearing loss
  - ◆ Intermittent – Meniere's disease
  - ◆ Pulsatile – vascular abnormality
- Exposure to ototoxic medications
- Noise exposure
- Ask about concurrent symptoms: e.g. vertigo, hearing loss

## 1.4 Focused Physical Exam[14]

### External Exam

- Inspection
  - Pinna for size, position, deformity, inflammation, symmetry, nodules, scars or lesions
    - e.g. microtia, macrotia, cauliflower ear
  - External auditory canal
  - Look for presence of ear discharge: color, consistency, clarity, presence or absence of an odor
- Palpation
  - Pinna, periauricular area, and mastoid process for tenderness, nodules
    - Pain elicited by tugging on pinna/tragus is associated with otitis externa
    - Pain over the mastoid process with an outward and inferior protrusion of the pinna and discharge is found in acute mastoiditis

**Table 3.** Auditory Acuity Testing[14]

| Procedure | Results |
|---|---|
| **Whisper Test**[15]: assessment of hearing impairment<br>• Lightly rub your fingers together next to the ear not being tested and ask the patient to repeat what you whisper into tested ear<br>• Repeat on other ear | • If the patient cannot hear, continue to increase the volume of your voice until it is heard by the patient<br>• 90-100% sensitivity<br>• 70-87% specificity |
| **Weber Test**: assessment of sound lateralization<br>• Place the base of the tuning fork on the center of the patient's forehead<br>• Ask the patient if he/she hears the sound louder on one side or if it is equal on both sides | • Normal hearing = no sound lateralization (patient hears sound or feels vibration in middle)<br>• Conductive hearing loss = sound lateralization to AFFECTED ear<br>• Sensorineural hearing loss = sound<br>• lateralization to NON-AFFECTED ear |
| **Rinne Test**: assessment of air vs. bone conduction<br>• Apply tuning fork against the patient's mastoid process, then place it<br>• still vibrating next to the patient's ear (abbreviated version)<br>• Ask the patient to identify which placement sounds louder<br>• Repeat with opposite ear | • Rinne positive (normal) = air> bone conduction<br>• Rinne negative* (conductive hearing loss) = bone> air conduction<br>• Partial sensorineural hearing loss = air> bone conduction (but both decreased)<br>• *Complete hearing loss in one ear in which patient may still process bone conduction that is picked up by contralateral cochlea is known as "false-negative Rinne" |

*For Weber and Rinne testing, strike a 512 Hz tuning fork on bony prominence (e.g. patella/ styloid process of radius). Do not place tuning fork over hair.

### Otoscopic Exam

- Techniques:
  - Use largest speculum that can be comfortably inserted to maximize visual field and to avoid irritation of bony canal
  - Adults & children: gently pull the pinna backward and upward
  - Stabilize otoscope by placing fifth digit against patient's cheek to protect against sudden movements (special attention with children)
- Examine:
  - External auditory meatus (foreign body, cerumen, inflammation, discharge)
  - Tympanic membrane (see **Table 6**)

## 1.5 Otoscopic Examination of Tympanic Membrane

**Table 4.** Otoscopic Examination of Tympanic Membrane

| Inspect | Normal | Abnormal |
|---|---|---|
| **Color** | Translucent and pearly gray | • **Red** (hyperemia due to inflammation, fever, Valsalva/crying/screaming)<br>• **Yellow** (pus in middle ear, suggests otitis media with effusion [OME])<br>• **Blue** (glomus jugulare, glomus tympanicum) |
| **Light Reflex** | Cone of light directed anteriorly and inferiorly | • Absent/distorted (abnormal geometry due to bulging or retraction, perforation, thickening) |
| **Anatomical Landmarks** | Pars flaccida, malleus (near center), incus (posterior to malleus) | • Obscured landmarks may indicate inflammation, fluid/pus in middle ear or membrane thickening |
| **Abnormal Margins** | Clear and tense margins | • Perforation (untreated ear infection, cholesteatoma, trauma [e.g. cotton swab use]) |
| **Mobility** | Brisk, equal movement with positive and negative pressure using pneumatic otoscopy | • Reduced/absent mobility: increased middle ear pressure (mucoid, serous or purulent effusion)<br>• Increased mobility: negative middle ear pressure (Eustachian tube dysfunction) |
| **Shape** | Drawn inwards slightly at center by handle of malleus | • Bulging: suggests pus/fluid in middle ear<br>• Retraction: Eustachian tube dysfunction resulting in negative middle ear pressure |

## 1.6 Common Investigations

**Table 5.** Common Investigations

| Test | Description | Results |
|---|---|---|
| **Pure Tone Audiogram** | • Tests forthreshold response at generated frequencies<br>• Tests both air and bone conduction | • Audiogram describes hearing deficits across all frequencies |
| **Otoacoustic Emissions**[16] | • Tests for presence and strength of sound generated by cochlea in response to a sound stimulus<br>• Part of screening for hearing loss in newborns | • Absence of emissions can, though not necessarily, be due to fluid or hearing loss in middle ear |
| **Tympanometry**[32] | • Applies positive<br>• and negative air pressure to eardrum and measures compliance<br>• of tympanic membrane | • Low compliance of tympanic membrane indicates fluid in middle ear or otosclerosis<br>• High compliance occurs in ossicularchain discontinuity |

# 2. NOSE

## 2.1 Essential Anatomy

HEAD, NECK & THROAT

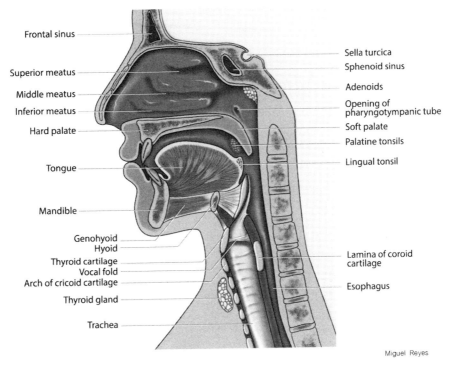

Frontal sinus

Superior meatus

Middle meatus

Inferior meatus

Hard palate

Tongue

Mandible

Genohyoid
Hyoid

Thyroid cartilage
Vocal fold
Arch of cricoid cartilage

Thyroid gland

Trachea

Sella turcica

Sphenoid sinus

Adenoids

Opening of
pharyngotympanic tube

Soft palate

Palatine tonsils

Lingual tonsil

Lamina of coroid
cartilage

Esophagus

Miguel Reyes

**Figure 3.** Anatomy of the right nasal cavity, oropharynx, and larynx (lateral aspect)

## 2.2 Common Chief Complaints and Differentials

**Table 6.** Differentials for Nasal Complaints[17-19]

| Chief Complaint | Differential Diagnosis | Differentiating Features |
| --- | --- | --- |
| **Anosmia (loss of smell)** | Inflammatory & obstructive disease | Rhinitis (allergic and nonallergic), rhinosinusitis, nasal polyps, enlarged turbinates, ethmoid tumor |
| | Post-viral olfactory dysfunction | Viral URTI causing damage to peripheral olfactory receptors (reversible, may persist for several months) |
| | Head trauma | Damage to nose/sinuses; fracture of cribriform plate; contusion injury to olfactory bulb or olfactory areas in cerebral cortex |
| | Neurodegenerative process | Alzheimer disease, Parkinson disease, dementia with Lewy bodies |
| | Autoimmune disease | Sjogren's syndrome, diabetes mellitus |
| | Intracranial pathology | Meningioma of olfactory groove, pseudomotor cerebri, frontal lobe tumor |
| | Congenital | Kallmann syndrome |
| | Environmental | Exposure to toxic agents |
| | Medications | Beta blockers, antithyroid drugs, calcium channel blockers, ACEi, intranasal zinc |
| **Facial/Sinus Pain** | Acute viral rhinosinusitis | <10 days of symptoms that are not worsening |
| | Acute bacterial rhinosinusitis | Persisting symptoms >10 days +/- fever >39C with purulent nasal discharge +/- facial pain for >3-4 consecutive days +/- overall worsening of symptoms after 5-6 days |
| | Acute invasive fungal rhinosinusitis | Rapidly progressive rhinosinusitis, often with extension outside sinuses; more common in diabetic and immunocompromised patients; rare in normal population |
| | Chronic sinusitis | >12wk, bacterial/fungal |
| | Other | Trigeminal neuralgia, TMJ disorder, dental infection, cancer pain |

HEAD, NECK & THROAT

| --- | --- | --- |
| **Rhinitis (sneezing, nasal discharge, nasal congestion, nasal pruritis)** | Allergic | Symptoms develop during childhood or young adult years; Occupational: workplace allergens (food proteins, organic dust, enzymatic proteins) |
| | Nonallergic | Onset at later age than allergic subtype; absence of pruritus; postnasal discharge Vasomotor: non-specific triggers (pollutants, temperature change Gustatory: food triggers (hot, spicy) |
| | Mixed | Combination of allergic & nonallergic |
| | Nasal decongenstant sprays (rhinitis medicamentosa) | Rebound congestion due to regular use of over-the-counter nasal sprays |
| | Nasal Obstruction | Septal deviation (unilateral rhinitis), adenoid hypertrophy, polyps, enlarged turbinates, tumours, foreign bodies, trauma |
| | Systemic disease (Granulomatous disease with polyangiitis, sarcoidosis, immotile cilia, hypothyroid) | Involvement of nose and sinuses; multi-organ involvement |
| | Other | Pregnancy Atrophic rhinitis caused by repeated sinus/nasal surgeries (atrophy of the nasal lining) |
| **Rhinorrhea (nasal discharge)** | Allergic, viral, vasomotor rhinitis | Watery/mucoid discharge |
| | CSF leak | Watery discharge, history of facial/head trauma |
| | Bacterial rhinitis | Purulent discharge |
| | Neoplasm | Serosanguinous discharge |
| | Other | Bloody discharge secondary to trauma, may be mixed with CSF |

| Chief Complaint | Differential Diagnosis | Differentiating Features |
|---|---|---|
| **Epistaxis (nosebleeds)** | Idiopathic | No identifiable trigger (most common) |
| | Systemic causes | Hemophilia, thrombocytopenia, chronic alcohol intake, hematologic disease |
| | Structural deformity | Septal deviations; chronic performations |
| | Inflammatory causes | URTI, allergies |
| | Irritants | Substance abuse (cocaine), foreign body reaction |
| | Trauma | Nose-picking (children), domestic violence |
| | Environmental | Cold, dry weather exposure |
| | Medications | Anti-coagulants, ginseng |

## 2.3 Focused Histories

- General characteristics to elicit on history:
- Unilateral vs bilateral symptoms
- Presence of neurological symptoms
- Characteristics of nasal fluid discharge
- Clear fluid discharge on pillow
- Changes in sense of smell
- Snoring/noisy breathing
- Facial pain
- Cough
- Fever
- Recent trauma
- Allergies
- Associated disease (ie. diabetes, coagulopathies)
- Follow OPQRSTUVW questions regarding each complaint

See **Figures 4** & **5** for guidelines regarding diagnosis & management of acute bacterial rhinosinusitis (ABRS) and chronic bacterial sinusitis (CBS)

# Acute Bacterial Rhinosinusitis (ABRS)

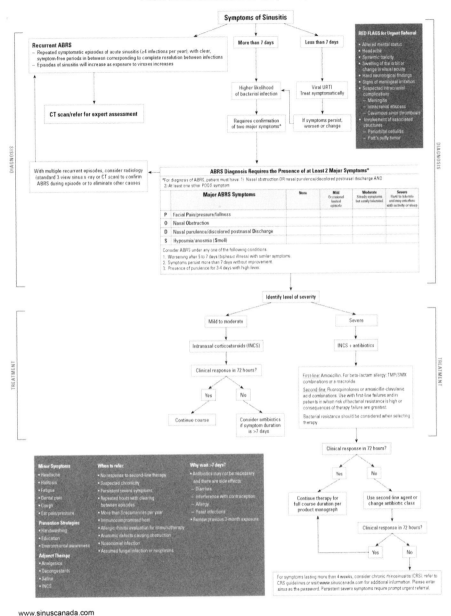

www.sinuscanada.com

**Figure 4.** Diagnosis & clinical management of ARBS (Canadian Rhinosinusitis guidelines[19])

# Chronic Rhinosinusitis

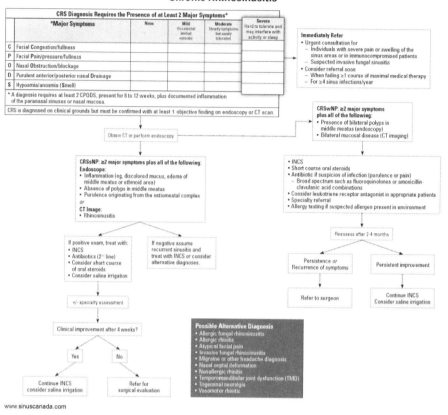

**Figure 5.** Diagnosis & clinical management of CRS (Canadian Rhinosinusitis guidelines[19])

## 2.4 Focused Physical Exam[19]

### External Exam
- Inspection
  - Note any swelling, trauma, deviation or congenital abnormalities o Extend patient's neck and examine the symmetry of the nares
- Palpation
  - Test airway patency: occlude one nostril and ask the patient to sniff then exhale and look for mirror fogging or movement of cotton wisp

### Internal Exam (Nasal Speculum)
- Hold speculum in nondominant hand and introduce horizontally, 1 cm into the vestibule. Place index finger of nondominant hand atop nose to anchor speculum
- **Note:** any swelling, trauma, deviation, masses, discharge or congenital abnormalities

### Inspection
- Septum for deviation or perforation
- Mucous membranes: normally pink, moist and smooth; blue/gray with allergies; red with inflammation
- Little's area for vascular engorgement or crusting (indicates recent epistaxis)

- Turbinates for size and color (black turbinates may indicate mucormycosis; pale turbinates commonly seen with allergies)
- Presence of nasal polyps (grayish color)
- Turbinates are rarely symmetric; asymmetry on inspection is frequently normal

### Olfactory Exam
- To assess CN I, perform the University of Pennsylvania Smell Identification Test (UPSIT) (standardized scratch and sniff test)

### Common Investigations
- Allergy testing
- IgE levels (for allergic patients)
- Endoscopic guided cultures (for sinusitis)
- β-2 transferrin of nasal fluid (if CSF leak suspected)
- CT (to confirm diagnosis or if complications suspected)

## 3. ORAL CAVITY AND PHARYNX

### 3.1 Essential Anatomy
See **Figure 3**

## 3.2 Common Chief Complaints and Differentials

**Table 7.** Differentials for Oral Cavity and Pharynx Complaints

| Chief Complaint | Differential Diagnosis | Distinguishing Features |
|---|---|---|
| Dysphagia[2,20,21] | **Oropharyngeal causes:** | Often presents with difficulty initiating swallow |
| | Structural: Peritonsillar abscess | Fever, malaise, sore throat, otalgia. Trismus (reduced jaw opening). Muffled voice. |
| | Pharyngitis | Sore throat, cold symptoms, hoarseness of voice. |
| | Tumor (e.g. squamous cell carcinoma) | Non-healing ulcer or mass in the oropharynx |
| | Zenker's diverticulum | Regurgitation of old food. Diverticulum seen on barium swallow. |
| | Neuromuscular (including lesions of CNS, cranial nerves, as well as systemic myopathies) | History of stroke. Cranial nerve deficits. Muscle weakness. Often slow progressive dysphagia |
| | Xerostomia | Dry mouth. Reduced saliva production |
| | **Esophageal causes:** See **The Gastrointestinal Exam** | |
| Oral ulcers/ lesions[22] | Aphthous ulcers (canker sores) | Well defined, painful, shallow ulcers. Self-limiting and heals in less than 2 weeks. |
| | **Infective ulcers:** Herpes simplex | Pro-drome of pain, burning, tingling followed by eruption of clusters vesicular lesions. |
| | Candida albican (thrush) | White plaques on buccal mucosa, palate, tongue, or oropharynx. Associated with immunodeficiency, inhaled glucocorticoid use. |
| | **Malignancy:** Squamous cell carcinoma | Non-healing papules, plaqaues, erosions, or ulcers. History of tobacco use. |
| | Melanoma | Oral pigmented lesions with features of asymmetry, irregular borders, variable color, or increasing diameter. |
| | **Other:** Systemic autoimmune disorders (e.g. Systemic lupus erythematosus, Crohn's disease) | Presence of systemic symptoms including but not limited to rash, arthritis, GI symptoms, kidney issue. |

| --- | --- | --- |
| Hoarseness[23] | Inflammatory or irritant: Vocal abuse | History of yelling or excess use of voice. |
| | Exposure to chemicals (e.g. smoke, tobacco) | Smoker. History of inhalation of irritant. Concurrent cough. |
| | Laryngitis/ upper respiratory tract infections | Associated with rhinorrhea, cough, sore throat. Self-limiting |
| | Neuromuscular or psychogenic Myasthenia gravis | Worse later in the day. Muscle weakness throughout rest of body |
| | Nerve injury (vagus or recurrent laryngeal nerve) | History of neck surgery or irradiation. Vocal cord paralysis on laryngoscopy |
| | Muscle tension dysphonia | Associated with stress and anxiety or recent upper respiratory illness. Strained effortful phonation. Vocal fatigue |
| | Parkinson | Associated with other motor symptoms including tremors, bradykinesia, impaired posture and balance |
| | ALS | Slurred speech, limb weakness, clumbsiness, tripping/falling. |
| | Neoplasms or cancer | May be associated with hemoptysis, dysphagia, weight loss. History of heavy smoke or alcohol use. Possible stridor and airway obstruction |
| Cough | See **Respiratory Exam** | |
| Sore throat | See **Infectious Diseases** | Often caused by upper respiratory tract infections. May have concurrent cough, rhinorrhea. |

HEAD, NECK & THROAT

## 3.3 Focused Histories
- See **General History and Physical Exam** for a detailed approach to history taking
- **OPQRSTUVW** questions regarding each complaint
- For all oral cavity and pharynx complaints, ask about
    - Hemoptysis
    - Constitutional symptoms
    - Lifestyle habits (smoking, alcohol)

## Complaint-specific questions

## Dysphagia[21]
- HPI
    - Onset, duration, severity of dysphagia
    - Problem initiating swallowing (oropharyngeal cause) or does food "stick" after swallow (esophageal cause)
    - Progressive or sudden
    - Affects solid food only? Or both solid and liquid?
    - Is it associated with coughing, choking or regurgitation?
    - Signs of infection such as cough, fever, rhinorrhea
    - Constitutional symptoms such as weight loss
    - Association with hoarseness

- PMH
  - History of stroke Parkinson's disease, or neuromuscular disorders.
- Medications:
  - Ask about medications that may cause mucosal injury
    - Antibiotics, NSAIDS
  - ACE inhibitors and antihistamines can cause xerostomia

## Oral ulcers[22,24]

- HPI:
  - Onset: Acute (more suggestive of trauma, infection) or progressive (malignancy)?
  - Duration: most benign lesions resolve in 2 weeks. Lesions lasting longer should be biopsied
  - Recurrence
  - Prodrome of tingling, numbness, burning – suggests Herpes simplex infection
  - Extra-oral symptoms: arthritis, GI symptoms, rash, kidney involvement – suggest systemic disease
- PMH:
  - Autoimmune disorders (Systemic lupus erythematosus, Crohn's, etc)
  - Diabetes, HIV or other immune compromised state

## Hoarseness[23]

- HPI
  - Onset, duration, and timing
  - Specific change in the quality of voice. Descriptors include: breathy, strangled, husky, muffled, honking, raspy, harsh, soft, strained.
  - Potential triggering factors
  - History of excessive voice use
  - Is it worse in the morning or worsens during the day?
  - Trouble or effort with phonation?
  - Constitutional symptoms
- PMH
  - Stroke
  - Neuromuscular disorders (e.g. Parkinson's, myasthenia gravis, multiple sclerosis)
  - History of neck surgery or irradiation
- Social history:
  - Ask about pattern of voice use or occupation (e.g. professional singer)
  - Tobacco and alcohol use

## 3.4 Focused Physical Exam

- Routine examination of the oral cavity is important as 30% of patients with oral carcinoma are asymptomatic

## Inspection (see Table 10)

- Adequate lighting is required
- Ask patient to remove dentures if present
- If discharge present, note volume, color, odor, consistency, and presence of blood
- For common signs of the mouth: see Table 11

**Table 8.** Inspection of Oral Cavity and Pharynx

| Anatomic Region | Inspection | Features to Assess |
| --- | --- | --- |
| **Oral Cavity** (lips, tongue, inside cheek, teeth, floor of mouth, gingivae, palate) | · Inspect entire oral cavity visually using two tongue depressors | · General (lesions, lumps, ulcers, purulence, blood, gum disease, xerostomia [dry mouth])<br>· Lips (color, pigmentation, symmetry, lesions, edema, ulcers, sores, lumps, fissures)<br>· Tongue (lesions, size, lumps, atrophy, fasciculations, symmetry)<br>· Teeth (number, size, wasting, pitting)<br>· Palate (perforation, edema, petechiae)<br>· Buccal mucosa (white lesions, leukoplakia) |
| **Palatine Tonsils** (between anterior and posterior pillars) | · Inspect visually using tongue depressor | · Enlargement, injection, exudate, ulcerations, crypts |
| **Salivary Apparatus** (parotid gland, submandibular gland) | · Direct: bimanual with two tongue depressors | · Gland enlargement<br>· Lumps, masses, lesions<br>· Painful or painless mass<br>· Discharge, salivary production<br>· Salivary stones<br>· Ranula |
| **Posterior Nasopharynx** (posterior nasal choanae, posterior nasopharyngeal wall, Eustachian tube orifices) | · Indirect laryngoscopy and tongue depressor<br>· Flexible nasopharyngoscopy | · Nasal polyps<br>· Lesions<br>· Ulceration<br>· Inflammation, edema<br>· Purulence, blood |
| **Hypopharynx/ Larynx** (posterior tongue, epiglottis, piriform fossa, vocal cords, false cords, posterior and lateral pharyngeal walls) | · Indirect laryngoscopy and tongue depressor<br>· Flexible nasopharyngoscopy | · Lesions, nodules<br>· Inflammation<br>· Ulceration<br>· Leukoplakia |

**HEAD, NECK & THROAT**

## Palpation

- With a gloved hand, palpate inside the mouth using one finger and use the opposite hand to follow alongside on the surface of the face
- Examine for texture, tenderness, masses, and lesions including plaques, vesicles, nodules, and ulcerations
- Follow a systematic approach: palpate the vermilion of lips, the inner mucosa of lips, mandible, cheeks, roof of mouth, floor of mouth, top of tongue, floor of mandible as far as the angle of the jaw, tonsils (ask patient not to bite)
- Salivary Apparatus
  - Parotid and submandibular glands (enlargement, masses, tenderness, salivary stones)
  - Examine the orifice of each gland:
    - Stenson's duct (parotid duct orifice) opposite upper second molar on buccal mucosa
    - Wharton's duct (submandibular duct orifice) lateral to frenulum of tongue on floor of mouth
  - Massage the gland and observe the discharge from each orifice:
    - Clear vs. cloudy
    - Pain on palpation of the gland

**Clinical Pearl: Parotid Gland Tumor**
Tumors of the parotid gland are the most common type of salivary gland tumor, which typically presents as a firm, nontender mass anterior to the ear with normal overlying skin.

**Motor Exam** (see The **Nervous Systems** chapter)
- Gag reflex (CN IX/X)
- Equal palatal elevation (CN X)
- Central tongue protrusion (CN XII)

**Table 9.** Common Signs of the Mouth

| Signs and Symptoms | Possible Causes |
|---|---|
| **Torus** | Benign congenital lesion |
| **Herpetic Lesions** | Fever, pneumonia, immunocompromised state |
| **Aphthous Ulcers (oral lesion)** | Associated with celiac disease or IBD |
| **Gum Hypertrophy** | Leukemia |
| **Leukoplakia** | Neoplasms, HIV |
| **Angular Stomatitis** | Vitamin B12 or folate deficiency |
| **Tongue Telangiectasias** | GI bleeding |
| **Peutz-Jeghers Spots (brown spots on lips and oral mucosa)** | Peutz-Jeghers syndrome, associated with intestinal polyps and GI bleeding |
| **Glossitis** | Vitamin B12 deficiency |

**Common Investigations**

**Table 10.** Investigations for Mouth and Throat Pathology

| Indication | Test |
|---|---|
| **Infection** | CBC and differential |
| **Sore Throat** with fever >38°C Swollen, red tonsils with exudate Peritonsillar abscess | Throat swab and culture (sensitivity for GAS 90-95%)[14] |
| **Suspected Neoplasm** (neck mass, salivary gland, thyroid) **Note:** diagnosis of follicular adenoma (thyroid) not possible with FNAB | FNAB |
| **Salivary Stone** >90% submandibular calculi are radiopaque >90% parotid calculi are radiolucent | Plain film X-ray, U/S, CT |
| **Neoplasm** (Hx smoking, smokeless tobacco, alcohol), salivary stone, abscess, branchial cleft cyst/sinus | CT/MRI Bone scan if mandible involved |

- McIsaac Modification of the Centor Strep Score (see **Infectious Disease**)

# 4. NECK & THYROID

## 4.1 Essential Anatomy

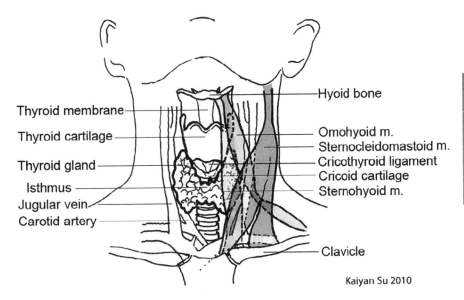

Thyroid membrane
Thyroid cartilage
Thyroid gland
Isthmus
Jugular vein
Carotid artery

Hyoid bone
Omohyoid m.
Sternocleidomastoid m.
Cricothyroid ligament
Cricoid cartilage
Sternohyoid m.

Clavicle

Kaiyan Su 2010

**Figure 6.** Anatomy of the Neck

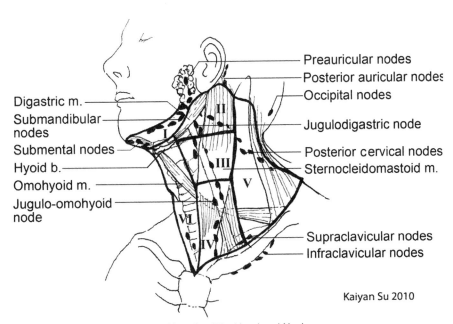

Digastric m.
Submandibular nodes
Submental nodes
Hyoid b.
Omohyoid m.
Jugulo-omohyoid node

Preauricular nodes
Posterior auricular nodes
Occipital nodes
Jugulodigastric node
Posterior cervical nodes
Sternocleidomastoid m.
Supraclavicular nodes
Infraclavicular nodes

Kaiyan Su 2010

**Figure 7.** Lymph Node Groups and Levels of the Head and Neck

**Table 11.** Lymph Node Groups and Levels of the Head and Neck (see **Figure 7**)

| Nodal Group/Level | Location | Drainage |
|---|---|---|
| Occipital | Base of skull, posterior | Posterior scalp |
| Posterior Auricular | Superficial to mastoid process | Scalp, temporal region, external auditory meatus, posterior pinna |
| Preauricular | Anterior Ear | External auditory meatus, anterior pinna, soft tissues of frontal and temporal regions, roof of nose, eyelids, palpebral conjunctiva |
| Submental (Level IA) | (Midline) Anterior bellies of digastric muscles, tip of mandible, and hyoid bone | Floor of mouth, anterior oral tongue, anterior mandibular alveolar ridge, lower lip |
| Submandibular (Level IB) | Anterior belly of digastric muscle, stylohyoid muscle, body of mandible | Oral cavity, anterior nasal cavity, soft tissues of the mid-face, submandibular gland |
| Upper Jugular (Levels IIA and IIB) | Skull base to inferior border of hyoid bone along sternocleidomastoid (SCM) muscle | Oral cavity, nasal cavity, naso/oro/hypopharynx, larynx, parotid glands |
| Middle Jugular (Level III) | Inferior border of hyoid bone to inferior border of cricoid cartilage along SCM muscle | Oral cavity, naso/oro/hypopharynx, larynx |
| Lower Jugular (Level IV) | Inferior border of cricoid cartilage to clavicle along SCM muscle | Hypopharynx, thyroid, cervical esophagus, larynx |
| Posterior Triangle* (Levels VA and VB) | Posterior border of SCM, anterior border of trapezius, from skull base to clavicle | Nasopharynx and oropharynx, cutaneous structures of the posterior scalp and neck |
| Anterior Compartment† (Levels VI) | (Midline) Hyoid bone to suprasternal notch between the common carotid arteries | Thyroid gland, glottic and subglottic larynx, apex of piriform sinus, cervical esophagus |

*Includes some supraclavicular nodes.
†Contains Virchow, pretracheal, precricoid paratracheal and perithyroidal nodes.

## 4.2 Common Chief Complaints and Differentials[25,26]

- Neck stiffness (nuchal rigidity)
- Neck mass
- Neck swelling
- Neck pain

**Table 12.** Lymph Node Groups and Levels of the Head and Neck (see **Figure 7**)

| Chief Complaint | Differential Diagnoses | Distinguishing Features |
|---|---|---|
| Neck mass/neck swelling | **Inflammatory/Infections:**<br>• Reactive adenopathy (abscess, tonsillitis, viral URTI, mononucleosis, HIV, Kawasaki's)<br>• Granulomatous disease (TB, sarcoidosis, syphilis, toxoplasmosis, cat scratch disease) | Fever, recent history of viral infection<br>Discrete, mobile, firm/rubbery, slightly tender, erythematous, asymmetric mass |
| | **Benign Neoplastic:**<br>• Salivary gland neoplasm (pleomorphic adenoma, Warthin's tumor)<br>• Vascular lesions (carotid body tumor, aneurysm)<br>• Hemangioma<br>• Lipoma<br>• Fibroma<br>• Nerve or nerve sheath tumor | Carotid body tumour/vagal schwannoma:<br>Firm, lateral neck mass which moves side-to-side (not up-down)<br><br>Vascular lesion: pulsatile, bruit |
| | **Malignant Neoplastic:**<br>• Primary: Hodgkin's or non-Hodgkin's lymphoma, salivary gland neoplasm (parotid, submandibular), thyroid, sarcoma<br>• Metastatic: head and neck (usually squamous cell carcinoma), thoracic, abdominal, leukemia | Rock-hard, fixed, nontender mass<br>Thyroid source: Immobile, midline, elevates with swallowing |
| | **Congenital:**<br>• Branchial cleft cyst<br>• Laryngocele<br>• Lymphatic malformation<br>• Thyroglossal duct cyst | Salivary gland, thyroid, thyroglossal, ranula:<br>midline mass in anterior neck |
| Neck pain | **Spinal causes:** | |
| | Degenerative disc disease | Radiologic diagnosis; axial pain; symptoms exacerbated by over-use |
| | Trauma | Whiplash injury |
| | Auto-immune disease (rheumatologic): Polymyalgia rheumatic Giant cell arteritis | Associated with headache, shoulder/hip girdle pain, visual symptoms |
| | Cervical myelopathy | Arm clumsiness, gait difficulty, bowel/bladder dysfunction |
| | Non-spinal causes: Infection/Tumour | Fever, chills, weight loss, IV drug use |
| | Thoracic outlet syndrome | Numbness, weakness, sensation of swelling in upper limbs |
| | Diabetic neuropathy | Neck, thoracic, scapular, extremity pain and weakness |

### 4.3 Focused Histories[25,26]

- See **General History and Physical Exam** for a detailed approach to history taking
- **Follow OPQRSTUVW** questions regarding each complaint

**Other features to investigate on history:**
- Headache
- Fever (if present, assess for meningitis - see The **Infectious Disease** chapter)
- Cardiovascular history (referred pain from angina or myocardial infarction)
- Focal neurological deficits (if present, suspect cerebrovascular accident (CVA))
- Travel history
- Neck masses:
  - Location: lateral vs. midline
  - Age of patient
  - Young (age <40 yr): congenital or inflammatory, neoplasms rare o Adult: neck mass malignant until proven otherwise15
  - Onset, tenderness, and rate of growth
  - A tender mass with rapid onset of swelling is suggestive of an inflammatory, acute infectious etiology or metastasis
  - A non-tender, slow-growing mass is suggestive of a malignancy
  - Constitutional symptoms (fever, chills, night sweats, weight loss)
  - Risk factors for cancer (e.g. tobacco use, alcohol, radiation)
  - Presence of recurrent head and neck infection (e.g. HPV, Epstein-Barr virus [EBV])
  - Cough, hemoptysis, bone pain
  - Dysphagia, odynophagia, hoarseness, dyspnea
  - Tooth abscess
  - For thyroid disorders - see the **Endocrine System** chapter

### 4.4 Focused Physical Examination
### General Head and Neck

*Inspection*
- Position of head, symmetry
- Hair quantity, quality, distribution
- Skin texture, color, moisture, scars
- Skin lesions (location, arrangement, color, size, type)
- Signs of muscle weakness/paralysis of CN VII, X, XII (e.g. facial drooping, flattened nasolabial fold)
- Neck masses (size, location, symmetry)
- Enlarged parotid or submandibular glands
- Trachea (should be in midline)

*Palpation*
- See **Lymphatic System and Lymph Node Exam**
- Have the patient sit with head slightly flexed forward and neck relaxed
- Use a consistent order when palpating lymph nodes (e.g. start with occipital nodes, move to posterior auricular and preauricular nodes and then palpate the levels of the neck in order)
- Use bimanual approach to examine Level I (submandibular and submental nodes) with one gloved finger in the floor of the mouth and fingers of other hand following along skin externally
- Note tenderness, size, consistency, mobility, level
- Palpate salivary glands

---

**Clinical Pearl: Supraclavicular Lymph Nodes[16]**
Left-sided enlargement of a supraclavicular node (Virchow's node) may indicate an abdominal malignancy; right-sided enlargement may
indicate malignancy of lungs, mediastinum or esophagus. Enlargement of occipital nodes may be a sign of rubella.

---

## Thyroid

*Inspection*
- Identify the thyroid and cricoid cartilages and the trachea (note any tracheal deviation)
- Visible thyroid is suspicious for enlargement (goiter)
- Look for systemic signs of thyroid disease (see **Essentials of Endocrinology**)

*Palpation*
- Patient's neck should be slightly flexed
- Anterior approach: position yourself in front and to the side of the patient
- Posterior approach: position yourself behind the patient's chair
- Examine one side at a time:
    - Relax the right sternocleidomastoid by turning patient's head slightly to right
- Landmark using thyroid and cricoid cartilages
- Displace trachea to right while palpating right side
    - Ask patient to swallow some water and feel for glandular tissue on right side rising under fingers
    - Repeat for left side
- The thyroid isthmus is often palpable
- Describe gland:
    - Shape/size: normal ~ size of an adult distal phalanx of thumb
    - Consistency:
        - Rubbery (normal)
        - Hard (associated with cancer or scarring)
        - Soft (associated with toxic goiter)
    - Nodules: size, consistency, number, tenderness (suggests thyroiditis)
- Pemberton's sign: a large goiter extending retrosternally may block the thoracic inlet and compress jugular veins, causing facial plethora when both arms are raised

*Auscultation*
- Auscultate over the lateral lobes to detect any bruits
- A localized systolic or continuous bruit may be heard in thyrotoxicosis (e.g. Graves' disease)

---

**Clinical Pearl: Thyroglossal Duct Cysts**
A thyroglossal duct cyst will elevate with tongue protrusion while a thyroid nodule will not.

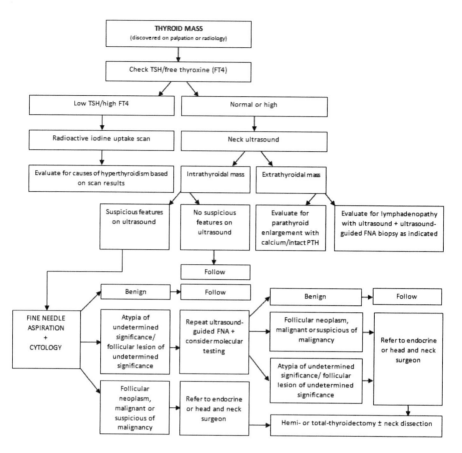

**Figure 8.** Investigations for thyroid mass. Reproduced with permisson from *Stack, BC. Assessment of Thyroid Mass. BMJ Best Practice. Jan 2017. http://bestpractice.bmj.com/best-practice/monograph/1200.html*

# 5. COMMON CLINICAL SCENARIOS

**Table 13.** Common clinical scenarios

| KEY SYMPTOMS / HISTORY | PHYSICAL EXAM | INVESTIGATIONS | MANAGEMENT |
|---|---|---|---|
| **Vertigo (Benign Positional Paroxysmal Vertigo – BPPV)[4,27,28]** | | | |
| Sensation that either the individual or surroundings are spinning<br><br>Acute onset vertigo that lasts several seconds<br><br>Precipitated by predictable head movements<br><br>Nausea, vomiting (occasionally) | Positive Dix Hallpike: Latency ~20; crescendo/decrescendo vertigo lasting 20; geotropic rotary nystagmus; reversal of nystagmus upon sitting up<br><br>Normal otoscopy<br><br>Normal cranial nerve & cerebellar exam | Brain MRI<br><br>Electronystagmography (ENG)<br><br>Videpnystagmography (VNG)<br><br>Audiometry<br><br>Brainstem evoked potentials | Particle repositioning maneuver (Epley, Semont)<br><br>Medications (betahistine may provide some relief)<br><br>Surgical options for refractory BPPV |
| **Hoarseness of Voice (Dysphonia) [21,23]** | | | |
| Abnormality of voice affecting: pitch, volume, resonance, quality<br><br>Often associated with viral URTI<br><br>Increased risk with smoking, alcohol use, radiation history to head & neck area, GERD | Palpate head and neck lymph nodes<br><br>Assess for laryngeal crepitus: normally felt when larynx is gently displaced laterally; absence of crepitus indicates mass in retropharyngeal space or hypopharynx<br><br>Examination of oral and nasal cavities for polyps or abnormal masses | Indirect laryngoscopy +/- flexible nasolaryngoscopy to rule out vocal cord nodules, laryngeal cancer<br><br>Chest X-Ray<br><br>CT +/- contrast<br><br>Endocrine testing& Inflammatory markers (TSH, ESR, CRP, RF)<br><br>If mass detected → biopsy | Voice Rest<br>Voice Therapy<br>Pharmacotherapy (limited use)<br><br>Surgery (open neck, microlaryngoscopy, injections, laser treatments) |

HEAD, NECK & THROAT

| KEY SYMPTOMS / HISTORY | PHYSICAL EXAM | INVESTIGATIONS | MANAGEMENT |
|---|---|---|---|
| **Epistaxis[29]** | | | |
| Bleeding from the nose | Vitals and volume status | Minor bleed: no investigations necessary | Lean forward, apply pressure to cartilaginous portion of nose for 20min |
| Key features on history: trauma, cocaine use, systemic coagulopathies | Speculum exam with topical anesthetic or decongestants to locate bleed | If recurrent and/or heavy: <br> • blood type, cross-match <br> • coagulation panel <br> • nasopharyngoscopy or CT/MRI if malignancy suspected | topical vasoconstrictor |
| | Flexible nasopharyngoscope for posterior bleeds | | silver nitrate cauterization (do NOT cauterize both sides of septum) |
| | | | Anterior packing with vasaline gauze or nasal tampons (Merocel) |
| | | | Posterior packing with foley with Foley cathether, gauze, Epistat balloon |
| | | | embolization by interventional radiology |
| **Acute Otitis Media** (See **Fig 8**) | | | |
| Acute onset otalgia, fever, hearing loss | Temperature <br> Otoscopic exam <br> – look for bulging, erythematous tympanic membrane | None | Observe if symptoms non-severe, onset <48-72h, >2yo <br> Otherwise, treat with antibiotics (amoxicillin) |
| **Otitis Media with Effusion[30,31]** | | | |
| Fluid in the middle ear without signs of acute infection. <br><br> History of upper respiratory infections or ear infections <br><br> Conductive hearing loss | Pneumatic otoscopy is primary diagnostic method – visualizing fluid behind tympanic membrane, and decreased tympanic membrane mobility | Tympanometry <br><br> Hearing test | May be safely observed for 3 months, unless child is a risk of speech development problems from hearing loss. Myringotomy and tympanostomy tube insertion may be considered after 3 months |

### Acute Sinusitis[19] (see **Figure 4**)

| KEY SYMPTOMS / HISTORY | PHYSICAL EXAM | INVESTIGATIONS | MANAGEMENT |
| --- | --- | --- | --- |
| PODS<br>• Facial Pain<br>• Nasal Obstruction<br>• Nasal purulent Discharge<br>• Decreased Smell<br><br>Symptoms lasting <4 weeks | Perform full head and neck exam<br><br>Nose exam with speculum or nasopharyngoscope<br><br>Examine for Red Flags: swelling of orbit, change in visual acuity, headaches, or altered mental status | None<br><br>CT sinuses for recurrent disease or suspected complications of acute sinusitis | Nasal steroids<br>Antibiotics (first line: amoxicillin) if severe or if no response to steroids |

### Chronic Sinusitis[19] (see **Figure 5**)

| KEY SYMPTOMS / HISTORY | PHYSICAL EXAM | INVESTIGATIONS | MANAGEMENT |
| --- | --- | --- | --- |
| CPODS<br>• Facial Congestion<br>• Facial Pain<br>• Nasal Obstruction<br>• Purulent Discharge<br>• Decreased Smell<br><br>Symptoms lasting 8-12 weeks | Perform full head and neck exam<br><br>Nose exam with speculum or nasopharyngoscope<br><br>Examine for Red Flags: swelling of orbit, change in visual acuity, headaches, or altered mental status | CT and nasopharyngoscopy | Saline Rinse<br>Intranasal steroids<br><br>Short course oral steroids (patients with polyps<br><br>Antibiotics (consider 2nd line and broad coverage e.g. fluoroquinolones or amoxicillin-clavulanic acid) |

**HEAD, NECK & THROAT**

**Clinical Pearl: Epistaxis**

Severe, unilateral epistaxis with no history of trauma in an adolescent male is juvenile nasopharyngeal angiofibroma until proven otherwise.

Recurrent epistaxis in older males of south-eastern Asian or southern Chinese descent is nasopharyngeal carcinoma until proven otherwise.

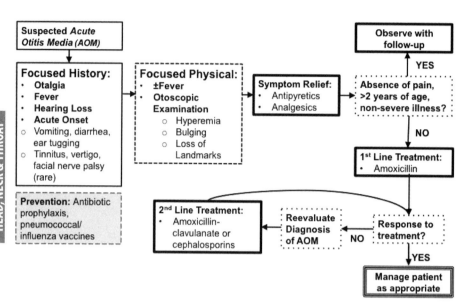

**Figure 9.** Clinical Evaluation and Management of Acute Otitis Media
American Academy of Pediatrics. 2004. Pediatrics 11 3(5):1451-1465.
Leach AJ, Morris PS. Cochrane Database of Systematic Reviews 2006, Issue 4. Art. No.:
CD004401.

# REFERENCES

1. Ely JW, Hansen MR, Clark EC. Diagnosis of ear pain. Am Fam Physician. 2008;77(5):621-628.
2. Hansen P, Mann K, Hauch S, et al. Objectives for the Qualifying Examination. Medical Council of Canada. http://apps.mcc.ca/Objectives_Online/objectives.pl?lang=english&loc=contents.
3. Isaacson JE, Vora NM. Differential diagnosis and treatment of hearing loss. Am Fam Physician. 2003;68(6):1125-1132.
4. Post RE, Dickerson LM. Dizziness: a diagnostic approach. Am Fam Physician. 2010;82(4):361-368, 369.
5. Harvey H. Diagnosing referred otalgia: the ten Ts. Cranio. 1992;10(4):333-334.
6. Roland P, Stewart MG, Hannley M, et al. Consensus panel on role of potentially ototoxic antibiotics for topical middle ear use: Introduction, methodology, and recommendations. Otolaryngol - Head Neck Surg. 2004;130(3):S51-S56. doi:10.1016/j.otohns.2003.12.010.
7. Curhan SG, Eavey R, Shargorodsky J, Curhan GC. Analgesic use and the risk of hearing loss in men. Am J Med. 2010;123(3):231-237. doi:10.1016/j.amjmed.2009.08.006.
8. Bisht M, Bist SS. Ototoxicity: the hidden menace. Indian J Otolaryngol Head Neck Surg. 2011;63(3):255-259. doi:10.1007/s12070-011-0151-8.
9. Prasher D. Heavy metals and noise exposure: health effects. Noise Health. 2009;11(44):141-144. doi:10.4103/1463-1741.53358.
10. Lee CA, Mistry D, Uppal S, Coatesworth AP. Otologic side effects of drugs. J Laryngol Otol. 2005;119(4):267-271. doi:10.1258/0022215054020485.
11. McGwin G. Phosphodiesterase type 5 inhibitor use and hearing impairment. Arch Otolaryngol Head Neck Surg. 2010;136(5):488-492. doi:10.1001/archoto.2010.51.
12. Tucci DL. Otorrhea - Ear, Nose, and Throat Disorders. Merck Manual Professional Version. https://www.merckmanuals.com/en-ca/professional/ear,-nose,-and-throat-disorders/approach-to-the-patient-with-ear-problems/otorrhea. Published 2016. Accessed November 20, 2016.
13. Crummer RW, Hassan GA. Diagnostic approach to tinnitus. Am Fam Physician. 2004;69(1):120-126.
14. Bickley LS, Szilagyi PG, Bates B. Bates' Guide to Physical Examination and History Taking. Wolters Kluwer Health/Lippincott Williams & Wilkins; 2009.
15. Pirozzo S, Papinczak T, Glasziou P. Whispered voice test for screening for hearing impairment in adults and children: systematic review. BMJ. 2003;327(7421):967. doi:10.1136/bmj.327.7421.967.
16. Meyer C, Witte J, Hildmann A, et al. Neonatal screening for hearing disorders in infants at risk: incidence, risk factors, and follow-up. Pediatrics. 1999;104(4 Pt 1):900-904.
17. Meltzer E, Hamilos D, Hadley J, et al. Rhinosinusitis: Establishing definitions for clinical research and patient care. Otolaryngol - Head Neck Surg. 2004;131(6):S1-S62. doi:10.1016/j.otohns.2004.09.067.
18. Rosenfeld RM, Piccirillo JF, Chandrasekhar SS, et al. Clinical Practice Guideline (Update): Adult Sinusitis. Otolaryngol -- Head Neck Surg. 2015;152(2 Suppl):S1-S39. doi:10.1177/0194599815572097.
19. Desrosiers M, Evans GA, Keith PK, et al. Canadian clinical practice guidelines for acute and chronic rhinosinusitis. Allergy, Asthma Clin Immunol. 2011;7(1):2. doi:10.1186/1710-1492-7-2.
20. Galioto NJ. Peritonsillar abscess. Am Fam Physician. 2008;77(2):199-202.
21. Spieker MR. Evaluating dysphagia. Am Fam Physician. 2000;61(12):3639-3648.
22. Goldstein BG, Goldstein AO. Oral lesions. In: Dellaballe RP, Deschler DG, Corona R, eds. UpToDate. Waltham, MA: Wolters Kluwer; 2015.
23. Feierabend RH, Shahram MN. Hoarseness in adults. Am Fam Physician. 2009;80(4):363-370.
24. Huber MA. Assessment of oral ulceration. BMJ Best Practice. http://bestpractice.bmj.com/best-practice/monograph/1119/diagnosis/step-by-step.html. Published 2016. Accessed November 20, 2016.
25. Alvi A, Johnson JT. The neck mass. A challenging differential diagnosis. Postgrad Med. 1995;97(5):87-90, 93-94, 97.
26. Weymuller EA. Evaluation of neck masses. J Fam Pract. 1980;11(7):1099-1106.
27. Furman JM, Cass SP. Benign paroxysmal positional vertigo. N Engl J Med. 1999;341(21):1590-1596. doi:10.1056/NEJM199911183412107.
28. Kim J-S, Zee DS, Zee DS. Clinical practice. Benign paroxysmal positional vertigo. N Engl J Med. 2014;370(12):1138-1147. doi:10.1056/NEJMcp1309481.
29. Melia L, McGarry GW. Epistaxis: update on management. Curr Opin Otolaryngol Head Neck Surg. 2011;19(1):30-35. doi:10.1097/MOO.0b013e328341e1e9.
30. Rosenfeld RM, Shin JJ, Schwartz SR, et al. Clinical Practice Guideline: Otitis Media with Effusion (Update). Otolaryngol Head Neck Surg. 2016;154(1 Suppl):S1-S41. doi:10.1177/0194599815623467.
31. Rosenfeld RM, Schwartz SR, Pynnonen MA, et al. Clinical practice guideline: Tympanostomy tubes in children. Otolaryngol Head Neck Surg. 2013;149(1 Suppl):S1-S35. doi:10.1177/0194599813487302.
32. Sensitivity, specificity and predictive value of tympanometry in predicting a hearing impairment in otitis media with effusion. MRC Multi-Centre Otitis Media Study Group. Clin Otolaryngol Allied Sci. 1999;24(4):294-300.

HEAD, NECK & THROAT

CHAPTER 6:

# The Lymphatic System

**Editors:**
Ahmed Zaki, BSc
Joel Gupta

**Resident Reviewer:**
Shohinee Sarma, MPH, MD

**Faculty Reviewers:**
Yoo-Joung Ko, MMSc, SM, MD, FRCPC
Sudhashree Rajagopal, MD, FRCPC

## TABLE OF CONTENTS

# 1. ANATOMY

**Figure 1.** Overview of Lymphatic System

**Figure 2.** Inguinal and Popliteal nodes

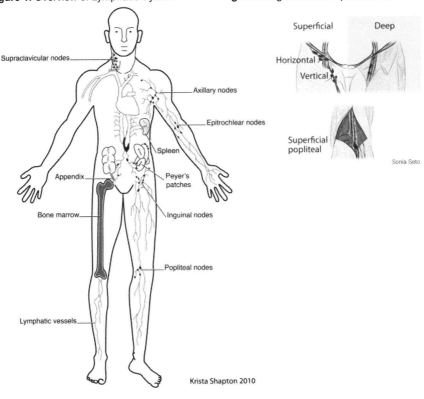

Krista Shapton 2010

**LYMPHATIC**

**Table 1.** Functional Overview of Lymph Tissues

| Lymphoid Tissue | Function | Site |
|---|---|---|
| **Lymph Nodes** | Lymphatic drainage | Located throughout body (see **Table 2**) |
| **Tonsils – lingual, palatine, tubal, adenoids (Waldeyer's)** | Protects respiratory passages | Tongue base, pharyngeal and nasopharyngeal walls |
| **Spleen** | RBC and platelet storage, defective RBC disposal, antibody formation by intrinsic B-lymphocytes | Left upper quadrant of abdomen |
| **Peyer's Patch** | IgA antibody formation by intrinsic B-lymphocytes | Ileal walls |
| **Appendix** | IgA immune response to ingested antigens | Lower cecal outpouching |

**Table 2.** Overview of Lymph Node Drainage[1]

| Lymph Node Groups | Location | Drainage |
|---|---|---|
| **Head and Neck Nodes** | | |
| **Supraclavicular** | Superior to clavicle | H&N and axillary nodes |
| **Infraclavicular** | Inferior to clavicle | H&N and axillary nodes |
| **Scalene** | Posterior to clavicle | H&N and axillary nodes |
| **Upper Extremities: Axillary** | | |
| **Apical Group** | Apex of axilla | All other axillary nodes |
| **Central Group** | High axilla; deep to pectoralis minor (often palpable) | Pectoral, lateral, and subscapular nodes |
| **Pectoral (Anterior) Group** | Inside anterior axillary fold, along lower border of pectoralis major | Anterior chest wall and breast |
| **Subscapular (Posterior) Group** | Deep posterior axillary fold, along lateral border of scapula | Anterior chest wall and breast |
| **Lateral Group** | Upper humerus | Most of arm |
| **Epitrochlear or Cubital** | Above medial epicondyle | Ulnar aspect hand and forearm |
| **Lower Extremities: Inguinal and Popliteal Nodes (see Figure 2)** | | |
| **Superficial Vertical Group** | Upper leg along proximal portion of great saphenous vein | Superficial tissue of upper leg |
| **Superficial Horizontal Group** | Just below inguinal ligament | Skin of lower abdominal wall, external genitalia (except testes), anal canal, lower third of vagina, gluteal region |
| **Superficial Popliteal** | Popliteal fossa (one) node | Heel and lateral aspect of foot |
| **Deep Inguinal femoral vein** | Deep medial aspect of | Popliteal and superficial inguinal regions |

LYMPHATIC

## 2. COMMON CHIEF COMPLAINTS[2]

**Table 3.** Chief complaints, differential diagoses, and clinical features of lymphadenopathy

| CC | Differential Diagnosis | Distinguishing Features |
|---|---|---|
| **Enlarged painless lymph node(s) e.g. "painLESS lumps & bumps"** | Malignancy | Lymph nodes that rapidly increase in size, are fixed, matted, persistent, confluent, >2 cm, supraclavicular, or are painless |
| | | Rapidly expanding lymph nodes can distend the capsule causing discomfort |
| | Lymphoma | Firm, rubbery, nontender |
| | Metastasis from carcinoma | Hard (often asymmetrical with unremarkable contralateral node), size >2 cm, nontender, fixed |
| **Enlarged painful lymph node(s) e.g. "painFUL lump or bump"** | Inflammation or infectious (CMV/EBV/TB) <br><br> *See **Infectious Disease** | Lymph nodes <2 cm in size, regularly bordered, tender to touch, soft or shotty, and mobile are likely inflammatory/infectious |
| | | CMV/EBV may present with mononucleosis type symptoms/serology |
| | | TB may present with respiratory manifestation |
| **Swollen extremity e.g. edema of arm, leg, ankle; +/- localized pain/ tenderness** | **Lymphatic Lymphedema:** | **Non-pitting Edema** |
| | 1. Resection of regional lymph nodes, chronic lymphangitis | Previous Hx of surgery/lymph node resection <br><br> Recurrent bacterial infections |
| | 2. Infectious e.g. filariasis | Travel to certain places in central Africa/ South Asia may suggest elephantiasis (edema with thickening of the skin and underlying tissues) <br><br> Associated with rash, arthritis and macules |
| | **Vascular:** <br><br> DVT, CHF, thrombophlebitis | **Pitting edema** <br> **RF:** <br> Smoking, blood clotting disorders, extended periods of immobility, medications (OCP/HRT) |
| | **Non-Vascular:** <br> Thyroid disease, cirrhosis, nephrotic syndrome | (For associated symptoms see CVS, Endo, GI, and Nephrosections) |

LYMPHATIC

**Clinical Pearl: Normal vs. Malignant Cervical Lymphadenopathy**
Cervical lymph node enlargement is common especially in children; > 90% are caused by benign enlargement secondary to infection/inflammation or physiological enlargement.

**Table 4.** Significance of Lymph Node Character and Location[2-4]

| Location of Enlarged Nodes | Indication |
| --- | --- |
| Occipital | Scalp infection, rubella |
| Cervical | URTI, oral or dental lesion, infectious mononucleosis (posterior) or other viral illness, metastases from H&N, lung, breast, or thyroid (refer to ENT section for locations) |
| Supraclavicular and Scalene (always abnormal) | Metastases:<br>• Virchow's (left supraclavicular): from gastrointestinal system, lungs, breast, testes, ovaries<br>• Right-sided Virchow's: from thoracic regions (mediastinal, lung, esophageal)<br>Non-neoplastic causes: TB, sarcoidosis, toxoplasmosis |
| Axillary | Infection/injury of ipsilateral upper extremity, metastases from breast, melanoma of upper extremity (refer to breast exam section for locations) |
| Epitrochlear | Syphilis, non-Hodgkin's lymphoma |
| Inguinal | Infection/injury of ipsilateral lower extremity, metastases from anal canal/genitalia (penile/scrotal or vulval/lower third of vaginal areas), melanoma of lower extremity, certain STIs (primarily syphilis) (refer to Part 1 – Essentials of Anatomy) |

**Note:** A normal (non-malignant) palpable lymph node is <1 cm in size, soft and nontender, with regular and discrete borders.

**Clinical Pearl: Distinguishing Lymph Nodes from Other Structures**
Cervical lymph node enlargement is common especially in children; > 90% are caused by benign enlargement secondary to infection/inflammation or physiological enlargement.

| Character | Lymph Node | Artery | Cyst | Muscle |
| --- | --- | --- | --- | --- |
| Rolls in 2 directions | ✓ | - | - | - |
| Pulsates | - | ✓ | - | - |
| Transilluminates with direct light | - | - | ✓ | - |

## 3. FOCUSED HISTORY[3]

### History of Present Illness
- Enlarged lymph node: "Do you have any bothersome lumps or bumps?"
    - Character: location, onset, duration, tenderness, number, generalized or localized.
    - Associated symptoms: pain, fever, erythema, warmth, itchiness, red streaks, weight loss, night sweats
    - Risk factors: infection, surgery, trauma
- Swollen extremity: "Do you have any leg or arm swelling?"
    - Character: unilateral/bilateral, intermittent/continuous, duration
    - Associated symptoms: warmth, erythema, discoloration, ulceration
    - Predisposing factors: cardiac and/or renal disorder, malignancy, surgery, infection,

trauma, venous insufficiency
- ◆ Alleviating factors: support stockings, elevation
- Red flags: Constitutional symptoms: fever, night sweats, weight loss, fatigue

### Past Medical History
- Surgeries/injuries (e.g. trauma to regional lymph nodes), medications (e.g. phenytoin, chemoradiation), malignancies, recurrent infections, chronic inflammatory diseases (e.g. SLE, RA), immunosuppression

### Family History
- Malignancies, recurrent infections, TB

### Social History
- Sexual behaviors STIs (e.g. syphilis, chlamydia, HIV), occupational/ travel (e.g. infectious or carcinogenic exposures)

## 4. FOCUSED PHYSICAL EXAM[3-6]

The lymphatic system examination consists primarily of inspection and palpation of lymph nodes. Consider regional drainage patterns and look for signs of local infection or malignancy. Distinguish between regional and generalized lymphadenopathy by assessing lymph nodes elsewhere.

### Screening Exam
- In an otherwise asymptomatic patient, or someone that presents with an unrelated chief complaint – inspect and palpate H&N, axillary and inguinal nodes, liver, and spleen

### Inspection
- Look for visible node enlargement, edema, muscle bulk/symmetry, color changes (e.g. erythema or red streaks) or ulceration

### Palpation
- Palpate lymph nodes in a firm, circular motion over the underlying tissues in each area, using the pads of the index and middle fingers; apply light pressure, then gradually increase the pressure and always evaluate for symmetry.

**Clinical Pearl:**
Excess pressure may displace or obscure nodes into deeper soft tissues before they are recognized. Ensure you palpate deeply enough to feel lymph nodes.

## For comparison, palpate right and left lymph nodes simultaneously and note:

- Location
- Size (<1 cm or >1 cm)
- Shape (regular or irregular borders)
- Delimitation (discrete or matted together)
- Mobility (fixed or mobile/tethered to skin or deeper tissues)
- Consistency (soft, shotty, rubbery, hard, or firm)
- Tenderness (tender or nontender)

**Clinical Pearl:**
A normal lymph node is <1 cm in size, feels soft and nontender, and has regular and discrete borders .

- If edema is noted, check for pitting edema to rule out lymphedema, which does not have the characteristic pitting associated with other causes of edema
- Approach an unexplained enlarged lymph node by examining
  - **PALS**: **P**rimary site, **A**ll associated nodes, **L**iver, **S**pleen

## 4.1 Head and Neck

Develop a systematic approach to palpating lymph nodes in the head and neck to ensure no groups are missed. A suggested practical approach is presented in groups of 3+3+3+1 sets of lymph nodes:

- Above the mandible
  - Pre-auricular: in front of the ears
  - Posterior auricular: behind the ears and superficial to the mastoid process
  - Occipital: posterior base of the skull
- At the mandible
  - Tonsillar: angle of the mandible
  - Submandibular: under the mandible between the angle and anterior tip
  - Submental: anterior tip of mandible
- Below the mandible
  - Superficial cervical: superficial to sternocleidomastoid (SCM)
  - Posterior cervical: in posterior triangle along border of trapezius
  - Deep cervical: deep to SCM; accessible by placing thumb on muscle belly of SCM and hooking fingers around the anterior border
- At the clavicle
  - Supraclavicular and infraclavicular: >1cm is significant
- Note: other structures such as salivary glands (parotid, sublingual, submandibular), arteries (carotid, temporal), or cysts can be present in these areas and may mimic lymph nodes

## 4.2 Upper Extremities

- **Axillary:** to examine the right axilla, support and slightly abduct the patient's flexed right arm with your right hand and palpate 5 regions with your left hand:
  - Anterior: pectoral muscles
  - Posterior: latissimus dorsi and subscapularis
  - Medial: rib cage
  - Lateral: upper arm
  - Apical: axilla
- Do vice-versa for the left axilla
- Epitrochlear: support patient's flexed elbow in one hand and palpate using the other hand in the depression above and posterior to the medial epicondyle of the humerus

## 4.3 Lower Extremities

- Inguinal: ask patient to lie supine with knee slightly flexed, roll fingers above and below inguinal ligament to access only the superficial nodes (small nodes of 0.5 cm are often found; deeper abdominal, pelvic, and para-aortic nodes that drain the testes and internal female genitalia are inaccessible by palpation)
- Popliteal: with both hands hooked around the patient's knee, place thumbs on tibial tuberosity and palpate deeply in popliteal fossa with 3-4 fingers from each hand (one node is occasionally palpable)

# 5. COMMON INVESTIGATIONS[5,7]

Use laboratory tests to confirm suspected diagnoses based on history and physical examination (e.g. infectious or malignant). If clinical evaluations are non-confirmatory, diagnostic work-up should consider if the adenopathy is localized or generalized.

- **Generalized (lymphadenopathy in more than one region):**
  - ◆ CBC, electrolytes, CXR (PA/AP and lateral views), urine routine and microscopy (R&M)/culture and sensitivity (C&S), throat and genital swabs
  - ◆ If normal, consider possible infections:
    - ▪ Tuberculin purified protein derivative test (PPD)
    - ▪ HIV antibody
    - ▪ Rapid plasma reagin (RPR) for syphilis
    - ▪ Antinuclear antibody (ANA) for autoimmune diseases
    - ▪ Heterophile/monospot for infectious mononucleosis due to Epstein-Barr virus
- • If uncertain: excisional biopsy of the most abnormal node (or supraclavicular, neck, axilla or groin in this order if a single node is unattainable) for abnormal cells and architecture, using local anesthesia.

> **Clinical Pearl: Inguinal Lymph Node Biopsies**
> Inguinal lymphadenopathy is relatively nonspecific and should be avoided for biopsy if there is another appropriate node to biopsy, given the frequency of lower extremity trauma and infection.

- **Localized (involving one region of lymph nodes):**
  - ◆ observe for 3-4 wk if history not suggestive of malignancy; if non-resolving adenopathy, consider open biopsy
    - ▪ Fine needle aspiration (FNA) for cytology (especially in HIV+ patients) and flow cytometry
    - ▪ Core needle biopsy for special studies and architecture
- **Imaging:**
  - ◆ CT, U/S, Doppler, or MRI are all modalities to distinguish enlarged lymph nodes from other structures – define pathological processes, stage malignancy and help guide fine needle aspiration

> **Clinical Pearl: Fluctuant Nodes**
> Incision and drainage of a fluctuant node is useful to help relieve pain and reduce infection, but not useful for diagnosis.

# 6. COMMON CLINICAL SCENARIOS[5-8]

**Table 5.** Common clinical scenarios in patients with lymphadenopathy

| Key Symptoms | Physical Exam Findings | Investigations | Management |
|---|---|---|---|
| **Acute Suppurative Lymphadenitis** | | | |
| • Sudden onset of swelling erythema, warmth and tenderness<br>• Abscess formation may also occur | • Assessment of the overall health of the patient and the presence of systemic signs of inflammation<br>• Firm and tender swollen nodes on palpation, possible erythema of overlying skin and tissue<br>• Enlarged lymph nodes may be unilateral or bilateral | • Utility of laboratory investigations depends on clinical assessment<br>• When suppurative lymphadenitis is cervical, percutaneous aspiration can provide diagnostic and therapeutic benefit<br>• Best diagnostic test is a contrast-enhanced computed tomography (CT) scan | • Broad-spectrum antibiotic PO<br>• If severe: Surgical consult, radiologic examination, IV antibiotics |
| **Epstein- Barr Virus Mono-nucleosis** | | | |
| • Prodrome: 2-3 d of malaise, anorexia<br>• Infants and young children: often asymptomatic or mild disease<br>• Older children and adolescents: malaise, fatigue, fever, sore throat, abdominal pain (LUQ), headache, myalgia | • Discrete and sometimes tender nodes with varying firmness on palpation (cervical nodes are especially affected)<br>• Classic triad: febrile, generalized nontender lymphadenopathy, pharyngitis/tonsillitis (exudative)<br>• hepatosplenomegaly<br>• periorbital edema,<br>• rash (urticarial, maculopapular, or petechial)<br>• any "-itis" (including arthritis, hepatitis, nephritis, myocarditis, meningitis, encephalitis, etc) | • Positive heterophilic antibody (monospot) test<br>• EBV titres<br>• CBC and differential, blood smear: atypical lymphocytes, lymphocytosis, Downey cells ± anemia<br>• ± thrombocytopenia | • Supportive: adequate rest, hydration, saline gargles, and analgesics for sore throat (e.g. Acetaminophen or NSAIDs)<br>• Splenic enlargement may not be clinically apparent -> avoid contact sports for all patients for 6-8 wk<br>• Airway obstruction secondary to nodal and/or tonsillar enlargement -> admit for steroid therapy<br>• Acyclovir does NOT reduce duration of symptoms or result in earlier return to school/work |

## HIV Sero Positivity

| Key Symptoms | Physical Exam Findings | Investigations | Management |
|---|---|---|---|
| • Acute infection: flu-like symptoms (fever, pharyngitis, lymphadenopathy, rash, ulcers, weight loss, etc.)<br>• Latent stage: asymptomatic<br>• AIDS: Severe fatigue, malaise, fever, weight loss, weakness, arthralgias, and persistent diarrhea. Mucocutaneous lesions, recurrent infections, tuberculosis, oral thrush, lymphoma | • Generally tender, discrete and freely mobile nodes on palpation; presence of small, ill-defined nodes may indicate disease progression, and/or treatment failure<br>• Persistent generalized lymphadenopathy for >3 mo and involving 2 or more extra-inguinal sites (may be first sign of initial infection and is part of the asymptomatic phase) | • CD4 count<br>• Anti-HIV antibodies<br>• ELISA for serum antibody to HIV<br>• Rapid point of care antibody tests (if positive, must do confirmatory test)<br>• Confirmatory test: western blot to confirm antibody detection | • Verify positive test<br>• Complete Hx and exam every 3-6 months<br>• Patient education<br>• Anti-retroviral treatment<br>• Health Maintenance (vaccines, screening e.g. pap smears, managing co-morbid conditions) |

## Hodgkin's lymphoma

| Key Symptoms | Physical Exam Findings | Investigations | Management |
|---|---|---|---|
| • Asymptomatic lymphadenopathy (70%): painless, nontender, firm, rubbery, enlargement of superficial lymph nodes, especially in cervical region<br>• B symptoms (can include fever, night sweats and pruritus) | • Complete Lymph node exam<br>• Abdominal exam looking for hepatosplenomegaly | • CBC, biochemistry (HIV serology to r/o infection, LFTs to check liver involvement<br>• CXR, CT for further lymph node involvement or mediastinal mass.<br>• Lymph node biopsy<br>• Bone marrow biopsy if indicated | • Chemotherapy and XRT<br>• For relapse, consider bone marrow transplant<br>• PET scans to follow Tx response (see oncology section for regimes) |

## Non-Hodgkin's lymphoma (most common)

| Key Symptoms | Physical Exam Findings | Investigations | Management |
|---|---|---|---|
| • Variable manifestations depending on location, tumor growth rate, affected organ<br>• Most patients present with painless slow growing peripheral lymphadenopathy that may spontaneously regress<br>• Constitutional symptoms e.g. fever, night sweats, weight loss, are not common (unlike in hodgkin's lymphoma)<br>• Fatigue and weakness are common at the end-stage.<br>• Patients with intermediate-high grade lymphoma are more likely to present with constitutional symptoms | • Painless superficial lymphadenopathy (usually >1 lymph node region) in the cervical, inguinal and/or axillary regions<br>• Lymphadenopathy may be rapidly growing depending on the grade<br>• Splenomegaly, hepatomegaly, large abdominal mass, testicular mass, and skin lesions may be present | • CBC<br>• Serum chemistry (including LDH)<br>• HIV serology<br>• CXR<br>• CT of neck, chest, abdomen, pelvis<br>• PET scan<br>• Excisional lymph node biopsy<br>• Bone marrow aspirate and biopsy<br>• Hep B testing | • Chemotherapy<br>• Surgical management is limited to selected situations e.g. GI lymphoma or testicular lymphoma |

LYMPHATIC

| Key Symptoms | Physical Exam Findings | Investigations | Management |
|---|---|---|---|
| **Acute Lymphangitis** | | | |
| • May occur with skin abrasion distally accompanied by lymphangitis<br>• Fine, red tender streaks along the lymphatic collecting ducts<br>• Regional lymphadenitis: Symptoms often include pain in affected extremity, malaise, and possibly fever (systemic symptoms) | • Inspect distally for sites of infection, especially for cracks in the interdigital spaces | • Swab (or biopsy/ aspirate) of the primary site for histology/microscopy/ culture | • Antimicrobial therapy (empiric then targeted) |
| **Lymphedema** | | | |
| • Painless, slowly progressive non-pitting swelling of ipsilateral extremity post lymph node dissection/radiation therapy, usually involves digits<br>• Over time, the skin becomes dry, firm, and fibrous to palpation | • Peripheral vascular, dermatological/ soft tissue exam, complete lymph node exam<br>• ⅔ cases are unilateral but depends on precipitating event<br>• Edema may initially be pitting but eventually becomes non pitting<br>• Stemmer's sign (thickened skin fold at the base of the second toe or finger)<br>• Limb circumference measurement/comparison | • Increased susceptibility to local infection or limb injury; evaluate for cellulitis from staphylococcal or streptococcal skin infection.<br>• Imaging: Lymphoscintigraphy, CT, MR/MR lymphography (not common)<br>• Genetic testing (e.g. Turner's - Note: also look for features on clinical exam) | • Conservative therapy: Self monitoring, limb elevation massage, healthy diet/exercise, compression therapies (bandaging, garments, intermittent pneumatic and physiotherapy (manual lymphatic drainage and complete decongestive therapy), avoiding infection/injury<br>• Surgical management: Lymphatic bypass procedure (not common), reductive techniques |

## Lymphatic Filariasis Elephantiasis

| Key Symptoms | Physical Exam Findings | Investigations | Management |
|---|---|---|---|
| • Initially similar to lymphedema;<br>• Skin texture becomes hyperkeratotic over time with verrucous and vesicular skin lesions<br>• May be asymptomatic<br>• Associated with: three distinct phases:<br>• asymptomatic microfilaremia,<br>• acute episodes of adenolymphangitis (ADL)<br>• chronic disease (irreversible lymphedema), (often superimposed upon repeated episodes of ADL)<br>• Major cause of disfigurement and disability in endemic areas, leading to significant economic and psychosocial impact | • Signs of unexplained eosinophilia (tropical) - e.g. nocturnal wheezing<br>• Acute manifestations: Acute adenolymphangitis, dermato lymphangio adenitis, filarial fever, and tropical pulmonary eosinophilia<br>• Chronic manifestations: Lymphedema, hydrocele, renal involvement | • Circulating antigen detection (filarial)<br>• Blood Smears<br>• PCR<br>• Circulating antibody detection<br>• Ultrasound + lymphoscintigraphy techniques can be used to detect the presence of adult worms in lymphatic vessels<br>• Evaluate for parasitic coinfection e.g. Loa Loa<br>• Screen for suicidality/depression | • Diethylcarbamazine (DEC) high single dose if monoinfection +/- doxycycline<br>• If concomitant loiasis and high microfilarial load, use low dose DEC over 21d<br>• If concomitant onchocerciasis use ivermectin +/- doxycycline |

## Systemic Lupus Erythematosus

| Key Symptoms | Physical Exam Findings | Investigations | Management |
|---|---|---|---|
| • Nodes are typically soft, nontender, discrete, variable in size, and usually detected in the cervical, axillary, and inguinal areas<br>• Associated with: the onset of disease or an exacerbation. Lymph node enlargement can also be the result of infection or a lymphoproliferative disease in SLE; when infections are present, the enlarged nodes are more likely to be tender<br>• Autoimmune disorder may present with multisystem involvement | • Multisystem involvement, dermatological, vascular/hemer, ophthalmologic symptoms etc (e.g. malar rash, purpura/petechiaekeratoconjunctivitis, etc) | • ANA, anti-dsDNA APA, ESR, CRP, C3, C4, etc | • Options include sun protection, antimalarials, steroids, immunosuppressants |

LYMPHATIC

**Mycobacterium Infection**

| Key Symptoms | Physical Exam Findings | Investigations | Management |
| --- | --- | --- | --- |
| • Nodes are typically nontender, enlarge over weeks to months without prominent systemic symptoms and can progress to matting and fluctuation<br>• Associated with lymphadenopathy alone, especially in the neck<br>• In patients with generalized lymphadenopathy, miliary tuberculosis should be considered | • Fever is most common finding on exam<br>• Clinical manifestations vary substantially, respiratory exam - symptoms in ⅓ of patients (cough, dyspnea, hemoptysis), mouth ulcers, muscle wasting/cachexia/anorexia | • CXR abnormalities<br>• Elevated CRP | • Antituberculous therapy (Isoniazid, rifampin pyrazinamide, ethambutol)- Intensive phase = 4 drugs x 2 months, Continuation phase 2 drugs x 4 months (total 6 months)<br>• Individual case management with Direct Observed Therapy (DOT) |

LYMPHATIC

# REFERENCES

1. Moore KL, Dalley AF, Agur AMR. *Clinically Oriented Anatomy,* 7th ed. Philadelphia: Lippincott Williams & Wilkins; 2013.
2. Porter RS (Editor). The Merck Manual of Diagnosis and Therapy, 19th ed. Whitehouse Station: Merck Research Laboratories; 2011.
3. Bickley LS, Szilagyi PG, Bates B. *Bates' Guide to Physical Examination and History Taking, 10th ed.* Philadelphia: Lippincott Williams & Wilkins; 2009.
4. Seidel HM, Ball JW, Dains JE, Flynn JA, Solomon BS, Stewart RW. *Mosby's Guide to Physical Examination,* 7th ed. St. Louis: Mosby Elsevier; 2011.
5. Longo DL, Fauci AS, Kasper DL, Hauser SL, Jameson JL, Loscalzo J (Editors). *Harrison's Online,* 19th ed. New York: McGraw-Hill; 2015.
6. Swartz MH. *Textbook of Physical Diagnosis: History and Examination,* 6th ed. Philadelphia: Saunders Elsevier; 2010.
7. Fletcher RH. *Evaluation of Peripheral Lymphadenopathy in Adults.* In TW Post, Boxer LA & Park L (Eds). UpToDate. 2014.
8. Simel D, Rennie D. *Jama Evidence: The Rational Clinical Examination.* United States of America: McGraw-Hill, American Medical Association; 2009.

LYMPHATIC

CHAPTER 7:

# The Musculoskeletal System

**Editors:**
Gillian Bedard, BSc
Ayan K. Dey, BSc
Aaron Gazendam, HBSc

**Resident Reviewer:**
Fahim Merali, MD, CCFP

**Faculty Reviewers:**
Anne Agur, PhD, MSc, BSc(OT)
Paul Kuzyk, MD, MASc, FRCSC

## TABLE OF CONTENTS

**MUSCULOSKELETAL**

# 1. MUSCULOSKELETAL HISTORY AND PHYSICAL EXAM

- See General History and Physical Exam for a detailed approach to history taking
- OPQRSTUVW questions regarding each complaint
- Hand dominance

## 1.1 Focused History

### Pain: OPQRST

- **O**nset (slow or sudden)
- **P**alliative factors, **P**rovocative factors (pain associated with rest, activity, certain postures, time of day), **P**rogression (of symptoms)
- **Q**uality
  - Nerve pain: sharp, burning, follows distribution of nerve
  - Bone pain: deep, localized
  - Vascular pain: diffuse, aching, poorly localized, may be referred to other areas
  - Muscle pain: dull and aching, poorly localized, may be referred to other areas
- **R**adiation, **R**eferred pain
- **S**ymptoms associated (joint locking, unlocking, instability; changes in color of limb, pins and needles)
- **T**iming (onset, duration, frequency)

### Referred Symptoms from other Joints/Organs

- Shoulder pain (from heart or diaphragm)
- Arm pain (from neck)
- Leg pain (from back)
- Knee pain (from hip or back)
- Hip (right iliac fossa) pain (from appendix)

### Inflammatory Symptoms

- Pain, erythema, warmth, swelling, morning stiffness (>30 min)
- Improves with activity
- Responds to NSAIDS
- Important to differentiate from mechanical/degenerative manifestations

### Mechanical/Degenerative Symptoms

- Pain is worse at end of day, better with rest, worse with exercise
- Ligament or meniscal symptoms (joint collapsing, clicking, locking, instability)

### Neoplastic and Infectious Symptoms

- Constant pain, night pain, fever, chills, weight loss, anorexia, fatigue, weakness
- History of prostate, thyroid, breast, lung or kidney cancer

### Neurological Symptoms

- Paresthesia, tingling, bowel and bladder complaints, headaches, weakness

### Vascular Symptoms

- Exercise-induced pain (usually in calf but can be in buttock, hip, thigh, or foot) that makes the patient stop exertion, no pain at rest, pain disappears within 10 min
- Differentiate vascular from neurologic claudication

## 1.2 Focused Physical Exam

- Always examine the joint above and below the site of interest
- If lower extremity complaint: examine lower back and perform complete neurological exam of lower limbs
- If upper extremity complaint: examine neck and perform complete neurological exam of upper limbs
- See **Examination of Specific Joints** for site-specific tests

## Inspection (Look)

In general, inspect each joint for the following: **SEADS**
- **S**welling, **E**rythema, **A**trophy of muscle
- **D**eformity (alterations in shape, bony alignment or posture)
- **S**kin changes (bruising, discoloration)

Remember to evaluate from front, side and back.

Also, inspect for the following while conducting the physical exam:
- Symmetry of the bony contours, soft tissues, limb positions
- Presence of scars to indicate recent injury/surgery
- Any crepitus or abnormal sound in joints when patient moves them
- Patient's attitude (apprehensiveness, restlessness)
- Patient's facial expression (indicating discomfort)
- Patient's willingness to move; normality of movements

## Palpation (Feel)

In general, palpate skin, soft tissues, bones, and joints while patient is as relaxed as possible. Palpation must be carried out in a systematic fashion to ensure that all structures are examined and any asymmetry is noted.

The following should be noted when palpating:
- Identify shapes, structures, tissue type, and detect any abnormalities
- Specifically, feel for **w**armth, **e**ffusion, **t**enderness, **c**repitus and **j**oint stability (WETCJ)
- Determine joint tenderness by applying firm pressure to the joint
- Palpate for variation in temperature, pulses, tremors, and fasciculations
- Take note of dryness or excessive moisture of the skin.

## Range of Motion (Move)

*Active Movements*
- Performed voluntarily by patient
- Abnormalities in active ROM result from either neurological problems or mechanical disruption of flexor/extensor mechanisms
- When testing active movements, note the following:
  - Pain; if present, note quality and amount of pain
  - Amount of observable restriction
  - Any limitation and its nature
  - Willingness of patient to move the joint
  - Quality of movement
  - Crepitus

*Passive Movements*
- Joint is moved through a range of motion by the examiner while the patient is relaxed
- Detect any limitation of movement (stiffness) or excessive range (hypermobility), and any associated pain
- Hypermobile joints: could be a result of ligament tears, collagen disorders, chronic pain, tendinitis, rheumatoid arthritis
- Hypomobile joints: could be a result of muscle strains, pinched nerve syndromes, tendinitis, osteoarthritis

*End Feel*
- Defined as the sensation felt in the joint as it reaches the end of its ROM
- In passive movement, the examiner should determine the quality of end feel
- Three normal types of end feel:
  1. Bone to Bone: a "hard" unyielding compression that stops further movement (e.g. elbow extension)
  2. Soft Tissue Approximation: a yielding compression that stops further movement (e.g. elbow and knee flexion where movement is stopped by muscles)
  3. Tissue Stretch: hard or "springy" (firm) movement with a slight give. There is a feeling of elastic resistance toward the end of the ROM with a feeling of "rising tension". Feeling depends on thickness of tissue and may be very elastic (i.e. Achilles tendon stretch) or slightly elastic (i.e. wrist flexion: lateral rotation of

MUSCULOSKELETAL

shoulder, extension of MCP joint)
- Abnormal end feel indicates pathology

## Power Assessment/Isometric Movements
- Type of movement that consists of strong, static, voluntary muscle contraction
- Examiner positions the joint in the resting position and asks the patient to maintain the position against an applied force
- Muscle weakness can be a result of:
  - Upper motor neuron lesion
  - Injury to peripheral nerve
  - Neuromuscular junction pathology
  - Pathology of muscles themselves
  - Disuse atrophy
  - Pain
- In certain anatomic sites (e.g. lumbar spine, cervical spine), isometric contractions are used to test for myotome function

## Functional Assessment
- Should always be performed on the joint during examination
- May involve task analysis or simply a history of patient's daily activities
- Assess limitations in activities of daily living (ADLs):
  - D = Dressing
  - E = Eating; feeding self.
  - A = Ambulation; getting up, sitting down, walking up stairs
  - T = Toileting
  - H = Hygiene: transferring from shower or bathtub, brushing teeth, combing hair.

## Reflexes
- Test reflexes to assess the nerve or nerve roots that supply the reflex (see **Neurological Exam**)

## Special Tests
- Refer to specific anatomic sites

## Other Considerations
- Gait Assessment
  - Walking: normal, heel-to-toe, heels only (dorsiflexor power), toes only (plantar flexor power)
  - Look for: Trendelenburg gait in hip disorders, high stepping (eg. drop-foot), circumduction, antalgic gait (due to pain)
- Peripheral Vascular Exam
  - Test peripheral pulses (see **Peripheral Vascular Exam**)
- Neurological Exam
  - Test power, sensation (see **Neurological Exam**)

# EXAMINATION OF SPECIFIC JOINTS
- Each joint should be inspected, palpated, put through the various range of motion maneuvers, have relevant reflexes examined, and put through special tests if appropriate
- Look for the symptoms listed above (see **Focused Physical Exam**, p. 166)

# 2. SHOULDER

## 2.1 Essential Anatomy

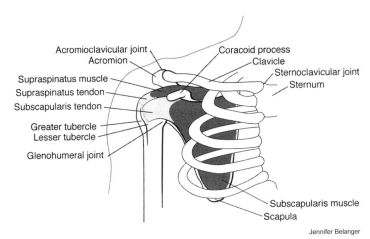

Figure 1. Anatomy of the Right Shoulder

## 2.2 Common Chief Complaints and Differentials

| Differential Diagnosis | Distinguishing Features |
| --- | --- |
| **Chief Complaint: Pain** | |
| **Impingement Syndrome** | Pain associated with past injury or degenerative shoulder, night pain, dull ache, weakness with drop arm test, atrophy of rotator cuff muscles. |
| **Rotator Cuff Tendinopathy/Tear** | Pain associated with past injury or degenerative shoulder, night pain, dull ache, weakness with drop arm test, atrophy of rotator cuff muscles |
| **Subacromial Bursitis** | Tenderness at anterior/inferior acromion. Limited active ROM but full passive ROM. Dull ache. Worse on exertion better with rest |
| **Bicipital Tendon Rupture (proximal)** | Often the result of acute trauma or force on muscle, worse with onset but improves over time, sharp ache. Asymmetry with bulge deformity |
| **Bicipital Tendonitis** | Often the result of overuse, worse with use and improves with rest, dull ache. Tenderness over bicipital groove. Often concurrent with impingement or subacromial bursitis |
| **Labral Tear** | Result of trauma (EG dislocation) or overuse (throwing athlete). Mimics rotator cuff pathology. Can cause instability. Should be suspected based on demographic, history and lack of response to conservative therapy |
| **Instability** | Result of trauma (dislocation) or congenital laxity. Often the cause of impingement-type symptoms in younger patients. |
| **Acromioclavicular pathology** | Painful arc. Painful and tender directly over ACJ. Can be concomitant with and contribute to impingement |
| **Adhesive Capsulitis** | Global restriction in active and passive ROM. Painful in early phase |
| **Chief Complaint: Weakness** | |

| Differential Diagnosis | Distinguishing Features |
|---|---|
| Axillary nerve mononeuropathy | Weakness affecting shoulder flexion, abduction and external rotation. Atrophy of deltoid and teres minor |
| Suprascapular nerve palsy | Weakness affecting overhead abduction and external rotation. Atrophy of infraspinatus and supraspinatus. Insidious onset, tenderness near suprascapular notch. Pain in lateral and posterior shoulder |
| Long thoracic nerve injury | Weakness affecting shoulder flexion and overhead motions. Scapular winging and atrophy of serratus anterior |
| Rotator cuff tear | Weakness or inability to raise the arm overhead. Positive drop arm test and/or empty can test |
| Cervical nerve root lesion | Weakness in myotome. Pain and sensation reduction in dermatome distribution. Reduced deep tendon reflexes |
| Spinal accessory nerve injury | Weakness in trapezius and sternocleidomastoid. Scapular winging. Reduced shoulder active flexion and abduction |

## 2.3 Focused History

- Onset of pain
- Location of pain (anterior, lateral, superior, posterior)
- History of trauma/surgery & mechanism of injury (if applicable)
- Radiation of pain
- Consider sources of referred pain
- Presence of night pain.
- Aggravating and alleviating factors.

## 2.4 Focused Physical Exam

### Physical Exam

*Inspection (Look)*
- Compare shoulder contours (anteriorly), alignment of the clavicles, symmetry of sternoclavicular and acromioclavicular joints, and scapulae (posteriorly) (see **Figure 1**)
- Note signs of "SEADS" around the shoulders
- Note any swelling, deformity, muscle atrophy, and asymmetry of the soft tissues and bones
- Note biceps tendon rupture by asking the patient to flex his/her arm and observe for a bulge of tissue ("Popeye sign")

*Palpation (Feel)*
- Palpate bones:
    - the ssternoclavicular joint and along the clavicle to the acromioclavicular joint to detect for asymmetry and/or discontinuity
- Palpate soft tissues:
    - The anterior and lateral aspects of the glenohumeral joint assessing the bicipital groove, subdeltoid bursa, AC joint and rotator cuff insertion (greater tuberosity) for tenderness
    - The glenohumoral joint for crepitus by placing your hand over the subacromial bursa and passively circumducting the arm
    - The deltoids to test axillary nerve sensation

*Range of Motion (Move)*
- Perform the following screening test by instructing your patients to do the following, noting any crepitus by cupping your hand over the shoulder joint during these movements (see **Table 1** for normal values):
    - Forward flexion: "Raise both your arms in front of you until they are straight above your head"
    - External rotation and abduction: "Place both your hands behind your neck with your elbows out to the sides"

- Hands should reach the neck base
  - Abduction and adduction: "Raise both arms from your sides straight over head, palms together; now bring them slowly down to your side again"
  - Extension and internal rotation: "Bring your arms toward your back and place your hands between the shoulder blades"
    - Hands should normally reach the inferior angle of the scapulae; record the level of the scapulae that can be reached
- Pain during motion can be localized
- Both shoulders can be assessed simultaneously
- If the screening tests above demonstrate any limitation of motion, assess the range of motion for passive movements as well

Table 1. Shoulder: Normal Ranges of Motion

| Movement | Range of Motion |
|---|---|
| Forward Flexion | 180° |
| Backward Extension | 60° |
| Abduction | 180° |
| Adduction | 50° |
| External Rotation (with elbows at sides) | 90° |
| Internal Rotation (with shoulder abducted to 90° and elbow flexed) | 70° |

*True glenohumeral abduction, with the scapula stabilized, is 110-120 degrees.
Gross G, Fetto J, Rosen E. Musculoskeletal Examination. Malden: Blackwell; 2002.

## Special Tests

Table 2: Special Tests for the Shoulder

| Special Test | Description | Rationale/Interpretation |
|---|---|---|
| **Tests For Shoulder Instability** | | |
| Anterior apprehension test | With the patient supine, passively abduct the arm to 90° (with elbow also flexed to 90°). Then hold the patient's wrist with one hand and externally rotate shoulder while the other hand applies anteriorly directed force to the humeral head. | Positive test: patient expresses anxiety that shoulder will dislocate or be painful. If the anterior structures are deficient, the humeral head may "pop" out or feel unstable. |
| Relocation test | With patient supine, patient's arm is passively abducted to 90° along with the elbow also to 90°. This is the same starting position as the apprehension test. Then apply posteriorly directed force to the humeral head. | Positive test: sensation of apprehension resolves. |
| Anterior release test (surprise) | At the end of the relocation test, the examiner's hand is suddenly removed from the proximal humerus. | Positive test: the test is positive in case of pain or apprehension when easing the pressure. |
| Load and shift | Stabilize the scapula with one hand and compress the humeral head into the glenoid (load) with the other. Then, translate the humeral heard anteriorly and posteriorly (shift) and compare with contralateral shoulder. | Positive test: >25% translation of humeral diameter anterior, >50% translation posteriorly. This test is specific for anterior/posterior instability. |

| Special Test | Description | Rationale/Interpretation |
|---|---|---|
| Sulcus sign | The patient stands or sits with the arm by the side and shoulder muscles relaxed. Arm is then pulled vertically downward. | Positive test: humeral head slides inferiorly or a gap is produced between the head of the humerus and the acromion.<br><br>May be indicative of instability of multiple ligaments. |

### Test For Glenoid Labral Pathology

| Special Test | Description | Rationale/Interpretation |
|---|---|---|
| O'brien's Sign/Test | The patient's arm is flexed to 90° with the elbow in full extension and then the arm is adducted 15° medial to sagittal plane; arm is then internally rotated (thumb pointing downward) and the patient resists the examiner's downward force.<br><br>The procedure is then repeated in supination | Positive test: if pain is elicited by the first maneuver and is reduced by the second maneuver.<br><br>Note: a false positive result may occur with rotator cuff or ac joint pathology. |
| Anterior Slide Test | Ask the patient to place hands on their waist with thumbs pointed posteriorly. The examiner from behind the patient stabilizes the scapula and clavicle and applies an anterosuperior force directed at the elbow. | Positive test: "pop" and/or anterosuperior pain. This suggests labral tear. |

### Tests For Rotator Cuff Tears

| Special Test | Description | Rationale/Interpretation |
|---|---|---|
| Drop Arm Test | The patient's arm is passively abducted to 90°with the elbow in full extension; the patient is then asked to slowly lower his/her arm back to the side. | Positive test: if arm drops suddenly or if patient has severe pain. This indicates rotator cuff tear.<br><br>This test assesses the <u>supraspinatus</u> <u>muscle</u> |
| Empty Can Test | The patient's shoulders are abducted to 45° and their hands are turned downward so that thumbs are pointing down (i.e. Emptying a can); patient is then asked to move their arm upward against <u>downward resistance</u>. (**Figure 3**) | Positive test: pain or weakness while resisting downward pressure.<br><br>This test assesses the <u>supraspinatus</u> <u>muscle</u> |
| External rotation resistance test | The patient's shoulders are abducted to 25° with elbows bent at 90°; patient is then asked to rotate his/her shoulders externally <u>as resistance is applied on their arms toward the midline</u> of their body. (**Figure 4**) | Positive test: sharp or dull pain with resistance; inability to externally rotate or the presence of muscle weakness.<br><br>This test assesses the integrity of the teres minor and infraspinatus muscles |
| Internal rotation lag sign | The patient's hands are placed behind their back with palms facing out, with forearms almost 90° to the length of the spine; hand is lifted off the back by the examiner, and patient is asked to maintain position. | Positive test: unable to maintain position. |

| Special Test | Description | Rationale/Interpretation |
|---|---|---|
| **Gerber lift-off test** | The patient's hands are placed behind their back with palms facing out, with forearms almost 90° to the length of the spine; patient is asked to lift hand off the back against <u>resistance toward their body</u>. (**Figure 5**). | Positive test: unable to lift arm toward posterior/ severe pain is indicative of a tear in the <u>subscapularis</u> muscle. |

### Test for Impingement Syndrome (Rotator Cuff Tendonitis)

| Special Test | Description | Rationale/Interpretation |
|---|---|---|
| **Neer's Test** | With the patient sitting or standing, the examiner stabilizes the patient's scapula and maximally forward flexes the patient's arm while internally rotating the shoulder. (**Figure 2**) | Positive test: anterolateral shoulder pain. Note: internal rotation should be more painful than external rotation.<br><br>This is suggestive of subacromial impingement. |
| **Hawkins-Kennedy Test** | With shoulder and elbow flexed at 90°, passively internally rotate the shoulder. | Positive: pain during internal rotation.<br><br>This is suggestive of supraspinatus impingement. |
| **Painful Arc Test** | With the patient sitting or standing, the patient actively abducts shoulder. Continue until arms are abducted directly above head. (**Figure 6**) | Positive test: pain during 60-120° abduction. |

### Acromioclavicular Joint Pathology

| Special Test | Description | Rationale/Interpretation |
|---|---|---|
| **Scarf (Cross Body Adduction) Test** | With the shoulder in 90° flexion, passively adduct the patient's arm in the horizontal plane. | Positive test: pain in the region of the ac joint.<br><br>May be due to compression of joint. |

### Bicipital Tendonitis

| Special Test | Description | Rationale/Interpretation |
|---|---|---|
| **Yergason Test** | Patient's elbow is flexed to 90 degrees with thumbs up. Examiner grasps the wrist, resisting attempts by the patient to actively supinate the arm and flex the elbow. | Positive test: pain is suggestive of biceps tendonitis. |
| Speed's Test | Patient flexes shoulder to 60° with elbow extended and forearm supinated. Examiner attempts to extend the arm by pushing down on the forearm | Positive test: pain in the bicipital groove. |

*Luime JJ, et al. 2004. JAMA 292(16):1 989-1999.*

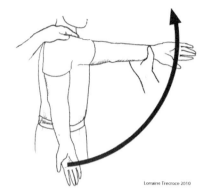

**Figure 2.** Neer's Test for Shoulder Impingement

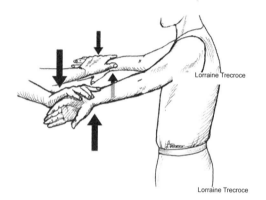

**Figure 3.** Empty Can (Jobe's) Test for Supraspinatus Tear

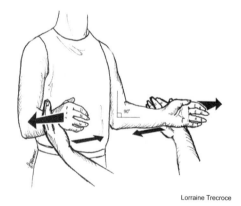

**Figure 4.** Infraspinatus and Teres Minor Strength Test

**Clinical Pearl: Shoulder Pain**

Shoulder pain (radiating down the arm to the elbow) when combing one's hair, putting on a coat, or reaching into a back pocket indicates supraspinatus inflammation.

Diffuse shoulder pain upon moving the humerus posteriorly (without radiation to the arm) indicates infraspinatus inflammation.

Discomfort and weakness of the upper extremity and "winging" of the ipsilateral scapula indicates a dysfunction of the serratus anterior or trapezius muscles often secondary to long thoracic or accessory nerve palsies.

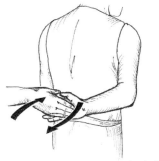

Lorraine Trecroce

**Figure 5.** Gerber's Lift-Off Test for Subscapularis Tear

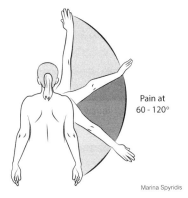

Pain at
60 - 120°

Marina Spyridis

**Figure 6.** Painful Arc Test

## 2.5 Common Clinical Scenarios

- Shoulder pain can be acute or chronic in nature and is commonly caused by soft tissue trauma/inflammation

| Key Symptoms | Physical Exam Findings | Investigations | Management |
|---|---|---|---|
| **Rotator Cuff Tendinopathies** | | | |
| • Shoulder pain on activity<br>• Sharp pain on elevation of arm into overhead position<br>• History of chronic usage (e.g. Throwing, swimming, overhead work) or trauma | • Inspect for muscle atrophy<br>• Palpate over glenohumeral joint<br>• Active & passive ROM<br>• Special tests:<br>  • Hawkins-kennedy test<br>  • Painful arc test<br>  • Empty can test<br>  • Resisted external rotation<br>  • Lift-off test | U/S for visualization of soft tissue if no response to conservative treatment | • Analgesic/NSAID<br>• Physical therapy to improve ROM (Codman exercises) and strength<br>• Steroid or hyaluronic acid injections may be indicated if no improvement.<br>• Surgical repair may sometimes be indicated |

## Rotator Cuff Tear/Rupture

| Key Symptoms | Physical Exam Findings | Investigations | Management |
|---|---|---|---|
| • Sharp pain after trauma<br>• Pain over greater tubercle<br>• Characteristic shoulder shrug and pain on attempted abduction<br>• Weakness on external rotation | • Inspect for muscle atrophy<br>• Palpate over glenohumeral joint<br>• Active and passive ROM<br>• Special tests:<br>  • Drop arm test<br>  • Empty can test<br>  • External rotation resistance test<br>  • Internal rotation lag sign<br>  • Gerber lift-off test | U/S for visualization of soft tissue if no response to conservative treatment | • Analgesic/NSAID<br>• Physical therapy to improve ROM (Codman exercises) & strength<br>• If no improvement, steroid or hyaluronic acid injections and referral to orthopedic surgeon may be indicated |

## Bicipital Tendonitis

| Key Symptoms | Physical Exam Findings | Investigations | Management |
|---|---|---|---|
| • Generalized anterior tenderness over bicipital groove<br>• Pain, esp at night<br>• Hallmark is reproduction of anterior shoulder pain during resistance to forearm supination | • Inspect for muscle atrophy<br>• Palpation over bicipital groove<br>• Active and passive ROM<br>• Special tesst:<br>  • Yergason test<br>  • Speed's test | U/S may be helpful | • Analgesic/NSAID<br>• Rest (avoid overhead reach)<br>• Local injection of an anesthetic & steroid may be indicated<br>• Consider orthopedic consultation if symptoms are persistent |

## Dislocation

| Key Symptoms | Physical Exam Findings | Investigations | Management |
|---|---|---|---|
| • Feeling of shoulder instability<br>• Poor ROM & shoulder pain on activity<br>• <u>Anterior dislocation</u>: present w/ slight abduction & internal rotation<br>• <u>Posterior dislocation</u>: present w/ slight adduction & exterrnal rotation | • Anterior apprehension test<br>• Relocation test<br>• Anterior release test<br>• Load and shift<br>• Sulcus sign | • X-ray or CT<br>• MRI may reveal damage to ligaments | • Reduction of dislocated joint with adequate analgesia and muscle relaxation<br>• Ex: Kocher Manoeuvre for anterior dislocation |

## Adhesive Capsulitis (Frozen Shoulder)

| Key Symptoms | Physical Exam Findings | Investigations | Management |
|---|---|---|---|
| • Progression of pain over several weeks from onset at night or with involved movements, to constant pain with any movement<br>• Pain at end of range of motion may be the only finding early in disease process | • Active and passive ROM (forward flexion, external rotation, abduction internal rotation)<br>• Rule out other shoulder pathology | • Consider fasting glucose test (high prevalence of diabetes in these patients)<br>• Imaging has limited diagnostic benefit; for ruling out other pathology, detecting concomitant issues | • Analgesic/NSAID for pain relief<br>• Glenohumeral steroid injection for pain relief<br>• Physical therapy<br>• Hydrodilation therapy<br>• Often self-limited condition, recovers w/ nonsurgical treatment<br>• Prognosis: 12-18 m/o<br>• Consider surgical options if no improvement with extensive therapy |

MUSCULOSKELETAL

### Clavicular fracture

| Key Symptoms | Physical Exam Findings | Investigations | Management |
|---|---|---|---|
| • MOA: fall onto outstretched upper extremity or shoulder, or direct trauma <br> • Inferior and anterior displacement of shoulder secondary to loss of support <br> • Tenderness, crepitus, edema, deformity | • Physical exam may show signs of ecchymosis, edema, focal tenderness, crepitation on palpation over clavicle <br> • Bone defects may be observed by visual inspection or localized by palpation | Standard AP X-ray + 45 degree cephalic tilt | • Immobilization (sling) <br> • ROM pendulum exercises <br> • Operative options include: open or closed reduction with plate fixation |

### Acromioclavicular Joint Pathology

| Key Symptoms | Physical Exam Findings | Investigations | Management |
|---|---|---|---|
| • Swelling, bruising, prominent clavicle depending on severity of sprain <br> • Acromio-clavicular joint separation is a common sports related injury <br> • Poor ROM and moderate pain when raising arm <br> • Reproduction of pain with adduction of elevated affected arm across the body | • Evaluate active and passive ROM <br> • Palpate bony structures of shoulder for fractures. <br> • Neurovascular exam to rule out brachial plexus injury (rare) | • X• rays (AP, lateral and axillary views) <br> • U/S may be helpful in assessing muscle detachment. <br> • MRI not routinely ordered; may help differentiate subtypes of acromio-clavicular injuries | • If Type I-II injury: analgesic & NSAID + ice & activity modification. Distal clavicle resection if no response to conservative management. <br> • Type III: consider reconstruction of the torn coracoclavicular ligaments <br> • Type IV: closed reduction <br> • Type V-VI: open reduction & internal fixation |

## 3. ELBOW

### 3.1 Common Complaints and Differentials

Table 3. Clinical Features Differentiating Diseases Affecting the Elbow

| Clinical Feature | Rheumatoid Arthritis | Psoriatic Arthritis | Acute Gout | Osteo-arthritis | Lateral Epicon-dylitis |
|---|---|---|---|---|---|
| Age | 3-80 | 10-60 | 30-80 | 50-80 | 20-60 |
| Pain Onset | Gradual | Gradual | Abrupt | Gradual | Gradual |
| Stiffness | Very Common | Common | Absent | Common | Occasional |
| Swelling | Common | Common | Common | Common | Absent |
| Redness | Absent | Uncommon | Common | Absent | Absent |
| Deformity | Flexion contractures, usually bi-laterally | Flexion contractures, usually bi-laterally | Flexion contractures, only in chronic state | Flexion contractures | None |

Swartz MH. Textbook of Physical Diagnosis: History and Examination, 6th ed. Philadelphia: Saunders Elsevier;

## 3.2 Focused History
- Location of pain (anterior, medial, lateral or diffuse)
- History of repetitive movements (occupation, hobby, sports)
- Timing (acute onset or insidious)
- Absence/presence of sensory changes
- Absence/presence of stiffness or swelling
- Functional limitations
- Constitutional symptoms

## 3.3 Focused Physical Exam
*Inspection (Look)*
- Inspect for swelling or masses (e.g. olecranon bursitis or rheumatic nodules)
- Ask the patient: "With your palms facing up, bend and then extend your elbow"
  - Note differences in carrying angles, flexion contractures, hyperextension

*Palpation (Feel)*
- Grasp the elbow with your fingers under the olecranon and your thumb next to the biceps tendon then passively flex and extend the elbow. Note any crepitus, tenderness or restricted movement.
- Anterior Surface:
  - Cubital fossa contents: Biceps tendon, brachial artery, median nerve
  - Muscles – biceps, pronator teres, flexor carpi radialis, palmaris longus, flexor digitorum superficialis, flexor carpi ulnaris.
- Medial Surface
  - Medial epicondyle, Medial (ulnar) Collateral Ligament, Ulnar nerve
- Lateral Surface
  - Lateral Epicondyle, Lateral Collateral Ligament, Radial head
- Posterior Surface
  - Olecranon, Olecranon bursa, Triceps

*Range of Motion (Move)*
- Ask the patient: "Bend your elbows until you can touch your shoulders (flexion) and then place your arms back down (extension)"
- With the patient's arms at sides and elbows flexed, ask patient to "Turn your palms up (supination) and down (pronation); hold a pencil in your fist" (may help with estimating the range of motion in degrees)
- Note any limitation of motion (see **Table 4**) or pain

**Table 4.** Elbow: Normal Ranges of Motion

| Movement | Range of Motion |
| --- | --- |
| Flexion | 150° |
| Extension | 0° |
| Supination | 80-90° from vertical (with pencil grasped in hand) |
| Pronation | 80-90° from vertical (with pencil grasped in hand) |

Gross G, Fetto J, Rosen E. Musculoskeletal Examination. Malden: Blackwell; 2002.

## Special Tests

| Special Test | Description | Rationale/ Interpretation |
| --- | --- | --- |
| Tinel Test | Tap the area of ulnar nerve between the olecranon process and medial epicondyle | Positive Test: Paresthesia in the ulnar nerve distribution of the hand may be suggestive of cubital tunnel syndrome or radial tunnel syndrome. |

MUSCULOSKELETAL

| Special Test | Description | Rationale/ Interpretation |
|---|---|---|
| **Active Resisted D3 Flexion ("middle finger test")** | Extend elbow and 3rd digit. Have patient actively resist (flex against resistance) while pressing down on the digit. | Positive Test: Pain at the medial epicondyle would be suggestive of flexor-pronator tendinopathy (medial epicondylitis). |
| **Test for Medial Epicondylitis** | Palpate the medial epicondyle. Passively supinate and extend elbow, then extend wrist. | Positive Test: Pain at the medial epicondyle. |
| **Active Resisted Wrist Extension** | Extend elbow and wrist in pronation. Have patient actively resist (extension against resistance) while trying to flex the wrist | Positive Test: Pain at the lateral epicondyle would be suggestive of extensor-supinator tendinopathy (lateral epicondylitis). |
| **Elbow abduction stress test** | Valgus stress applied against an elbow held in 20-30 degrees of flexion. | Positive Test: Absence of a firm end-point and movement of the articular surfaces of the medial epicondyle and ulna may be suggestive of ulnar collateral ligament injury. |
| **Hook Test** | Shoulder actively abducted to 90° with elbow in 90° flexion. Then examiner attempts to hook the distal biceps tendon with their fingertips to confirm whether tendon is intact. | Positive Test: If examiner's finger does not meet resistance this may be suggestive of distal biceps tendon rupture. Pain can indicate a partial injury. |

Kane SF, Lynch JH, & Taylor JC. Evaluation of Elbow Pain in Adults, American Family Physician, 2014

## 3.4 Common Clinical Scenarios

| Key Symptoms | Physical Exam Findings | Investigations | Management |
|---|---|---|---|
| **Olecranon Bursitis (student's elbow)** | | | |
| • Hx of minor trauma to elbow common; focal swelling at posterior elbow<br>• Aseptic – gradual irritation Absence of redness, warmth or other signs of infection<br>• Septic – sudden onset pain, swelling, warmth, erythema over the olecranon<br>• Pain often exacerbated by pressure | Palpation over the olecranon process of the ulna | Bursal fluid analysis | If aseptic – activity modification, ice and compressive dressing. Aspiration if persistent If septic – activity modification, aspiration, and systemic oral or IV antibiotics informed by bursal fluid culture |

MUSCULOSKELETAL

| Key Symptoms | Physical Exam Findings | Investigations | Management |
|---|---|---|---|
| **Medial Epicondylitis (Golfer's elbow)** | | | |
| • Insidious onset of pain in the region of the medical epicondyle of the humerus, radiating down the surface of the forearm<br>Resisted wrist flexion • and pronation produces pain (turning a door knob or holding a glass)<br>• Flexor• pronator mass is tender to palpation | While palpating the medial epicondyle, patient's forearm is supinated and the elbow & wrist are extended - pain over the medial epicondyle is diagnostic | Primarily a clinical diagnosis Plain radiography following acute injury or MRI for chronic elbow pain may be indicated | • Relative rest, ice, bracing, NSAIDS (topical or oral)<br>• Stretching and strengthening exercises<br>• Corticosteroid injection if pain is persistent |
| **Lateral Epicondylitis (tennis elbow)** | | | |
| • Common form of epicondylitis with insidious onset due to increased activity<br>• Pain and decreased strength with resistant gripping and with wrist supination and extension<br>• Common extensor tendon is tender to palpation | While palpating the lateral epicondyle, pronate the patient's forearm, flex the wrist fully, and extend the elbow – pain over the lateral epicondyle is diagnostic | Primarily a clinical diagnosis Plain radiography following acute injury or MRI for chronic elbow pain may be indicated | • Relative rest, ice, bracing, NSAIDS (topical or oral)<br>• Stretching and strengthening exercises<br>• Corticosteroid injection if pain is persistent |
| **Ulnar nerve subluxation** | | | |
| Medial elbow pain and snapping sensation Can be associated with ulnar distribution paresthesiae in hand | Reproduce snapping by ranging elbow through flexion-extension in pronation, applying light pressure over the cubital tunnel Sensory and motor exam of upper extremity | Clinical diagnosis | Nighttime elbow splinting in extension, rest/ice/analgesics; nerve decompression +/- nerve transposition |
| **Fracture** | | | |
| Acute injury such as FOOSH | Unable to extend elbow fully, unable to pronate/supinate without pain | AP + Lateral XRay | Cast immobilization vs. ORiF |

Kane SF, Lynch JH, & Taylor JC.  Evaluation of Elbow Pain in Adults, American Family Physician, 2014. - modified

# 4. WRIST

## 4.1 Common Chief Complaints and Differentials

| Chief Complaint | Differential Diagnosis | Distinguishing Features |
|---|---|---|
| Pain | Fracture | Trauma, and identifiable mechanism of injury |
| | Repetitive stress injury | Overuse of joint |
| | Systemic Illness | Not associated with trauma or overuse. Also will likely have constitutional symptoms |
| Numbness/ Tingling | Carpal Tunnel syndrome | Symptoms in the median nerve distribution (generally worse at night) |
| | Guyon's ulnar nerve entrapment | Symptoms in ulnar nerve distribution |
| | Referral from proximal lesions (c-spine, brachial plexus, elbow) | Symptoms and findings proximal to wrist and hand |
| | Systemic disease | Systemic findings with non-specific MSK findings |

## 4.2 Focused History
- See General History and Physical Exam for a detailed approach to history taking
- OPQRSTUVW questions regarding each complaint
- Associated features – swelling, stiffness, clicking, instability
- Occupational History
- Constitutional symptoms (fever, night sweats)
- Hobbies, sports and recreation
- Hand dominance

## 4.3 Focused Physical Exam

*Inspection*
- Inspect the palmar and dorsal surfaces of the wrist for swelling over the joints or deformities

*Palpation*
- Palpate the distal radius and ulna on the lateral and medial surfaces
- Palpate the groove of each wrist joint with your thumbs on the dorsum of the wrist, while your fingers support the wrist from beneath
- Note any tenderness, swelling, warmth or redness
- Palpate the anatomical snuffbox (a hollowed depression just distal to the radial styloid process formed by the abductor and extensor tendons of the thumb)
  - Tenderness over the snuffbox suggests a scaphoid fracture or carpal arthritis

*Range of Motion*
- **Extension:** ask the patient to press the palms of the hands together in the vertical plane and to bring the forearms into the horizontal plane (see **Figure 7**)
- **Flexion:** ask the patient to put the backs of the hands in contact and then to bring the forearms into the horizontal plane (see **Figure 7**)
- Note any asymmetry and limitation of motion (see **Table 5**)
- Test active ulnar and radial deviation
- Test active pronation and supination (having a patient hold a pencil in his/her fist may help with estimating the range of motion in degrees)

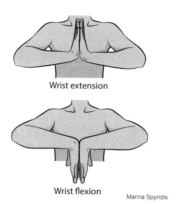

Wrist extension

Wrist flexion

Marina Spyridis

**Figure 7:** Wrist Extension and Flexion Range of Motion

**Table 5.** Wrist: Normal Ranges of Motion

| Movement | Range of Motion |
|---|---|
| Flexion | 80° |
| Extension | 70° |
| Radial Deviation | 20° |
| Ulnar Deviation | 30° |
| Supination | 80-90° from vertical (with pencil grasped in hand) |
| Pronation | 80-90° from vertical (with pencil grasped in hand) |

Gross G, Fetto J, Rosen E. Musculoskeletal Examination. Malden: Blackwell; 2002.

## 4.4 Common Clinical Scenarios

### Wrist: Neurologic

| Key Symptoms | Physical Exam Findings | Investi-gations | Management |
|---|---|---|---|
| **Carpal Tunnel Syndrome** | | | |
| Burning, tingling (pins and needles), and numbness in median nerve distribution (generally worse at night)

Often due to fluid retention (common in pregnancy), hypothyroidism, DM, and overuse (work or recreation) | Ask patient to indicate location of sensory symptoms on hand or arm.

Compare ability to perceive painful stimuli applied along palmar aspect of index finger compared with ipsilateral little finger (decreased sensitivity to pain in index finger suggests diagnosis).

-Tinel's Sign: see below

-Phalen's Sign: see below | EMG may be considered but is often not helpful | Night splint

Corticosteroids

Decompression surgery of carpal tunnel if unmanageable by nonsurgical interventions |

- Tinel's Sign: sharp tap given with fingers directly over median nerve.
    - Positive if tingling, paresthesia or pain in the median nerve distribution
- Phalen's Sign: patient puts dorsal aspects of hands in contact so that wrists are maximally flexed.
    - Positive if paresthesia or numbness in median nerve distribution after holding the position for 60s or less

## Wrist: Tendon

| Key Symptoms | Physical Exam Findings | Investigations | Management |
|---|---|---|---|

### De Quervain's Tenosynovitis

| Key Symptoms | Physical Exam Findings | Investigations | Management |
|---|---|---|---|
| Weakness of grip and pai at the base of the thumb which is aggravated by certain movements of the wrist | Swelling of wrist, hand or thumb Cervical spine screen and neurological screen Range of motion of joints | Finkelstein Test: Patient to flex thumb and close fingers over it; then attempt to move the hand into ulnar deviation. Pain is a positive test | Rest Thumb splint Modification of daily activities Exercises of thenar muscle group and forearm extensors/ flexors; physical therapy |

### Extensor Carpi Ulnaris (ECU) tendinopathy or snapping

| Key Symptoms | Physical Exam Findings | Investigations | Management |
|---|---|---|---|
| Can tear the ECU subsheath, causing instability/subluxing of the tendon Causes pain at dorsoulnar wrist | ECU Synergy Test: – patient puts both thumbs together w palms facing outward and pushes distal aspects together to reproduce ulnar sided pain Actve ulnar and radial deviation in wrist flexion can reproduce snapping | Dynamic U/S, can consider MRI | Wrist splint, immobilize in pronation/radial deviation ECU sheath reconstruction for refractory cases |

### Ganglion Cyst

| Key Symptoms | Physical Exam Findings | Investigations | Management |
|---|---|---|---|
| Dorsal (most common) or volar hand mass, may be painful | Palpable firm and regular mass, Transilluminates, vascular exam to exclude arterial impingement | U/S | Monitor/allow to self-resolve Aspiration (high recurrence) Resection |

## Wrist: Ligament

| Key Symptoms | Physical Exam Findings | Investigations | Management |
|---|---|---|---|

### TFCC injury

| Key Symptoms | Physical Exam Findings | Investigations | Management |
|---|---|---|---|
| Traumatic injury, (usually fall on extended wrist in pronation) vs. degenerative process; pain with turning key/ door handle | Positive fovea sign (soft spot just volar to ulnar styloid), pain with ulnar deviation (compression) or radial deviation (extension) | XR usually normal, MRI | 1st line: Immobilization, NSAiDs 2nd line, for refractory cases: arthroscopy |

MUSCULOSKELETAL

## Wrist: Bones

| Key Symptoms | Physical Exam Findings | Investi-gations | Management |
|---|---|---|---|
| **Keinbock's Disease (lunate AVN)** | | | |
| Progressive dorsal wrist pain, worse with activity, history of wrist trauma | Decreased ROM and grip strength, effusion, tender radiocarpal joint | XR, MRI | Immobilization, NSAIDs for early disease. Operative treatment for progressive or refractory disease |
| **Ulnocarpal Abutment Syndrome (lunate or triquetrum)** | | | |
| Dorsal ulnar sided wrist pain, worse with ulnar deviation and grip | Limited ROM, tender distal ulna/styloid, painful Ulnar dorsal and palmar displacement, painful ulnar deviation with axial loading | XR to look for ulnar variance | Modify activity, NSAIDs Ulnar shortening osteotomy |
| **OA/OCD** | | | |
| Local or diffuse pain around radiocarpal joint, gradually progressive, worse with activity, history of prior remote trauma | Carpal deformity, decreased ROM, crepitus, | XR | Modify activity, analgesic, brace, steroid injection Operative management |
| **Rheumatoid Arthritis** | | | |
| Pain and wrist deformity, inflammatory pain and swelling, Concomitantly affected hand with DiP sparing, FHx of inflammatory disorders | Observable deformity (radial deviation, supination), nodules Joint effusion | Labs (ant-CCP, ESR, RF), XR | NSAID, injection, steroids, methotrexate, DMARDs and biologics |
| **Gout/Pseudogout** | | | |
| Episodic acute monoarthritis (usually), pain and decreased ROM | Can have observable tophi Joint effusion, warm/red over joint | Joint aspirate cytology | NSAIDs, colchicine, steroids Dietary modifications Allopurinol for prevention |

## Wrist: FOOSH*-Related Injuries (*Fall on outstretched hand)

| Key Symptoms | Physical Exam Findings | Investigations | Management |
|---|---|---|---|
| **Distal Radius Fracture (Colles' Fracture)** | | | |
| Pain, possible "fork-like" deformity | Inspect for swelling, deformity and possible open fracture Assess neurovascular status, ROM | XR | Reduction of fracture Immobilization (splint) Surgery (displaced fractures) |

MUSCULOSKELETAL

### Distal Radioulnar Joint (DRUJ) Subluxation

| | | | |
|---|---|---|---|
| Pain and instability of DRUJ | Snapping and crepitus | XR | Immobilization, rest, NSAIDs |
| Dorsal wrist pain Limited pronation/ supination | Pronation with compression of the ulna against the radius results in pain Decreased grip strength | MRI | Surgery if conservative treatment fails. |

### Scaphoid Fracture

| | | | |
|---|---|---|---|
| "Snuffbox" pain/ tenderness | Palpate the anatomic snuffbox by bringing the patient's wrist into ulnar deviation and slight flexion | Mainly clinical diagnosis in acute setting; Often unable to acutely detect on X-ray X-ray 7-10 days post injury may reveal lesion *If missed, can lead to avascular necrosis - important to have high index of suspicion | Immobilization (thumb spica/cast), NSAIDs Surgery (displaced fractures) |

### Scaphoid AVN

| | | | |
|---|---|---|---|
| Chronic dorsal radial wrist pain, history of prior trauma with or without diagnosed fracture | Snuffbox tenderness, painful radiocarpal and 1st CMC ROM | XR, MRI | Immobilization Operative treatment if conservative treatment fails |

**Clinical Pearl: Carpal Tunnel Syndrome**

Findings that **favour** diagnosis of Carpal Tunnel Syndrome (CTS) when present in patients who present with hand dysesthesias:
- Hypalgesia in median nerve territory (LR, 3.1; 95%CI, 2.0-5.1)
- Classic or probable Katz hand diagram results (LR, 1.8; 95% CI, 1.4-2.3)

Findings that **argue against** diagnosis of CTS:
- Katz diagram results classified as unlikely (LR, 0.2; 95%CI, 0.0-0.7)
- Normal thumb abduction strength (LR, 0.5; 95%GI, 0.4-0.7)

Findings that are **not useful** in distinguishing those with CTS from those without:
- Age
- Thenar atrophy
- Other sensory abnormalities (2-point discrimination, vibration, monofilament)
- Tinel sign, Phalen sign

## 5. HAND

### 5.1 Essential Anatomy – Nerves of the Hand

| Nerve | Sensory | Motor |
|---|---|---|
| Radial | Dorsum of first web space | Extension of fingers, thumb and wrist |

| Nerve | Sensory | Motor |
|---|---|---|
| Posterior Interosseous Branch | None | Extension of fingers, thumb and wrist |
| Median | Tip of index/middle/lateral half of ring finger (dorsum) Index/middle/lateral half of ring finger (palmar) | Thumb IP flexion, index/middle finger flexion, wrist flexion |
| Anterior Interosseous Branch | None | Flexion of index/middle finger |
| Recurrent Terminal Branch | None | Thumb opposition |
| Ulnar Nerve | Anterior and posterior 5th digit and ulnar half of 4th | Finger ab/adduction |

IP = interphalangeal

Gross G, Fetto J, Rosen E. Musculoskeletal Examination. Malden: Blackwell; 2002

## 5.2 Common Chief Complaints and Differentials

| Chief Complaint | Differential Diagnosis | Distinguishing Features |
|---|---|---|
| Pain | Osteoarthritis | Over age of 40, joint pain exacerbated by activity, relieved by rest |
| | Rheumatoid arthritis | Insidious onset, pain, stiffness and swelling of multiple joints |
| | Trigger finger | Snapping and locking of finger during flexion Palpable thickened flexor tendon |
| Swelling | Rheumatoid arthritis | See above |
| | Ganglion cyst | Overlays joint or tendon sheath |

## 5.3 Focused History
- See General History and Physical Exam for a detailed approach to history taking OPQRSTUVW questions regarding each complaint
- Hand dominance
- Location of pain (which fingers)
- Absence/presence of sensory changes (establish patterns in relation to nerve distribution)
- Absence/presence of stiffness or swelling
- History of repetitive movements (occupation, hobby, sports)
- Functional limitations

## 5.4 Focused Physical Exam

*Inspection*
- Carefully inspect for deformities, cuts, scars, and wounds with special emphasis on possible damage to nerves and tendons (see **Table 6** and **Figure 8**)
- Note any tenderness, redness, or swelling

**Table 6.** Common Deformities of the Hand

| Name of Deformity | Interpretation |
|---|---|
| Mallet Finger/Thumb | Trauma or RA |
| Swan Neck Deformity | RA, but has many other causes |
| Boutonnière Deformity | Trauma or RA Occurs when the central slip of the extensor tendon detaches from the middle phalanx |

| Name of Deformity | Interpretation |
|---|---|
| **Dupuytren's Contracture** | Nodular thickening in the palm and fingers. Associated with DM, epilepsy, alcoholism, and hereditary tendencies |
| **Heberden's Nodes** | OA often associated with a deviation of the DIPs |
| **Bouchard's Nodes** | Similar to Heberden's nodes, but affects the PIPs |

OA = osteoarthritis, RA = rheumatoid arthritis
Swartz MH. Textbook of Physical Diagnosis: History and Examination, 6th ed. Philadelphia: Saunders Elsevier; 2010.

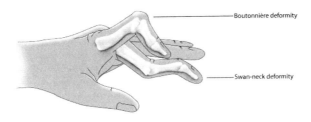

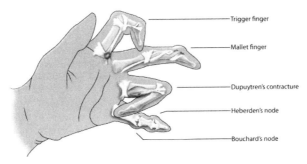

Caitlin C. Monney

**Figure 8.** Common Deformities of the Hand

### Palpation
- Compress the metacarpophalangeal (MCP) joints by squeezing the patient's hand between your thumb and index finger
  - If this causes pain, use your thumb to palpate the dorsal side of each MCP joint while using your index finger to feel the heads of the MCPs on the palmar side
- Palpate the medial and lateral aspects of each PIP and DIP joint (dorsal and volar surfaces) with your index finger and thumb

### Range of Motion
- Check for smooth, coordinated, and easily performed movements (see **Table 7**)
- Ask the patient: "Make a fist with each hand with your thumb across the knuckles, and then open your hand and spread your fingers" and assess
  - During flexion:
    - Normal fingers should flex to the distal palmar crease
    - Thumb should oppose the DIP joints
  - During extension:
    - Each finger should extend to the zero position in relation to its metacarpal upon opening
- Assess motion of the thumb: flexion, extension, abduction, adduction, opposition (movement of the thumb across the palm)

**Table 7.** Hand: Normal Ranges of Motion

| Movement | Joint | Range of Motion |
|---|---|---|
| Fingers | MCPs | 80° |
| | PIPs | 110° |
| | DIPs | 90° |
| Thumb | MCP | 0° extension; 50° flexion |
| | IP | 20° extension; 90° flexion |

IP = interphalangeal, MCP = metacarpophalangeal

Gross G, Fetto J, Rosen E. Musculoskeletal Examination. Malden: Blackwell; 2002

## Special Tests

- For intact flexor digitorum superficialis: restrict motion of 3 out of 4 fingers by holding down distal phalanges with the dorsum of the patient's hand (palm up) rested on a table; ask the patient to flex the free finger and look for PIP flexion
- For intact flexor digitorum profundus: hold down both the proximal and middle phalanges and ask the patient to flex fingers; look for DIP flexion

## 5.5 Common Clinical Scenarios

| Key Symptoms | Physical Exam Findings | Investi-gations | Management |
|---|---|---|---|
| **Cubital Tunnel Syndrome** | | | |
| Pain and paresthesia to ulnar 1½ digits, often from prolonged compression, can be sensory and/or motor | Intrinsic muscle weakness, ulnar distribution diminished sensation, | Nerve conduction studies | Modify activity, NSAIDS, splint, Operative decompression |
| **Trigger Finger** | | | |
| Finger clicking and locking in flexion (usually ring finger), pain at distal palm | Tender over distal palm near MCP, may be able to demonstrate triggering | Clinical dx | Night splint, steroid injection Surgical release |
| **Ligamentous Injury** | | | |
| Acute pain and swelling +/- deformity after acute trauma | Decreased ROM | XR if concerned about concomitant avulsion or fracture | Splint, rest, therapy for ROM |
| **Long flexor tendon avulsion (FDP)** | | | |
| Pain after forced eccentric DIP flexion | Finger rests at slight extension relative to other fingers, unable to actively flex DIP, tender volar distal finger | XR | First line: operative management |

### Arthritis (see Table 8)

| | | | |
|---|---|---|---|
| Joint pain (see chart below) developing slowly over several years, exacerbated with use | Deformity, nodes Muscle atrophy Range of motion testing Crepitus Palpate for osteophytes | Typically, a clinical diagnosis, but can use X-ray to confirm | Analgesics Physical therapy Exercise |

### Fracture

| | | | |
|---|---|---|---|
| Acute mechanism (FOOSH). Hand/ wrist pain. Need high suspicion of scaphoid fracture and scapholunate ligament injury. | Hand ROM, point tenderness (snuffbox), axial loading and circumduction of 1st CMC for scaphoid | AP, lateral, scaphoid views +/- CT | Cast immobilization vs ORIF; immobilize thumb for suspected scaphoid injury |

**Table 8.** Arthritis in the Hand and Wrist

| Joint | Osteoarthritis | Rheumatoid |
|---|---|---|
| **DIP** | Very common | Rare |
| **PIP** | Common | Very common |
| **MCP** | Rare | Very common |
| **Wrist** | Rare* | Very common |

MCP = metacarpophalangeal
*Osteoarthritis will sometimes affect only the carpometacarpal joint of the thumb Swartz MH. Textbook of Physical Diagnosis: History and Examination, 6th ed. Philadelphia: Saunders Elsevier; 2010.

## 6. SPINE
### 6.1 Essential Anatomy

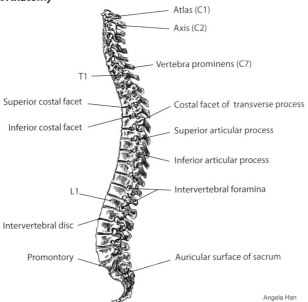

Atlas (C1)
Axis (C2)
Vertebra prominens (C7)
T1
Superior costal facet
Inferior costal facet
Costal facet of transverse process
Superior articular process
Inferior articular process
Intervertebral foramina
L1
Intervertebral disc
Promontory
Auricular surface of sacrum

Angela Han

**Figure 9.** Anatomy of the Vertebral Column

MUSCULOSKELETAL

## 6.2 Common Chief Complaints and Differentials

| Chief Complaint | Differential Diagnosis | Distinguishing Features |
|---|---|---|
| Pain (see Table 10) | **Degenerative disease (90% of all back pain)[10]** | Often non-specific pain |
| | **Mechanical problem (degenerative, facet)** | Difficulty with specific movements |
| | **Spinal stenosis (congenital, osteophyte, central disc)** | Neural involvement of a particular root |
| | **Peripheral nerve compression (disc herniation)** | Numbness/tingling throughout peripheral nerve distribution |
| | **Less commonly[10]:** | |
| | **Infection** | Fever |
| | **Cauda equina syndrome** | Acute weakness, loss of bladder and bowel function |
| | **Neoplastic (primary or metastatic)** | Constitutional symptoms |
| | **Fracture** | Trauma |
| | **Spondyloarthropathies (e.g. ankylosing spondylitis)** | Other joint involvement (ie. Hip and shoulder) |
| | **Referred (aorta, renal, ureter, pancreas)** | Often have other accompanying symptoms |

**Table 9.** Common Patterns of Back Pain[9-11]

| Etiology | Clinical Features |
|---|---|
| **Intervertebral Discs or Adjacent Ligament Involvement** | • Back dominant (back, buttock)<br>• Pain: worse with flexion<br>• Pattern: constant or intermittent |
| **Posterior Joint Complex Involvement** | • Back dominant<br>• Pain: worse with extension (never worse with flexion)<br>• Pattern: intermittent |
| **Radiculopathy: L4, L5, S1, S2** | • Leg dominant (below buttock)<br>• Pain: worse with back movement<br>• Pattern: previously or currently constant |
| **Neurogenic Claudication due to Nerve Compression** | • Leg dominant<br>• Pain: worse with activity and better with rest<br>• Pattern: intermittent (short duration) |

## 6.3 Focused Histories
* See General History and Physical Exam for a detailed approach to history taking
* OPQRSTUVW questions regarding each complaint
* Constitutional symptoms (e.g. Unintentional weight loss, fever, night sweats)
* Neurologic symptoms (e.g. weakness, falls, instability, numbness, bladder/bowel changes)
* Use of injected drugs, corticosteroids
* Recent procedures/surgeries

## Lumbar Spine
* There are 5 key questions that should be asked of patients who present with low back

MUSCULOSKELETAL

pain.
- Where is your pain the worst? (This will determine if the pain is leg or back dominant)
- Is your pain constant or intermittent?
- Does bending forward make your typical pain worse? (Alternatively, what are the aggravating movements and positions for your pain?)
- Since the start of your pain has there been any change in your bladder or bowel function? (cauda equina syndrome can present with bowel incontinence and bladder retention)
- What can't you do now that you could do before your pain developed and why?

## 6.4 Focused Physical Exam

### Cervical Spine
*Inspection*
- May be examined with the patient seated; in general, check for deformity, unusual posture, physical asymmetries, and guarding
- In normal sitting posture, nose should be in line with manubrium and xiphoid process of sternum; from side, ear lobe should be in line with acromion process
- Check for head tilting or lateral rotation; indicates possible torticollis
- Check for Klippel-Feil syndrome (fusion of the cervical vertebrae resulting in a short and relatively immobile neck; congenital)
- Check for venous obstruction in the upper limbs
  - Note any temperature changes, sensory changes, altered coloration of the skin, ulcers, or vein distension

*Palpation*
- Palpate for any tenderness, trigger points, muscle spasms, skin texture and bony/soft tissue abnormalities on the posterior, lateral, and anterior aspects of the neck
- Posterior aspect: external occipital protuberance, spinous processes and facet joints of cervical vertebrae, mastoid processes
- Lateral aspect: transverse processes of cervical vertebrae, lymph nodes and carotid arteries, temporomandibular joints, mandible, and parotid glands
- Anterior aspect: hyoid bone, thyroid cartilage, supraclavicular fossa

*Range of Motion: Active Movements*
- Ask the patient to perform the movements in **Table 10** below

**Table 10.** Active Movements of the Cervical Spine: Normal Ranges of Motion

| Maneuver | Range of Motion |
| --- | --- |
| Flexion ("Touch your chin to your chest") | 80-90° |
| Extension ("Put your head back") | 70° |
| Side Flexion* ("Touch each shoulder with your ear without raising your shoulders") | 20-45° |
| Rotation* ("Turn your head to the left and right") | 70-90° |

*Look for symmetrical movements
Gross G, Fetto J, Rosen E. Musculoskeletal Examination. Malden: Blackwell; 2002. Magee DJ. Orthopedic Physical Assessment. St. Louis: Saunders Elsevier. 2008.

*Range of Motion: Passive Movements*
- Flexion, extension, side flexion, and rotation should all be tested with passive movements to test the "end feel" of each movement (tissue stretch)

*Power Assessment/Isometric Movements*
- Flexion, extension, side flexion, and rotation should all be tested with isometric movements
- Determine muscle power and possible neurological weakness originating from the nerve roots in the cervical spine by testing the myotomes with isometric movements (each contraction should be held for ≥5 s) (see **Table 11**)

**Table 11.** Cervical Spine Movements and their Respective Myotomes

| Movement | Myotome |
|---|---|
| Neck Flexion | C1-C2 |
| Neck Side Flexion | C3 |
| Shoulder Elevation | C4 |
| Shoulder Abduction | C5 |
| Elbow Flexion and/or Wrist Extension | C5-C6 |
| Elbow Extension and/or Wrist Flexion | C7 |
| Thumb Extension and/or Ulnar Deviation | C8 |
| Abduction and/or Adduction of Hand Intrinsics | T1 |

Magee DJ. Orthopedic Physical Assessment. St. Louis: Saunders Elsevier; 2008

*Reflexes*
- Biceps (C5, C6)
- Triceps (C6, C7, C8)
- Brachioradialis (C5, C6)
- (see **Neurological Exam**)

*Tests for cervical radiculopathy*
- Wainner's clinical prediction rule*
    - At least 3/4 positive tests to rule in
        - Cervical rotation <60 degrees
        - Spurling's test (side flex neck toward affected side, compress in the directed of side flexion; positive test is reproduction of radicular symptoms)
        - Distraction test (patient is symptomatic at rest; while supine, cradle chin and occiput and apply distracting force; positive test is relief of symptoms)
        - Upper limb tension sign (while supine, stabilize the scapula, abduct shoulder to 110 degrees, supinate forearm, extend and ulnarly deviate wrist and fingers, extend the elbow and laterally flex the neck away – perform in this exact order while looking for reproduced symptoms)

*Cook, C., Hegedus,E. Orthopedic Physical Examination Tests: An Evidence Based Approach 2nd edition, Pearson Education Inc New Jersey 2008

## Thoracic Spine
*Inspection*
- Examine with the patient standing
- SEADS
- Inspect for
    - Kyphosis, scoliosis (an imaginary line drawn down from T1 should fall through the gluteal cleft)
    - **Adam's Forward Bend Test:** have the patient bend forward to see if there is a rib prominence (rib hump) on one side (an indication of scoliosis)
- Inspect for chest deformities
    - E.g. pectus carinatum, pectus excavatum, barrel chest
    - Note asymmetry
    - Look for symmetrical folds of skin on either side of the spine
- Look for differences in height of shoulders and iliac crests

*Palpation*
- Palpate for tenderness, muscle spasm, altered temperature, swelling
    - Usually done with patient sitting
- Anterior aspect: sternum, ribs and costal cartilages, clavicles, abdomen
- Posterior aspect: scapulae, spinous processes of the thoracic spine

*Percussion*
- Percussion of spine performed to examine for tenderness and irritability

MUSCULOSKELETAL

- Ask patient to stand and bend forward
- Lightly percuss spine with fist in an orderly progression from root of neck to sacrum
- Significant pain is a feature of TB and other infections, trauma (especially fractures), and neoplasms

### Range of Motion: Active Movements
- Ask the patient to perform the movements in **Table 12**

### Range of Motion: Passive Movements
- Flexion, extension, side flexion, and rotation should all be tested with passive movements to test the "end feel" (tissue stretch) of each movement

### Power Assessment/Isometric Movements
- Performed with patient sitting
- The examiner is positioned behind the patient and instructs the patient to resist movements of forward flexion, extension, side flexion, and rotation of the spine

## Special Tests
### Tests for Thoracic Outlet Syndrome (see p. 192 for definition)
- Look for evidence of ischemia in one hand (coldness, discoloration, trophic changes)
  - Bilateral changes are more suggestive of Raynaud's disease[10]
- Palpate radial pulse and apply traction to arm; obliteration of pulse is not diagnostic, but a normal pulse present on opposite arm may suggest thoracic outlet syndrome
- Paresthesia in the hand is usually severe
- May have hypothenar wasting; thenar wasting less common

### Reflexes
- Patellar (L3, L4), medial hamstring (L5, S1), and Achilles reflex (S1, S2) need assessment since pathology of thoracic spine can affect these reflexes
- Abdominal reflexes should also be tested to assess the mid-thoracic cord (see **The Nervous System** Chapter)

**Table 12.** Thoracic and Lumbar Spine: Normal Ranges of Motion

| Maneuver and Instruction to Patient | Range of Motion | |
|---|---|---|
| | **Thoracic Spine** | **Lumbar Spine** |
| **Forward Flexion: "Bend forward and touch your toes"*** | 20-45° | 40-60° |
| **Extension: Standing behind the patient at an arm's length, stabilize pelvis to prevent patient from falling; then ask: "Arch your back"** | 25-45° | 20-35° |
| **Side Flexion: For each side, ask patient to: "Slide your hand down your leg"*** | 20-40° | 15-20° |
| **Rotation: With the patient seated, ask the patient to: "Rotate toward each side"** | 35-50° | 3-18° |
| **Chest Expansion: Place a tape measure around patient's chest; note difference between rest and full inspiration** | Normal is >5 cm | N/A |

*With forward flexion, the distance from the fingers to the ground is measured; majority of patients can reach the ground within 7 cm. Other methods are:
  1) Examiner first measures the length of the spine from the C7 spinous process to the T12 spinous process with the patient standing. The patient is asked to bend forward, and the spine is measured again: a 2-7 cm difference in tape measure length is considered normal
  2) Examiner compares the length of the spine from the C7 spinous process to the S1 spinous process with the patient standing and with the patient bent forward: a 10 cm difference in tape measure length is considered normal. This measures thoracic and lumbar movement, but with most movement, 7.5 cm occurs between T12 and S1.
**With side flexion, distance from fingertips to floor is measured and compared with other side – should be same

Gross G, Fetto J, Rosen E. *Musculoskeletal Examination*. Malden: Blackwell; 2002.
Magee DJ. *Orthopedic Physical Assessment*. St. Louis: Saunders Elsevier; 2008.

## Special Tests
### Slump Test (Sitting Dural Stretch Test)
- The patient sits and is asked to "slump": spine flexes and shoulders sag while head and chin are held erect by examiner
  - If no symptoms (e.g. pain) are produced, examiner flexes the neck and applies a small amount of pressure
  - If no symptoms are produced, one knee is extended passively
  - If no symptoms are produced, the foot on the same side is dorsiflexed
- Process is repeated with other leg
- Positive test: reproduction of patient's symptoms (pain) may indicate possible impingement of the dura, spinal cord or nerve roots[10]

## Lumbar Spine
### Inspection
- Deformities or swelling
- Inspect for scoliosis, lumbar lordosis (see **Thoracic Spine**)
- Check body type of patient
  - ectomorphic (very little body fat)
  - mesomorphic (square body type, heavily muscled, minimal body fat)
  - endomorphic (large amount of body fat)
- Inspect gait
- Inspect total spinal posture (waist angles should be equal, "high" points on iliac crest should be the same height, leg length should be equal)
- Inspect for skin markings: café-au-lait spots may indicate neurofibromatosis or collagen disease
- Check for dimples and scars

### Palpation
- Tenderness, altered temperature, muscle spasm
- Palpate the paravertebral muscles
- Anterior aspect: with patient supine, palpate umbilicus, inguinal areas (look for hernia, abscess, infection), iliac crests, symphysis pubis
- Posterior aspect: with patient prone, palpate spinous processes of lumbar vertebrae and at the lumbosacral junction, sacrum, sacroiliac joints, coccyx, iliac crests, ischial tuberosities

### Percussion
- Same procedure as percussion for thoracic spine

### Range of Motion
- See **Table 12** for directions and normal ROM

### Power Assessment/Isometric Movements
- As described in thoracic spine isometric movement exam
- Myotomes are tested with the examiner placing the test joint or joints in a neutral or resting position and then applying a resisted isometric pressure that is held for ≥5 s (see **Table 13**)

**Table 13.** Lower Limb Movements and their Respective Myotomes

| Movement | Myotome |
|---|---|
| **Hip Flexion** | L2 |
| **Knee Extension** | L3 |
| **Ankle Dorsiflexion** | L4 |
| **Great Toe Extension** | L5 |
| **Ankle Plantar Flexion, Ankle Eversion, Hip Extension** | S1 |

MUSCULOSKELETAL

Magee DJ. Orthopedic Physical Assessment. St. Louis: Saunders Elsevier; 2008.

*Reflexes*
- Patellar (L3, L4), medial hamstring (L5, S1), and Achilles reflex (S1, S2) need assessment since pathology of lumbar spine can affect these reflexes

## Special Tests
*Straight Leg Raise (Lasègue) Test* (see **Figure 10**)
- The patient is in the supine position with the hips in a neutral position
- The examiner, ensuring the patient's knee remains extended, supports and raises the leg until radicular pain (back or leg) is felt
- This maneuver stretches the sciatic nerve
- Note the degree of elevation (pain usually occurs at <60° if there is an abnormality, as well as quality and distribution of the pain)
- Back pain suggests a central disc prolapse while leg pain suggests a lateral protrusion (ensure that pain is not due to hamstring tightness)
- The leg is lowered in increments until pain is relieved
- If dorsiflexion of the ankle results in a return of the pain, it is an indication of nerve root irritation (positive Lasègue sign)
- Paresthesia or radiating pain in the distribution of the sciatic nerve (L4-S3) suggests nerve root irritation/tension
- ***Note:*** the pain must be below the knee if the roots of the sciatic nerve are involved
- Compare with the other leg (with central disc protrusions, crossover pain may occur: e.g. straight leg raising on one side may cause pain down the opposite leg)

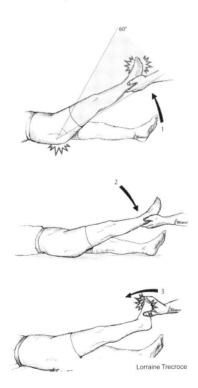

Lorraine Trecroce

**Figure 10.** Straight Leg Raise (Lasègue) Test for Nerve Root Irritation

MUSCULOSKELETAL

MUSCULOSKELETAL

> **Clinical Pearl:** Reproducibility of Physical Exam Findings for Lumbar Disc Herniation
> • Straight Leg Raise - 0.78-0.97 (*r*)
> • Neurological Exam:
>    • Ankle dorsiflexion (tested with the patient supine, they then dorsiflex the ankle against resistance. This is more precise than the patient's ability to heel stand) – 1.00 (*K*)
>    • Calf wasting – 0.80 (*K*)
>    • Note: 98% of clinically important lumbar disc herniations occur at L4 to L5 or L5 to S1 intervertebral levels, causing neurologic impairments of L5 and S1 nerve roots

### Femoral Stretch Test (Reverse Lasègue)
- With the patient lying prone, stretch the femoral nerve roots (L2-L4) by extending the hip (lift the thigh with one hand and use the other hand to maintain full extension of the knee)
- Limited hip extension due to pain radiating into the thigh suggests nerve root irritation

### Rib-Pelvis Distance
- Assesses height loss (due to vertebral compression fractures)
- Examiner's hands are inserted into the space between inferior margin of the ribs and superior surface of pelvis in the mid-axillary line while the patient is standing
- The rib-pelvis distance is determined in fingerbreadths to the closest whole value
- Normal distance is at least 3 fingerbreadths

### Screen the Hips
- Both osteoarthritis of the hip and a prolapsed intervertebral disc (at L2-L3 or L3-L4) are often confused with spinal stenosis

### Peripheral Vascular System
- Crucial to obtain a thorough history to distinguish between claudication due to vascular insufficiency versus spinal stenosis
   - i.e. vascular claudication versus neurogenic claudication
- **Claudication due to Vascular Insufficiency:** constant pain, worse with walking, occurs after walking a very consistent distance; involves stocking type of sensory loss; peripheral pulses usually absent; is rapidly relieved by rest
- **Claudication due to Spinal Stenosis:** relieved by changes in posture (sitting, bending, flexing spine) and rest; slower to be relieved of pain than claudication due to vascular insufficiency

## 6.5 Common Clinical Scenarios

| Key Symptoms | Physical Exam Findings | Investi-gations | Management |
|---|---|---|---|
| **Cauda Equina Syndrome (EMERGENCY)** | | | |
| Saddle anesthesia Fecal incontinence Urinary retention Bilateral lower leg weakness | Saddle sensation Decreased anal tone and reflex Muscle testing in lower limb – bilateral weakness | MRI spine (urgent) | Surgical intervention |
| **Thoracic Outlet Syndrome** | | | |
| Neck, shoulder and arm pain Numbness and weakness in arm, hands or fingers | Evaluation of cyanosis or edema of upper limb Palpate supraclavicular fossa for pain Inspect cervical spine and shoulders Neurological testing, including upper limb tension testing | X-ray MRI EMG | Physical therapy, stretching Nerve block Surgery if conservative treatment fails |

| Key Symptoms | Physical Exam Findings | Investigations | Management |
|---|---|---|---|
| **Sciatica** | | | |
| Pain, burning, or aching in buttocks radiating down posterior thigh to posterolateral aspect of calf<br>Pain is worse with sneezing, laughing or straining during bowel movement | Straight leg test (see **Figure 10**)<br>Neurological testing | Clinical diagnosis<br>Imaging only in patients with "red flags" | NSAIDs<br>Exercise<br>Heat/cold packs<br>Surgery if conservative treatment fails |
| **Cervical Spondylosis** | | | |
| Cervical pain – chronic suboccipital headache<br>Cervical radiculopathy – sensory dysfunction and/or motor dysfunction | Neurological testing<br>Palpation for pain | X-ray<br>MRI | NSAIDs<br>Physical therapy |
| **Whiplash** | | | |
| Suboccipital headache<br>Progressive onset of neck pain (peak at 12-72 hrs. post-trauma) | Range of motion testing (decreased active and passive)<br>Palpation for rigidity in neck | X-ray to rule out fracture | Exercises<br>Analgesics |
| **Scoliosis** | | | |
| Spinal twist<br>Back pain | Inspection of spine<br>Adam's forward bend test – if scoliosis, will have a thoracic or lumbar prominence unilaterally) | Primarily clinical | Surgery if severe |
| **Kyphosis** | | | |
| Back pain<br>Stiffness of spine | Inspection of spine | Primarily clinical | Surgery if severe |
| **Ankylosing Spondylitis** | | | |
| Insidious onset of low back pain (>3mo) in patients <40<br>Pain worse in the morning, improves with exercise and NSAIDs | Range of motion testing<br>Palpation of SI joints | Blood work for inflammatory markers<br>X-ray | Physical therapy and exercise<br>NSAIDs<br>Corticosteroids |
| **Prolapsed Intervertebral Disc (Herniated Disc)** | | | |
| Back pain<br>Movement restriction<br>Sensory changes | Range of motion testing<br>Palpation for pain<br>Neurological exam | Clinical diagnosis<br>Imaging to rule out red flags (CT or MRI) | Analgesics<br>Surgery if conservative treatment fails or symptoms worsen |

MUSCULOSKELETAL

| Key Symptoms | Physical Exam Findings | Investigations | Management |
|---|---|---|---|
| **Spinal Stenosis** | | | |
| Back pain with walking or standing, relieved with sitting or flexed position<br>Focal weakness or sensory changes | Range of motion<br>Palpation<br>Neurological exam | X-Ray | Analgesics,<br>NSAIDs<br>Physcial therapy, exercise<br>Bracing<br>Surgery if conservative treatment fails |
| **Neural Foraminal Narrowing and Radiculopathy** | | | |
| Pain, weakness and loss of sensation following a particular nerve root | Palpation for pain<br>Neurological Exam | EMG, CT or MRI | NSAIDs, steroids<br>Surgery if conservative treatment fails |

# 7. HIP

## 7.1 Essential Anatomy

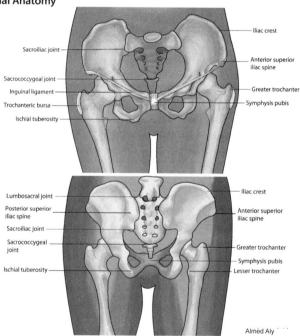

Sacroiliac joint
Sacrococcygeal joint
Inguinal ligament
Trochanteric bursa
Ischial tuberosity

Iliac crest
Anterior superior iliac spine
Greater trochanter
Symphysis pubis

Lumbosacral joint
Posterior superior iliac spine
Sacroiliac joint
Sacrococcygeal joint
Ischial tuberosity

Iliac crest
Anterior superior iliac spine
Greater trochanter
Symphysis pubis
Lesser trochanter

Almèd Aly

**Figure 11.** Anterior (A) and Posterior (B) Anatomy of the Pelvis and Hip Joint

## 7.2 Common Chief Complaints and Differentials

| Chief Complaint | Differential Diagnosis | Distinguishing Features |
|---|---|---|
| | Bursitis | Exacerbated by movement of gluteus medius tendon and tensor fascia lata |

| Pain | Osteoarthritis | Patient age over 40. Exacerbated by activity, relieved by rest |
| | Fracture | Trauma, severe pain when weight bearing |
| | Referred pain from LS Spine or SI joint | Accompanied by back symptoms |

## 7.3 Focused History
- See General History and Physical Exam for a detailed approach to history taking OPQRSTUVW questions regarding each complaint
- Functional limitations
- Specific inquiry regarding ability to get in/out of car, pain with putting on socks or tying shoes may point to intra-articular pathology
- Occupational History
- Constitutional symptoms (fever, night sweats)
- Trauma
- Hobbies, sports and recreation

## 7.4 Physical Exam
*Inspection*
- With Patient Standing
  - Inspect from the front and from behind for any pelvic tilting or rotational deformity
  - Note any abnormalities of bony or soft tissue contours (see **Figure 11**)
  - From the side, note presence of lumbar lordosis that may indicate a fixed flexion deformity
  - Observe the contour of the buttock for any abnormality (gluteus maximus atrophy or atonia)
- Examine Gait
  - Note antalgic gait (to avoid pain, time spent on injured limb during stance phase is minimized)
  - Note Trendelenburg gait (dropping of the pelvis on the unaffected side during the stance phase of the affected side)
- Trendelenburg Test
  - Ask the patient to stand on one leg
  - Pelvis on non-weight bearing side should not drop, indicating functioning abductors on the weight bearing leg
  - If the pelvis drops, it is a positive test
    - Can be caused by gluteal muscle weakness (mainly gluteus medius), inhibition from pain, or a hip deformity
- Measurement of Leg Length
  - True leg length: pelvis must first be set square and feet placed 15-20 cm apart; measure each leg from anterior superior iliac spine (ASIS) to the medial malleolus
  - Apparent leg length: apparent shortening (e.g. uncorrectable pelvic tilting) may also be assessed by comparing the distances between the umbilicus and each medial malleolus
  - Acceptable leg length discrepancy: ± 1 cm13

*Palpation*
- Anterior Aspect
  - Palpate the iliac crest, greater trochanter and trochanteric bursa, ASIS, inguinal ligament, femoral triangle, and symphysis pubis (see **Figure 11**)
  - Palpate the hip flexors, adductor and abductor muscles for signs of pathology
  - Palpate for crepitus by placing your fingers over the femoral head (which is just lateral to the femoral artery below the inguinal ligament)
  - Roll the relaxed leg medially and laterally to detect any crepitus
- Posterior Aspect
  - Palpate the iliac crest, posterior superior iliac spine (PSIS), ischial tuberosity, greater trochanter, sacroiliac, lumbosacral, and sacrococcygeal joints (see **Essential Anatomy**)

MUSCULOSKELETAL

*Range of Motion*

**Table 14.** Hip: Maneuvers and Normal Range of Motion

| Maneuver | Range of Motion |
|---|---|
| Flexion: with patient lying supine, have patient pull knee to chest; knee is also flexed | 120° |
| Extension: with patient lying on side, palpate the ASIS and PSIS and have patient fully extend the leg until pelvis shifts | 30° |
| Abduction: place one hand on the contralateral ASIS and with the other hand, grasp the heel and abduct the patient's leg until the pelvis shifts | 45° |
| Adduction: place one hand on the ipsilateral ASIS and with the other hand, grasp the heel and adduct the patient's leg until the pelvis shifts | 30° |
| Rotation: flex knee and hip to 90°, grasp the lower leg and move medially (external rotation) and laterally (internal rotation) OR with patient lying supine with the leg fully extended, roll the leg medially and laterally | External Rotation in extension: 45° External Rotation at 90° flexion: 45° Internal Rotation in extension: 45° Internal Rotation at 90° flexion: 45° |

ASIS = anterior superior iliac spine, PSIS = posterior superior iliac spine
Gross G, Fetto J, Rosen E. Musculoskeletal Examination. Malden: Blackwell; 2002

*Power Assessment/Isometric Movements*
- Performed with patient in supine position (except for hip extension where patient is on his/her side), noting which movements cause pain or show weakness
- Since hip muscles are strong, instruction of "Don't let me move your leg" ensures that the movement is isometric
- All active movements performed should be tested isometrically
- Sciatic nerve function (motor and sensation) should also be assessed

## Special Tests

*Patrick's Test (FABER (Flexion Abduction External Rotation) or Figure Four Test)*
- Patient lies supine, with both knees flexed
- The foot of the test leg is placed on top of the knee of the opposite leg
- Gently press down on the knee of the test leg, lowering it toward the examining table
- Test is negative when test leg is at least parallel with the opposite leg
- Test is positive when the leg remains above the opposite leg
- Positive test indicates an affected hip or sacroiliac joint, or that iliopsoas spasms exist
- Pain indicates early osteoarthritic changes

*Thomas Test*
- Used to assess hip flexion contracture (fixed flexion deformity), the most common contracture of the hip
- With the patient supine, place your hand under the lumbar spine
- Reduce lumbar lordosis by passively flexing the hip by bringing the patient's knee to his/her abdomen (or ask the patient to hold his/her leg against his/her abdomen)
- Elevation of the opposite thigh suggests a loss of extension in that hip (tight hip flexors) and a fixed flexion deformity
- Useful observations to accompany this test:
  - Note the degree of knee flexion in the free leg (knee flexion <90° suggests tight quadriceps)
  - Note the degree of leg abduction in the free leg (abduction of the leg suggests tight abductors and/or tight iliotibial band)

*Anterior Impingement Test (FADIR)*
- Used to assess for femoroacetabular impingement syndrome[14]
- Sensitive for intraarticular pathology, however not specific
- With patient supine, the hip and knee of affected limb are flexed to 90°

- The leg is adducted and internally rotated
- Sudden onset of pain, typically in the groin, is considered a positive test

## Ober's Test
- Used to assess for tight/short Tensor Fascia Lata and IT Band
- Patient lies on unaffected side with same hip and knee flexed to 90 degrees to stabilize the pelvis
- Examiner uses 1 hand to stabilize the pelvis and with the other hand under the top knee, flexes the hip 5 degrees, then abducts the hip fully and finally extends the hip, thereby hooking the ITB over the greater trochanter
- Next, the examiner releases the extremity and allows it to fall toward the table (adduct) with the force of gravity
- If the ITB is tight, the knee and ankle will stay suspended in the air

## 7.4 Common Clinical Scenarios

### Hip: Intra-articular/Anterior

| Key Symptoms | Physical Exam Findings | Investigations | Management |
|---|---|---|---|
| **Hip Fracture** | | | |
| Unable to weight bear Sharp pain in groin and down thigh | Injured leg is shorter, classically externally rotated Pain on palpation | X-Ray | Surgical intervention |
| **Avascular Necrosis** | | | |
| Joint pain Limited range of motion due to pain | Tenderness on palpation Limited range of motion | X-ray | Analgesics Assistive devices Arthroplasty |
| **Septic Arthritis/Transient Synovitis** | | | |
| Acute, atraumatic, unable to weight bear, fever/otherwise unwell, recent surgery or joint prosthesis | Unable to WB, looks sick | WBC, ESR, CRP, Arthrocentesis for gram stain and cytology | Surgical irrigation and antibiotics |
| **Femoroacetabular Impingement** | | | |
| Young, active patient, atraumatic groin pain worse with flexion and adduction type activities (sitting, tying shoes) | Obligate external rotation, decreased internal rotation +FABER, + FADDIR | XR (Dunn view for subtle lesions) Image guided anesthetic injection | Modify activity, steroid injection 2nd line: Operative removal of bony deformity |
| **Hip OA** | | | |
| Gradual onset deep pain and stiffness, worse with activity and weight bearing | Decreased and painful ROM (internal rotation), positive FADDIR | XR | Modify activity, analgesics, steroid injection Arthroplasty |

MUSCULOSKELETAL

| Key Symptoms | Physical Exam Findings | Investi-gations | Management |
|---|---|---|---|
| **Labral Tear** | | | |
| Deep groin pain, can have catching or clicking with activity | FABER + FADDIR (for intra-articular pathology) | XR, MRI, MRA | Modify activity, analgesics, rehab, steroid injection Labral debridement vs. repair |

## Hip: Extra-articular/Anterior

| Key Symptoms | Physical Exam Findings | Investi-gations | Management |
|---|---|---|---|
| **Snapping Hip (Iliopsoas bursitis)** | | | |
| Audible snap/clunk at inguinal crease when extending hip from flexed position, can be painful if bursa is involved | Patient can often reproduce problem by actively extending and internally rotating hip | Dynamic U/S MRI to r/o other intra-articular pathology | Activity modification, stretching Surgical release of iliopsoas tendon |
| **Pubic Symphysitis (osteitis pubis)** | | | |
| Midline pubic pain, worse with movement, especially stride and changing directions | Painful resisted adduction, tender over symphysis pubis | XR, bone scan | Rest, NSAIDs, activity modification |
| **Muscle and Tendon Injuries** | | | |
| Overuse vs acute pain, worse with specific activity | Observation for ecchymoses, Pain with active resisted contraction and opposite passive stretch, test specific muscles individually, focal tenderness to palpation | Clinical dx, U/S, MRI | Modify activity, analgesics, eccentric strengthening |

## Hip: Posterolateral

| Key Symptoms | Physical Exam Findings | Investi-gations | Management |
|---|---|---|---|
| **Greater Trochanteric Pain Syndrome** | | | |
| Lateral hip pain at or around greater trochanter, difficulty sleeping on affected side, tender to self-palpation | Palpation, Ober's maneuver (check ITB tightness/shortening), observe double and single leg squat mechanics (dynamic valgus and adduction = weak glutes) | Clinical diagnosis | Rest, NSAIDS, Stretch IT Band, Gluteus Medius strengthening, Consider steroid injection into bursa |

MUSCULOSKELETAL

| Key Symptoms | Physical Exam Findings | Investi- gations | Management |
|---|---|---|---|

**Piriformis Syndrome**

| | | | |
|---|---|---|---|
| Leg and buttock pain with radiation to lower extremity consistent with sciatic nerve impingement | Decrease in hip internal rotation | Clinical diagnosis MRI to r/o lumbar pathology if unclear | Modify activity, NSAIDs, rehab for strengthening, steroid injection Surgical Piriformis release |

**Hamstring Strain/Tear**

See "Muscle and Tendon Injuries" above

**Clinical Pearl: Referred Pain**
Pain referred to groin and thigh is HIP pain.
Pain referred to buttocks is BACK pain.

## 8. KNEE

### 8.1 Common Chief Complaints and Differentials

| Chief Complaint | Differential Diagnosis | Distinguishing Features |
|---|---|---|
| Pain | Ligamentous Injury | If acute, identifiable mechanism of injury If chronic, often associated with locking, catching or clicking |
| | Osteoarthritis | Pain with movement and pain on palpation. Decreasing joint ROM, grinding (crepitus), swelling and stiffness (Section 10.4) |
| | Systemic Illness | Not associated with trauma or overuse. Also will likely have constitutional symptoms |
| Instability | Ligamentous Injury | See Above |
| Effusion | Ligamentous Injury | See Above |
| | Systemic Illness (ie Rheumatoid Arthritis) | See Section 10.5 |
| | Meniscal Injury | Associated joint line tenderness, locking and clicking |
| | Infection | Constitutional symptoms. Recent TKA. |

### 8.2 Focused History
- See General History and Physical Exam for a detailed approach to history taking OPQRSTUVW questions regarding each complaint
- Occupational History
- Constitutional symptoms (fever, night sweats)
- Hobbies, sports and recreation

### 8.3 Focused Physical Exam
*Inspection*
- SEAD
    - **S**welling: note any swelling in knees; specifically, look at the medial fossa and any

bulging on the sides of the patellar ligament (indicative of small effusion)
- ♦ **A**trophy: inspect quadriceps for muscle atrophy (vastus medialis)
- ♦ **D**eformity: ask the patient to stand with his/her feet together; inspect for genu valgum (knock-knee), genu varum (bow-leg), genu recurvatum (hyperextended knee) or flexion contracture
- Gait
  - ♦ Patient will limit extension and flexion of a painful knee and minimize time spent on the injured knee while walking (antalgic gait)

*Palpation*
- Anterior palpation with knee extended
  - ♦ With the back of the hand, palpate the knee for temperature; compare both sides proximal to the joint, over the patella, and distal to the joint; normally, the patella is the coolest area of the knee
  - ♦ Palpate the anatomical structures noting tenderness, swelling or nodules; patellar tendon, tibial tuberosity, suprapatellar pouch (check for thickening or swelling of the suprapatellar pouch starting 10 cm proximal to the superior border of the patella), quadriceps muscles, medial collateral ligament
- Anterior palpation with knee flexed
  - ♦ Using thumbs, palpate the tibiofemoral joint line; noting the lateral aspect for swelling (meniscal cysts), tibial condyles, femoral condyles
- Posterior palpation with knee flexed
  - ♦ Palpate the popliteal fossa (for a Baker's cyst), hamstrings, and gastrocnemius muscles
- ROM: active movement
  - ♦ Flexion – 135 degrees
  - ♦ Extension – 0 degrees

*Range of Motion*
- While patient is lying prone, have him/her actively flex and extend knee
- With the patient supine, passively flex and extend the patient's knee by placing one hand over the joint, and one hand on the lower leg
  - ♦ Note any crepitus, clicking, and end feel of the motion
- Passive, medial and lateral movement of patella is also tested for mobility, symmetry:
  - ♦ Normally, patella should move half of its width laterally and medially
  - ♦ Note whether patella tilts, rotates or stays parallel to femoral condyles

## Special Tests: Tests for Effusion
*Patellar Tap Test*
- Place hand on the top of the femur, about 15 cm proximal to the patella, with index finger and thumb placed on either side
- Displace fluid from the suprapatellar pouch by sliding hand distally to just above the patella
- While maintaining pressure with the left hand, push down quickly on the patella with the tips of your thumb and 3 fingers of free hand
- In the presence of an effusion, a palpable tap (click) will be transmitted and felt by index finger and thumb on either side of the patella
- If the effusion is slight, the exam will be negative

*Fluctuation/Ballotment Test*
- Compress suprapatellar pouch back against the femur with your left hand as above
- With your right hand placed just below the patella, feel for fluid entering the patellar fossae, spaces next to the patella, with your right thumb and index finger
- If you feel fluid, confirm its presence by pushing the fluid between the medial and lateral fossae
  - ♦ **Note:** do not move the patella itself back and forth
  - ♦ Press the patella backward against the femur with your right hand and feel fluid returning to the suprapatellar pouch

MUSCULOSKELETAL

*Fluid Displacement/"Milk" Bulge Test (for detecting small effusions)*
- Place hand on the top of the femur, about 15 cm proximal to the patella, with index finger and thumb placed on either side
- Displace fluid from the suprapatellar pouch by sliding hand distally to just above the patella
- With the back of the hand, stroke upward on the medial side of the knee to milk fluid into the lateral compartment
- Stroke downward on the lateral side of the knee and observe for fluid returning to the medial compartment, distending the medial fossa
- The wave of fluid may take up to 2 s to appear
- Normally, the knee contains 1-7 mL of synovial fluid
- This test shows as little as 4-8 mL of extra fluid in knee
- This test is positive if the effusion is small and negative if the effusion is large

## Special Tests: Ligament Tests
*Anterior Drawer Test for Anterior Cruciate Ligament (ACL) Tear*
- With the patient supine, flex the hips to 45° and flex both knees to 90°
- Inspect the joint lines of both knees; a false positive can occur if the tibia was initially subluxed posteriorly due to a torn posterior cruciate ligament (PCL) (see **Posterior Sag Sign**, p. 201)
- Sit close to the foot to steady it, grasp the leg just below the knee with both hands, ensure the hamstrings are relaxed, and pull the tibia forward (see **Figure 12**)
- Compare both knees, noting any abnormal forward displacement of the tibia
- Movement ≥1.5 cm is indicative of an ACL tear (sensitivity 62%)[10]

*Lachman Test for ACL Tear*
- Relax the knee in 15° of flexion
- Grasp the distal femur with one hand and the upper tibia with the other
- With the thumb of the tibial hand resting on the joint line to detect movement, simultaneously pull the tibia forward and push the femur back
- This exam is the most sensitive test (84%) for ACL insufficiency[10]
- A positive test shows anterior tibial movement and a spongy end point

*Posterior Drawer Test for Posterior Cruciate Ligament (PCL) Tear*
- Perform the same maneuver as the anterior drawer test, including inspection for subluxed tibia, but push the tibia backward instead (see **Figure 12**)
- Movement of >1.0 cm is indicative of a complete PCL tear (sensitivity 55%)[10]

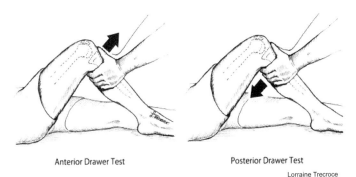

Anterior Drawer Test          Posterior Drawer Test

Lorraine Trecroce

**Figure 12.** Anterior and Posterior Drawer Tests for ACL and PCL Tears

*Posterior Sag Sign*
- Patient is supine with hips flexed to 45° and test knee flexed to 90°
- If the PCL is torn, the tibia drops back or sags on the femur; compare to the other knee

*Medial Collateral Ligament (MCL)*
- With knee extended, place one hand on the lateral aspect of the knee at the level of the joint

- Pull the lower leg laterally with the other hand, applying a valgus force  at the knee
- A positive test is indicated by pain and laxity on the inside of the knee
- Perform at 0 and 30 degrees of knee flexion
- Laxity at 0degrees indicates concomitant injury of other medial stabilization structures such as the medial capsule or cruciate ligaments

### Lateral Collateral Ligament (LCL)
- Place one hand on the medial aspect of the knee at the level of the joint
- Push the lower leg medially with the other hand, applying a varus force at the knee
- A positive test is indicated by pain on the outside of the knee

## Special Tests: Menisci Tests
### General Examination of the Meniscus
- Examine for joint line tenderness
- Discern if there is a springy block to full extension
- These two signs in association with quadriceps wasting are the most consistent and reliable signs of a meniscus tear
- Knee may also lock and click on movement

### McMurray Maneuver for Medial Meniscus
- Fully flex the knee and place the thumb and index finger along the joint line with the palm of the hand resting on the patella
- Externally rotate the foot and extend the knee joint smoothly with the other hand
- A meniscal tear is suggested if the patient's pain is reproduced or if a click accompanies the pain
- Asymptomatic, nonpathological clicks may be caused by tendons or other soft tissues snapping over bony prominences

### McMurray Maneuver for Lateral Meniscus
- Similar to the test above, but with the foot internally rotated

## 8.4 Common Clinical Scenarios

### Knee: Anterior

| Key Symptoms | Physical Exam Findings | Investi-gations | Management |
|---|---|---|---|
| **Patellofemoral Syndrome (Runner's knee)** | | | |
| Pain is a dull ache at the anterior surface of the knee. Worse when going downstairs, while squatting, or after getting up after sitting for prolonged periods | Valgus static and dynamic alignment, can have underdeveloped quads (especially VMO) No effusion, normal ROM, painful compression of patella | Clinical Dx, XR | Strengthen quads, glutes and other hip external rotators, stretch IT Band |
| **Patellar Tendinopathy (Jumper's knee)** | | | |
| Overuse mechanism, Anterior pain with jumping, localized to patellar tendon between inferior patella and tibial tuberosity | Painful resisted knee extension, tender patellar tendon | U/S | Modify activity, eccentric and ballistic quads strengthening, quads stretching |

### Quadriceps Tendinopathy

| | | | |
|---|---|---|---|
| Overuse mechanism, Anterior pain with jumping, localized to superior border of patella | Painful resisted knee extension, tender superior border of patella/ distal quads tendon | U/S, MRI | Modify activity, eccentric and ballistic quads strengthening, quads stretching |

### Pre-patellar Bursitis

| | | | |
|---|---|---|---|
| Anterior knee pain and swelling, directly over patella, excessive kneeling | Prepatellar swelling and tenderness, no true knee effusion | Aspiration if suspected septic | Modify activity, ice, NSAIDs,, compression wrap |

## Knee: Posterior

| Key Symptoms | Physical Exam Findings | Investi-gations | Management |
|---|---|---|---|

### Distal Hamstrings Tendinopathy

| | | | |
|---|---|---|---|
| Posterolateral or posteromedial pain with sprinting, knee flexion | Painful resisted knee flexion localized to area of pain, tender semimembranosus tendon or biceps femoris tendon +/-proximal tib/ fib joint | U/S if uncertain | Modify activity, NSAIDs, eccentric strengthening |

### Ruptured Baker's Cyst

| | | | |
|---|---|---|---|
| Acute posterior knee pain with radiation and occasionally swelling into the calf, can mimic s/s DVT | R/O DVT using clinical decision aids and physical exam may have knee effusion | XR, U/S, Doppler U/S, ABI | Rest, analgesics |

## Knee: Medial/Lateral

| Key Symptoms | Physical Exam Findings | Investi-gations | Management |
|---|---|---|---|

### Pes Anserine Bursitis

| | | | |
|---|---|---|---|
| Gradual onset anteromedial knee pain below joint line, can be painful with running or changing directions | Pain provoked by passive hip flexion + knee extension (semitendinosus), hip abduction + external rotation (gracilis), hip internal rotation + knee extension (Sartorius) Tender at pes insertion and along distal pes mass at medial knee | U/S | Modify activity, NSAIDs (topical or oral), Hamstring stretching and strengthening Steroid injection |

| Key Symptoms | Physical Exam Findings | Investigations | Management |
|---|---|---|---|

**Iliotibial Band Friction Syndrome**

| | | | |
|---|---|---|---|
| Lateral knee pain over lateral femoral condyle due to repetitive knee flexion/extension, exacerbated to activity, relieved by rest | Varus alignment, dynamic hip adduction, positive Ober's test, tender over ITB | Clinical dx | Modify activity, analgesics (oral or topical), stretch ITB, strengthen quads, hip abductors |

**MCL/LCL**

See below

## Knee: Intra-articular

| Key Symptoms | Physical Exam Findings | Investigations | Management |
|---|---|---|---|

**Ligamentous Injury**

| | | | |
|---|---|---|---|
| Acute and severe pain Acute ACL (tibial external rotation mechanism) injuries are commonly seen with MCL (valgus force) and lateral meniscus injuries | Effusion or hemarthrosis, instability,,bruising, limited ROM due to muscle spasm Positive Lachman, anterior drawer (ACL), Laxity on valgus stress (MCL) | MRI | ACL reconstruction if unstable MCL – rest, analgesics, ice, surgical management if refractory |

**Meniscal Injury**

| | | | |
|---|---|---|---|
| Pain localized to medial or lateral side Locking and clicking on flexion and extension Knee flexion/twisting mechanism (acute) vs degenerative meniscus (atraumatic, associated with OA) | Joint line tenderness on palpation + McMurray's test Effusion | X-Ray and MRI | Rest and NSAIDs Steroid Injection Surgical Management for mechanical symptoms Concomitant management of OA |

**Osteoarthritis**

| | | | |
|---|---|---|---|
| Gradual onset knee pain/ stiffness, intermittent swelling and functional disturbance, worse with activity, may have had a remote knee trauma history | Knee alignment (varus more common due to high incidence of medial compartment OA), gait assessment, effusion, decreased ROM due to pain or swelling, joint line tenderness, +/- baker's cyst | Weight-bearing XR | Modify activity, analgesics, general muscle strengthening, weight loss Steroid (or other) injection Offloader Brace Arthroplasty |

**Gout**

| | | | |
|---|---|---|---|
| Acute episodic knee pain and inability to weight bear, history of gout, history of renal stones | Decreased ROM, difficulty weight bearing, effusion | Arthro-centesis | NSAIDs vs colchicine, ice, rest |

**Septic Arthritis**

| | | | |
|---|---|---|---|
| Acute knee pain and inability to weight bear | Decreased ROM, difficulty weight bearing, effusion, systemically unwell | Arthro-centesis | IV antibiotics, emergent incision and drainage |

## 9. ANKLE AND FOOT

### 9.1 Common Common Chief Complaints and Differentials

| Chief Complaint | Differential Diagnosisx | Distinguishing Features |
|---|---|---|
| **Pain** | Ligamentous Injury | Identifiable mechanism of injury. Swelling, hematoma, loss of ROM, and inability to bear weight. |
| | Osteoarthritis | Chronic pain with weight bearing. Loss of range of motion. Often post-traumatic. |
| | Fracture | Similar to ligamentous injury. Pain over palpation of bony surfaces (see Figure 13). |
| **Instability** | Ligamentous Injury | See Above |
| **Effusion** | Ligamentous Injury | See above |
| | Fracture | See above |

### 9.2 Focused History
- See General History and Physical Exam for a detailed approach to history taking
- OPQRSTUVW questions regarding each complaint
- Occupational History
- Hobbies, sports and recreation

### 9.3 Focused Physical Exam
*Inspection*
- SEADS
  - Inspect the feet and ankles with and without weight bearing
  - Inspect bony and soft tissue prominences, noting any deformities or asymmetries, edema, scars, bruising, toe alignment, skin, or nail changes
  - Inspect the plantar surface of the foot for ulcerations, fungal infection, excess callous formation
- With the patient weight bearing
  - Inspect the posture of the ankle and foot anteriorly, posteriorly, and laterally, noting any splaying of the forefoot
  - With the patient standing, assess, from behind, for pronation (valgus) deformity of subtalar joint
  - Slip fingers under the arch to detect pes cavus (high arch) or pes planus (flatfoot)
  - Have patient stand on toes to differentiate between a flexible and fixed flatfoot
- Assess gait with and without shoes
  - Note the posture of the foot during walking (e.g. pronation of the ankle during the stance phase)

*Palpation*
- Palpate the feet and ankles
  - Palpate the bony prominences for tenderness and swelling
  - Note any temperature differences that exist between the feet
  - Place one hand over the anterior surface of the ankle and passively plantar flex and dorsiflex the ankle, noting any crepitus
  - Examine the pedal pulses and the more proximal pulses if required

- Screen for tenderness of the metatarsophalangeal (MTP) joints by compressing the forefoot between thumb and fingers
- To evaluate joints individually, firmly palpate the metatarsal heads and grooves between them with thumbs and index fingers

*Range of Motion: Active Movements*
- Ankle (Tibiotalar) Joint
  - Dorsiflex and plantar flex the foot
  - Invert and evert the foot; note that these motions involve the transverse tarsal and subtalar joints
- MTP joints
  - Ask the patient to flex and extend the toes
  - See **Table 15** for the complete list of active movements to be examined

**Table 15.** Ankle: Normal Ranges of Motion

| Maneuver | Range of Motion |
|---|---|
| Plantar Flexion | 50° |
| Dorsiflexion | 20° |
| Inversion of Heel | 35° |
| Eversion of Heel | 15° |
| Supination of the Forefoot | 35° |
| Pronation of the Forefoot | 15° |
| Toe Extension | Lateral Toes: (MTP: 40°, PIP: 0°, DIP: 30°)<br>Great Toe: (MTP: 70°, IP: 0°) |
| Toe Flexion | Lateral Toes: (MTP: 40°, PIP: 0°, DIP: 60°)<br>Great Toe: (MTP: 45°, IP: 40°) |

IP = interphalangeal, MTP = metatarsophalangeal
Gross G, Fetto J, Rosen E. Musculoskeletal Examination. Malden: Blackwell; 2002.

*Range of Motion: Passive Movements*
- Ankle (Tibiotalar) Joint
  - Test passive dorsiflexion and plantar flexion by grasping the foot proximal to the subtalar joint (or lock the subtalar joint in inversion) as subtalar dorsiflexion may be confused with ankle dorsiflexion
- Subtalar Joint
  - Stabilize the ankle with one hand, grasp the calcaneus with the other hand, and invert and evert the forefoot
  - This should be done with the ankle in dorsiflexion to lock the ankle joint
- MTP Joints
  - Steady the heel with one hand and flex and extend the MTP and interphalangeal (IP) joints of the great toe and lesser toes

## Special Tests
*Anterior Drawer for Ankle Stability (ATFL + CFL)*
- With the knee at 90° and the foot flat on the table, stabilize the tibia and pull the foot forward to detect abnormal movement
- Alternatively, immobilize the foot and shift the tibia backward

*Ligament Tests*
- When testing the integrity of each ligament, it is important to stabilize the lower leg
- Each ligament is preferentially stressed passively as follows:
  - Anterior talofibular ligament (ATFL): plantar flexion and inversion
  - Calcaneofibular ligament (CFL): inversion at 90°
  - Posterior talofibular ligament (PTFL): dorsiflexion and inversion
  - Deltoid ligament: eversion

## Ottawa Ankle Rules (*Figure 13*)

- The purpose is to discern the need for X-ray
- Rules do not apply to patients <16 yr
- Palpation of bone, not the soft tissue
- An X-ray is indicated in the presence or absence of bone pain if the patient cannot walk
- During palpation, note the presence of isolated medial tenderness
  - Palpate the proximal fibula to rule out a Maisonneuve's fracture (fracture of the fibular head and disruption of the interosseous membrane secondary to an ankle fracture)
- Sensitivity is 100%, negative predictive value is 1 (i.e. by applying the rules, no significant ankle fractures are missed)[17]

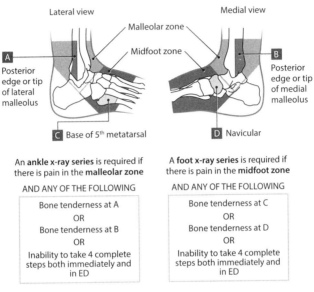

Marina Spyridis

**Figure 13.** Ottawa Ankle Rules

## 9.4 Common Clinical Scenarios

### Ankle

| Key Symptoms | Physical Exam Findings | Investigations | Management |
|---|---|---|---|
| **Ankle Sprain** | | | |
| Acute and localized pain with clear pattern of injury | Swelling, hematoma, loss of ROM, inability to bear weight | See Ottawa Ankle Rules for X-ray | Generally non-operative. Compression and rest followed by ROM and strengthening exercises |
| **Syndesmotic Injury (High ankle sprain)** | | | |
| External rotation mechanism, anterolateral and medial ankle pain, trouble weight-bearing | Painful passive external rotation, painful tibfib (At mid-calf) squeeze test, tender over syndesmosis | XR, CT | Stable: Non-weight bearing in boot x 2-4 weeks or until pain-free weight bearing Unstable: operative fixation |

**MUSCULOSKELETAL**

### Tibialis Posterior Dysfunction

| Key Symptoms | Physical Exam Findings | Investigations | Management |
| --- | --- | --- | --- |
| Medial ankle and foot pain with progressive loss of arch. Risk factors include age, pes planus, HTN, DM and local steroid injections[18] | Collapse of medial longitudinal arch. Swelling and tenderness behind and below medial malleolus. Weakness and pain with foot inversion. Persistent valgus hindfoot with heel raise.<br><br>Too many toes sign (foot pronation): more than normal (1.5-2) toes are seen along lateral border of the foot when examining patient from behind | U/S | Nonoperative: activity modification, rehab, ankle/foot orthosis; immobilization is controversial<br>Operative: based on stage of disease |

### Peroneal Tendon Subluxation

| Key Symptoms | Physical Exam Findings | Investigations | Management |
| --- | --- | --- | --- |
| Dorsiflexion injury followed by clicking/popping or sensation of instability at lateral ankle | Swelling and tenderness posterior to lateral malleolus, reproducibility of subluxation, apprehension with active resisted dorsiflexion and eversion | MRI | Immobilization and protected weight-bearing; majority need operative repair of torn superior retinaculum |

### Flexor Hallucis Longus Tendinopathy

| Key Symptoms | Physical Exam Findings | Investigations | Management |
| --- | --- | --- | --- |
| Plantar flexion injury or overuse followed by posteromedial ankle pain and locking of great toe | Painful resisted plantar flexion of IP joint of great toe, non-tender toe painful dddwewewewewe | Clinical Dx, MRI | Activity modification, NSAIDs, rehab, arch support<br>Operative: 2nd line |

### Achilles Tendinopathy/Bursitis

| Key Symptoms | Physical Exam Findings | Investigations | Management |
| --- | --- | --- | --- |
| Posterior heel pain, swelling, stiffness with activity (running/walking) or pain with shoe wear | Tender at insertion site or along distal Achilles tendon, painful passive dorsiflexion or resisted active plantarflexion<br><br>Thompson calf squeeze positive in full tear | Clinical Dx, XR, MRI | Activity and shoe wear modification, eccentric and ballistic rehab (heel drop protocol), NSAIDs, injections (still controversial)<br>Operative: for refractory cases |

| Key Symptoms | Physical Exam Findings | Investigations | Management |
|---|---|---|---|
| **Tarsal Tunnel Syndrome** | | | |
| Vague medial foot pain with plantar sharp/burning pain or numbness | Tinel's sign in tibial tunnel (posterior to medial mal), compression through plantar flexion/inversion, pain with passive ankle dorsiflexion/eversion, sensory changes, wasting of intrinsic toe muscles | EMG | Footwear changes and neuropathic agents Tarsal tunnel release after 3-6 months of failed conservative therapy |
| **Posterior impingement** | | | |
| Overuse or acute plantar flexion mechanism, posterolateral pain with active and passive plantar flexion | Tender or swollen posterolateral ankle, pain with both active and passive plantar flexion | XR, MRI | NSAIDs, activity modification, surgical excision of Os Trigonum as second line |
| **OCD** | | | |
| Traumatic or atraumatic, chronic ankle pain and swelling, sensation of instability | Effusion, tender to palpation, no ligamentous laxity | XR, CT, MRI | Immobilization and non-weight bearing 6 weeks vs operative (arthroscopy or ORIF/graft) |
| **OA** | | | |
| Stiffness, pain with weight bearing, reduced range of motion | Effusion, painful and restricted ROM | XR | Activity modification, NSAIDs, bracing/special footwear, intra-articular injection Operative management based on disease stage and patient factors |

## Foot

## Hindfoot

| Key Symptoms | Physical Exam Findings | Investigations | Management |
|---|---|---|---|
| **Plantar Fasciitis** | | | |
| Gradual onset posteromedial heel pain with chronic overuse, worst when getting out of bed and at the end of the day | Pes planus, Tight heel cord, tender medial calcaneal tuberosity | Clinical Dx | Stretching, analgesics, brace, shockwave, injections |
| **Heel Pad Syndrome** | | | |
| Obese patients, runners; plantar heel pain, painful heel strike | Tender heel | Clinical Dx | Activity modification, heel insert, injection |

## Midfoot

| Key Symptoms | Physical Exam Findings | Investi-gations | Management |
|---|---|---|---|
| **Tarsometatarsal Fracture/Dislocation (Lisfranc Injury)** | | | |
| High force trauma through hyperplantarflexed forefoot, resultant pain and inability to weight bear. Chronic injury results in foot deformity and chronic pain | Medial plantar bruising and midfoot swelling, tender tarsometatarsal joints, dorsal subluxation of TMT joint, | XR, CT, MRI | Immobilization 8 weeks if no instability or bony injury Operative management |
| **Midfoot Arthritis (various joints)** | | | |
| Midfoot and arch pain with toe-off | Antalgic gait, deformity, acquired arch collapse, tender midfoot and arch | XR | Activity modification, NSAIDs, footwear modification, injection Operative management |

## Forefoot

| Key Symptoms | Physical Exam Findings | Investi-gations | Management |
|---|---|---|---|
| **Turf Toe** | | | |
| Hyperextension injury to 1st MTP followed by pain, swelling and painful toe-off | Plantar swelling and ecchymosis, painful hyperextension of MTP, dorsal-plantar or varus-valgus instability | XR, MRI | Rest, NSAID, stiff-soled shoe, delayed rehab Surgical repair for severe injuries or failed conservative management |
| **Morton's Neuroma** | | | |
| Pain between 2nd and 3rd metatarsal heads, web space paresthesia, worse with tight shoes | MTP squeeze, palpable neuroma | Clinical Dx, U/S, common digital nerve block | Footwear modification, steroid injectionsurgical neurectomy |
| **Bunion (Hallux Valgus)** | | | |
| Difficulty wearing shoes due to medial eminence. Pain over the MTP joint | Proximal phalanx of the great toe is drifted, creating a valgus deformity. Gross deformity, pain and stiffness are seen. | XR | Nonoperative management with shoe modification. Surgical correction if conservative management fails |

MUSCULOSKELETAL

THE ESSENTIALS OF CLINICAL EXAMINATION HANDBOOK, 8TH ED.

## Other

**Charcot Foot**

| Key Symptoms | Physical Exam Findings | Investigations | Management |
|---|---|---|---|
| Progressive foot and ankle swelling, can be painless | Warm, swollen, erythematous, deformity (rocker bottom), sensory deficit | XR, MRI, ESR, WBC | Cast, footwear modification, analgesics, orthotics Operative management |

**Stress fractures**

| | | | |
|---|---|---|---|
| Navicular, 5th metatarsal, calcaneus, talus | | | See Orthopedics |

# 10. GENERAL MSK CLINICAL SCENARIOS

## 10.1 Fracture
"SAMPLE" Hx
- Signs/Symptoms
- Allergies
- Medications
- Past Medical Hx
- Last Meal
- Events
    - Mechanism of injury
    - High vs. low energy

Physical Exam
- Inspection
    - SEADS
    - Joint above and below
- Palpation
    - Swelling, deformity, temperature change, localized pain and severity
    - Neurovascular exam examining for paresthesia or loss of pulse
- Range of Motion
- Inspection of joint above and below the fracture
- Fracture Description (on imaging)
    - Open/closed
    - Involvement of joint (intra-/extra-articular)
    - Part of bone (epiphyseal, metaphyseal, diaphyseal – proximal, middle, distal)
    - Pattern
        - Transverse: fracture line is perpendicular to long axis
        - Oblique: fracture at 30-60
        - Spiral: fracture line is greater than 60
        - Comminuted: bone is separated into >2 components
    - Displacement
        - Angulation: distal fragment position relative to proximal fragment; orientation (degrees) of the distal bone fragment toward (valgus) or away (varus) from the midline
        - Translation: "sliding" (percentage) of distal bone fragment in relation to proximal fragment
        - Rotation: movement of distal fragment (longitudinal axis) in relation to proximal fragment
        - Impaction: bone ends are compressed together

## 10.2 Compartment Syndrome

- Increased tissue pressure decreases the perfusion and function of the tissues and nerves within the compartment
- Associated hx of trauma, hemorrhage, fracture or surgical procedure, external compression (cast)
- Perform motor and sensory exams, note 6 **P**'s:
    - **Pain** (most important clinical feature)
        - out of proportion to the injury
        - with passive stretch
        - with muscle contraction
    - **Pallor**
    - **Paresthesia** (late)
    - **Paralysis** (late)
    - **Pulselessness** (very late)
    - **Poikilothermia**

## 10.3 Osteoporosis

- Systemic disease characterized by low bone mass and micro- architectural deterioration of bone tissue
- Leads to increased risk of fragility fractures
- May present with height loss and a history of fragility fractures
- Diagnosed through Bone Mineral Density (BMD) testing
- Indications for BMD testing
    - Age (>65 yr)
    - History of fragility fractures
    - Family history of osteoporotic fracture
    - Vertebral fracture or osteopenia identified on X-ray
    - Systemic glucocorticoid therapy of >3 mo duration
    - Early menopause (age <45 yr)
    - Dietary calcium intake
    - Weight <60kg
    - Current smoker
    - High alcohol intake

---

**Clinical Pearl: Fragility #**

Refers to a fracture resulting from minimal or no trauma such as a fall from standing height or less. Common fragility fractures are distal radius, hip, vertebral and proximal humerus fractures

---

## 10.4 Osteoarthritis

- Degeneration of cartilage within joints, damage to underlying bone, and new bone formation at joint margins
- Disease occurs most commonly in weight-bearing joints
- Patient complains of pain with movement and pain on palpation
- Decreasing joint ROM, grinding (crepitus), swelling and stiffness, bony enlargement of joint, fixed flexion deformity, generally worse with activity, better with rest
- Hip OA
    - Pain most commonly in the groin, also presenting in the outer thigh, buttocks and knee
    - Decreased internal rotation and flexion
    - Leg length discrepancy is common
- Knee OA
    - Pain in the knee, thigh, or lower leg
    - Reduced flexion and extension
    - Varus or valgus malalignment

## 10.5 Rheumatoid Arthritis

- Systemic inflammatory disorder characterized by destructive hypertrophic synovitis
- Symptoms include:
    - Symmetrical peripheral polyarthritis causing pain and stiffness that is most

prominent in the morning and lasts >30 min
- ◆ Insidious onset with involvement of an increasing number of joints including wrists, elbows, shoulders, ankles, knees, and hips
- ◆ Systemic features such as malaise, weight loss, and low-grade fever
- ◆ Soft tissue problems such as carpal tunnel syndrome and flexor tenosynovitis
- Physical signs include:
    - ◆ Soft tissue swelling, tenderness, stiffness, erythema, and increased temperature of affected synovial joints (often peripheral joints)
    - ◆ Synovial effusions
    - ◆ Raynaud's phenomenon, tenosynovitis, carpal tunnel syndrome
    - ◆ Swan-neck and boutonnière deformities of the fingers, volar and ulnar subluxation of the fingers at the MCP joints
    - ◆ Diagnosis is made if ≥4 of the American College of Rheumatology 1987 Criteria are met: morning stiffness (>1 h, >6 wk), arthritis in at least three areas (>6 wk), arthritis of hands or wrists (>6 wk), symmetrical arthritis (>6 wk), rheumatoid nodules, positive rheumatoid factor, radiographic changes in wrists/hands10

**Table 17.** Inflammatory vs. Non-inflammatory arthritis

| Inflammatory | Non-inflammatory |
|---|---|
| **Major Types** ||
| Rheumatoid Arthritis | Osteoarthritis |
| Lupus | |
| Vasculitis | |
| Spondyloarthritis | |
| **Features** ||
| Painful joints | Painful joints |
| Joint effusion | Minimal swelling/effusion |
| Joint space warmth and redness | Minimal joint space warmth and redness |
| Morning stiffness >30 min | Stiffness after prolonged immobilization (ie |
| Improvement with NSAIDs | sitting) |

MUSCULOSKELETAL

# REFERENCES

1. O'Brien SJ, Pagnani MJ, Fealy S, McGlynn SR, Wilson JB. 1998. The active compression test: A new and effective test for diagnosing labral tears and acromioclavicular joint abnormality. Am J Sports Med. 26(5):610-613.
2. Michener LA, Walsworth MK, Doukas WC, Murphy KP. Reliability and diagnostic accuracy of five physical examination tests and combination of tests for subacromial impingement. Arch Phys Med Rehabil 2009; 90(11 ):1898-1903.
3. Gerber C, Krushell RJ. Isolated rupture of the tendon of the subscapularis muscle. Clinical features in 16 cases. J Bone Joint Surg Br. 1991; 73(3):389-394.
4. Bickley LS, Szilagyi PG, Bates B. Bates' Guide to Physical Examination and History Taking, 10th ed. Philadelphia: Lippincott Williams & Wilkins; 2009.
5. Swartz MH. Textbook of Physical Diagnosis: History and Examination, 6th ed. Philadelphia: Saunders Elsevier; 2010.
6. McRae R. Clinical Orthopaedic Examination. Edinburgh: Churchill Livingstone; 2004.
7. Foye PM, Stitik TP, Sinha D. Olecranon Bursitis. Medscape Reference. Available from: http:// emedicine.medscape.com.
8. D'Arcy CA, McGee S. The rational clinical examination. Does this patient have carpal tunnel syndrome? JAMA. 2000; 283(23):3110-3117.
9. Engstrom JW, Deyo RA. Back and Neck Pain. In: Longo DL, Fauci AS, Kasper DL, Hauser SL, Jameson JL, Loscalzo J (Editors), Harrison's Principles of Internal Medicine, 18th ed. New York: McGraw-Hill; 2011. Available from: http://www.accessmedicine.com.
10. Magee DJ. Orthopedic Physical Assessment. St Louis: Saunders Elsevier; 2008.
11. Vroomen PC, de Krom MC, Knottnerus JA. Diagnostic value of history and physical examination in patients suspected of sciatica due to disc herniation: A systematic review. J Neurol 1999; 246(10):899-906.
12. Storm PB, Chou D, Tamargo RJ. Lumbar spinal stenosis, cauda equina syndrome, and multiple lumbosacral radiculopathies. Phys Med Rehabil Clin N Am. 2002; 13(3):713-733.
13. Harvey WF, Yang M, Cooke TD, Segal NA, Lane N, Lewis CE, et al. Associations of leg length inequality with prevalent, incident, and progressive knee osteoarthritis: A cohort study. Ann Intern Med. 2010; 152(5):287-295.
14. Dooley PJ. Femoroacetabular impingement syndrome: Nonarthritic hip pain in young adults. Can Fam Physician. 2008; 54(1 ):42-47.
15. Karachalios T, Hantes M, ZibisAH, Zachos V, KarantanasAH, Malizos KN. Diagnostic accuracy of a new clinical test (the Thessaly test) for early detection of meniscal tears. J Bone Joint Surg Am. 2005; 87(5):955-962.
16. Juhn MS. Patellofemoral pain syndrome: A review and guidelines for treatment. Am Fam Physician. 1999; 60(7):2012-2018.
17. Stiell IG, McKnight RD, Greenberg GH, McDowell I, Nair RC, Wells GA, et al. Implementation of the Ottawa Ankle Rules. JAMA. 1994; 271(11):827-832.
18. Kohls-Gatzoulis J, Angel JC, Singh D, Haddad F, Livingstone J, Berry G. Tibialis posterior dysfunction: A common and treatable cause of adult acquired flatfoot. BMJ. 2004' 329(7478):1328-1 333.
19. What is Osteoporosis? Osteoporosis Canada Website. http://www.osteoporosis. ca/osteoporosis-and-you/what-is-osteoporosis/. No datheue.
20. Vath SA, Owens BD, & Stoneman P. Insidious Onset of Shoulder Girdle Weakness. Journal of Orthopaedic & Sports Physical Therapy. 2007; 37(3): 140-147.
21. Dandy DJ, Edwards DJ. Essential Orthopaedics and Trauma. Edinburgh: Churchill Livingstone/Elsevier; 2009.
22. Kane SF, Lynch JH, & Taylor JC. Evaluation of elbow pain in adults. Am Fam Physician. 2014; 89(8): 649-657.
23. Cook C, Hegadus E. Orthopedic Physical Examination Tests: An evidence based approach, 2nd edition. New Jersey: Pearson Education Inc.; 2008

# CHAPTER 8:

# The Nervous System

**Editors:**
Tiffanie Tse, BSc
Jeremy Zung, HBSc, MD
Brian Tsang, BSc

**Resident Reviewer:**
Fahim Merali, MD, MSc, CCFP

**Faculty Reviewers:**
Esther Bui, MD, FRCPC
Catherine Maurice, MD, FRCPC

## TABLE OF CONTENTS

# 1. COMMON CHIEF COMPLAINTS

**Table 1.** Common Chief Complaints[1,2]

| Symptom | Common Etiologies | Differential Diagnoses | Clinical Pearls |
|---------|-------------------|------------------------|-----------------|
| **Headache** | • Tension headache<br>• Migraine<br>• Cluster headache<br>• Neck pain<br>• Occipital neuralgia | • Trauma (Head/neck injury)<br>• Intracranial hemorrhage (ruputured aneurysm, spontaneous subarachnoid hemorrhage, hemorrhagic stroke)<br>• Neoplasm<br>• Other (pregnancy, idiopathic) | Rule out red flag diagnosis:<br>• Venous thrombosis<br>• Meningitis<br>• SAH ("thunderclap" headache)<br>• Reversible cerebral vasoconstriction syndrome (RCVS)<br>• Vascular dissection<br>• Vasculitis<br>• Intracranial hypertension |
| **Imbalance/Gait Disorders** | • Orthostatic hypotension<br>• Myopathy<br>• Radiculopathy<br>• Sensory ataxia<br>• Vestibular imbalance<br>• Spastic gait<br>• Cerebellar disorder<br>• Parkinsonism | • Supratentorial or cerebellar lesion<br>• spinal cord compression cauda equina syndrome (bowel/bladder dysfunction, severe back pain, sensory/motor symptoms). | Extensive differential diagnosis, therefore detailed history and physical examination is necessary for formulating diagnosis and management plan |
| **Monoplegia/ Hemiplegia** | • Cerebral lesions: stroke/TIA, migraine, seizure, MS, tumor<br>• Peripheral lesions: neuropathy or pressure palsies (trauma, DM, infection, neoplasm). | • brainstem lesions (stroke, tumours)<br>• spinal cord compression (cauda equina syndrome: bowel/bladder Sx, severe back pain, sensory/motor level). | Should first determine if the lesion is "upper motor neuron" vs "lower motor neuron" |
| **Muscle Pain and Cramps** | • Systemic disorder (dehydration, hypo $Na^+Mg^{2+}$-$Ca^{2+}$, uremia, TSH changes)<br>• Drug induced (hydralazine, penicillamine, alcohol)<br>• Denervation (radiculopathy)<br>• Familial (dystrophy)<br>• Myokimia | • myositis<br>• fasciitis<br>• rhabdomyolysis<br>• ischemia<br>• electrolytes abnormalities<br>• drugs/medication-induced | Blood work: TSH, CK, lactate. Look at vitals (fever), disproportionate pain (fasciitis, ischemia) |
| **Lower Back Pain** | • Mechanical: facet, bony destruction, osteomyelitis, spondylosis<br>• Neuropathic: DM, zoster, hematoma, autoimmune, abscess<br>• Non-neurologic: see clinical pearls section. | • cauda equina syndrome (assess for bowel/bladder function, saddle sensation)<br>• polyradiculopathy<br>• plexopathy | Rule-out non-neurologic etiologies such as: urolithiasis, retroperitoneal mass, ovarian cyst, endometriosis.<br><br>The localization can be difficult if there are multiple lesions |

NERVOUS

| Symptom | Common Etiologies | Differential Diagnoses | Clinical Pearls |
|---|---|---|---|
| **Visual Loss** | · Migraine<br>· Hypotension<br>· Seizure<br>· Uhthoff effect (MS)<br>· Refraction error<br>· Dry eyes | · Occipital lobe lesion/stroke<br>· Glaucoma<br>· Retinal detachment<br>· Occlusion of central vein/artery of retina<br>· Giant cell arteritis<br>· Intracranial hypertension | In order to best establish a differential dx, ask if symptoms are:<br>· Mono/Binocular<br>· Transient/sustained<br>· Acute/progressive |
| **Diplopia** | · Strabismus<br>· Orbital apex lesion<br>· Myasthenia gravis<br>· Cranial nerve palsy (III, IV, VI)<br>· Brainstem lesion<br>· Cavernous sinus lesion | · Brainstem lesions<br>· Cavernous sinus lesions<br>· Abducens nerve palsy<br>· Myasthenia gravis | Cavernous sinus lesions can also involve ophthalmoplegia, chemosis, proptosis, Horner syndrome, or trigeminal sensory loss<br><br>Non-localizing lesion such as intracranial hypertension can be associated with abducens palsy<br><br>Myasthenia gravis is associated with fatigability |
| **Speech Disturbance** | · Aphasia<br>· Dysarthria<br>· Apraxia<br>· Neuromuscular disease<br>· Extra-pyramidal disease | · Stroke<br>· Intracranial hemorrhage, other intracranial mass effect (tumour, cyst, infection)<br>· Broca's aphasia<br>· Dyspnea | In an acute presentation, consider stroke, especially if presentation is within thrombolysis window. |
| **Tremor** | · Parkinsonism<br>· Physiological<br>· Drug-induced (sympathetic stimulants)<br>· Metabolic abnormality | · Parkinson disease<br>· Wilson's disease<br>· Cerebellar lesion (tumour, infarct, abscess)<br>· Midbrain/rubral tumour<br>· Hepatic encephalopathy, hypocalcemia<br>· Hypoglycemia<br>· Hyponatremia,<br>· Hypomagnesemia,<br>· Hyperthyroidism,<br>· Hyperparathyroidism<br>· Vitamin B12 deficiency | Rest tremor is separate from other tremors and commonly found in Parkinson's disease<br><br>3rd ventricle lesions may present with head bobbing |

NERVOUS

| Symptom | Common Etiologies | Differential Diagnoses | Clinical Pearls |
|---------|-------------------|------------------------|-----------------|
| **Dizziness** | • Vestibular neuritis<br>• BPPV<br>• Meniere disease<br>• Stroke/TIA<br>• Migraine<br>• MS<br>• Perilymph fistula | • Vestibular neuritis<br>• BPPV<br>• Meniere disease<br>• Stroke/TIA<br>• Migraine<br>• MS<br>• Perilymph fistula | The clinical exam should include: gaze, smooth pursuit, saccades, OKN, vestibule-ocular reflex, vestibular nerve, position, gait, fistula testing, auditory exam.<br><br>CNS lesions often associated with: ocular motor abnormalities, ataxia, decreased level of consciousness |
| **Syncope** | • Cardiac (arrhythmia, cardiomyopathy)<br>• Hypovolemic<br>• Cerebrovascular<br>• Metabolic<br>• Hyperventilation<br>• Seizures | • Cardiac etiology (highly suspected if there is rapid onset, presence of palpitations, family history of sudden death [eg. long QT syndrome])<br>• Carotid artery stenosis<br>• Vaso-vagal episode | Ask for precipitating factors, posture, abrupt vs gradual onset, position of head/neck, presence/ duration of associated neurologic Sx, loss of consciousness, rate of recovery, sequela. |

CNS = central nervous system, DM = diabetes mellitus, Dx = diagnosis, MS = multiple sclerosis, OKN = optokinetic nystagmus RCVS = reversible cerebral vasoconstriction syndrome, SAH = subarachnoid hemorrhage, Sx = symptoms, TIA = transient ischemic attack

## 2. FOCUSED HISTORY[2,3]
• See General History and Physical Exam for a detailed approach to history taking

### Approach to a Neurological Problem
1. What is the chief complaint?
2. Where are possible lesions? (anatomical diagnosis)
3. What are the possible lesions? (pathological diagnosis)
4. Physical examination to help confirm or disconfirm hypotheses
5. Investigations (labs, imaging, others) to rule out localizations and etiologies.
6. Establish a diagnosis or review all the potential differential diagnosis again if a clear diagnosis cannot be made at this point.

### History-Taking

1. Chief complaint: Describe the presenting symptom (e.g. diplopia), do not make a premature diagnosis (e.g. 3rd nerve palsy).
2. History of present illness:
   ◆ OPQRSTUVWX (onset, palliating/exacerbating factors and precipitants, quality, radiation and distribution, severity, timing, effect on 'you' the patient, previous similar episodes (déjà vu), what does the patient think it is?, associated sx) regarding each complaint
   ◆ Focal vs diffuse symptoms
      ▪ Focal/asymmetrical--> traumatic, neoplastic, vascular
      ▪ Diffuse/symmetrical--> infectious, autoimmune, nutritional/toxic, metabolic, degenerative
   ◆ Complaint-specific questions
      ▪ Associated risk factors for diseases (e.g. stroke: hypercholesterolemia, hyperlipidemia, HTN, family history of stroke, etc.)

NERVOUS

3. Review of systems
4. Past Medical History: Medical, surgical, obstetric, psychiatric
5. Family history: Especially if hereditary condition is suspected.
6. Social history: Marital status, employment, toxin exposure, travel, animals at home, hobbies, exercise.

**Table 2.** What is the Lesion?[3,4]

| Type of Lesion | Signs and Symptoms | Examples |
| --- | --- | --- |
| **V**ascular | Acute (seconds) with focal deficits, HTN, fibrillation, bruit | TIA, infarction, SAH, ICH, vasculitis, vasopasm |
| **I**nfectious | Subacute (days, weeks), diffuse, headache, fever, nuchal rigidity, back pain | Meningitis, encephalitis, osteomyelitis, discitis |
| **T**raumatic | Identifiable event, focal, pain, tenderness, confusion, nausea/vomiting | concussion, SDH, SAH, vertebral fracture |
| **T**oxic / Nutritional | Acute/chronic, diffuse | Medications, substance abuse, pernicious anemia |
| **A**utoimmune / Inflammatory | Subacute, relapsing, multifocal/diffuse | Polymyositis, myasthenia gravis, GBS, MS |
| **M**etabolic | Acute/chronic, diffuse | electrolyte disturbances, uremia, cirrhosis, myxedema, sepsis |
| **I**atrogenic / Idiopathic | Error, known complication | embolization from coronary or carotid stent |
| **N**eoplastic / Paraneoplastic | Progressive, accelerating, focal, headache, back pain | Primary or metastatic tumor |
| **C**ongenital | Early onset, static, suggestive habitus | Hydrocephalus, cerebral palsy |
| **D**egenerative | Chronic, diffuse, familial | DMD, CMT, ALS, Parkinson's, Alzheimer's |
| **E**ndocrine | Past medical history | T2DM, hypoglycemia, uremia thyroid |

*Mnemonic: **VITAMIN CDE**
ALS = amyotrophic lateral sclerosis, CMT = Charcot-Marie-Tooth disease, DMD = Duchenne muscular dystrophy, GBS = Guillain-Barré syndrome, ICH = intracerebral hemorrhage, SAH = subarachnoid hemorrhage,
SDH = subdural hematoma, T2DM = Type 2 Diabetes Mellitus

## 3. FOCUSED PHYSICAL EXAM
- For a general approach to the neurological physical exam, see ("General approach to the neurological history")

### 3.1 Mental Status Examination (MSE)
The mental status exam can help identify neurological disease and help distinguish focal deficits from diffuse processes. Before making judgments about a patient's mental status, the examiner should ensure the patient is alert, cooperative, attentive, and has no language impairment.

- Mnemonic for MSE: ORAL
  - **O**rientation (place, time, person)
  - **R**egistration / recall (5min)
  - **A**ttention (WORLD backward, serial 7's)
  - **L**anguage testing (reading, writing, naming, copying, 3 step commands)
- For more detail on the complete MSE, see **Psychiatry**

**Table 3.** Chief complaints, differential diagoses, and clinical features of lymphadenopathy[5]

| Altered states of Consciousness | Description |
|---|---|
| **Clouding of consciousness** | Minimally reduced wakefulness/awareness, including irritability/agitation (especially at night) alternating with drowsiness. Patient inattentive and disoriented. |
| **Delirium** | More profound abnormal mental state characterized by fluctuations, disorientation, misperception of sensory stimuli and delusions/hallucinations. |
| **Obtundation** | Mild/Moderate reduction in alertness, less interest in the environment, slower psychologic responses to stimulation. |
| **Stupor** | Deep sleep or state of unresponsiveness from which the patient can be aroused with sustained and vigorous stimulation. |
| **Coma** | State of unresponsiveness, the patient cannot be aroused with sustained and vigorous stimulation. The patient may grimace in response to painful stimuli. |
| **Locked-in syndrome** | Paralysis of the 4 limbs and lower cranial nerves. Often caused by a lesion of the midpons, disrupting descending cortical pathways involved in motor functions. |

NERVOUS

**Table 4.** Language Exam[2]

| Components of the Exam | Examples | Aphasias in which Impairment is Expected |
|---|---|---|
| **Spontaneous speech** | Articulation, Content, Fluency, Prosody, Grammar | Global, Broca, Motor TC, Mixed TC |
| **Naming** | Nouns and objects with visual confrontation naming | Global, Broca, Motor TC, Mixed TC, Wernicke, Sensory TC, Conduction, Anomic |
| **Comprehension** | Simple to complex commands, Yes/No questions, multiple choices questions | Global, Wernicke, Sensory TC, Mixed TC |
| **Repetition** | From simple words to complex sentences, Concrete and abstract words | Global, Broca, Wernicke, Conduction |
| **Reading** | Including aloud reading, verify the understanding of the content | Global, Broca, Wernicke, Motor TC, Sensory TC, Mixed TC |
| **Writing** | Dictated and spontaneous words and sentences, including atypical and abstract words | Global, Broca, Wernicke, Motor TC, Sensory TC, Mixed TC |

TC: Transcortical

**Table 5.** Common clinical scenarios in patients with lymphadenopathy[1,6]

| Subtypes | Can the patient... | | | Where is the lesion? (Dominant Hemisphere) |
|---|---|---|---|---|
| | Speak fluently? | Comprehend? | Repeat? | |
| Global | N | N | N | Large MCA stroke |
| Mixed TC | N | N | Y | Watershed ACA-MCA + MCA-PCA |
| Broca | N | Y | N | Broca's area, frontal lobe |
| Motor TC | N | Y | Y | Watershed ACA-MCA |
| Wernicke | Y | N | N | Wernicke's area, temporal lobe |
| Sensory TC | Y | N | Y | Watershed MCA-PCA |
| Conduction | Y | Y | N | Arcuate fasciculus |
| Anomia | Y | Y | Y | Cortical/subcortical lesion or recovery from other aphasias |

ACA: Anterior cerebral artery, MCA: Middle cerebral artery, N: No, PCA: Posterior cerebral artery, TC: Transcortical, Y: Yes

## Glasgow Coma Scale (GCS)[7,8]

- Used to assess the patient's level of consciousness (originally created to assess traumatic brain injury)
- Scored as a total between 3 -15, assessing: eye opening (E), verbal response(V), motor response (M)
- As a general rule, a score of ≤8 indicates coma
- When testing response to pain, apply central pressure to the supraorbital region (deep pinching of the skin) or the sternum (firm twisting pressure applied with the examiner's knuckles) because spinal reflexes may occur with peripheral stimulation
- When testing motor function, use the score of the higher-scoring limb if patients have asymmetric motor abilities
- The GCS can reliably predict the outcome for head trauma, nontraumatic coma, ischemic stroke, subarachnoid and intracerebral hemorrhage, and meningitis[1,2]. However, it has some limitations:
  - An examiner cannot perform a full assessment in aphasic or aphonic patients, as well as those who have craniofacial trauma or are sedated
  - The GCS does not directly assess brainstem function

**Table 6.** Language Exam[2]

| Best Eye Response (E) | Best Verbal Response (V) | Best Motor Response (M) |
|---|---|---|
| 1. No eye opening | 1. No verbal response | 1. No motor response |
| 2. Eye opening to pain | 2. Incomprehensible sounds | 2. Extension to pain (Decerebrate) |
| 3. Eye opening to verbal command | 3. Inappropriate words | 3. Flexion to pain (Decorticate) |
| 4. Eyes open spontaneously | 4. Confused | 4. Withdraws from pain |
| | 5. Oriented | 5. Localizes pain (hand crosses midline or clavicle to remove stimulus) |
| | | 6. Obeys commands |

## 3.2 Cranial Nerve Examination[2]
- Cranial nerves may have sensory function, motor function, or both (see **Table 7**)

**Table 7.** The Cranial Nerves

| Nerve | Name | Function | S/M/B |
|---|---|---|---|
| **CN I** | Olfactory | • Smell | S |
| **CN II** | Optic | • Vision<br>• Accommodation<br>• and pupillary light reflex (afferent limb) | S |
| **CN III** | Oculomotor | • Innervates medial/superior/inferior rectus, inferior oblique, and levator palpebrae superioris<br>• Accommodation and pupillary light reflex (efferent limb) | M |
| **CN IV** | Trochlear | • Innervates superior oblique | M |
| **CN V** | Trigmerinal<br>V1 = ophthalmic | • Forehead, vertex of head, and tip of nose (see Figure 1)<br>• Corneal reflex (afferent limb) | S |
| | V2 = maxillary | • Lower eyelid, cheek, and upper lip | S |
| | V3 = mandibular | • Sensory from chin, except angle of the jaw (C2-C3)<br>• Innervates jaw muscles<br>• Jaw-jerk reflex | B |
| **CN VI** | Abducens | • Innervates lateral rectus | M |
| **CN VII** | Facial | • Innervates muscles of facial expression<br>• Taste to anterior 2/3 of tongue<br>• Sensory from skin posterior to ear, external acoustic meatus<br>• Corneal reflex (efferent limb)<br>• Lacrimation and salivation (except parotid gland)<br>• Stapedius tympanum | B |
| **CN VIII** | Vestibulocochlear (Acoustic) | • Hearing and balance | S |
| **CN IX** | Glossopharyngeal | • Innervates stylopharyngeus (swallowing and articulation)<br>• Gag reflex<br>• Taste to posterior 1/3 of tongue<br>• Salivation (parotid gland) | B |
| **CN X** | Vagus | • Swallowing<br>• Phonation and articulation<br>• Gag reflex<br>• Sensory from skin posterior to ear, external acoustic meatus, dura in posterior cranial fossa | B |
| **CN XI** | Spinal Accessory | • Innervates sternocleidomastoid and trapezius | M |
| **CN XII** | Hypoglossal | • Innervates tongue muscles | M |

S/M/B = Sensory/Motor/Both

## CN I
- *Sensory Testing*
  - **Smell Test**: test each nostril separately using cloves, coffee, mint; patient closes eyes and occludes one nostril; note unilateral vs. bilateral loss
- *Common Pathologies*
  - Nasal disease, head trauma, smoking, aging, cocaine use, congenital, chronic sinusitis, skull-base surgery

**Clinical Pearl: CN I Dysfunction**
The common cold is the most common cause of loss of smell.

## CN II
- *Reflexes*
  - **Pupillary Light Reflex** (see CN III/CN IV/CN VI)

- *Sensory Testing*
  - **Visual Acuity** (tests central acuity)
    - Test each eye separately for best corrected vision using a Snellen chart or near card (use a pinhole card if patient's glasses are not available); patient covers other eye with palm of hand, avoiding pressure on the covered eye; estimate best corrected vision
    - Snellen chart: numerator = distance patient can read chart, denominator = distance normal eye can read chart (e.g. 20/200: what the normal eye can see at 200 ft, this patient reads at 20 ft) (see the Eye Chart at the back of the handbook)
  - **Visual Fields by Confrontation**:
    - Face patient; patient closes left eye and looks into the examiner's left eye (examiner closes right eye)
    - Test using "counting" or "object" method in each of 4 quadrants (upper and lower temporal, upper and lower nasal)
      - **Counting method**: hold up 1 or 2 fingers in quadrant being tested and ask patient, "How many fingers?"
      - **Object method**: bring finger or a pen tip slowly toward the quadrant being tested; ask patient to "Tell me when you first notice the object"
      - Repeat for the other eye
  - **Visual extinction**: patient looks with both eyes uncovered into examiner's eyes; simultaneously hold up fingers to both sides of the visual field and ask "How many fingers?"
    - Neglect of visual field can suggest a parietal lesion (see Ophthalmological Exam, Figure 3, p.236)
  - **Color Test**: have patient read Ishihara plates

- *Fundoscopic Exam* (see Ophthalmological Exam, p.241)

- *Common Pathologies*
  - optic neuropathy, papilledema

## CN III/CN IV/CN VI
- *Visual Inspection:*
  - **General**: ptosis, pupil size/shape/asymmetry, eye position, resting nystagmus; defects may help localize lesions
  - **Eye Alignment**: hold penlight in front of patient; patient looks straight ahead into the distance; normal: location of light in center of both pupils

- *Motor Testing*
  - **Smooth pursuit:** patient tracks a target without moving his/her head; move the target through an "H" pattern, pausing at the ends to observe for endpoint

nystagmus; normal if absent binocular diplopia and absent nystagmus
- ◆ **Saccades:** patient shifts gaze quickly between two closely placed targets (e.g. examiner's nose and index finger) in the horizontal then vertical directions; normal if eyes move together and find targets quickly

- *Reflexes*
  - ◆ **Accommodation reflex:** patient alternates between focusing on a distant object and an object held 10-15 cm from the nose; normal if eye convergence and pupil constriction observed at the near object
  - ◆ **Pupillary Light Reflex**: dim lights; as the patient looks into the distance, shine light obliquely into pupils; normal if direct and consensual responses present

- *Sensory Testing*
  - ◆ **Swinging Light Test[3]:**
    - ▪ Shine light in eye A, then swing light to eye B
    - ▪ If CN II of B is damaged, A and B will paradoxically dilate when light is swung to B
      - Neither A or B will constrict when light is at B, but both will constrict when light is at A
      - B will have more consensual response (when light is at A) than direct response (when light is at B)
      - This describes a relative afferent pupillary defect (RAPD) or a "Marcus Gunn pupil" in eye B
    - ▪ If CN III of B is damaged but CN II is intact, no pupillary constriction in B will be observed
      - Light at B will cause a consensual response in A
      - Light in A will cause a direct response in A

- *Common Pathologies*: see Table 9

>
> **Clinical Pearl: RAPD and MS**
> RAPD is an important finding in optic neuritis, which is common in MS.

**Table 8.** Afferent and efferent limbs of common reflexes[2,9]

| Reflex | Afferent limb | Efferent limb |
|---|---|---|
| **Pupillary light reflex** | CN II (Optic) | CN III (Oculomotor) |
| **Corneal reflex** | CN V1 (Trigeminal) | CN VII (Facial) |
| **Jaw jerk reflex** | CN V3 (Trigeminal) | CN V3 (Trigeminal) |
| **Gag reflex** | CN IX (Glossopharyngeal) | CN X (Vagus) |

**Table 9.** Defects of CN III, IV, VI

| Presentation | Location of Lesion |
|---|---|
| Eye position down and out, ptosis, mydriasis | CN III palsy (complete) |
| Ptosis, miosis, anhydrosis, pseudoenophthalmosis (Horner's syndrome) | Sympathetic pathway |
| Vertical diplopia on down and medial gaze (e.g. walking down stairs) | CN IV palsy |
| Difficulty looking laterally | CN VI palsy |
| Impaired adduction of ipsilateral eye and nystagmus in abduction of contralateral eye | Medial longitudinal fasciculus (MLF) internuclear ophthalmoplegia (can suggest MS) |

## CN V

- *Visual Inspection:* temporal wasting, jaw alignment with open mouth (jaw deviates toward side with lower motor neuron [LMN] lesion)

> **Clinical Pearl: Congenital Horner's**
> Congenital Horner's associated with additional iris depigmentation (i.e. blue coloured iris on affected side.

- *Motor Testing:* ask patient to
  - "Clench your teeth": palpate masseter and temporalis muscles
  - "Open your mouth against resistance": lateral pterygoids
  - "Divert your jaw to the side against resistance": medial and lateral pterygoids

- *Reflexes*
  - **Corneal reflex**: patient looks up and away as examiner approaches with a piece of cotton/tissue from side; touch sclera avoiding the eyelashes or conjunctiva; normal if direct and consensual blink response is observed
  - **Jaw jerk reflex**: patient opens mouth slightly; place finger over patient's chin and tap downward with reflex hammer; normal if elevation is minimal; increased reflex = pseudobulbar palsy

- *Sensory Testing* over areas innervated by V1, V2, V3
  - **Light touch**: patient closes eyes; apply tip of cotton wool at single spot and have patient respond with "yes" when contact is made; compare both sides of forehead (V1), upper lip/cheeks (V2), and lower lip/chin (V3);
    - avoid nose (V1) and angle of jaw (C2-C3) (see Figure 1 for trigeminal dermatomes)
    - avoid multiple swipes in the same spot, as this can result in summation and underappreciation of subtle regions of hypoesthesia
  - **Pain**: patient closes eyes; vary application of end of broken tongue depressor vs. rounded end in same distribution as for light touch; have patient respond with "sharp" or "dull" when contact is made
  - **Temperature**: use a cold tuning fork (if necessary run it under cold water) and apply it to the same distribution as for light touch and pain; have patient respond with "cold" when contact is made

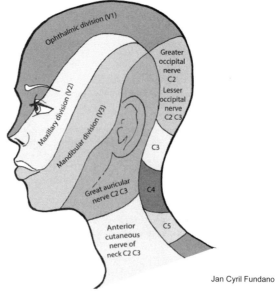

Jan Cyril Fundano

**Figure 1**. Trigeminal Dermatomes

# CN VII

- *Visual Inspection*: nasolabial fold (e.g. flattened), palpebral fissure (e.g. eyelid retracted), mouth (e.g. drooping), involuntary facial movements

- *Motor Testing*
  - "Raise your eyebrows": frontalis
  - Close your eyes tight and don't let me open them": orbicularis ocul
  - "Show me your teeth": buccinator
  - "Puff your cheeks out and don't let me pop them": orbicularis oris
  - "Show me your bottom teeth only": platysma

- *Reflexes*
  - **Corneal Reflex** (see above)

- *Sensory Testing*
  - **Taste**: patient sticks out tongue; touch each side of tongue on anterior 2/3 (CN VII) and posterior 1/3 (CN IX) with 4 primary tastes (sweet = sugar, salty = salt, sour = vinegar, bitter = quinine); keeping tongue protruded, ask patient to point to taste perceived on card displaying taste options; provide sip of water between test

- *Common Pathologies*
  - **LMN lesion** (e.g. Bell`s palsy): ipsilateral facial paralysis, including forehead
  - **UMN lesion** (e.g. cortex, corticobulbar tract): contralateral partial facial paralysis; forehead relatively spared

# CN VIII

- *Visual Inspection*
  - Mnemonic SEADS: Scarring, Erythema, Atrophy / Asymmetry, Deformity / Discharge, Swelling

- *Sensory Testing*
  - **Whisper Test**: mask sounds entering one ear by rubbing tragus or snapping fingers; whisper numbers/letters into other ear and ask patient to repeat
  - **Rinne Test**: strike 512 Hz tuning fork and place on patient's mastoid process; ask patient to indicate when sound disappears; immediately place tines of fork in front of auditory canal without touching ear; normal if patient notes the reappearance of sound (air > bone conduction)
  - **Weber Test**: strike 512 Hz tuning fork and place on patient's forehead in midline; normal if there is an absence of sound lateralization (equal on both sides)
    - Rinne and Weber tests can be used to differentiate between conductive and sensorineural hearing loss (see Table 10)

- *Vestibular Function*: not usually tested in office setting except for
  - **Romberg test** (see Sensory Examination, p.191)
  - **Positional nystagmus**: induced with changes in head position
  - **Gaze-evoked nystagmus**: induced at extreme eccentricities of gaze (see CN III/CN IV/CN VI, p.177)

- *Common Pathologies*: see Table 10

**Table 10.** Defects of CN VIII

| Pathology | Rinne (affected ear) | Weber |
|---|---|---|
| **Normal** | Air > Bone Conduction | No lateralization |
| **Conductive Loss** | Bone > Air Conduction | Lateralization to affected ear |
| **Sensorineural Loss** | Air > Bone Conduction | Lateralization to unaffected ear |

NERVOUS

**Clinical Pearl: Conductive Deafness**
Wax is the most common cause of conductive deafness.

## CN IX/CN X

- *Visual Inspection*
  - ◆ Mnemonic SEADS: Scarring, Erythema, Atrophy / Asymmetry, Deformity / Discharge, Swelling

- *Motor Testing*
  - ◆ **Palatal Elevation**: depress patient's tongue with tongue depressor; ask patient to "Say Ahh"; normal if elevation of soft palate and uvula is symmetrical (uvula deviates to unaffected side)
  - ◆ **Swallowing**: ask patient to swallow a sip of water; normal if there is no retrograde passage of water through nose after the nasopharynx is closed off
  - ◆ **Articulation**: ask patient to say "Pa Pa Pa" (labial), "La La La" (lingual), "Ka Ka Ka" (palatal), "Ga Ga Ga" (guttural)
    - ▪ Note that CN V, VII, IX, X, XII are all involved in articulation; CN IX and X are specifically involved in guttural and palatal articulation

- *Reflexes*
  - ◆ **Gag Reflex:** touch posterior wall of pharynx with tongue depressor; normal if palate moves up, pharyngeal muscles contract, uvula remains midline, and palatal arches do not droop
    - ▪ Note: CN IX is the afferent limb, CN X is the efferent limb of this reflex
    - ▪ The gag reflex is normally only tested in patients with suspected brainstem pathology, impaired consciousness, or impaired swallowing
    - ▪ Note: an absent gag reflex can be normal

- *Sensory Testing*
  - ◆ **Taste:** (see CN VII, p.179)

**Clinical Pearl: Deviations of Uvula and Tongue**
Uvula deviates to the unaffected side; jaw and tongue deviate to the affected side.

## CN XI

- *Visual Inspection:* neck and shoulder; look for fasciculations, atrophy, asymmetry

- *Motor Testing*
  - ◆ "Shrug your shoulders" (with and without resistance): trapezius
  - ◆ "Turn your head to the side" (with and without resistance): sternocleidomastoid

- *Common Pathologies*
  - ◆ Weak trapezius: shrugging of shoulders on the ipsilateral side is impaired
  - ◆ Weak sternocleidomastoid: turning head to the contralateral side is impaired

## CN XII

- *Visual Inspection:* tongue at rest in the floor of the mouth; look for fasciculations, atrophy, asymmetry

- *Motor Testing*
  - ◆ "Stick your tongue out and move it side-to-side"; normal if protrusion of tongue is symmetrical (tongue deviates to affected side)
  - ◆ "Push your tongue into your cheek" (with and without resistance)

**Table 11.** Causes of Multiple CN Abnormalities

| CN Combination | Likely Cause |
|---|---|
| Unilateral III, IV, V1, V2, VI | Cavernous sinus lesion |
| Unilateral V, VII, VIII | Cerebellopontine angle lesion |
| Unilateral IX, X, XI | Jugular foramen syndrome |
| Bilateral X, XI, XII | Bulbar palsy (LMN), pseudobulbar palsy (UMN) |

**Clinical Pearl: Correcting for Facial Weakness**
If there is facial weakness, support the upper lip on the side of weakness; otherwise, the tongue may erroneously appear to deviate. Once the facial weakness is corrected for, the tongue will no longer appear to deviate.

### 3.3 Motor and Reflexes Examination
- Considerations for pathology:
  - UMN vs. LMN pattern (see Table 12)
  - Pyramidal (corticospinal tract) vs. extrapyramidal tract lesion
  - Localization to specific root or peripheral nerve

**Table 12.** Pattern of Upper and Lower Motor Neuron Lesions

**Table 12a.** Upper Motor Neuron Lesions

| Level of Lesion | Signs and Symptoms |
|---|---|
| Cortex | Seizures, hemianopsia, aphasia, hemineglect, forced eye deviation, contralateral hemiparesis, cortical sensory loss, disordered consciousness |
| Thalamus | Hemisensory change, may mimic cortex-level symptoms, |
| Basal Ganglia | Tremor, bradykinesia, rigidity, involuntary movements (chorea, dystonia) |
| Brainstem | Cranial nerve deficits (diplopia, dysphagia, dysarthria, hearing loss, vertigo), crossed hemiplegia or sensory loss (ipsilateral face, contralateral body) |
| Cerebellum | Ipsilateral ataxia, dysmetria, intention tremor, dysdiadochokinesia, wide-based gait, staggering, lurching, scanning speech (explosive with pauses), nystagmus |
| Spinal Cord | Bilateral distal motor/sensory deficits sparing face, sensory level, bowel/bladder incontinence, sexual dysfunction, saddle anesthesia |

**Table 12b.** Lower Motor Neuron Lesions

| Level of Lesion | Signs and Symptoms |
|---|---|
| Lower Motor Neuron (anterior horn) | Diffuse weakness, fasciculations, atrophy |
| Nerve Root | Myotomal/dermatomal deficits, radiating back/neck pain |
| Plexus | Muscle weakness, atrophy, sensory loss, pain |
| Peripheral Nerve | Glove/stocking paresthesia, distal paresis e.g. footdrop, areflexia |
| Neuromuscular Junction | Fatigable muscle weakness (e.g. upgaze), bulbar (fluctuating diplopia, ptosis, dysphagia, nasal speech) |
| Muscle | symmetric proximal weakness (e.g. climbing stairs, combing hair), myalgia, usually preserved reflexes |

NERVOUS

**Table 12c.** Comparing Upper and Lower Motor Neuron Lesions

| | UMN Lesion | LMN Lesion |
|---|---|---|
| **Appearance** | Atrophy of disuse, arms flexsed, legs extended | Atrophy, fasciculations |
| **Power** | Extensors < Flexors in upper extremities Extensors > Flexors in lower extremities | Weak / absent in myotomal pattern |
| **Tone** | Increased / spastic | Decreased |
| **Coordination** | Limited assessment due to weakness | |
| **Reflexes** <br> • Superficial <br> • Deep <br> • Plantar[10] | • Absent <br> • Increased clonus <br> • Upgoing (dorsiflexion of big toe) | • Absent <br> • Decreased <br> • Downgoing (plantar flexion of big toe) |

## Inspection[1, 11-13]

- *Muscle bulk* (atrophy, hypertrophy, abnormal bulging/depression); distribution of muscle wasting can suggest possible causes (see **Table 12c**)
- *Symmetry*
- *Fasciculations:* quivering of the muscle under skin; typically benign, may be associated with LMN lesion (e.g. ALS)
- Abnormal movements and positioning (see **Table 14**)

**Table 13.** Distribution of Muscle Wasting or Weakness

| Pattern | Possible Causes |
|---|---|
| **Focal (one limb)** | Nerve root or peripheral nerve pathology |
| **Proximal (bilateral)** | Myopathy (no sensory loss) |
| **Distal (bilateral)** | Peripheral neuropathy (distal sensory loss) |

**Table 14.** Abnormal Movements and Positioning[14]

| Movement | Description | Possible Causes |
|---|---|---|
| **Asterixis** | Brief, jerky downward movements of the wrist when patient extends both arms with wrists dorsiflexed, palms forward and eyes closed | • Toxic/metabolic encephalopathies <br> • Electrolyte disturbances <br> • Wilson's disease |
| **Tics** | nvoluntary contractions of single muscles or groups of muscles, suppressive, associated with sense of relief | • Tourette syndrome |
| **Myoclonus** | Sudden, rapid muscle jerk; may be focal, unilateral or bilateral | • Epilepsy <br> • CNS injury/infection <br> • Neurodegenerative disease |
| **Athetosis** | Repetitive, involuntary, slow, sinuous, writhing movements, especially severe in the hands | • Perinatal hypoxia <br> • Kernicterus <br> • Huntington's disease <br> • Antipsychotics/antiemetics |
| **Dystonia** | Muscle contraction that is more sustained or prolonged than athetosis and results in spasms and distorted positions of limbs, trunk or face | • Basal ganglia disorders (Parkinson's/Huntington's/Wilson's diseases) <br> • Anoxic brain injury <br> • Infections (TB/encephalitis) |

NERVOUS

| Movement | Description | Possible Causes |
|---|---|---|
| **Tremor** | Rhythmic / semi-rhythmic oscillating movements; can be fast or slow; both agonist and antagonist muscles simultaneously activated (unlike in myoclonus or asterixis); classified as resting, postural, and intention (ataxic) | • Physiological tremor<br>• Parkinson's disease (resting tremor)<br>• Essential tremor (postural tremor)<br>• Hyperthyroidism (postural tremor)<br>• Cerebellar appendicular ataxia (intention tremor |
| **Chorea** | "Dance" - fleeting random involuntary movements that affect multiple joints; may be fluid or jerky and varying in quality | • Huntington's disease<br>• SLE/Sydenham's chorea<br>• Chorea gravidarum<br>• Tardive dyskinesia (levodopa/antipsychotics/antiemetics) |
| **Hemiballismus** | Violent flinging movement of half of the body | • Lesions of the subthalamic nucleus |
| **Seizure Automatisms** | Stereotyped semi-purposeful movements; repeated eye blinks, tonic or clonic motor activity | • Seizures |

## Muscle Tone

- Slight residual tension in a normal muscle when it is relaxed voluntarily: test by flexion/extension, pronation/supination of joint through its ROM
- *Hypotonia (decreased tone)* is seen in LMN lesions, acute stroke, spinal shock, some cerebellar lesions
- *Hypertonia (increased tone)* may manifest as spasticity or rigidity
- Patterns of tone: the characteristic of abnormal tone suggests possible causes (see **Table 15**)
  - *Spasticity (velocity-dependent)*: limb moves, then catches, and then goes past catch (spastic, clasp-knife); best appreciated during rapid supination of forearm or flexion of knee; pyramidal lesion
  - *Rigidity (velocity-independent)*: increased tone through range of movement (cogwheeling, lead-pipe); best detected with circumduction of the wrist; extrapyramidal lesion

**Table 15.** Causes of Abnormal Tone

| Characteristic | Possible Causes |
|---|---|
| **Decreased Tone: Flaccidity** | LMN lesion, cerebellar; rarely myopathies, "spinal shock" (e.g. early response after a spinal cord trauma) |
| **Increased Tone: Spasticity ("clasp-knife", velocity-dependent)** | UMN lesion: corticospinal tract (commonly late or chronic stage after a stroke) |
| **Increased Tone: Rigidity ("lead-pipe", "cogwheeling")** | Extrapyramidal tract lesion: parkinsonism, phenothiazines |
| **Increased Tone: Paratonia (inconsistently increased tone of limb tested)** | Ability for patient to relax can vary with distraction |

## Power

- Measure active motion of the patient against resistance; compare both sides; grade power on a standard scale (see **Table 16**)
- Ensure all muscle groups are tested (see **Table 17**)

**Table 16.** MRC Scale for Grading Muscle Strength

| Grade | | Assessment |
|---|---|---|
| 0 | Absent | No contraction detected |
| 1 | Trace | Slight contraction detected but cannot move joint |
| 2 | Weak | Movement with gravity eliminated only |
| 3 | Fair | Movement against gravity only |
| 4 | Good | Movement against gravity with some resistance |
| 5 | Normal | Movement against gravity with full resistance |

Note: Since this rating scale is skewed toward weakness and "4" is the category with greatest variability, many clinicians further subclassify their finding by adding a (+) or a (-) to a grade of 4, e.g. 4- or 4+.

**Table 17.** Muscle Groups to Test (Myotomal Distribution)

| Muscle | Movement | Nerve | Spinal Roots |
|---|---|---|---|
| **Deltoid** | Arm abduction | Axillary | C5, C6 |
| **Triceps** | Forearm extension | Radial | **C6, C7,** C8 |
| **Biceps** | Forearm flexion | Musculocutaneous | C5, C6 |
| **Wrist Extensors** | Wrist extension | Radial | C7, C8 |
| **Wrist Flexors**<br>· Flexor carpi radialis<br>· palmaris longus | Wrist flexion | Median | <br>· C6, C7<br>· **C7, C8,** T1 |
| **Flexor Pollicis Longus** | Thumb DIP flexion | Median (anterior interosseous branch) | C7, **C8** |
| **Interossei of Hand** | Fingers abduction/adduction | Ulnar | **C8, T1** |
| **Iliopsoas**<br>· Iliacus<br>· Psoas | Hip flexion | Femoral | **L1, L2,**<br>**L3**<br>**L2, L3, L4** |
| **Hip Adductors** | Hip adduction | Obturator | **L2, L3, L4** |
| **Hip Abductors** | Hip abduction (and medial rotation) | Superior gluteal | **L4, L5,** S1 |
| **Quadriceps** | Knee extension | Femoral | L2, **L3, L4** |
| **Hamstrings** | Knee flexion | Sciatic | **L5, S1,** S2 |
| **Tibialis Anterior** | Foot dorsi-flexion and inversion | Deep peroneal (branch of sciatic) | L4, L5 |
| **Tibialis Posterior** | Foot plantar flexion and inversion | Tibial (branch of sciatic) | L4, L5 |
| **Gastrocnemius, Soleus** | Foot plantar flexion | Tibial (branch of sciatic) | S1, S2 |
| **Peroneus (Fibularis) Longus and Brevis** | Foot plantar flexion and eversion | Superficial peroneal (branch of sciatic) | L5, S1 |
| **Extensor Hallucis Longus** | Great toe extension | Deep peroneal (branch of sciatic) | **L5, S1** |

## Pronator Drift

- Have the patient stand or sit with his/her eyes closed and arms held straight out from his/her body with hands supine
- Pronator drift is positive if patient cannot maintain position; may be due to:
  - Muscle weakness (may see pronation and outward drift of arm and hand)
  - UMN lesion (may see pronation and downward drift of arm and hand)

NERVOUS

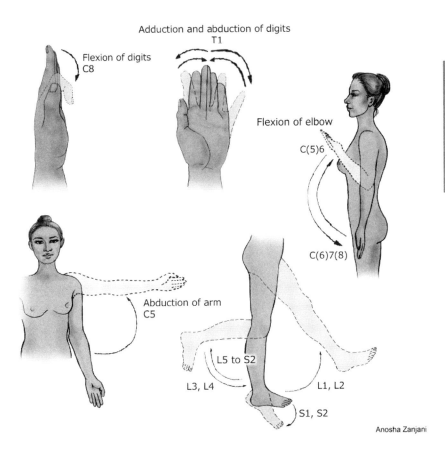

**Figure 3**. Myotomes of the Upper and Lower Limbs

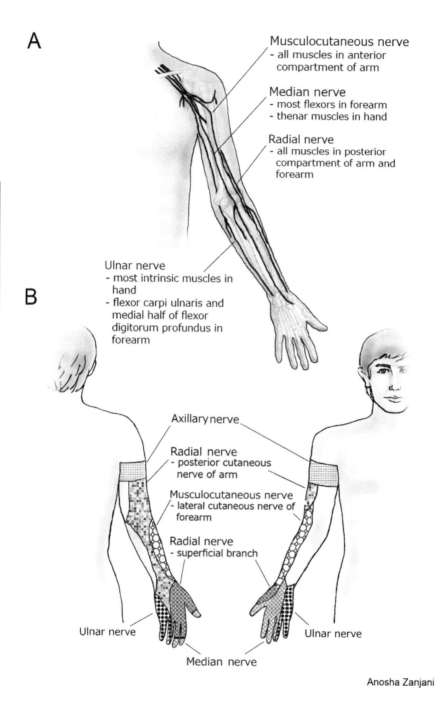

**A**

Musculocutaneous nerve
- all muscles in anterior compartment of arm

Median nerve
- most flexors in forearm
- thenar muscles in hand

Radial nerve
- all muscles in posterior compartment of arm and forearm

Ulnar nerve
- most intrinsic muscles in hand
- flexor carpi ulnaris and medial half of flexor digitorum profundus in forearm

**B**

Axillary nerve

Radial nerve
- posterior cutaneous nerve of arm

Musculocutaneous nerve
- lateral cutaneous nerve of forearm

Radial nerve
- superficial branch

Ulnar nerve

Median nerve

Ulnar nerve

Anosha Zanjani

**Figure 4**. Motor (A) and Cutaneous (B) Distribution of Upper Limb

NERVOUS

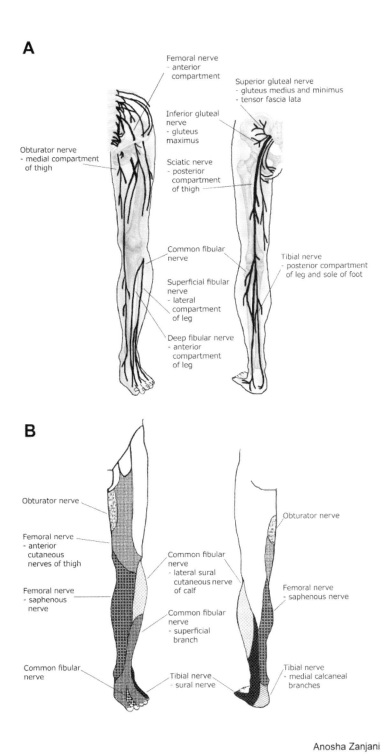

**A**

Femoral nerve
- anterior
compartment

Superior gluteal nerve
- gluteus medius and minimus
- tensor fascia lata

Inferior gluteal
nerve
- gluteus
maximus

Obturator nerve
- medial compartment
of thigh

Sciatic nerve
- posterior
compartment
of thigh

Common fibular
nerve

Tibial nerve
- posterior compartment
of leg and sole of foot

Superficial fibular
nerve
- lateral
compartment
of leg

Deep fibular nerve
- anterior
compartment
of leg

**B**

Obturator nerve

Obturator nerve

Femoral nerve
- anterior
cutaneous
nerves of thigh

Common fibular
nerve
- lateral sural
cutaneous nerve
of calf

Femoral nerve
- saphenous nerve

Femoral nerve
- saphenous
nerve

Common fibular
nerve
- superficial
branch

Common fibular
nerve

Tibial nerve
- sural nerve

Tibial nerve
- medial calcaneal
branches

Anosha Zanjani

**Figure 5**. Motor (A) and Cutaneous (B) Distribution of Lower Limb Nerves

NERVOUS

## Deep Tendon Reflexes

- Monosynaptic spinal segmental reflexes
- Patient should be relaxed with muscle mildly stretched
- Strike tendon briskly and compare both sides
- Make sure that you watch or feel muscle for contraction
- If reflexes appear to be hyperactive, examine for clonus at the ankle and knee (patella)
- If reflexes are absent, have patient use reinforcement:
  - For upper body reflexes: clench teeth or push down on bed with thighs
  - For lower body reflexes: lock fingers and try to pull hands apart (Jendrassik maneuver)
- Graded on a standard scale (see **Table 18**)

**Table 18.** Grading Reflexes

| Grade | Response |
|-------|----------|
| 0 | Absent |
| 1+ | Hypoactive, or seen only with reinforcement |
| 2+ | Normal |
| 3+ | Brisk (no clonus) |
| 4+ | Hyperactive (associated with clonus; always pathological) |

- *Biceps Tendon Reflex* (C5, C6):
  - Have patient relax arm and pronate forearm midway between flexion and extension
  - Place your thumb on the tendon and strike the hammer on your thumb
  - Observe for contraction of the biceps followed by flexion at the elbow

- *Brachioradialis Tendon Reflex* (C5, C6):
  - Have patient rest forearm on the knee in semiflexed, semipronated position
  - Strike hammer on stylus process of radius about 2.5-5 cm above wrist
  - Observe for flexion at elbow and simultaneous supination of the forearm

- *Triceps Tendon Reflex* (C6, C7, C8):
  - Have patient partially flex his/her arm at the elbow and pull toward his/her chest
  - Alternatively, allow patient's arm to hang relaxed while supporting anterior arm
  - Strike hammer on tendon above insertion of the ulnar olecranon process (2.5-5 cm above the elbow)
  - Observe for contraction of triceps with extension at the elbow

- *Finger Flexor Reflex* (C7, C8):
  - Have patient curl their fingers
  - Place your fingers against the palmar surface of their fingers
  - Strike your fingers with the reflex hammer
  - Observe for flexion of the fingers

- *Patellar Tendon Reflex* = knee jerk (L3, L4):
  - Bend the knee to relax the quadriceps muscle
  - With your hand on the quadriceps, strike the patellar tendon firmly
  - Observe for extension at the knee and contraction of the quadriceps

- *Achilles Tendon Reflex* = ankle jerk (S1, S2):
  - Place your hand under the foot to dorsiflex the ankle; strike the tendon
  - Observe for plantar flexion at the ankle and contraction of the calf muscle

- *Mnemonics for major myotomal levels*
  - C5, C6: pick up sticks (biceps)
  - C6, C7, C8: lay them straight (triceps)

- L3, L4: kick the door (quadriceps)
- S1, S2: buckle my shoe (ankle plantarflexion)

## Clonus
- *Ankle*: with knee flexed, quickly dorsiflex foot and maintain flexed position
- *Knee*: with knee extended, grasp quadriceps muscle just proximal to patella and exert sudden downward force
- Clonus is present if sudden movements elicit rhythmic involuntary muscle contractions; suggests UMN lesion

**Table 19.** Interpreting Deep Tendon Reflexes

| Characteristic | Possible Causes |
|---|---|
| **Increased Reflexes or Clonus** | UMN lesion above root at that level |
| **Absent Reflex** | Generalized: peripheral neuropathy<br>Isolated: peripheral nerve or root lesion |
| **Reduced Reflex** (insensitive) | Peripheral neuropathy<br>Cerebellar syndrome<br>(reflexes may also be absent in early phases of UMN lesion, e.g. "spinal shock") |
| **Inverted** (reflex tested is absent [e.g. biceps], but there is spread to lower or higher level [e.g. produces a triceps response]) | LMN lesion at level of the absent reflex, with UMN below (spinal cord involvement at the level of the absent reflex) |
| **Pendular** (reflex continues to swing for several beats) | Cerebellar disease |
| **"Hung"** (slow to relax, especially at ankle) | Hypothyroidism |

## Primitive Reflexes
- Generally not present in adults: when present, they may signify diffuse cerebral damage, particularly of the frontal lobes (e.g. "frontal lobe release") (see **Pediatric Exam**, p.258 for further details)
  - *Glabellar*: tap forehead and watch if eyes blink. Abnormal if individual cannot overcome the reflex and continues blinking as long as the tapping continues[7]
  - *Snout and Pout*: tap filum (above upper lip) and watch for protrusion of lips[7]
  - *Palmo-Mental*: scrape palm over thenar muscles and watch for chin muscle contraction on the ipsilateral side[7]
  - *Grasp*: place fingers in palm to see if grasp reflex is elicited[7]
  - *Rooting reflex:* head turn and suck by stroking side of mouth/cheek

## Superficial and Other Reflexes
- *Abdominal Reflex:* stroke abdomen toward umbilicus along the diagonals of the four abdominal quadrants
  - Normal: ipsilateral muscles contract, umbilicus deviates toward the stimulus
  - Above umbilicus tests T8-T10
  - Below umbilicus tests T10-T12

- *Cremasteric Reflex*: draw line along medial thigh
  - Normal: elevation of ipsilateral testis in the scrotum
  - Spinal roots involved are L1-L2
  - Abdominal and cremasteric reflexes may be absent on the side of a corticospinal tract lesion

- *Plantar Response*[16] (Babinski's sign, L5-S1): stroke the sole from the heel to the ball of the foot curving medially across the heads of the metatarsal bones
  - Normal (downgoing): plantar flexion of big toe, curling of the other toes

NERVOUS

- Abnormal (upgoing): dorsiflexion of the big toe, fanning of the other toes; associated with UMN lesion
  - Stroking the lateral aspect of the foot (Chaddock's sign) and downward pressure along the shin (Oppenheim's sign) can elicit the same reflex

- *Anal Reflex* (anal wink): stroke perianal skin
  - Normal: contraction of the muscles around the rectal orifice
  - Loss of reflex signifies lesion in S2-S3-S4 reflex arc (e.g. cauda equina lesion)

## 3.4 Sensory Examination

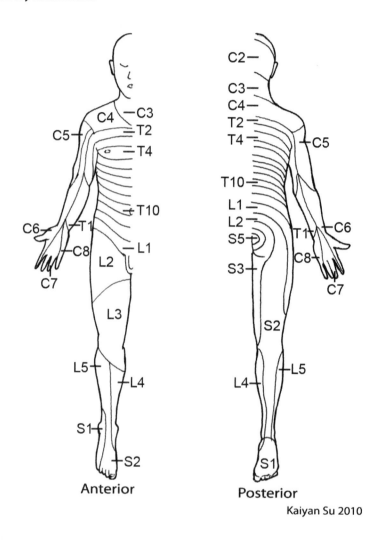

Anterior          Posterior

Kaiyan Su 2010

**Figure 6**. Map of Dermatomes

- Primary sensory exam (see below): tests peripheral sensory nerves and primary modalities
- Secondary sensory exam (see below): tests sensory cortices; perform only after confirming that primary modalities are intact

- *Tips for the Sensory Exam*:
  - Explain and demonstrate the test beforehand so patients understand how to respond (i.e. run a sample test with the patient's eyes open)
  - Have the patient close his/her eyes before testing
  - Test both sides of the body and ask the patient to compare the sensations
  - Begin testing distally at fingers and toes; if abnormal, continue proximally to map out the abnormality
  - If sensory deficits are found, note the location, magnitude, and quality
  - Because there is considerable overlap and variation in peripheral nerve distribution, a deficit in one area may be compensated by another
  - Distribution of sensory loss can suggest location of lesion (see Table 20)
  - Compare sensory function from right to left, distal to proximal, and peripheral nerve to spinal nerve dermatome (see Figure 4, 5, 6)

## Primary Sensory Exam
- Aspects of touch sensation are carried by both the dorsal column pathway (fine, discriminative touch) and the spinothalamic pathway (crude touch/pain); touch sensation is not eliminated by isolated lesions to either pathway

- *Fine Touch*[17]: dorsal column pathway (see **Figure 7**)
  - Use cotton or tissue paper tip to touch skin; ask patient to say "yes" if touch is felt

- *Pain*[17]: spinothalamic pathway (see **Figure 7**)
  - Alternate between sharp and dull touches (and false touches to see if the patient is using other cues)
  - Ask the patient to identify sensation as sharp or dull

- *Temperature*: spinothalamic pathway (often not done if pain sensation is normal)
  - Run your tuning fork under cold water
  - Ask the patient to identify whether the tuning fork feels cold, and compare to the other side

- *Vibration:* dorsal column pathway
  - Place a 128 Hz tuning fork on joint (e.g. DIP) and ask the patient when the 'buzzing' stops and compare to control (i.e. examiner)
  - If the patient is unable to feel any vibrations, move proximally and repeat testing (e.g. from DIP to PIP to MCP joint, to wrist, to elbow, to shoulder) until a level with normal vibration relative to control is established

- *Proprioception* (position sense): dorsal column pathway
  - Hold the patient's joint (e.g. DIP) from the sides so he/she does not get cues from the pressure of your hand
  - Begin with the joint in the neutral position; raise or lower the digit and ask the patient to state the direction of movement ('up' or 'down'); increment 1-2 mm in upper limbs and 2-3 mm in lower limbs
  - Return the digit to the neutral position before moving it in another direction

.
- *Romberg Test*[18]: tests proprioception and vestibular sense in the absence of visual input
  - Have the patient stand in front of you with his/her feet together; be prepared to catch or support patient if he/she falls
  - Ask the patient to close both eyes and stand still for one minute o Positive Romberg sign if the patient falls in any direction without being aware of the fall
  - If the patient sways, ask him/her to stand perfectly still: this is NOT a positive Romberg sign
  - This test has low specificity - positive test may be present in peripheral sensory denervation, vestibular dysfunction, or cerebellar disease

- *Note:* if there is a more serious proprioceptive or vestibular lesion (or a midline cerebellar lesion causing truncal instability), the patient will be unable to maintain his/her position even with his/her eyes open

NERVOUS

**Table 20.** Lesions Involving Sensory Modalities

| Location of Lesion | Distribution of Sensory Loss | Examples |
|---|---|---|
| **Single Nerve** | Within distribution of single nerve; commonly median, ulnar, peroneal, lateral cutaneous nerve of the thigh | Entrapment, most commonly in carpal tunnel syndrome, rheumatoid arthritis, and hypothyroidism; mononeuritis multiplex |
| **Root(s)** | Confined to single root or roots in close proximity; commonly C5, C6, C7 in arm and L4, L5, S1 in leg | Compression by disc prolapse |
| **Peripheral Nerves** | Distal glove and stocking deficit | DM, alcohol-related, B1 2 deficiency, drugs |
| **Spinal Cord** | Depends on level of lesion and complete vs. partial lesion | Trauma, spinal cord compression by tumor, cervical spondylitis, MS |
| **Brainstem** | Loss of pain and temperature sensation in ipsilateral face and contralateral body | Demyelination (young) Brainstem stroke (older) |
| **Thalamic Sensory Loss** | All modalities; contralateral hemisensory loss (face, body) and pain - dysesthesia (e.g. burning feeling) | Stroke, cerebral tumor, MS, trauma |
| **Cortical** (parietal) | Hemianesthesia | Stroke, cerebral tumor, trauma |

## Secondary Sensory Exam
- Must first confirm that primary modalities are intact
- Inability to perform the following tests suggests a lesion in sensory cortex

- *Neglect and Extinction*: parietal lobe
  - Touch right hand, left hand, and then both hands
  - Patients with parietal lobe lesions can identify when each side is touched independently, but will neglect the side contralateral to the lesion when both sides are touched
  - Can also test extinction using visual and less commonly, auditory stimuli
  - For hemineglect, draw a line and ask the patient to bisect the line in the middle; patient with neglect will bisect the line away from the middle toward the affected side (usually right side)

- *Two-Point Discrimination*: parietal lobe
  - Ask patient if he/she feels two stimuli or one (use an untwisted paper clip)
  - Normal minimum values for discrimination are 2 mm on fingertips, 3-8 mm on toes, 8-12 mm on palms, 40-60 mm on back

- *Stereognosis*[11]: integration between parietal and occipital lobes
  - Place objects in the patient's hand one at a time and ask the patient to recognize them by feeling the object (e.g. a coin, pen, key, paperclip) o Patient must only use one hand to feel object, and must have eyes closed
  - Tactile agnosia: inability to recognize objects by touch; suggests a parietal cortex lesion

- *Graphesthesia*[11]: parietal lobe
  - Use a blunt object to write numbers on a patient's hand in the correct orientation to the patient; patient tries to identify the numbers

- *Point Localization*: sensory cortex
  - Touch the patient and ask him/her to point to the area touched

## 3.5 Coordination and Gait Examination
- Assess speech, nystagmus, tremor, head titubation (i.e. "to and fro" movements)
- Inspect limbs for erratic nonrhythmic movements; movements should normally be rapid, smooth, and accurate

### Coordination Testing
- *Finger-To-Nose Test:*
  - Ask the patient to alternate between touching his/her nose and your finger (held at an arm's length from the patient)
  - Make sure that your finger is far enough away from the patient in order to stress the system; keeping your finger too close makes the test too easy
  - Watch for:
    - "Past pointing" where patient persistently overshoots target » Tremor as the finger approaches the target
    - Inability to perform test (dysmetria) may indicate cerebellar disease

- *Heel-To-Shin Test:*
  - Have patient slide the heel of one foot down the opposite shin, starting at knee
  - Watch for wobbling of the heel from side-to-side

- *Rebound Test:*
  - Have the patient close his/her eyes, extend his/her arms and maintain that position; push the arms down and out of position; examine if there is asymmetry in the degree of compensation

- *Rapid Alternating Movements (RAM):*
  - Dysdiadochokinesia: an abnormality in doing RAM (may be due to cerebellar lesion)

- *Upper Extremities:*
  - Pronate and supinate one hand on the other hand rapidly
  - Touch the thumb to each finger as quickly as possible

- *Lower Extremities:*
  - Tap toes of foot and then heel of foot to floor in rapid alternation

### Gait
- Ask patient to:
  - "Walk straight ahead"
  - "Stop and return to me, now on tiptoe" (also tests strength of plantar flexors)
  - "Walk away again but this time on your heels" (also tests strength of dorsiflexors)
  - "Stop, return by walking in tandem gait with one foot placed in front of the other (like walking on a tightrope)"
- Pathologic pattern of gait may suggest possible causes (see **Table 21**)

**Table 21.** Pathologic Patterns of Gait

| Gait Pattern | Possible Causes |
| --- | --- |
| **Hemiplegic** | Unilateral UMN lesion due to stroke, MS |
| **Parkinsonian** (shuffling) | Parkinson's, extrapyramidal effects of antipsychotics, tranquilizers |
| **Spastic or Scissor** (legs held in adduction at the hip, thighs rub together, knees slide over each other) | Cerebral Palsy, MS |
| **Cerebellar Ataxia** (spreads legs wide apart to provide wider base of support – veers toward side of lesion) | Drugs (e.g. phenytoin), alcohol, MS, cerebrovascular disease |
| **Foot Drop/Steppage** (takes high steps as if climbing a flight of stairs) | Unilateral: common peroneal palsy, corticospinal tract lesion, L5 radiculopathy |

Summarized version of the extra-pyramidal assessment based on the UPDRS (Unified Parkinson's Disease Rating Scale)

**Table 22.** Extrapyramidal Examination

| Assessment | Examples |
|---|---|
| Mentation, behavior and mood | Mentation, thought disorder, depression, motivation and initiative |
| Activities of daily living | Speech, salivation, swallowing, handwriting, cutting food, dressing, hygiene, turning in bed, falling, walking, freezing |
| Motor exam | 1. Speech<br>2. Facial expression<br>3. Tremor (rest, posture, action)<br>4. Rigidity (axial and appendicular)<br>5. Bradykinesia (finger tapping, pronation-supination, opening/closing hand, heel tapping)<br>6. Ambulation (rising from a chair, posture, gait, stability) |
| Complications from treatment | Dyskinesias, clinical fluctuations, sleep disturbances, autonomic symptoms |

**Table 23.** Tremor Classification[19]

| Tremor Type | Description | Pathologies |
|---|---|---|
| Resting tremor | • Evident when body part is supported and completely at rest<br>• Diminishes with voluntary activity<br>• Can be enhanced with voluntary movement of the opposite limb, or during walking | • Parkinson Disease 4-6 Hz |
| Postural / Action tremor | • Elicited when arms are suspended against gravity, or during goal-directed activity<br>• Typically remains constant throughout the range of motion (in contrast to intention tremors) | • Physiologic tremor<br>• Essential tremor |
| Intention tremor | • I.e. kinetic tremor<br>• Typically increases in severity as the hand approaches the target (in contrast to postural or action tremors)<br>• Due to disturbances along the outflow path from the cerebellar dentate nucleus to the motor division of the thalamus | • Multiple sclerosis<br>• Midbrain trauma<br>• Stroke |
| Functional tremor | • I.e. psychogenic tremor<br>• Complex resting, postural, action tremor with abrupt onset<br>• Inconsistent or variable display | |

## 4. COMMON INVESTIGATIONS

• See the **Medical Imaging** chapter for a detailed approach to neuroimaging

**Table 24.** Common neurologic investigations and their indications

| Investigation | Indications |
|---|---|
| Lumbar Puncture | • Urgent: suspected CNS infection, suspected subarachnoid hemorrhage with negative CT scan<br>• Commonly used to diagnose or exclude meningitis, measures opening pressure |
| Computerized Tomography (CT) | • Recent head trauma, especially fracture and hemorrhage |

NERVOUS

| Investigation | Indications |
|---|---|
| Magnetic Resonance Imaging (MRI) | Soft tissue, spinal cord, postoperative back or leg pain, unclassified headache, Chiari 1 malformation<br>• T1-weighted: useful to visualize anatomical details<br>• T2-weighted: useful to identify pathology<br>• FLAIR (fluid attenuated inversion recovery): useful to identify pathology, particularly if adjacent to fluid (fluid brightness is attenuated in FLAIR) |
| Positron Emission Tomography (PET) | • Workup of dementias, epilepsy |
| Conventional Angiography | • Suspected large vessel occlusion, aneurysms, arterial thrombosis, arteriovenous (AV) malformations |
| CT/MR Angiogram | • Ischemic stroke, blunt cerebrovascular injury, noninvasive alternative to conventional angiography |
| Electroencephalography (EEG) | • Epilepsy, seizures; sleep deprived EEG can improve sensitivity |
| Electromyography (EMG) | • EMG: neuropathies, myopathies, neuromuscular disease |
| Nerve Conduction Studies | • Entrapment neuropathies, polyneuropathies, conduction block<br>• Perform & interpret with EMG |
| Evoked Potentials | • Neuromonitoring during surgeries, neuroprognostication in anoxic brain injury |

**Table 25.** Common MRI Scans and the Appearance of Tissues[6]

| Tissue Type | T1-Weighted | T2-Weighted | FLAIR |
|---|---|---|---|
| Gray Matter | Gray | Light gray | Light gray |
| White Matter | White | Dark gray | Gray |
| CSF or Water | Black | White | Dark gray |
| Fat | White | White* | White* |
| Air | Black | Black | Black |
| Bone or Calcification | Black | Black | Black |
| Edema | Gray | White | White |
| Demyelination or Glyosis | Gray | White | White |
| Ferritin Deposits | Dark gray | Black | Black |
| Proteinaceous Fluid | White | Variable | Variable |

Note: While fat appears dark on T2 and FLAIR images using spin echo (SE) imaging, subcutaneous and epidural fat appears bright with the commonly used fast spin echo (FSE) imaging, unless fat saturation is applied.

## 5. COMMON CLINICAL SCENARIOS

**Table 26.** Common Stroke Syndromes[20]

| Type of Stroke | Clinical Findings |
|---|---|
| Anterior Cerebral Artery (ACA) | • Frontal lobe dysfunction (disinhibition, speech perseveration, presence of primitive reflexes, altered mental status, impaired judgment)<br>• Contralateral weakness (greater in legs than arms)<br>• Contralateral cortical sensory deficits<br>• Gait apraxia<br>• Urinary incontinence |

NERVOUS

| Type of Stroke | Clinical Findings |
|---|---|
| **Middle Cerebral Artery (MCA)** | • Contralateral hemiparesis (greater in face and arms than legs)<br>• Contralateral sensory loss<br>• Contralateral hemianopsia<br>• Gaze preference toward the side of the lesion<br>• If stroke is in dominant hemisphere, also agnosia, receptive/expressive aphasia<br>• If in nondominant hemisphere, neglect, inattention, and extinction |
| **Internal Carotid Artery (ICA)** | • Contralateral MCA and ACA signs<br>• May also have ipsilateral transient monocular blindness (amaurosis fugax) |
| **Posterior Cerebral Artery (PCA)** | • Contralateral homonymous hemianopsia<br>• Cortical blindness<br>• Visual agnosia<br>• Altered mental status<br>• Impaired memory |
| **Vertebrobasilar Artery** | • Posterior circulation strokes can present with ipsilateral CN deficits and contralateral motor deficits. Findings include:<br> ○ Vertigo<br> ○ Nystagmus<br> ○ Diplopia<br> ○ Visual field deficits<br> ○ Dysphagia<br> ○ Dysarthria<br> ○ Facial hyperesthesia<br> ○ Syncope<br> ○ Ataxia |
| **Lacunar** | • Pure contralateral motor weakness<br>• Pure sensory loss<br>• Ataxic hemiparesis |
| **Left-Sided** | • Aphasia<br>• Right hemiparesis or hemiplegia<br>• Impaired memory |

**Table 27.** Common Headache Syndromes

| Type | Characteristics |
|---|---|
| **Tension** | • Lasts 30 min-7 d<br>• Nonpulsating, mild-moderate in intensity, bilateral<br>• Not aggravated by exertion, not associated with N/V or sensitivity to light, sound, or smell |
| **Migraine** | • Lasts 4-72 h<br>• Throbbing, moderate to severe intensity, unilateral (not always same side)<br>• Worse with exertion<br>• Associated with photophobia, phonophobia, N/V<br>• May be preceded by short prodromal period of depression, irritability, restlessness, or anorexia; 10-20% of occurrences associated with an aura: transient, reversible visual, somatosensory, motor, and/or language deficit – usually precedes headache by ≤1 h, can be concurrent |
| **Cluster** | • Lasts 15-180 min, occurs up to 8 times/d<br>• Severe, unilateral, located periorbitally and/or temporally associated with at least one of: tearing, red eye, stuffy nose, facial sweating, ptosis, miosis |
| **Subarachnoid Hemorrhage** | • Acute, severe, "thunderclap"<br>• May have neurologic deficits or changes in level of consciousness |

NERVOUS

**Table 28.** Common Neurological Tumours

| Neurological Tumours | Commonly present with progressive focal neurological deficits<br>May be associated with headache: worse in the morning, improves during the day, worse when lying down or with Valsalva maneuver, may be associated with signs of increased intracranial pressure (e.g. N/V, blurry vision, papilledema, transient visual obscuration)<br>May be present with seizures, cognitive deficits, focal motor deficits |
| --- | --- |
| **Astrocytoma** | Seizures, headache |
| **Oligodendroglioma** | Seizures |
| **Ependymoma** | Headache, vomiting, ataxia |
| **Meningioma** | Commonly in middle aged females<br>Problematic due to mass effect |
| **Schwannoma (eg. Acoustic neuroma)** | Often manifests as unilateral tinnitus and/or hearing loss |

**Clinical Pearl: False lateralizing signs**
**CN VI palsy** can be elevated in high ICP and does not always imply a specific localization

**Clinical Pearl: Syncope vs Seizure**
**Syncope** is associated with lightheadedness, diaphoresis, positional change, tunnel vision.
**Seizure** is associated with déjà vu, epigastric rising sensation, auditory or visual hallucination, fear/anxiety

**Table 29.** Seizure Classification[3]

| Partial seizure | · i.e. focal seizure<br>· onset involves regions of one hemisphere only |
| --- | --- |
| **Simple partial seizure** | · Motor, sensory, visual, auditory, or psychomotor phenomena without loss of consciousness/awareness of surroundings<br>· Seizures can begin in one part of the body and spread to other parts |
| **Complex partial seizure** | · May be preceded by an aura (sensory or psychic manifestations that represent seizure onset)<br>· Staring, performing automatisms (automatic purposeless movements), uttering unintelligible sounds, resisting aid<br>· Motor, sensory, or psychomotor phenomena<br>· Post-ictal confusion<br>· An EEG may be needed to distinguish from absence seizures |
| **Generalized seizure** | · Onset involves regions of both hemispheres<br>· Often has loss of consciousness/awareness |
| **Tonic-clonic seizure** | · Formerly known as grand mal seizures<br>· Tonic phase: stiffening of limbs<br>· Clonic phase: jerking of limbs<br>· Respiration may decrease during tonic phase but usually returns during clonic phase, although it may be irregular<br>· Incontinence may occur<br>· Postictal confusion |
| **Atonic seizure** | · Brief, primarily generalized seizures in children<br>· Complete loss of muscle tone, resulting in falling or pitching to the ground<br>· Risk of serious trauma, particularly head injury |

NERVOUS

| Absence seizure | · Formerly known as petit mal seizures<br>· Brief, primarily generalized attacks manifested by a 10-30 s loss of awareness of surroundings<br>· Eyelid fluttering<br>· No loss of axial muscle tone<br>· No postictal symptoms<br>· An EEG may be needed to distinguish from complex partial seizures |
|---|---|
| Status epilepticus | · A medical emergency!<br>· Repeated seizures lasting >5-10 min with no intervening periods of normal neurologic function<br>· Generalized convulsive status epilepticus may be fatal |

**Table 30.** Spinal Cord Disorders and Key Signs and Symptoms

| Spinal Cord Disorder | · Stage 1: spinal shock<br>  ◦ Loss of all reflex activity below level of lesion<br>  ◦ Atonic bladder/bowel with overflow incontinence<br>  ◦ Gastric dilatation<br>  ◦ Loss of vasomotor control<br>· Stage 2: heightened reflex activity<br>  ◦ Hyperactive tendon reflexes<br>  ◦ Frequency and urgency of urination, automatic emptying of bladder<br>  ◦ Hyperactive vasomotor and sweating reactions |
|---|---|
| Central Cord Syndrome | · More often in older patients or patients with cervical spondylosis<br>· Weakened hands with impaired pain sensation<br>· Hyporeflexia in areas with impaired pain sensation<br>· May have bladder symptoms, and spared vibration and proprioception sense |
| Anterior Cord Syndrome | · Paraplegia or quadriplegia<br>· Urinary retention<br>· Bilateral loss of pain and temperature sensation below the lesion<br>· Sparing of vibration and proprioception sense |
| Conus Medullaris (CM) and Cauda Equina (CE) Syndrome | · Pain localized to the lower back, with radiation to legs<br>· Bowel and bladder dysfunction (eg. Urinary retention, laxity of anal sphincter)<br>· Erectile dysfunction<br>· Loss of sensation in sacral segments (saddle paresthesia)<br>· Leg weakness with upper and lower motor neuron signs (usually asymmetric in CE)<br>· Leg atrophy more common in CE<br>· Knee jerk reflexes preserved in CM, but absent in CE<br>· Ankle jerk reflexes absent in both |

**Table 31.** Other Common Neurological Scenarios

| Scenario | Key Signs and Symptoms |
|---|---|
| Diabetic Neuropathy | · Peripheral neuropathy<br>· Autonomic neuropathy (eg. Orthostatic hypotension, gastroparesis)<br>· Sensory ataxia<br>· Motor weakness<br>· Pain, paresthesia, hyperesthesia<br>· Loss of deep tendon reflexes<br>· Impotence<br>· Pupil abnormalities |

| Scenario | Key Signs and Symptoms |
|---|---|
| **Alzheimer's Disease** | • Anterograde amnesia, and at least one of: aphasia, apraxia, agnosia, executive function deficits<br>• As disease progresses, may also notice: halting speech, slower comprehension, calculation errors, defective visuospatial orientation, disorientation, amnesia<br>• Later stages: involuntary primitive reflexes, significant cognitive impairment |
| **Parkinson's Disease** | • Mnemonic: TRAP<br>• Tremor (resting tremor, pill rolling)<br>• Rigidity (lead-pipe with cogwheeling)<br>• Akinesia / bradykinesia<br>• Postural instability<br>• Other findings may include: fixed facial expression, shuffling gait with reduced arm swing, micrographia, dysarthria, hypophonia, cognitive decline |
| **Multiple Sclerosis** | • Typical age of onset: 20-30 years old<br>• Most common presenting symptom: optic neuritis (partial/total loss of vision, pain with eye movement)<br>• Dx requires dissemination of neuronal dysfunction in time and space<br>• Brainstem signs: dipolopia, internuclear opthalmoplegia, trigeminal neuralgia, Bell's palsy<br>• Cerebellar signs: ataxia, nystagmus, intention tremor, gait disturbances<br>• Spinal cord signs: weakness, spasticity, hyperreflexia/clonus, upgoing toes, bladder/bowel dysfunction, sexual dysfunction, paraparesis, Lhermitte's sign |
| **Traumatic Brain Injury** | • Loss of consciousness (lasting seconds-minutes)<br>• Headache<br>• Nausea/vomiting<br>• Fatigue/drowsiness<br>• Blurred vision<br>• Dizziness/loss of balance/tinnitus<br>• Photophobia, phonophobia<br>• Memory or concentration problems<br>• Depression, anxiety |
| **Lumbar disc prolapse** | • May be caused or exacerbated by trauma<br>• Burning, tingling pain in the distribution of the irritated/compressed root<br>• Restricted spinal movement<br>• Loss of reflexes<br>• Decreased motor strength<br>• Diminished sensation |

**Table 32.** Lumbar Disc Prolapse Patterns and Physical Findings

| Disc | Root | Motor Weakness | Sensory Loss | Reflex Affected |
|---|---|---|---|---|
| **L3/L4** | L4 | Quadriceps<br>Hip adductors | Medial leg / foot | Patellar (knee jerk) |
| **L4/L5** | L5 | Foot dorsiflexors, EDL, EHL, foot evertors / invertors<br>Hip abductors | Lateral calf, dorsum of the foot, big toe | None |
| **L5/S1** | S1 | Foot plantar flexors<br>Hip extensors | Lateral foot, sole | Achilles tendon (ankle jerk) |

EDL = extensor digitorum longus, EHL = extensor hallucis longus

NERVOUS

**Table 33.** Common Scenarios, Physical Exam Maneuvers, Investigations, and Management

| Physical Exam | Investigations | Management |
|---|---|---|
| **Stroke** | | |
| • Signs of trauma (especially head and neck)<br>• Retinal changes (hypertensive changes, cholesterol crystals, papilledema)<br>• PVS (bruits, decreased pulses, skin changes)<br>• CVS (murmurs)<br>• Neurologic findings (to localize lesion) | • CT scan (to determine if hemorrhagic | • tPA considered for ischemic stroke within time window 4.5h from symptom onset<br>• Consider moderate BP control or decompressive neurosurgery in hemorrhagic |
| **Headache** | | |
| • Scalp tenderness<br>• Jolt accentuation sensitive but nonspecific<br>• Fundoscopy to check for optic disc swelling<br>• See Table 27 for subtypes | • Neuroimaging (see Figure 8) | • Non-pharmacologic: diet, rest, exercise<br>• Pharmacologic: Early abortive therapy for migraine, prophylactic |
| **Neurological Malignancies** | | |
| • Focal neurologic deficits<br>• Fundoscopy to check for optic disc swelling<br>• See Table 28 | • Neuroimaging (see Figure 8) | • Dexamethasone<br>• Neurosurgery<br>• Radiation therapy for diffuse disease |
| **Diabetic Neuropathy** | | |
| • Sensory exam (sensory ataxia indicates large fiber involvement)<br>• Motor exam (weakness typically begins distally)<br>• Deep tendon reflexes (may be lost)<br>• Pupil abnormalities | • HbA1C, fasting BG<br>• NCS | • BG management<br>• Footwear and foot hygiene to avoid trauma and secondary infection |
| **Alzheimer's Disease** | | |
| • Note whether patient accompanied by caregiver, tidiness, and whether patient turns head to another when asked a question<br>• Sequential MoCA/MMSE | • TSH<br>• B12<br>• (MRI head if rapid progression dementia) | • Acetylcholineste-rase inhibitors may slow progression |
| **Seizures** | | |
| • Video recording<br>• Focal neurologic deficit<br>• See **Table 29** | • EEG (to distinguish between types of seizures) earlier is higher yield<br>• Sleep-deprived EEG<br>• Continuous EEG monitoring<br>• MRI head to rule out structural cause | • General: adequate rest, hydration, feeding, avoidance of triggers<br>• Pharmacologic: Antiepileptic drugs<br>• Surgical: epilepsy surgery for definable focus |
| **Parkinson Disease** | | |
| • Motor exam: rest tremor, tone (axial neck and trunk rigidity and limb), fatiguing decrementing finger oppositions<br>• Narrow based bradykinetic shuffling gait<br>• Failed pullback test<br>• Extraocular movements (esp. vertical)<br>• MoCA, orthostatic vitals | • MRI brain | • Levodopa<br>• Dopamine agonists<br>• DBS |

### Multiple Sclerosis

| | | |
|---|---|---|
| • Painful extraocular movements<br>• INO<br>• UMN signs | • MRI (T2-weighted or FLAIR scans show hyperintense plaques, enhanced with gadolinium contrast)<br>• Oligoclonal bands from CSF protein electrophoresis<br>• CT (oligoclonal IgG banding)<br>• Evoked potentials (abnormal visual, brainstem, auditory, somatosensory evoked potentials) | • Steroids for acute flares<br>• Disease-modifying immunomodulators, biologics |

### Traumatic Brain Injury

| | | |
|---|---|---|
| • Focal neurologic deficit<br>• CSF leak<br>• Depending on extent of injury, may be asymptomatic initially<br>• MoCA | • CT head<br>• Inspect for basal skull fracture | • Brain rest for concussion<br>• Arrange for scheduled follow-up |

### Lumbar Disc Prolapse

| | | |
|---|---|---|
| • Reflexes (lost in radicular distribution)<br>• Motor exam (decreased strength)<br>• Sensory exam (decreased sensation; note: testing with pinprick is more sensitive than touch)<br>• Straight leg raise test (reproduction of pain and paresthesias)<br>• See Table 32 for patterns of findings that can help localize the level of disc prolapse | • MRI spine | • Watchful waiting<br>• Remain active<br>• Pain management |

### Spinal Cord Disorders

| | | |
|---|---|---|
| • Reflexes (can be hypo- or hyperreflexive)<br>• Sensory-level changes<br>• Weakness<br>• Bowel/bladder function<br>• Anal tone | • CT/MRI spine | • Spinal surgery or radiation<br>• Analgesia<br>• Steroids |

NERVOUS

# REFERENCES

1. Greenberg MS. Handbook of Neurosurgery, 8th Edition. New York: Thieme Medical Publishers; 2016.
2. Bickley LS, Szilagyi PG, Bates B. Bates' Guide to Physical Examination and History Taking, 10th ed. Philadelphia: Lippincott Williams & Wilkins; 2009.
3. Campbell WW. DeJong's the Neurological Examination, 6th ed. Philadelphia: Lippincott Williams & Wilkins; 2005.
4. Benarroch EE. Medical Neurosciences: An Approach to Anatomy, Pathology, and Physiology by Systems and Levels. Philadelphia: Lippincott Williams & Wilkins; 1999.
5. Posner JB, Saper CB, Schiff ND, Plum F. Plum and Posner's Diagnosis of the Stupor and Coma, 4th edition. Contemporary Neurology Series. Oxford University Press; 2007
6. Blumenfeld H. Neuroanatomy Through Clinical Cases, 2nd ed. Sunderland: Sinauer Associates; 2010
7. Stevens RD, Bhardwaj A. 2006. Approach to the comatose patient. Crit Care Med 34(1 ):31-41.
8. Young GB. Stupor and Coma in Adults. Waltham: Wolters Kluwer Health. 2012. Available from: http://www.uptodate.com/contents/stupor-and-coma-in-adults.
9. Wilhelm H. 1998. Neuro-ophthalmology of pupillary function--practical guidelines. J Neurol 245(9):573-583.
10. Kumar SP, Ramasubramanian D. 2000. The Babinski sign--a reappraisal. Neurol India 48(4):314-318.
11. Bird TD, Miller BL. Alzheimer's Disease and Other Dementias In: Hauser S, Josephson S (Editors). Harrison's Neurology in Clinical Medicine, 2nd ed. New York: McGraw-Hill; 2010.
12. Ross RT. How to Examine the Nervous System. Totowa: Humana Press; 2006.
13. Zigmond MJ. Fundamental Neuroscience. San Diego: Academic Press; 1999.
14. Yaman A, Akdeniz M, Yaman H. 2011. J Fam Pract 60(12):721-725.
15. Ivanhoe CB, Reistetter TA. 2004. Spasticity: The misunderstood part of the upper motor neuron syndrome. Am J Phys Med Rehabil 83(10 Suppl):S3-9.
16. Walterfang M, Velakoulis D. 2005. Cortical release signs in psychiatry. Aust N Z J Psychiatry 39(5):31 7-327
17. Walk D, Sehgal N, Moeller-Bertram T, Edwards RR, Wasan A, Wallace M, et al. 2009. Quantitative sensory testing and mapping: A review of nonautomated quantitative methods for examination of the patient with neuropathic pain. Clin J Pain 25(7):632-640
18. Lanska DJ, Goetz CG. 2000. Romberg's sign: Development, adoption, and adaptation in the 19th century. Neurology 55(8):1201-1206.
19. Daroff RB, Fenichel GM, Jankovic J, Mazziotta JC. Bradley's Neurology in Clinical Practice, 6th Edition, Edition Elsevier Saunders, Volume 1: Principles of Diagnosis and Management, Chapter 21: Movement Disorders: Diagnosis and Assessment, 2012, P 235-238.
20. Cruz-Flores S. Ischemic Stroke. New York: WebMD LLC. 2013. Available from: http:// emedicine.medscape.com/article/1916852-overview.

# FURTHER READING:

1. Tesfaye S, Boulton AJ, Dyck PJ, Freeman R, Horowitz M, Kempler P, et al. 2010. Diabetic neuropathies: Update on definitions, diagnostic criteria, estimation of severity, and treatments. Diabetes Care 33(10):2285-2293.
2. Levine AM. Spine Trauma. Philadelphia: Saunders; 1998.
3. Agur AMR, Dalley AF. Grant's Atlas of Anatomy. Philadelphia: Wolters Kluwer Health/Lippincott Williams & Wilkins; 2009.
4. Kandel ER, Schwartz JH, Jessell TM. Principles of Neural Science. New York: McGraw-Hill, Health Professions Division; 2000.

# The Breast Exam

**Editor:**
Erica Pascoal, BSc

**Resident Reviewer:**
Anjali Kulkarni, MD, MSc

**Faculty Reviewers:**
Dr. Frances Wright MD, MEd, FRCPSC

REPRODUCTIVE

## TABLE OF CONTENTS

# 1. ESSENTIAL ANATOMY

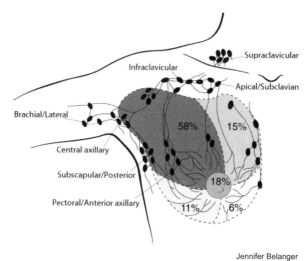

Jennifer Belanger

**Figure 1:** Location of primary breast cancer and lymph node drainage by breast quadrant.

# 2. COMMON CHIEF COMPLAINTS

**Table 1.** Evaluation of common chief complaints relating to the breast exam[1]

| Chief Complaint | Chief Complaint | Typical Presentation |
|---|---|---|
| **Breast Pain/ Tenderness (Mastalgia)** | Cyclic mastalgia | Younger women, bilateral, poorly localized, general heaviness or soreness pre-menstrually, relieved with menses, resolves spontaneously |
| | Mastitis | Unilateral erythema, swelling, tenderness, warmth, often associated with breast feeding |
| **Breast Mass** Benign | Fibroadenoma | Age <30 yr, unilateral, solitary, discrete, fluctuating with menses, round, firm and rubbery |
| | Fibrocystic breasts | Women 40-50 years, unilateral or bilateral, fluctuating with menses, varying from rice-like nodularity to ropey thickening, often associated with mastalgia peri-menopausally |
| | Breast cyst | Age 30-50, unilateral or bilateral, firm, often fluctuating with menses well-demarcated. Can be confused with malignancy until aspirated. |
| | Fat necrosis | Often a result of trauma to the breast, firm, round, often non-tender, associated nipple changes and/or skin erythema |
| Malignant | Breast carcinoma | Solitary, discrete, hard, irregular shape, often non-tender, maybe associated skin and nipple changes |

| Chief Complaint | Chief Complaint | Typical Presentation |
| --- | --- | --- |
| Nipple discharge | *Physiologic* | Non-spontaenous, bilateral, non-bloody (green/ grey/ white in colour) |
| | *Malignancy (e.g. ductal carcinoma in situ)* | Unilateral, spontaneous, bloody, associated with breast mass or nipple changes (Paget disease) |
| Nipple changes (retraction, ulceration, scaling) | *Duct ectasia* | Bilateral and symmetrical nipple inversion (usually easily everted), green nipple discharge, noncyclical mastalgia, |
| | *Periductal mastitis* | Inverted nipple, patients who smoke are at increased risk |
| | *Subareolar abscess* | Inverted nipple, subareolar mass, pus discharge, fever |
| | *Paget Disease* | Unilateral, red, scaly, raw, vesicular or ulcerated lesion on the nipple and areola, pain, burning, pruritus; commonly associated with ductal carcinoma in situ (DCIS) or invasive ductal carcinoma |
| | *Carcinoma* | Asymmetric nipple inversion, areolar retraction |
| Breast skin changes | *Mastitis* | Lactational if breastfeeding, nonlactational if not, erythema, breast pain, fever, myalgia |
| | *Breast cellulitis* | Pain, diffuse erythema, tenderness, warmth, edema, axillary nodes may be enlarged and tender |
| | *Breast cancer* | Erythema, peau d'orange appearance, skin thickening due to edema, may or may not be associated with a mass |

## 3. FOCUSED HISTORIES

### Breast pain (mastalgia)
- **HPI:** onset (sudden or gradual, when it was first noticed) bilateral or unilateral, location, characterization of pain (heaviness, general soreness, sharp, burning), progression over time, intermittent or constant, changes with menstrual cycle, recent trauma
- **Associated signs and symptoms:**
  - Skin changes: erythema, local swelling, warmth
  - Nipple changes: inversion, non spontaneous discharge
  - Other: fever, myalgia
- **Risk Factors:**
  - Mastitis: breastfeeding and smoking

### Breast mass:
- **HPI:** onset (sudden or gradual, when it was first noticed), location, bilateral or unilateral, progression (worse, better, same), changes with menstrual cycle, recent trauma
- **Associated signs and symptoms:**
  - Changes in skin of breast: colour, induration
  - Nipple changes: retraction, ulceration, scaling (Paget's Disease)
  - Nipple discharge: spontaneous or upon compression, bloody, unilateral or bilateral, uniductal or multiductal

- ◆ Lymph node enlargement: axillary, supraclavicular,
- ◆ Constitutional symptoms: weight loss, night sweats

- **Risk Factors for Breast Cancer[2]:**
  - ◆ Major Risk Factors
    - ▪ Age >50 yr
    - ▪ Female
    - ▪ Personal history of breast or ovarian cancer
    - ▪ Maternal or paternal family history of breast and/or ovarian cancer in 1st or 2nd degree relatives, especially if early onset (<50 yr)
    - ▪ Genetics: mutations in the tumor suppressor genes BRCA1, BRCA2
    - ▪ History of atypical ductal hyperplasia or lobular carcinoma in situ (LCIS)
    - ▪ History of high-dose radiation (e.g. mantle radiation for Hodgkin's)
    - ▪ Hormone replacement therapy if used for extended period (>10 years)
  - ◆ Minor Risk Factors
    - ▪ Nulliparity
    - ▪ First full term pregnancy after age 30
    - ▪ Menarche <12 yr
    - ▪ Menopause >55 yr
    - ▪ Hormone replacement therapy
    - ▪ Obesity in postmenopausal women
    - ▪ Excessive alcohol intake (>2 drinks/d)
    - ▪ Previous history of breast biopsy regardless of findings

**Table 2.** Breast cancer screening recommendations according to risk stratification categories[3,4,5]

| Category | Category | Screening Modality | | |
| --- | --- | --- | --- | --- |
| | | Clinical Breast Exam | Mammogram | MRI |
| **Average Risk** | • No personal or family history of breast cancer in 1st degree, pre-menopausal relatives<br>• No known BRCA1 or BRCA2 mutation<br>• History<br>• No history of chest wall irradiation | No | q 3 years, starting at age 50 and until age 74 | No |
| **Moderate Risk** | • Personal or family history of breast cancer<br>• Past premalignant biopsy (atypical hyperplasia, lobular carcinoma in situ [LCIS]) | No | q 1 year, age to start depends on degree of risk/ clinical assessment | No |
| **High Risk** | • BRCA mutation carriers<br>• Family history of breast cancer or BRCA mutation in a first degree relative<br>• History of chest wall irradiation before age 30 and at least 8 years previously<br>• Multiple major risk factors for breast cancer<br>• Are determined to be have ≥25% lifetime risk of breast cancer (must have been assessed using either the IBIS or BOADICEA risk assessment tools at a genetics clinic) | No | q 1 year starting at age 30 until age 69 | q 1 year, starting at age 30 until age 69 |

REPRODUCTIVE

**Clinical Pearl: Breast Cancer Risk**
Validated tools of estimating breast cancer risk:
- BOADICEA Model http://ccge.medschl.cam.ac.uk/boadicea/
- IBIS Breast Cancer Risk Evaluation Tool
  www.ems-trials.org/riskevaluator.

## 4.FOCUSED PHYSICAL EXAM

### The Clinical Breast Exam (CBE)[6]
- Purpose: identify features that distinguish malignant vs. benign lumps (see **Table 3**)
- May be used for screening purposes in patients at increased risk
- Sensitivity of 54% and specificity of 94%
- CBE contributes to cancer detection independent of mammography, however CBE used in conjunction with mammography achieves the greatest reduction in breast cancer mortality
- Cancer may be difficult to rule out on the basis of clinical exam alone; other diagnostic tests often performed (see **Common Investigations**)[2]
- The patient must be draped appropriately
- If male doctor is performing the exam, ask the patient if they would like a female witness to accompany in the room
- Always examine both breasts, even if complaints are localized to one side
- Breast exam is usually more comfortable for women 7-10 days after the start of their periods
- If a mass is detected:
  - Document which breast, quadrant, and location it is found in
  - Document qualities of mass: size, shape, consistency, delineation of borders, tenderness, mobility, and if impacted by menstrual changes (see **Table 3**)

**Clinical Pearl: Clinical Breast Exam**
- Clinical breast examination (CBE) can detect up to 50% of cancers not detected by mammography alone
- Cancer cannot be ruled out on the basis of clinical exam alone; other diagnostic tests must be performed (see **Common Investigations**)
- Increase in breast size, density, nodularity, and tenderness occur 3-5 d prior to menses: the most appropriate time for a breast exam is 7-10 d post menses
- Breasts normally become less firm and full following menopause due to replacement of glandular tissue with fat tissue

**Table 3.** Interpretation of Findings[7,8]

|  | Carcinoma | Fibroadenoma | Breast Cyst |
|---|---|---|---|
| **Location of Mass** | Usually unilateral and solitary | Usually unilateral and solitary | Unilateral or bilateral |
| **Size** | Variable | 1-3 cm (may be larger) | Variable Fluctuating with menses (increased size premenstrually) |
| **Shape** | Irregular | Round | Variable (may have regions of thickening or discrete mass) |
| **Consistency** | Firm or hard | Firm and rubbery | Fluid filled sac |
| **Delineation** | Ill-defined | Discrete | Well demarcated |
| **Tenderness** | Nontender | Nontender | Occasionally tender |
| **Mobility** | May be tethered | Mobile | Mobile |

| | Carcinoma | Fibroadenoma | Breast Cyst |
|---|---|---|---|
| **Menstrual Changes** | No | May change in size with menstrual cycle | Increased tenderness premenstrually |
| **Age Group** | 80% ≥40 yr | Usually <30 yr | 30-50 yr |
| **Investigations** | Mammography, U/S for palpable findings or to evaluate mammography findings further, core biopsy for definitive diagnosis | U/S, mammography if ≥30 yr, core biopsy or FNAB to confirm benign | Mammography if ≥30 yr, U/S for discrete masses, FNAB of dominant or symptomatic cysts to rule out carcinoma |

FNAB = fine needle aspiration biopsy
Morrow M. 2000. *Am Fam Physician* 61(8):2371-2378.

## 4.1 Inspection

- With patient seated upright, lower the drape to the patient's waistline to reveal both breasts
- Inspect both breasts with the patient in each of the following positions: o Patient sitting with hands resting on thighs
    - ◆ Patient sitting with arms raised above head
    - ◆ Patient sitting with hands pressed against hips
    - ◆ Patient sitting and leaning forward
- The clinician should note movement of the breast tissue as she does this and observe for any tethering of tissue to the chest wall

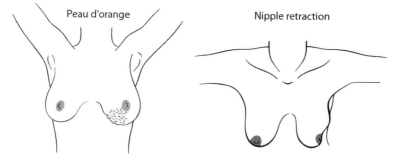

Jennifer Belanger

**Figure 2. The Clinical Breast Exam** – Inspection with arms raised above the head (left) and arms stretched out (right)

- Inspection of the breast: **4 S**'s
    1. **Size** of each breast
    2. **Symmetry** of two breasts (some variability is normal)
    3. **Shape** and contour: bulges, flattening, skin dimpling, retraction
    4. **Skin changes:**
        - Inflammation
        - Erythema
        - Peau d'orange (edema in skin: may be indicative of advanced cancer or postoperative/postradiation edema) (see **Figure 2**)
        - Abnormal vascularity (increased visibility of blood vessels)
        - Thickening

- Inspection of nipple: **5 S**'s (see **Figure 3**)
  1. **Size**
  2. **Symmetry**
     - Ask patient to raise arms: one nipple may be retracted due to a small cancer in breast (caused by tethering) (see **Figure 2**)
  3. **Skin changes**: eczema or ulceration/scaling
  4. **Spontaneous nipple discharge**: serous, bloody, or colored, from one or more ducts (discharge with expression only is usually benign)
  5. **Supernumerary nipple**: rare, insignificant finding along milk line

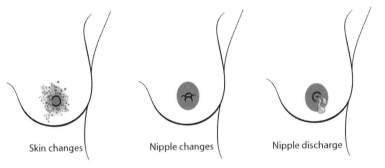

Skin changes   Nipple changes   Nipple discharge

Jennifer Belanger

**Figure 3.** Visible Signs of Breast Disease

**Clinical Pearl: Palpation**
- Always palpate both breasts.
- Palpation in supine position with arm above head allows breast tissue to stretch more evenly across the chest wall for easier deep palpation. For large breasts or more effective deep palpation, the breast can be palpated in oblique position.

## 4.2 Palpation

### Axillae and Supraclavicular Area
- Three key groups of lymph nodes: axillary, supraclavicular, and infraclavicular (see **Figure 1**)
  - With the patient sitting up with arms at her sides palpate above and below clavicle with patient's arms resting on thighs
  - Partially abduct patient's arm and support it on your arm to assess axilla
  - Palpate deeply into axilla, along posterior surface of pectoralis muscles, and up along inferior surface of upper arm
  - Check for size, location, consistency, and mobility

### Palpation of Breasts
- Positioning
  - Patient should be lying down flat
  - Lower the drape on one side to reveal the breast you are examining
  - Have the patient raise their arm to rest their hand behind their head on the same side of the body as the breast you will be examining
  - Both breasts are to be examined to compare findings or lack thereof on both sides
  - Examine the unaffected breast first
  - Before beginning, ask the patient to point with one finger where their area of concern is
- Use fleshy pads of three middle fingertips
  - Systematically cover entire breast area: from clavicle to below the infra-mammary fold and sternum to mid-axillary line
  - At each new point of contact, first use light, then increasingly stronger pressure

REPRODUCTIVE

- Two possible patterns of palpation (see **Figure 4**):
  1. **Radial vector pattern**
     - Palpation at each location in small circular motion
     - Begin at "12 o'clock" position at outer edge of breast and move inwards along all "spokes of wheel" with nipple as central point; end with palpation of areolar area and nipple
     - Continue with next vector, partially overlapping with previous one, and work inwards to nipple
  2. **Vertical strip pattern**
     - Palpate each location with small circular motions
     - Mentally divide breast area into a series of vertical regions, and palpate each one thoroughly from top to bottom
     - Begin at axilla and palpate downward along midaxillary line to 6th rib » For next strip, work upward from 6th rib to top of breast and partially overlap with first strip
     - Continue in this antiparallel fashion until the entire breast is examined
     - Do not lift hand entirely off the breast as you move along, to avoid missing any part of the breast (i.e. "walk" the fingers to the next area")

REPRODUCTIVE

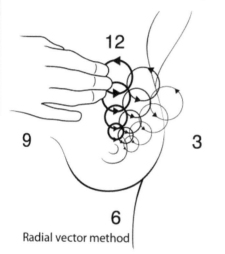

Radial vector method

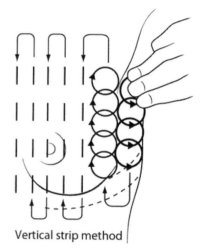

Vertical strip method

Jennifer Belanger

**Figure 4.** Common Approaches to Breast Palpation

- The preferred technique for CBE includes:
  - Use of a vertical-strip search pattern
  - Proper position and movement of fingers (3 fingers, finger pads, circular motion, varying palpation pressure)
  - CBE duration of at least 3 minutes per breast
  - Distinguish between abnormal mass and normal compressed tissue ridge (inframammary fold) which may be found along lower border of breast, particularly with large breasts
- If a mass is detected:
  - Determine distance from nipple
  - Gently elevate breast near the mass and watch for dimpling (suggests an underlying cancer)
  - Nipple distortion may be a sign of underlying cancer

## 5. COMMON INVESTIGATIONS
- Refer to **Figure 5** on p. 258 for application and summary

## Mammogram
- Low dose X-ray to examine breast
- Digital mammography is standard practice (rather than screen film)
- Indication:
  - Evaluation of new or worrisome palpable mass in any woman >30 yr
  - Best modality for picking up ductal carcinoma in situ (DCIS, earliest stage of breast cancer), often before a mass is palpable (usually presents with microcalcifications)3
- Nonpalpable malignancies <1 cm in size may be detected
  - 1/3 of all malignancies detected by mammography are nonpalpable Note: negative mammogram does not rule out breast cancer, however false positives can generate significant anxiety

## MRI[9]
- For high-risk women
- For further evaluation of undifferentiated abnormalities on mammogram/ U/S

## Ultrasound[3]
- Indication:
  - First method of investigation in women <30 with a breast mass
  - Evaluate palpable/nonpalpable masses or mammographic abnormalities
  - Differentiate cystic masses from solid masses
- Highly operator-dependent, requires special breast expertise
- False positives can generate significant anxiety
- False negatives can miss malignancy
- Most solid-dominant palpable masses need a biopsy

## Fine Needle Aspiration Biopsy (FNAB)
- Indication:
  - To determine if breast mass or cystic or cancerous
  - To determine if malignant cells are present in lymph nodes
- Smears prepared from aspirate for cytologic evaluation
- If aspirated fluid is bloody or if lesion biopsied was solid, send aspirate for cytology
- Simple cyst: non-bloody aspirate followed by resolution of mass, no cytological evaluation required (follow-up in 4-6 wk to ensure no reoccurrence; if reoccurs, re-aspirate and send fluid to cytology)3
- A negative FNAB does NOT rule out cancer[3]

## Core Needle Biopsy
- Preferred method for tissue diagnosis[3]
- Better sample and pathology (tissue architecture, staining, hormone receptor status)
- Provides more information for planning surgery (DCIS vs. invasive cancer)

## Excisional Biopsy/Lumpectomy
- When core biopsy is not concordant or clinical suspicion is high, even if core biopsy is negative
- When core biopsy is not possible or available
- To treat/rule out cancer

REPRODUCTIVE

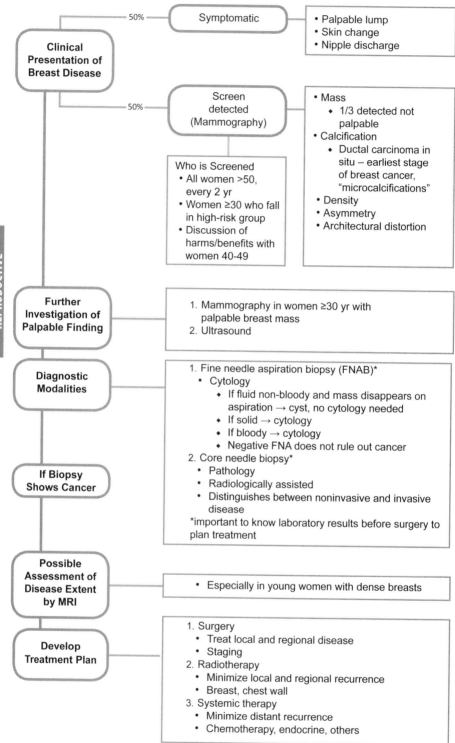

**Clinical Presentation of Breast Disease**

— 50% — **Symptomatic**
- Palpable lump
- Skin change
- Nipple discharge

— 50% — **Screen detected (Mammography)**
- Mass
  - 1/3 detected not palpable
- Calcification
  - Ductal carcinoma in situ – earliest stage of breast cancer, "microcalcifications"
- Density
- Asymmetry
- Architectural distortion

**Who is Screened**
- All women >50, every 2 yr
- Women ≥30 who fall in high-risk group
- Discussion of harms/benefits with women 40-49

**Further Investigation of Palpable Finding**
1. Mammography in women ≥30 yr with palpable breast mass
2. Ultrasound

**Diagnostic Modalities**
1. Fine needle aspiration biopsy (FNAB)*
   - Cytology
     - If fluid non-bloody and mass disappears on aspiration → cyst, no cytology needed
     - If solid → cytology
     - If bloody → cytology
     - Negative FNA does not rule out cancer
2. Core needle biopsy*
   - Pathology
   - Radiologically assisted
   - Distinguishes between noninvasive and invasive disease

**If Biopsy Shows Cancer**

*important to know laboratory results before surgery to plan treatment

**Possible Assessment of Disease Extent by MRI**
- Especially in young women with dense breasts

**Develop Treatment Plan**
1. Surgery
   - Treat local and regional disease
   - Staging
2. Radiotherapy
   - Minimize local and regional recurrence
   - Breast, chest wall
3. Systemic therapy
   - Minimize distant recurrence
   - Chemotherapy, endocrine, others

REPRODUCTIVE

**Figure 5.** Breast Screening Flow Chart[4,5]

## 6. COMMON CLINICAL SCENARIOS

**Table 4.** Common breast-related disorders [1,6]

| Key Signs/Symptoms | Physical Exam | Investigations | Management |
|---|---|---|---|
| **Fibroadenoma** | | | |
| • Single nontender lump<br>• 15% are multiple, especially on U/S<br>• Usually develop in young women (<30 yr)<br>• About 1/3 get smaller, 1/3 stay the same, 1/3 grow<br>• May regress with menopause<br>• New mass at an older age requires work-up to rule out malignancy or phyllodes tumour (average age 45 yrs). | • Palpable breast lump 1-2 cm in size.<br>• Well-defined, nontender, round or lobulated, with firm or rubbery consistency<br>• No tethering to underlying tissue, very mobile | • U/S or core needle biopsy for tissue diagnosis | • Consider excision if >4-5 cm, if enlarging >5mm every 6 months (pathology required to rule out Phyllodes tumor) or if diagnosis not conclusive from FNAB/core biopsy<br>• Repeat U/S q6 mo x 2 yr |
| **Breast Cyst** | | | |
| • Cysts may increase in size rapidly, may decrease or disappear<br>• Bilateral, with occasional non-spontaneous multi-ductal nipple discharge, color can be murky or greenish-black<br>• Affected females often 30-50 yr<br>• Estrogen therapy may cause cyst development in menopausal women | • Firm, smooth, tender, mobile, and well-defined mass | • Mammography, U/S ± FNAB ± cytological studies<br>• U/S or FNAB are the best ways to differentiate cystic from solid masses | • Aspirate dominant or bothersome cysts<br>• Cysts determined to be complicated cysts on U/S followed with repeat U/S at 6 mo<br>• Those determined to be complex cysts require FNAB and tissue diagnosis (identified as complex on U/S or clinically by not resolving completely with aspiration) |
| **Mastalgia** | | | |
| **Cyclic:**<br>• Common in premenopausal females<br>• Bilateral, poorly localized, variable duration, heaviness or soreness that radiates to axilla and arm, etiology unknown, relieved with menses, and resolves spontaneously<br>**Noncyclic:**<br>• More common in women between 40-50 yr, unilateral, described as sharp, burning pain localized in breast, usually caused by cyst or costochondritis | • Nonspecific, look for mass.<br>• Check for pain with palpation over the ribs secondary to costochondritis. | • If normal physical exam and breast pain is cyclic, no investigations warranted<br>• If physical exam findings in women ≥30, mammography to rule out cancer<br>• U/S or FNAB is the best way to differentiate cystic from solid masses6 | • If physical exam and investigations are negative, then reassure given high rate of spontaneous remission (60-80%)6<br>• Other non-pharmacological treatments: evening primrose oil, sports bra, TylenolTM, reassurance |

REPRODUCTIVE

**Mastitis/Superficial Cellulitis of the Breast**

| | | | |
|---|---|---|---|
| • Fever, unilateral breast tenderness and inflammation<br>• Occurs around the time of childbirth, in nursing mothers, or after injury | • Unilateral erythema, swelling, tenderness, and warmth<br>• Distinct from Paget's disease, which may appear as scaly skin with p'eau d'orange and generally involves the nipple | • In non-lactating women, need imaging to rule out cancer<br>• *S. aureus* almost always the etiologic agent[5] | • Drain and aspirate/ incise abscess if present<br>• Antibiotics<br>• Continue breast feeding<br>• If no resolution, investigate further |

REPRODUCTIVE

## REFERENCES

1.  Morrow M. The evaluation of common breast problems. Am Fam Physician. 2000; 61 (8):2371- 2378.
2.  Bilimoria MM, Morrow M. The woman at increased risk for breast cancer: Evaluation and management strategies. CA Cancer J Clin. 1995; 45(5):263-278.
3.  Ontario Breast Screening Program (OBSP) Guidelines Summary. Cancer Care Ontario. www. cancercare.on.ca. Published 2015. Accessed August 31, 2016.
4.  Warner E, Heisey R, Carroll J. Primer: Applying the 2011 Canadian guidelines for breast cancer screening in practice. CMAJ. 2012; 184(16):1803-1807.
5.  Tonelli M, Gorber SC, Joffres M. The Canadian Task Force on Preventive Health Care. Recommendations on screening for breast cancer in average-risk women aged 40-74 years. CMAJ. 2011; 183(17):1991-2001.
6.  Barton MB, Harris R, Fletcher SW. The rational clinical examination. Does this patient have breast cancer? The screening clinical breast examination: should it be done? How? JAMA. 1999; 282(13):1270-1280.
7.  Pruthi S. Detection and evaluation of a palpable breast mass. Mayo Clin Proc. 2001; 76(6):641- 648.
8.  Klein S. Evaluation of palpable breast masses. Am Fam Physician. 2005; 71(9):1731-1 738.
9.  Lehman CD, Blume JD, Weatherall P, Thickman D, Hylton N, Warner E, et al. Screening women at high risk for breast cancer with mammography and magnetic resonance imaging. Cancer 2005; 108(9):1898-1 905.

REPRODUCTIVE

REPRODUCTIVE

CHAPTER 9B:

# The Gynecological Exam

**Editors:**
Erica Pascoal, BSc
Priyanka Patel, MSc

**Resident Reviewer:**
Anjali Kulkarni, MD, MSc

**Faculty Reviewers:**
Elyse Levinsky, MD, MHSc, FRCSC
Richard Pittini, MD, MEd, FACOG, FRCSC

## TABLE OF CONTENTS

# 1. ESSENTIAL ANATOMY AND PHYSIOLOGY

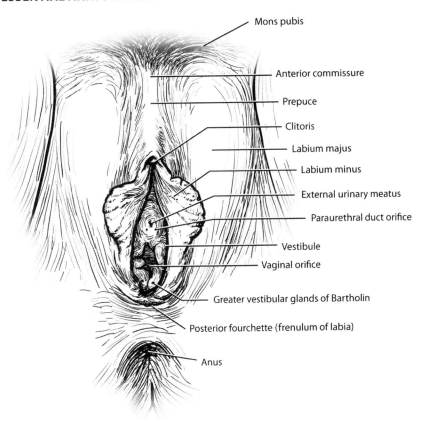

**Figure 1.** External Female Genitalia

Diana Kryski

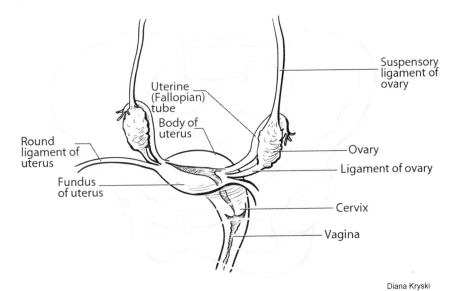

**Figure 2.** Female Reproductive Tract

Diana Kryski

## 1.2 Physiology[1]

### The Menstrual Cycle
The average adult menstrual cycle lasts approx. 28d (range of 'normal' is q21-q35d)
- By convention, the first day of menses represents the first day of the cycle (Day 1)
- The proliferative phase begins following menses and ends on the
- day of the luteinizing hormone (LH) surge.
- The LH surge may occur on any day between day 7 and day 21 of the menstrual cycle. Therefore, the length of the proliferative is variable.
- The secretory phase begins on the day of the LH surge and ends at the onset of the next menses
- The LH surge always occurs 14 days prior to the onset of menses. Therefore, the length of the secretory phase is fixed at 14 days

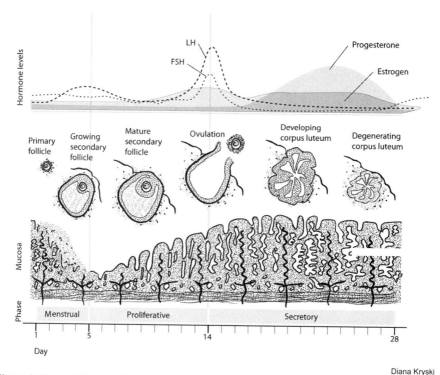

**Figure 3.** Normal Menstrual Cycle

Diana Kryski

### Menarche
- Onset of menarche (normally between 9-16 yr, mean 12.5 yr)
- Refer to the Tanner stages of development for males and females (see **The Pediatrics** chapter)

### Menopause
- Retrospective diagnosis based on the lack of menses for 12 mo,
- Average age for menopause is 51 yr (in Canada), with 95% of women experiencing it between the ages of 44 and 55 yr
- 60% of menopausal women are relatively asymptomatic, while 15% experience moderate or severe symptoms

REPRODUCTIVE

## 2. COMMON GYNECOLOGICAL CHIEF COMPLAINTS

**Table 1.** Common presentations in gynecology[2,3]

| Chief Complaints | Etiology | Differential Diagnosis |
|---|---|---|
| **Abdominal or pelvic pain** | Uterine: | Fibroids (degeneration), endometritis (pelvic inflammatory disease – PID), miscarriage |
| | Ovarian: | Cysts, ruptured cyst, torsion, tubo-ovarian abscess |
| | Fallopian Tube: | Salpingitis (PID), ectopic pregnancy |
| | Peritoneal: | Endometriosis, PID, adhesions |
| **Abnormal vaginal bleeding** | Premenarchal: | Vulvovaginitis, trauma, foreign body, urethral prolapse, sexual abuse, hormonally active tumour |
| | Premenopausal: | Endometriosis, dysfunctional uterine bleeding, uterine fibroid/polyp, pelvic inflammatory disease |
| | Peri and postmenopausal: | Endometrial hyperplasia/cancer, anticoagulant medications, hormonal medications, underlying coagulopathy |
| | Pregnancy-related: | Ectopic pregnancy, placental (see Obstetrics chapter) |
| **Absence/ cessation of menses (amenorrhea)** | Hypothalamus: | Anorexia nervosa, stress, significant weight changes, sleep disturbances, female athlete triad, Kallman's syndrome, pregnancy |
| *Always rule-out pregnancy before undergoing further investigations.* | Pituitary: | Prolactinoma, Sheehan's syndrome |
| | Thyroid: | Hyperthyroidism |
| | Adrenal Gland: | Cushing's disease, adrenal tumor, congenital adrenal hyperplasia |
| | Ovary: | Polycystic ovarian syndrome, premature ovarian failure, ovarian neoplasm |
| | Outflow tract: | Absence of uterus, outflow tract obstruction (imperforate hymen, vaginal septum, stenotic cervix, Asherman's syndrome) |

REPRODUCTIVE

| Chief Complaints | Etiology | Differential Diagnosis |
|---|---|---|
| Painful intercourse (dyspareunia) | Introital: | Inadequate lubrication unrelated to hypoestrogenism, vaginismus, vulvovaginitis |
| | Midvaginal: | Anatomical abnormalities (short vagina, congenital differences i.e. vaginal septum), urinary tract disease |
| | Deep: | Endometriosis, uterine retroversion, pelvic inflammatory disease |
| | Other: | Postpartum, postoperative, psychogenic, pelvic organ prolapse |
| Vaginal discharge/ itchiness | Inflammatory: | Vulvovaginitis, genital tract infection/ inflammation, neoplasia |
| | Infectious: | Chlamydia, gonorrhoea |
| | Hormonal: | IUD, OCP (secondary to progesterone) |
| Difficulty getting pregnant (infertility) | Refer to page 278 | |
| Symptoms of menopause | Refer to page 278 | |

## 3. COMMON DISORDERS[2,3]

Disorders marked with (P) are discussed in **Common Clinical Scenarios**

- Endometriosis (P)
- STIs (P)
- Infertility (P)
- Pelvic Inflammatory disease (PID) (P)
- Polycystic ovarian syndrome
- Ectopic pregnancy

- Endometriosis (P)
- STIs (P)
- Infertility (P)
- Pelvic Inflammatory disease (PID) (P)
- Polycystic ovarian syndrome
- Ectopic pregnancy

## 4. FOCUSED GYNECOLOGICAL HISTORY

**Menstrual History**
1. **Age at menarche**
2. **Last menstrual period (LMP):** specify first day of last menses
3. **Pattern of Menstruation**
   - Duration of menses (normally between 3-7d)
   - Presence or absence of dysmenorrhea (pain associated with menses)
   - Cycle regularity, intermenstrual bleeding
   - Cycle length (measured as interval between first day of menses to first day of menses in subsequent month; normally 21-35d)
   - Flow (normally heaviest on days 1-2; dark red discharge suggest normal flow; bright red blood ± clots may suggest excessive flow; pad/tampon count and saturation can help quantify)

4. **Perimenopause/menopause** (onset normally between 44-55 yr; mean 51.2 yr)
   - Symptoms of premenstrual syndrome (PMS) (4-10d before menses): (anxiety, nervousness, mood swings, irritability, food cravings, change in libido, difficulty sleeping, breast tenderness, headaches, and fluid retention)
   - Symptoms (hot flashes, flushing, sweating, sleep disturbances, vaginal dryness, vulvovaginal atrophy, mood changes, dysuria/ frequency)
   - Hormonal therapy use
   - Postmenopausal bleeding (bleeding after 1 year without periods warrants further investigation)
5. **Investigate abnormal menstrual bleeding** (see **Table 1**)

**Table 2.** Types of Abnormal Uterine Bleeding (AUB)[1]

| Type | Definition |
|---|---|
| **Dysmenorrhea** | Painful menstruation (OPQRST), amount of disability, current treatment |
| **Amenorrhea** | Absence of periods (primary vs. secondary) |
| **Polymenorrhea** | Increased frequency |
| **Oligomenorrhea** | Decreased frequency (menstrual cycle >35 d) |
| **Menorrhagia** | Increased duration or flow |
| **Metrorrhagia** | Irregular bleeding |
| **Menometrorrhia** | Heavy and irregular bleeding |
| **Contact Bleeding** | Postcoital, post-douching |

## Gynecological History

*Common Symptoms:*

- Pelvic pain
- Vaginal bleeding
- Vaginal discharge/itching
- Vaginal sores/lumps
- Menstrual irregularities
- Dysuria/hematuria
- Dyschezia/hematochezia
- Infertility

*Previous Diagnoses*
- Previous infections: STIs, pelvic inflammatory disease (PID), vaginitis, vulvitis, UTI; include treatment and complications
- History of infertility: duration, cause (if known), previous treatments (if applicable) (See **The Obstetrics Exam** chapter)

*Investigations and Procedures*
- Last known Pap smear (result, follow-up)
- Past history of abnormal Pap smears (results, treatments)
- Previous gynecological or abdominal surgery (e.g. laparoscopy, hysteroscopy, hysterectomy)

*Medications and Substance Use*
- Use of prescription/OTC medications and herbal remedies (Note exogenous hormones)
- Use of cigarettes, alcohol, or recreational drugs

*Family History*
- History of breast cancer, ovarian cancer, endometrial cancer, or colon cancer

*Review of Systems*
- Breast: History (see **The Breast Exam** chapter)
- Urological: day/night urinary frequency, pain, urge/stress incontinence, hematuria
- Gastrointestinal: changes in bowel movements (eg. regularity, pain, bleeding), use of laxative

REPRODUCTIVE

*Sexual and Contraceptive History (5 P's)* (see **The General History and Physical** chapter)

*Obstetrical History* (see **The Obstetric Exam** chapter)

## 5. FOCUSED GYNECOLOGICAL EXAM[4]

### 5.1 Breast Examination (see **Breast Exam** chapter)

### 5.2 Pelvic Examination

#### Preparing for the Examination
- Explain each step in advance
- Encourage questions and feedback about comfort and pain
- Advise patient to avoid intercourse, douching, or use of vaginal suppositories for 24 to 48 h prior to examination
- Ask patient to empty bladder and remove all clothing below waist
- Avoid terminology that can be misinterpreted
  - "Let your knees fall apart" not "spread your legs"
  - "Removing the speculum" not "pulling out"
- Monitor comfort level of examination by observing patient's face

#### Lithotomy Positioning
- Drape cover sheet from lower abdomen to knees; depress drape between knees to provide eye contact
- Patient lies supine, with head and shoulders elevated, arms at sides or folded across chest to enhance eye contact and reduce tightening of abdominal muscles
- Ask patient to place heels in foot rests and slide down table until buttocks align with table edge
- Ensure hips flexed, abducted, and externally rotated

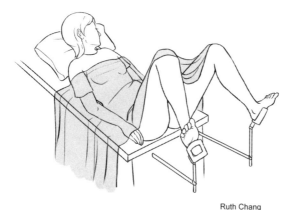

Ruth Chang

**Figure 4.** Lithotomy Position

#### Inspection of External Genitalia
*Mons Pubis, Labia, Perineum, and Perianal Area*
  - Inspect for masses, nodules, pubic lice, lesions, scars, fistulas, blisters, ulcers, hemorrhoids, inflammation, discharge, pigmentation, asymmetry, varicosities

*Vagina and Vulva*
  - Note masses and lesions for signs of vaginal carcinoma and vulvar intraepithelia neoplasia

## Speculum Examination

*Preparation*
- Have all equipment ready and within reach (Pap smear kit, endocervical brush, vaginal culture medium, glass slide, gonococcal or chlamydia sterile cotton swab, and collection tube)
- Warm speculum under running water, test temperature on inside of patient's thigh
- Use water to lubricate the speculum if necessary, not gel (interferes with Pap smear and culture test results)

*Insertion of Speculum*
- Use index and middle finger to separate labia and expose vaginal opening
- Insert speculum aiming for posterior fornix, avoiding contact with urethra
- Slide speculum inward along posterior wall of vagina, applying downward pressure to keep the vaginal introitus relaxed
- Open blades slowly
- Locate cervix by adjusting the angle of the speculum; lock speculum in open position once it is well exposed

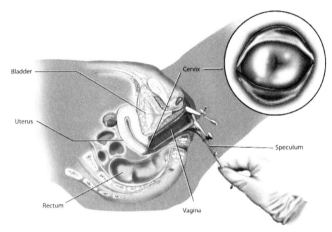

Caitlin C. Monney

**Figure 5.** Insertion of the Speculum in Lithotomy Positioning

*Inspection of Cervix*
- Note cervical color, shape of os, discharge, polyps, lesions, ulcerations, or inflammation
- Deviation of cervix from midline may indicate pelvic mass, uterine adhesions, or pregnancy
- Note position of cervix
  - Anterior cervix: retroverted uterus
  - Posterior cervix: anteverted uterus

*± Gonococcal (GC) or Chlamydial Culture*
- Introduce sterile cotton swab through open speculum and insert into os
- Hold in place for 10-30 s (45 s for chlamydia)
- Remove swab and insert into collection tube (PCR media for both GC and chlamydia)
- Note: urine samples are now commonly used to screen for GC and chlamydia (74% sensitivity, 96% specificity)

*± Pap Smear*
- For best results, patient should not be menstruating
- Inform patient she may feel an uncomfortable scraping sensation

- Most centers use the liquid based ThinPrep® technology that provides an improvement in detection over other methods[5]
  - Insert the central bristles of the broom into the endocervical canal
  - Maintaining gentle pressure, rotate the brush five revolutions in a clockwise direction
  - Twirl brush in ThinPrep® solution to loosen cells from broom and discard broom or detach tip of broom into solution

## ± Vaginal Culture
- Introduce sterile cotton swab through open speculum
- Collect any obvious secretions
- Remove swab and insert into collection container or perform a wet mount where vaginal discharge is placed on a glass slide, mixed with salt solution and viewed under microscope

## Removal of Speculum and Inspection of Vaginal Walls
- Unlock speculum and remove slowly, rotating to inspect vaginal walls (careful not to pinch mucosa)
- Gradually bring blades together while simultaneously withdrawing speculum; blades should be completely closed by the time the tip of the speculum is removed
- Maintain downward pressure of speculum to avoid injuring urethra o Assess support of vaginal walls. Separate labia with middle and index fingers, ask patient to bear down. Look for any bulging of vaginal walls (cystocele or rectocele)
  - Cystocele: bulging of upper two-thirds of anterior vaginal wall
  - Rectocele: herniation of rectum into posterior wall of vagina

**Clinical Pearl: STI Co-Infection[6]**
If one STI is detected, other pathology or diseases may co-exist. If gonococcal infection is suspected, simultaneous treatment for chlamydia should be given. Both partners must be treated for an STI to prevent recurrence.

**Clinical Pearl: Reportable Infections[6]**
*Chlamydia trachomatis* and *Neisseria gonorrhoeae* infections are reportable according to certain provincial/territorial public health acts. Contact tracing, the process of informing all sexual partners within 60 d of onset of symptoms, is recommended by the Canadian Guidelines on Sexually Transmitted Infections. Contact tracing may be done by the patient or confidentially by a healthcare provider or public health officials without naming the index case.

**Clinical Pearl: HPV Vaccination[7]**
There are currently 3 HPV vaccines available in Canada: Gardasil, Cervarix and Gardasil 9 which all protect against HPV-16 and HPV-18 (account for 70% of cervical cancers). In addition, Gardasil protects against HPV-6 and HPV-11 and Gardasil 9 protects against HPV-6, 11, 16, 18, 31, 33, 45, 52, and 58. Note: HPV-6 and HPV-11 account for 90% of genital warts. The National Advisory Committee on Immunization recommends Gardasil or Cervarix to females aged 9-26 (most effective before sexually active), females aged 15-26 who have been sexually active or have a history of abnormal Pap tests or genital warts. Similarly, Gardasil is most effective when given to males prior to any sexual activity. It is recommended for males between the ages of 9 and 26, and males aged 9 or older who have sex with other males.

## Palpation of External Genitalia
### Labia
- Spread labia majora laterally to see labia minora, introitus, and outer vagina[1]
- Palpate labia majora between thumb and second finger to feel for masses or tenderness
- Separate labia minora and palpate as above; palpate introitus and perineum
- Note: any fusion of minora to majora, or other distortion of anatomy

*Vagina*
- Place forefinger 2-3cm into vagina
- Assess vaginal muscles by asking patient to squeeze vaginal opening around your finger (usually better in nulliparous women)
- Note: avoid contact with antero-superior aspect of labia including the clitoris

## Palpation of Internal Genitalia (Bimanual Examination)
- Lubricate index and middle finger of gloved examining hand
- Separate labia with non-examining hand and insert examining fingers into vaginal opening, pressing downward against perineum to help muscles relax
- Keep fourth and fifth fingers flexed into palm, thumb extended
- Palpate vaginal walls and fornices as fingers are inserted1
- Normally smooth, homogenous, and nontender with no masses/ growths

## Examination of the Cervix
- Locate cervix with palmar surface of fingers
- Feel its end and circumference for size, length, and shape
- Consistency: hard suggests nonpregnant, soft suggests pregnant
- Position: anterior/posterior as discussed in speculum exam
- Gently move cervix side-to-side between fingers
  - Should move 1-2 cm each way without discomfort (watch for grimace)
  - Cervical motion tenderness suggests inflammatory process
  - Evaluate os patency by trying to insert fingertip 0.5 cm

**Table 3.** Methods for Examination of the Uterus: Positions of the Uterus

| Position | Examination Method |
|---|---|
| Anteverted (most common) | <ul><li>Press down with palmar surface of free hand on abdomen, between umbilicus and pubic symphysis</li><li>Place intravaginal fingers in posterior fornix and elevate cervix and uterus to abdominal wall</li><li>If fundus is felt by abdominal hand, uterus is anteverted</li></ul> |
| Retroverted | <ul><li>As above; if fundus is best felt by intravaginal fingers as</li><li>opposed to abdominal hand, uterus is retroverted</li></ul> |
| Midposition | <ul><li>As above; if fundus not felt well by either hand, uterus is midposition</li></ul> |

## Examination of the Uterus
- Once position established, assess:
  - Size (normal is approximately that of a closed fist; larger in multiparous women and those with fibroids)
  - Shape (usually pear-shaped; globular with adenomyosis)
  - Contour (rounded and smooth if nulliparous; irregular with fibroids) » Mobility in AP plane (absence indicates adhesions)
  - Mobility tenderness (pelvic inflammatory process, ruptured tubal pregnancy, endometriosis)
  - Consistency (soft if pregnant; firm with fibroids)

## Examination of the Adnexa
- Shift abdominal hand to right lower quadrant (RLQ) and press inward and obliquely downward toward pubic symphysis
- With intravaginal fingers in the right lateral fornix, elevate lateral
- fornix up toward abdominal hand o Assess if ovaries are palpable
- If ovaries palpable, assess:
  - Size (normally 3 x 2 x 1 cm)
  - Shape (normally ovoid)
  - Consistency (normally firm, smooth)
  - Tenderness (moderately sensitive to compression)
  - Mobility
- Normal fallopian tube is not palpable
- Repeat on left; exam more difficult due to sigmoid colon

REPRODUCTIVE

## 5.3 Rectovaginal Examination

- Warn patient of possible sensation of having a bowel movement
- Inspect anus for lesions, hemorrhoids, or inflammation
- Insert lubricated index finger in vagina and lubricated middle finger of same hand against anus (insert fingertip into rectum just past sphincter)
- Note sphincter tone
  - Tight: anxiety, scarring, fissures, lesions, inflammation
  - Lax: neurological deficit
  - Absent: improper repair of childbirth tear or trauma
- Slide both fingers forward; rotate rectal finger to assess rectovaginal septum and posterior vaginal wall
  - Note any tenderness, thickening, nodules, polyps, or masses
- Body of a retroflexed uterus may be palpable with rectal finger
  - Assess with intravaginal finger in posterior fornix; push up against cervix and press down with abdominal hand just above pubic symphysis
- Assess cul-de-sac and uterosacral ligaments for nodularity or tenderness
  - Possible endometriosis, PID, or metastatic carcinoma
- Repeat adnexal exam (using same maneuvers as above) if palpation difficult or questionable on bimanual examination
- Gently withdraw fingers and note any blood, secretions, or stool

# 6. COMMON INVESTIGATIONS

**Table 4.** Common diagnostic investigation in gynaecology

| Investigations | Details |
| --- | --- |
| Blood Work | • CBC: done preoperation or to evaluate abnormal uterine bleeding, anemia, or infection<br>• β-hCG: to investigate possible pregnancy/ectopic pregnancy<br>• LH, FSH, TSH, prolactin (PRL), DHEAS, testosterone, estradiol: to investigate menstrual irregularities, menopause, infertility |
| Imaging | • U/S: transvaginal and transabdominal examination of pelvic structures<br>• Sonohysterogram: U/S of saline-infused, expanded uterus; visualizes uterine mass, abnormalities of uterine cavity (such as a uterine septum), tubal patency<br>• Hysterosalpingography (HSG): X-ray of contrast-injected uterus and tubes (rarely done now with availability of sonohysterography) |
| Colposcopy | • Endoscopic exam of vagina and cervix<br>• Acetic acid allows visualization of areas to biopsy for identification of dysplasia and/or neoplasia |
| Genital Tract Biopsy | • Vulvar, vaginal, cervical, endometrial (endometrial biopsy performed in all post-menopausal bleeding to exclude endometrial cancer) |

## 7. COMMON CLINICAL SCENARIOS[1,3]

**Table 5.** Common clinical scenarios in gynaecology

| Definition | Key Signs and Symptoms | Diagnosis | Management |
|---|---|---|---|
| **MENARCHE** | | | |
| Onset of menses (normally between 9-16 yr, mean 12.5 yr)<br><br>Average cycle of 28 +/- 7d with 1-6d of bleeding | Premenstrual syndrome (PMS):<br>• Breast tenderness or swelling<br>• Headache<br>• Acne<br>• Fatigue<br>• Cramping (abdomen, back, legs)<br>• Mood changes, irritability<br>• Appetite changes | Clinical | N/A |
| **MENOPAUSE** | | | |
| Retrospective diagnosis based on the lack of menses for 12 mo, age >40yr | **Symptoms** (mainly associated with estrogen deficiency)<br>• Menstrual cycle alteration: cessation of menses for >12 mo due to ovarian failure<br>• Vasomotor instability (aka "hot flushes")<br>• Sleep disturbances (night sweats)<br>• Dyspareunia, vaginal dryness/pruritus, genital tract atrophy, vaginal bleeding<br>• Increased frequency of urination, urgency, incontinence<br>• Fatigue, irritability, mood changes, memory loss, decreased libido<br>• Increased frequency of urination, urgency, incontinence<br>• Fatigue, irritability, mood changes, memory loss, decreased libido<br><br>**Signs:**<br>• Skin thinning, decreased elasticity, increased facial hair, thin and brittle nails, vaginal dryness, pale tissues, loss of rugae, less distensible | **Diagnosis**<br>• Increased levels of FSH (>40 IU/L)<br>• Decreased levels of estradiol (15-350 pg/mL) | • Hormone replacement therapy (HRT): estrogen, progestin<br>• Selective estrogen receptor modulators (SERMs)<br>• Calcium, vitamin D supplements (to decrease bone loss)<br>• Selective serotonin reuptake inhibitors, clonidine, herbal remedies (soy and black cohosh) (for hot flushes)<br>• Local estrogen cream/vaginal suppository/ring, lubricants (for vaginal atrophy)<br>• Nonmedical (complementary medicine, exercise, counseling, healthy diet, other lifestyle modifications)<br>• Counselling and monitoring to prevent osteoporotic changes |

**REPRODUCTIVE**

| Definition | Key Signs and Symptoms | Diagnosis | Management |
|---|---|---|---|

## PELVIC INFLAMMATORY DISEASE[6]

| Definition | Key Signs and Symptoms | Diagnosis | Management |
|---|---|---|---|
| Inflammatory disorder of the uterus, fallopian tubes, and adjacent pelvic structures caused by direct spread of microorganisms ascending from the vagina and cervix<br><br>Common organisms: *Neisseria gonorrhoeae, Chlamydia trachomatis,* genital mycoplasmas<br><br>**Risk factors:** Young age at first intercourse, multiple partners, uterine instrumentation, smoking | **Symptoms**<br>• Low abdominal or pelvic pain of recent onset that may be bilateral<br>• Vaginal discharge<br>• Irregular vaginal bleeds (irregular menstrual cycle and/or intermittent bleeds)<br>• Deep dyspareunia<br><br>**Signs**<br>• Fever<br>• Abdominal tenderness; signs of peritoneal irritation<br>• Cervical motion tenderness<br>• Cervical discharge<br>• Adnexal mass and/or tenderness on bimanual examination<br>• Pelvic heat | **On abdominal exam:** look for focal tenderness/ peritoneal signs<br><br>**On speculum:** look for mucopurulent discharge<br><br>**On pelvic exam:** look for adnexal masses, cervical motion tenderness, adnexal tenderness | **Outpatient Rx:** PO/IM antibiotics (e.g. ceftriaxone IM + doxycycline PO +/- metronidazole PO x 14 d)<br><br>**Inpatient Rx:** IV antibiotics with step-down to PO antibiotics 24 h after clinical improvement (e.g. cefoxitin IV + doxycycline IV/PO)<br><br>**Complications:** Infertility, ectopic pregnancy, chronic pain |

## CANDIDIASIS[6]

| Definition | Key Signs and Symptoms | Diagnosis | Management |
|---|---|---|---|
| Overgrowth of yeast in the vagina<br><br>Common organisms: Candida albicans (90%), Candida tropicalis, Candida glabrata<br><br>**Risk factors:** Immunosuppression, antibiotic use, pregnancy | **Asymptomatic** (20%)<br><br>**Symptoms**<br>• Itching, burning<br>• White, lumpy, "cottage cheese" discharge | **pH test:** pH <4.7<br><br>**Wet mount:** 50-60% sensitive; can see budding yeast, hyphae, pseudohyphae<br><br>**Culture:** higher sensitivity than wet mount; can identify species of yeast | Topical azole drugs most effective (available as ovules and creams for 1, 3, or 7 d)<br><br>Oral therapy also available<br><br>Treat male partner only if yeast balanitis present |

## BACTERIAL VAGINOSIS[6]

| Definition | Key Signs and Symptoms | Diagnosis | Management |
|---|---|---|---|
| Replacement of normal vaginal flora with other organisms<br><br>Common organisms: *Gardnerella vaginalis, Mycoplasma hominis,* certain anaerobes | Symptoms:<br>• Malodorous<br>• Thin, white/gray adherent discharge<br>• Possible itching | **pH Test:** pH > 4.5<br><br>**Wet mount:** clue cells with adherent coccoid bacteria<br><br>**KOH whiff test:** fishy odor | Metronidazole<br><br>No treatment for male partner |

| Definition | Key Signs and Symptoms | Diagnosis | Management |
|---|---|---|---|

### ENDOMETRIOSIS[9]

| Definition | Key Signs and Symptoms | Diagnosis | Management |
|---|---|---|---|
| Affects 5-10% of reproductive-age women and 25-35% of women with infertility History of cyclic pelvic pain and dysmenorrhea supports the diagnosis, but needs to be distinguished from chronic pelvic pain | **Symptoms:**<br>• pelvic pain<br>• dysmenorrhea (worsens with age)<br>• infertility<br>• deep dyspareunia<br>• premenstrual and postmenstrual spotting<br>• increased frequency of urination, dysuria, hematuria, dysuria<br>• diarrhea, constipation, hematochezia, dyschezia<br><br>**Signs:** tender nodularity of uterine ligaments and cul-de-sac, fixed retroversion of the uterus, firm, fixed adnexal mass (endometrioma) | **Diagnosis:** responds to medical treatment (presumptive), laparoscopy ± histology (definitive) | **Medical**<br>*1st line:* NSAIDs, OCP (cyclic/continuous), progestin therapy (oral, injection or progestin IUD)<br><br>*2nd line:* antiestrogen agents (e.g. Danazol), gonadotropin releasing hormone agonists<br><br>**Surgical:** laparoscopic resection/vaporization/ ablation of implants, removal of adhesions, Mirena IUD, definitive therapy (hysterectomy, bilateral salpingo-oophorectomy) |

**Table 6.** Common clinical scenarios in gynaecology: benign neoplasms

| Definition | Key Signs and Symptoms | Diagnosis | Management |
|---|---|---|---|

### LICHEN SCLEROSUS

| Definition | Key Signs and Symptoms | Diagnosis | Management |
|---|---|---|---|
| Site: vulva Description: Benign, inflammatory, immune-mediated skin disease Most common in postmenopausal women | **Symptoms:**<br>• Pruritus<br>• Dyspareunia<br>• Burning | **Diagnosis:** Silvery or ivory white tissue on examination and shiny or crinkly, with areas of purpura or ecchymosis | Topical steroids |

### ENDOCERVICAL POLYPS & UTERINE FIBROIDS

| Definition | Key Signs and Symptoms | Diagnosis | Management |
|---|---|---|---|
| Site: cervix, uterus (leiomyomata [fibroids]) Description: growth from smooth muscle (monoclonal); can be submucosal, intramural, subserosal, or pedunculated | Asymptomatic (60%), abnormal uterine bleeding (30%; most often from submucosal fibroid), pressure/bulk symptoms (20-50%), acute pelvic pain, infertility | **Diagnosis:** bimanual exam, CBC (anemia), ultrasound, sonohys-terogram/saline infusion hysterography | **Conservative:** useful if minimal symptoms, size <8 cm or stable<br>**Medical:** ibuprofen, tranexamic acid, OCP/Depo-Provera®, GnRH agonists<br>**Interventional radiology:** uterine artery embolization<br>**Surgical:** myomectomy (hysteroscopic if intracavitary, laparoscopic, or laparotomy), hysterectomy |

| Definition | Key Signs and Symptoms | Diagnosis | Management |
|---|---|---|---|

### HYDATIDIFORM MOLE

**Description:**
Benign form of gestational trophoblastic neoplasm; includes complete and partial mole

| Definition | Key Signs and Symptoms | Diagnosis | Management |
|---|---|---|---|
| **Complete mole:** 2 sperm fertilize empty egg or 1 sperm with duplication<br><br>**Risk factors:** maternal age >40yr, low beta carotene diet, vitamin A deficiency | **Clinical features:** vaginal bleeding, excessive uterine size, hyperemesis gravidum | **Diagnosis:** Diagnosis often based on pathology from D&C, β-hCG >100,000, no fetal heart detected<br>*Additional supportive findings:* theca-lutein cysts <6cm, hyperthyroidism, preeclampsia | **Treatment:** D&C; watch out for thyroid storm and be prepared to treat appropriately (rare complication)<br>Avoid pregnancy for 6-12mo |
| **Partial mole:** single ovum fertilized by 2 sperm; often associated with fetus that is growth restricted and has multiple congenital malformations | **Clinical features:** similar to spontaneous abortion (spontaneous loss of a fetus before the 20th wk) | **Diagnosis:** diagnosis often based on pathology from D&C, ultrasound showing abnormal placental features, β-hCG high for early pregnancy | **Treatment:** D&C with sharp curettage and oxytocin, hysterectomy if future fertility not desired, prophylactic chemotherapy (controversial); RhoGAM® if patient is Rh negative<br>Avoid pregnancy for 6-12mo |

**Table 7.** Common clinical scenarios in gynaecology: malignant neoplasms

| Definition | Key Signs and Symptoms | Diagnosis | Management |
|---|---|---|---|

### VULVULAR CANCER

| Definition | Key Signs and Symptoms | Diagnosis | Management |
|---|---|---|---|
| Description: 90% squamous cell carcinoma<br><br>Risk Factors: HPV infection (HPV-16, HPV-18), vulvar intraepithelial neoplasia | **Clinical Features:** asymptomatic, localized pruritus, lump, or mass, raised red, white or pigmented plaque, ulcer, bleeding, discharge, pain, dysuria | | |

### CERVICAL CANCER

| Definition | Key Signs and Symptoms | Diagnosis | Management |
|---|---|---|---|
| Description: 95% squamous cell carcinoma<br><br>Risk Factors: HPV infection (HPV-16, HPV-18), smoking, high risk sexual behavior | **Clinical Features:**<br>• Early: asymptomatic, discharge (watery, becoming brown or red), postcoital bleeding<br>• Late: bleeding (postcoital, postmenopausal, irregular), pelvic or back pain, bladder/bowel symptoms | Diagnosis: Pap screening, colposcopy, endocervical curettage, cervical biopsy, cone biopsy | Prevention (secondary): regular Pap smears |

REPRODUCTIVE

## ENDOMETRIAL CARCINOMA

**Description:** most common gynecological malignancy

**Clinical Features:** postmenopausal bleeding, abnormal uterine bleeding

**Diagnosis:** endometrial biopsy, if endometrial biopsy unsuccessful (I.e. cervical stenosis), consider D&C ± hysteroscopy

Stage 1: Grade A and B: total abdominal hysterectomy (TAH)/bilateral salpingo-oophorectomy (BSO) and washings; Grade C: requires nodal dissection
Stages 2 and 3: TAH/BSO, washings, and nodal dissection
Stage 4: nonsurgical
• Adjuvant radiotherapy: based on myometrial penetration, tumor grade, lymph node involvement
• Hormonal therapy: progestins for distant or recurrent disease
• Adjuvant chemotherapy: based on disease progression

## OVARIAN CANCER

**Description:**
3 types: epithelial (80-85%), germ cell (10-15%), and stromal cell (3-5%); 4th leading cause of cancer death in women
**Risk Factors:** white race, late age at menopause, family history of ovarian, breast or bowel cancer, prolonged intervals of ovulation uninterrupted by pregnancy

**Clinical Features:** usually asymptomatic until advanced (Stage III)
• Early: vague abdominal symptoms (nausea, bloating, dyspepsia, anorexia, early satiety), postmenopausal or irregular bleeding (rare)
• Late: increased abdominal girth, urinary frequency, constipation, ascites

**Diagnosis:** bimanual exam, CBC, LFTs, electrolytes, creatinine, CA-125, CXR, abdominal/pelvic U/S ± transvaginal U/S

Early: TAH/BSO, infracolic omentectomy, and thorough surgical staging
Late: cytoreductive surgery ("debulking") and chemotherapy

## GESTATIONAL TROPHOBLASTIC NEOPLASMS

**Description:** includes invasive mole (a locally invasive lesion) and choriocarcinoma (a frankly malignant form; may follow any type of pregnancy, highly anaplastic )

**Risk factors:** preceding molar pregnancy

**Clinical features:** symptoms of metastatic disease, vaginal bleeding, hemoptysis, cough or dyspnea, headaches, dizzy spells, "blacking out" or rectal bleeding

**Diagnosis:**
i. Invasive mole
Increase or plateau in β-hCG following treatment of molar pregnancy, molar tissue on histology

ii. Choriocarcinoma: CBC, electrolytes, creatinine, β-hCG as above, TSH, LFTs, CXR, pelvic U/S, CT abdomen/pelvis, CT head

**Treatment:**
i. invasive mole: chemotherapy (single agent or combination), radiation for metastases to brain or liver

ii. Choriocarcinoma: chemotherapy

REPRODUCTIVE

## Infertility[3]

*Description*
- Failure to conceive after 1 year of unprotected sexual intercourse

*Etiology*
- Approximately 40% due to a male factor, 40% due to a female factor, and 20% due to both male and female contributing causes, 10-15% unexplained

*Symptoms/signs:*
- Often asymptomatic
- Not recognized until pregnancy attempts unsuccessful

**Table 8.** Common causes of female infertility

| Localization | Diagnosis |
| --- | --- |
| **Ovulatory dysfunction** (20-40% of cases)<br><br>Hyperprolactinemia, thyroid disease, PCOS, luteal phase defects, certain systemic diseases, congenital diseases, poor nutrition, stress, excessive exercise, eating disorder, hypothalamic-pituitary dysfunction | Serum PRL, TSH, LH, FSH, history of cycle patterns, basal body temperature, mucus quality, endometrial biopsy for luteal phase defect, serum progesterone level, karyotype, liver and renal function |
| **Tubal factors** (20-30% of cases)<br><br>PID, adhesions, tubal ligation, previous gynecological surgery | Hysterosalpingogram, sonohysterogram, laparoscopy with dye |
| **Cervical factors** (<5% of cases)<br><br>Structural abnormalities, antisperm antibodies, hostile acidic cervical mucus, glands unresponsive to estrogen | Postcoital test |
| **Uterine factors** (<5% of cases)<br><br>Polyps, infection, intrauterine adhesions, congenital anomalies, leiomyomata, endometriosis | Hysterosalpingogram, sonohysterogram, hysteroscopy |

**LH = LUTEINIZING HORMONE**
**PCOS = POLYCYSTIC OVARIAN SYNDROME**
**PID = PELVIC INFLAMMATORY DISEASE**
**PRL = PROLACTIN**

**Clinical Pearl: Vaginal Bleeding**
Vaginal bleeding in postmenopausal women is endometrial cancer until proven otherwise.

REPRODUCTIVE

## Contraception

**Table 9.** Contraceptive Methods[11-14]

| Type (Effectiveness*: perfect use, typical use) | Side effects | Contraindications |
| --- | --- | --- |
| **Barrier Methods** | | |
| **Spermicide Alone** (82%, 71%) | | Latex allergy, past expiry date |
| **Spermicide Alone** (82%, 71%) | Vaginal irritation may promote HIV transmission, messy, tastes bad, costly | |
| **Sponge** Parous (80%, 68%) Nulliparous (91%, 84%) | Vaginal irritation or dryness, toxic shock syndrome | Sulfa, polyurethane, or spermicide nonoxynol-9 sensitivity or allergy |
| **Diaphragm with Spermicide** (94%, 84%) | Diaphragm: UTI, vaginal irritation, toxic shock syndrome | Latex allergy |
| **Female Condom** (95%, 79%) | | |
| **Cervical Cap** Parous (74%, 68%) Nulliparous (91%, 84%) | Vaginal irritation, urinary tract infection | Silicone or spermicide sensitivity or allergy |
| **Hormonal Methods** | | |
| **Oral Contraceptive Pill (OCP)** (99.7%, 92%) | Breakthrough bleeding, nausea, headache, depression, bloating, decreased libido, increased venous thromboembolism (VTE) risk, increased stroke or MI risk in smokers and those with other risk factors | Known/suspected pregnancy, undiagnosed abnormal vaginal bleeding, thromboembolic disorders, cerebrovascular or coronary artery disease7, estrogen dependent tumors, impaired liver function with acute liver disease, smoker > 35 yr, migraines with focal neurological symptoms, uncontrolled HTN |
| **Progestin-Only Pill (Micronor®)** (90-99%) | Irregular menstrual bleeding, weight gain, headache, breast tenderness, mood changes, functional ovarian cysts, acne/oily skin, hirsutism | Refer to OCP contraindications |
| **Nuva Ring®** (99.7%, 92%) | Vaginal infections/irritation, vaginal discharge | Refer to OCP contraindications |

REPRODUCTIVE

| Type (Effectiveness*: perfect use, typical use) | Side effects | Contraindications |
|---|---|---|
| **Transdermal (Ortho Evra®)** (99.7%, 92%) | Breakthrough bleeding, breast symptoms, headaches, nausea, application site reactions, dysmenorrhea | Refer to OCP contraindications |
| **Depo Provera®** (99.7%, 97%) | Irregular bleeding, weight gain, mood changes, decreased bone density, delay in return of fertility (average 9 mo) | |
| **Implant Methods** | | |
| **IUD** | Intermenstrual bleeding, expulsion, uterine wall perforation possible, greater chance of ectopic if pregnancy does occur, increased risk of PID in first 30d after insertion | Known or suspected pregnancy, undiagnosed genital tract bleeding, acute or chronic PID, lifestyle risk for STIs |
| *Types: Nonhormonal* **Copper** (99.3%) | Increased blood loss and duration of menses, dysmenorrhea | Known allergy to copper, Wilson's disease |
| *Hormonal* **Mirena® IUD** (99.9%) | Bloating, headache, unpredictable bleeding especially in first 4-6mo | |
| **Jaydess® IUD** (99%) | Missed menstrual periods, cysts on ovary | |
| **Surgical Methods** | | |
| **Tubal Ligation** (99.7%) | Invasive, generally permanent, surgical risk | |
| **Vasectomy** (99.9%) | As above | |
| **Emergency Contraception** | | |
| **Yuzpe® Method** (OCP 2 tabs 12h apart) (98% in 24h, decreases by 30% at 72h) | Nausea, spotting | Pre-existing pregnancy, caution in women with contraindications to OCP |
| **"Plan B" Levonorgestrel Only** (98% in 24h, decreases by 70% at 72h) | See above | See above |
| **Postcoital (Copper) IUD** (99.9%) | See above | See above Copper allergy, Wilson's Disease |

*Effectiveness: percentage of women reporting no pregnancy after 1yr of use

REPRODUCTIVE

## Physiological Methods
- **Withdrawal/Coitus Interruptus** (77%)
- **Rhythm Method/Calendar/Mucus/Symptothermal** (98%, 76%)
- **Lactational Amenorrhea** (98% - first 6 months   postpartum)
- **No Method Used** (10%)
- **Abstinence of All Sexual Activity** (100%)

## REFERENCES

1. Glass, K 2015, 'Menstrual Cycle & Disorders of Menstruation', Mechanisms, Manifestations, and Management of Disease, Toronto, Canada, 2 Nov.
2. Pittini, R 2015, 'Acute & Chronic Pelvic Pain', Mechanisms, Manifestations, and Management of Disease, Toronto, Canada, 4 Nov.
3. Hacker NF, Gambone JC, Moore JG. Essentials of Obstetrics and Gynecology. Philadelphia: Saunders; 2009.
4. Edelman A, Anderson J, Lai S, Braner DAV, Tegtmeyer K. 2007. Pelvic examination. N Engl J Med 356(26):e26.
5. Dawson AE. 2004. Can we change the way we screen?: The ThinPrep Imaging System. Cancer 102(6):340-344.
6. MacDonald N, Wong T. 2007. Canadian guidelines on sexually transmitted infections, 2006. CMAJ 176(2):175-176.
7. HPV vaccines, Canadian Cancer Society, July 2016, <http://www.cancer.ca/en/cancer-information/cancer-101/what-is-a-risk-factor/viruses-bacteria-and-other-infectious-agents/hpv-vaccines/?region=mb>.
8. Ontario Cervical Screening Cytology Guidelines, May 2012, <http:www.cancercare.on.ca>.
9. Leyland N, Casper R, Laberge P, Singh SS, SOGC. 2010. Endometriosis: Diagnosis and management. J Obstet Gynaecol Can 32(7 Suppl 2):S1-32.
10. DeCherney AH, Nathan L, Laufer N, Roman AS. Current Diagnosis & Treatment Obstetrics & Gynecology, 11th ed. McGraw-Hill Medical; 2013.
11. Black A, Francoeur D, Rowe T, Collins J, Miller D, Brown T, et al. 2004. SOGC clinical practice guidelines: Canadian contraception consensus. Part 1. J Obstet Gynaecol Can 26(2):143-156.
12. Black A, Francoeur D, Rowe T, Collins J, Miller D, Brown T, et al. 2004. SOGC clinical practice guidelines: Canadian contraception consensus. Part 2. J Obstet Gynaecol Can 26(3):219-296.
13. Black A, Francoeur D, Rowe T, Collins J, Miller D, Brown T, et al. 2004. SOGC clinical practice guidelines: Canadian contraception consensus. Part 3. J Obstet Gynaecol Can 26(4):347-387.
14. Boroditsky R, Fisher WA, Sand M. 1995. The Canadian contraception study. J Obstet Gynaecol Can 1 7(Suppl):S1-28.

# The Obstetrical Exam

**Editors:**
Erica Pascoal, BSc
Priyanka Patel, MSc

**Resident Reviewer:**
Anjali Kulkarni, MD, MSc

**Faculty Reviewers:**
Rory Windrim, MD, FRCSC
Adrian Brown, MD, FRCSC

## TABLE OF CONTENTS

REPRODUCTIVE

# 1. ESSENTIAL PHYSIOLOGY

**Table 1.** Physiological Changes During Pregnancy[1]

| Parameter | Changes | Comments |
|---|---|---|
| **General** | | |
| Weight | Increase | Generally recommend 11kg to 16kg weight gain for non-twin pregnancy. More weight gain recommended if low BMI, and less weight gain if high BMI. 0.5 kg /wk in second half of pregnancy |
| Energy needs | ↑15% | Increased due to fetal growth, and fat deposition. |
| **Respiratory** | | |
| Arterial Blood Gases | pCO2 98% (28-32 mmHg) | pCO2 in maternal blood facilitates placental pCO2 transfer |
| Tidal Volume | ↑40% | Increased due to progesterone effects. Results in increased minute ventilation. |
| **Cardiovascular** | | |
| Plasma Volume | ↑45% | Plasma volume must increase to supply the fetus and placenta with more circulating blood |
| Cardiac Output | ↑ 30-50% (6.0 L/min) | Cardiac output peaks at 24 weeks due to increase in stroke volume |
| Heart Rate | ↑15-20bpm | The increase in plasma volume results in increased heart rate |
| Blood Pressure | Systolic: ↓5-10 mmHg Diastolic: ↑10-15 mmHg | Overall vasodilation caused by elevated progesterone. BP lowest at 20-26 wks and then gradually increases to pre-pregnancy levels by 36 weeks. |
| **Hematologic** | | |
| Hemoglobin (Hb) | Apparent decrease | In pregnancy, the RBC volume does not increase to the same extent as plasma volume. Consequently, Hb levels decrease on lab value. This is not an absolute decrease, but rather due to dilution. |
| WBC | ↑3.5 x 1 09 /L | Leukocytosis is increased in pregnancy due to physiologic stress induced by pregnancy. |
| Coagulation | ↑Factor VII to X ↑venous stasis | 1.8-fold ↑ risk of thromboembolism |
| **Renal** | | |
| GFR | ↑50% | No change in urine output due to tubular reabsorption |

## 2. COMMON CHIEF COMPLAINTS

**Table 2.** Common Chief Complaints in Pregnancy

| Chief Complaint | Trimester | Possible Causes |
|---|---|---|
| Breast Tenderness/ Heaviness | 1 | Growth of breast tissue ↑blood flow to breast |
| Fatigue | 1 | Multifactorial |
| Nausea/vomiting | 1 | ↑estrogen and β-hCG ↑gastric motility |
| Weight Loss | 1 | Decreased appetite from nausea/vomiting |
| Heartburn | 1, 2, 3 | Relaxation of lower esophageal sphincter increases risk of reflux from stomach |
| Backache | 1, 2, 3 | Relaxation of joints and ligaments Growth of uterus Weight of fetus |
| Amenorrhea | 1, 2, 3 | ↑estrogen, progesterone, β-hCG |
| Constipation | 1, 2, 3 | Decreased peristalsis |
| Pelvic Girdle Pain | 2, 3 | Pain in the front or back of pelvis. Caused by increased stress on the sacroiliac and symphysis pubis joints, ligaments, and muscles of the pelvis |
| Round Ligament Pain | 2 | Pain in the right/ left lower quadrant that's worse with walking and improves with rest. Caused by increased stress on the round ligament |
| Urinary Frequency | 1, 2, 3 | ↓plasma osmolality ↑vascularity, pressure of enlarged uterus Pressure of fetal head on bladder |
| Leukorrhea | 1, 2, 3 | Hormonal effects of pregnancy lead to increased blood flow to vagina resulting in increased white/yellow mucous discharge from the vagina |

**Clinical Pearl: Hyperemesis Gravidarum**
Severe nausea/ vomiting in pregnancy leading to weight loss, dehydration, and electrolyte disturbances. Often resolving by 20 weeks, and occasionally lasting the entire pregnancy. Treatment may include anti-nausea medications and oral/IV fluids.

REPRODUCTIVE

**Table 3.** Chief Complaints in Pregnancy Indicative of Potential Pathological Processes

| Chief Complaint | Differential Diagnosis | Typical Presentation |
|---|---|---|
| Vaginal bleeding | Spontaneous Abortion (Miscarriage) | Before 20 wks GA<br>+/- Painful uterine cramps/ contractions, +/- dilated cervix, presence of gestational tissue at cervical os, falling β-hCG levels |
| | Abnormal Pregnancy (ectopic/molar) | 1st, 2nd Trimester<br>Abdominal/ pelvic pain, cervical motion tenderness, adnexal tenderness/ mass, β-hCG >1500 mIU/mL, presence of adnexal mass and lack of intrauterine pregnancy on transvaginal ultrasound |
| | Placenta Previa | After 20 wks GA<br>Usually **painless** bright red bleeding, diagnosed by ultrasound<br>Sudden onset |
| | Abruptio Placentae | After 20 wks GA<br>Sudden onset abdominal pain, back pain, rapid uterine contractions, fetal distress |
| | Labour | Scant blood/ blood-tinged mucous ("bloody show") preceding the onset of labour by as much as 72 h |
| | Trauma | History of physical trauma |
| Decreased Fetal Movements (DFM) | Fetal Distress | 2nd, 3rd Trimester<br><6-10 kicks perceived by mother in 2 consecutive hours, fetal tachycardia/ bradycardia, repetitive variable decelerations and/ or late deceleration on non-stress testing, low biophysical profile |
| | Fetal Demise | Sudden DFM or absence of fetal movements, lack of fetal cardiac activity on auscultation and ultrasound |
| Contractions | Normal Labour | >37 wks GA; Regular contractions increasing in frequency, intensity and duration. Associated with cervical changes (effacement, dilation, softening, movement to an anterior position) |
| | Preterm Labour | As above, occurring at <37 wks GA |
| | Braxton Hicks Contractions (False Labour) | Mild irregular contractions that do not result in cervical changes |
| Abdominal Pain | Urinary tract Infection | Suprapubic pain and abdominal cramps. Often associated with dysuria, frequency urgency. |
| | Appendicitis | May present as right upper quadrant pain rather than right lower quadrant in late pregnancy. |

REPRODUCTIVE

| Chief Complaint | Differential Diagnosis | Typical Presentation |
|---|---|---|
| Leakage of Fluid | Amniotic Fluid (Rupture of Membranes) | Spontaneous gush or slow trickling of clear fluid. Confirmed as amniotic fluid by visualization of pooling fluid, nitrazine paper test, ferning on light microscopy. In labour, associated with contractions and cervical changes. |
| | Yeast or other infection | Purulent or odorous discharge, pruritus |
| | Urine | History of urinary incontinence, tests for amniotic fluid are negative |

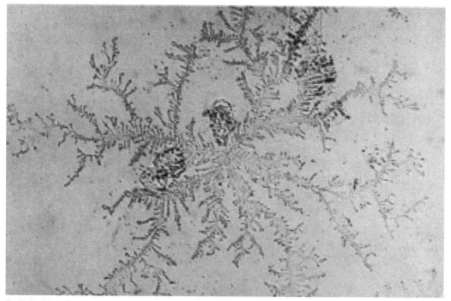

Duff, P, Glob. libr. women's med., (ISSN: 1756-2228) 2016; DOI 10.3843/GLOWM.10119

**Figure 1.** Ferning of amniotic fluid, as visualized on light microscopy

---

**Clinical Pearl: Previa or Abruption?**
PainLESS bleeding vs. PainFUL bleeding may help differentiate between placenta previa and placental abruption respectively.

---

**Clinical Pearl: 3 Cardinal Signs of Rupture of Membranes[2]**
1. Visualization of pooling fluid in the posterior fornix
2. Positive nitrazine paper test (paper turns from yellow to blue)
3. Ferning visualized on light microscopy (Figure 1)

# 3. PRECONCEPTION MANAGEMENT

### 3.1 Preconception Counseling
Routine Objectives in Preconception Care

## A) Risk Assessment
1. Genetic Screening and Family History
   - Assess based on age, ethnic background, family history
2. Nutritional Assessment
   - Assess anthropometric (BMI), biochemical (anemia), clinical and dietary risks
3. Substance Abuse
   - Assess tobacco, alcohol, and drug use
4. Infections and Immunizations
   - Screen for periodontal, urogenital and sexually transmitted infections as indicated
   - Update immunization for hepatitis B, rubella, varicella, Tdap, HPV, and influenza as needed
5. Toxins and Teratogens
   - Review exposures at home, neighbourhood, and work (e.g. chemical/radiation exposure)
6. Past Medical History
   - Assess for diseases that could affect future pregnancy (see **Gynecological Exam**)
7. Medications
   - Review current medications
   - Avoid use of FDA category X and D drugs
8. Psychosocial concerns
   - Screen for depression, anxiety, intimate partner violence and major psychosocial stressors

## B) Health Promotion
1. Healthy Weight and Nutrition
   - Promote healthy pre-pregnancy weight through exercise, nutrition
   - Discuss nutrient intake including intake of a prenatal multivitamin (PNV) with a minimum of 0.4 mg of folic acid. Women at increased risk of neural tube defects should begin taking 4.0 mg of folic acid.
   - All women should begin PNV after discontinuation of birth control and for 10-12 week after last menstrual period.
2. Health Behaviours
   - Promote nutrition and exercise
   - Discourage risky behaviors such as smoking, alcohol consumption, and substance abuse

### 3.2 Diagnosis of Pregnancy

**Table 4.** Signs and Symptoms of Pregnancy

| Diagnosis of a New Pregnancy | |
|---|---|
| **History** | Amenorrhea<br>Nausea/vomiting<br>Fatigue<br>Breast tenderness<br>Urinary frequency |
| **Physical Exam** | Signs on pelvic examination = **CHUG**<br>**C** = Chadwick's sign: bluish discoloration of cervix and vagina (9-12 wk)<br>**H** = Hegar's sign: softening of lower segment of uterus (6 wk)<br>**U** = Uterine enlargement<br>**G** = Goodell's sign: softening of cervix and vagina (8 wk) |

| **Investigations** | Serum β-hCG follow the Rule of 10's |
| --- | --- |
| | **10 IU** at time of missed menses (double every 1-2 d) |
| | **100,000 IU** at **10 wk** (peak) |
| | **10,000 IU** at term |

*Note:* Confirmation of pregnancy with fetal heart rate can be heard via transvaginal ultrasound as early as 5 wk gestational age (GA).

# 4. FOCUSED HISTORY, PHYSICAL EXAM, AND COMMON INVESTIGATIONS

## 4.1 Initial Prenatal Assessment

### A. Focused History
*Patient Identification*
- Age, occupation, and marital status

*Fertility Summary*
- Menstrual history (see **Gynecological Exam**)
    - Date of last menstrual period (LMP), last cycle frequency
    - Estimated date of birth (EDB)
        - By date of LMP using Naegele's rule:
            - 1st day of LMP + 7 days -3 months (if cycle is not 28 d, add number of additional days, i.e. add 4 if 32-day cycle)
        - By ultrasound (most accurate in first trimester); once established by U/S, EDB does not change
- Contraception
    - Type, duration of use, last use
- History of current pregnancy
    - Physiologic symptoms (see Table 1 and Table 2)
    - Potentially harmful exposures: smoking, alcohol, radiation, etc.
    - Nutritional assessment: diet, calcium, folate; avoid unpasteurized milk products, raw meats, and sushi
    - Red flags: bleeding (duration, amount, any clots), discharge/leaking fluid, cramping/ contractions, abdominal pain
- GTPALM status or GPA Status

    i.GTPALM
| | |
| --- | --- |
| **G**ravida | # of pregnancies regardless of outcome, current pregnancy included, twin pregnancy counted as 1 |
| **T**erm | # of deliveries at 37-42 wk gestation |
| **P**remature | # of deliveries <37 wk gestation |
| **A**bortion | # of abortions (spontaneous and therapeutic) |
| **L**ive | # of live deliveries |
| **M**ultiples | # of multiple pregnancies |

    ii.GPA Status
| | |
| --- | --- |
| **G**ravidity | # of pregnancies regardless of outcome, current pregnancy included, twin pregnancy counted as 1 |
| **P**arity | # of pregnancies reaching viable gestational age (including live births and stillbirths). Twin pregnancy counted as 1. |
| **A**bortus | # of abortions (spontaneous, ectopics, and therapeutic) |

*Obstetrical History*
- Year, place of birth
- Sex, gestational age, birth weight of baby
- Abortion (medical vs. surgical dilatation/curettage)

- Labor duration, type of delivery (vaginal, forceps, vacuum, Cesarean section [important to characterize direction of scar on the uterus])
- Pregnancy/delivery/perinatal/postpartum complications (e.g. preeclampsia, gestational hypertension, gestational DM, pulmonary embolism, postpartum depression)
- Health status of previous children (alive, well, illnesses)

*Medical History*
- Including, but not limited to:
  - Infections
    - TORCH infections: Toxoplasmosis, Other (Syphilis, VZV, Parvovirus B19), Rubella, Cytomegalovirus, Herpes Infections
    - HIV, STIs/HSV/bacterial vaginosis, TB risk
  - Psychiatric history
  - Transfusion history
  - Surgical history
  - Anesthesia complications
  - Allergies and medications

*Other Discussion Topics*
- Exercise: encourage regular low-moderate physical activity with a target HR of 3/4 of their non-pregnant target HR; discourage high impact activities (e.g. scuba diving, horseback riding)
- Coitus: safe during pregnancy (except placenta previa)
- Prenatal classes
- Avoiding cat litter boxes (risk of toxoplasmosis)
- Home pregnancy tests: accuracy depends on number of days since missed menstrual period and ease of use of test

## Focused Physical Exam
*Baseline Physical Assessment*
- Height
- Pre-pregnancy weight and current weight
- Blood pressure
- Bimanual pelvic exam (uterine size and adnexa)

*Systematic Assessment* (see **Table 1** for description of expected changes)
- Thyroid (see **The Head, Neck, and Throat** chapter)
- Cardiovascular (see **The Precordial Exam** chapter)
- Breasts (see **The Breast Exam** chapter)
- Abdominal (see **The Gastrointestinal System** chapter): may be able to palpate the uterine fundus if pregnancy is 12 wk or further along
- Auscultate for fetal heart rate

## Common Investigations
*Blood Work*
- CBC (Hemoglobin [Hb], mean corpuscular volume [MCV])
- Blood group and type, Rh status
- Rubella titer
- Venereal disease research laboratory (VDRL) test
- Hepatitis B surface antigen
- HIV serology
- TSH

*Urinalysis*
- Routine and microscopy
- Urine dipstick for glucosuria, proteinuria, ketones
- Culture and sensitivity: for asymptomatic bacteriuria
- Urine for gonorrhea and chlamydia

*Cervix*
- Pap smear
- Culture for chlamydia and gonorrhea

## 4.2 Subsequent Prenatal Assessments
*Recommended frequency of prenatal visits is outlined in* **Table 5**

**Table 5.** Schedule for Uncomplicated Pregnancies

| Gestational Age | Usual Frequency of Visit |
|---|---|
| **Up to 32 wk** | Every 4 weeks |
| **32-36 wk** | Every 2 weeks |
| **36 wk to Delivery** | Every week |

### Focused History
Note any changes from the initial assessment
- Ask about the **ABCDE**s
  - **A**ctivity (of the fetus)
  - **B**leeding
  - **C**ontractions
  - **D**ripping (discharge or fluid)
  - **E**stimated date of birth
- Other discussion topics:
  - Diet/nutrition, rest
  - Signs of labor, premature labor
  - Prenatal education classes
  - Review labor and delivery plans (e.g. supports, pain relief) o Breastfeeding

### Focused Physical Exam
- Height, Weight (see table 6)
- Blood pressure
- Bimanual pelvic exam (see **Gyencological Exam**)
  - Not done at every visit
  - Do NOT perform if known placenta previa or patient has undiagnosed vaginal bleeding

**Table 6.** Appropriate Weight Gain in Pregnancy

| Expected Weight Gain | |
|---|---|
| **BMI (kg/m2)** | **Weight (kg)** |
| **<19** | 12.7-18.2 |
| **19-25** | 11.3-15.9 |
| **>25** | 6.8-11.3 |

**General Rule:** 1-3 kg/wk during T1, then 0.45 kg/wk until delivery

*Other Physical Assessments*
- Abdominal Exam
  - Symphysis-fundal height (SFH) (see **Table 7** and **Figure 2**)
  - From 20-37 wk, SFH = GA ± 2 cm e.g. 30 weeks = 28-32 cm
- Fetal Heart Rate Assessment
  - Every visit beginning at 12 wk with doppler U/S or fetoscope
  - Normal FHR is between 120-160 bpm, decreasing through pregnancy
- Leopold's Maneuvers (see Table 8)
  - Done in T3 to identify lie, presentation, and position of the fetus

**Table 7.** Symphysis-Fundal Height

| Symphysis-Fundal Height Reference Chart | |
|---|---|
| **Weeks** | **Top of Uterus** |
| **12** | Pubic symphysis |
| **20** | Umbilicus |
| **36** | Just below xiphoid |
| **Term** | No longer reliable due to engagement and descent |

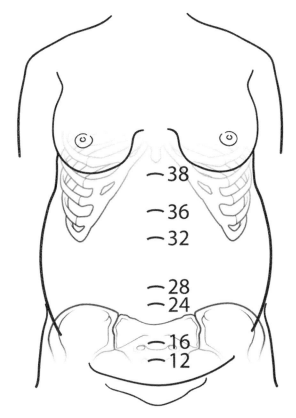

Caitlin O'Connell 2010

**Figure 2.** Expected Symphysis-Fundal Height by Gestational Age (weeks)

**Table 8.** Leopold's Maneuvers

| Maneuver | Purpose | How to Perform | Findings |
|---|---|---|---|
| **First** | Determines which part of the fetus occupies the fundus | Face patient's head and palpate the fundal area. | Buttocks at fundus/ vertex: soft or irregular<br><br>Head at fundus/ breech: round, hard, ballotable. |
| **Second** | Determines side on which fetal back lies | Place hands on lateral sides of the abdomen and palpate. | Back: linear and firm<br><br>Extremities: multiple parts ("small parts"). |
| **Third** | Determines the presenting part | Place one hand just above the symphysis and grasp the presenting part between the thumb and third finger. | Unengaged head/ vertex: round, firm, and ballotable<br><br>Breech: irregular and nodular |
| **Fourth** | Determines head flexion | Face patient's feet and place hands on either side of lower abdomen just above inlet. Exert pressure in direction of inlet; one hand will usually descend further than the other. | Head flexed: cephalic prominence prevents descent of one hand, which is on the same side as the small parts (suggests occiput presentation).<br><br>Head extended: occiput is felt prominently on the same side as the back (suggests face presentation) |

REPRODUCTIVE

## Routine Investigations

**Table 9.** Gestational Age-Dependent Tests

| Gestational Age (wk) | Tests |
|---|---|
| **All Visits** | Urine dip for proteinuria, glucosuria, ketones |
| **18-20** | U/S (transabdominal or transvaginal anatomical scan). May be indicated at other points in pregnancy to assess for intrauterine growth restriction, in setting of preeclampsia, or to investigate other abnormalities. |
| **24-28** | Oral glucose challenge test (50 g load) |
| **26** | Screen for Rh and give RhoGAM® at 28 weeks to Rh negative women |
| **28-32** | Repeat CBC to determine need for iron supplementation |
| **36-37** | Group B *Streptococcus* culture (anovaginal) |

CVS = chorionic villus sampling, MSS = maternal serum screen, Rh = Rhesus factor

*Genetic Screening Tests*
- Offered to all pregnant women

**Table 10.** Genetic Screening Tests[3]

| Test | Purpose/ Indication | Measurements | Accuracy |
|---|---|---|---|
| FTS: First Trimester Screening (11-14 weeks GA) | Estimates risk of Down Syndrome (Trisomy 21) | • Nuchal Translucency (U/S)<br>• β-hCG<br>• Pregnancy-associated plasma protein (PAPP-A) | • 78-85% sensitivity for Down Syndrome<br>• 8-9% false positive rate |
| MSS: Maternal Serum Screen (16 weeks GA) | Estimates risk of Trisomy 21, 18 and neural tube defects (NTDs) | • Maternal serum α-fetoprotein (MSAFP)<br>• β-hCG<br>• Estriol (µE3) | • 75-85% sensitivity for down syndrome<br>• 5-10% false positive rate |
| IPS: Integrated Prenatal Screen | Integrates part of FTS and MSS. More specific estimated risk of trisomies 21 and 18 and NTDs. | Part 1: 11-14 week GA:<br>• Nuchal Translucency (U/S)<br>• PAPP-A<br><br>Part 2: 15-18 week GA:<br>• MSS markers | • 85-90% sensitivity for Down Syndrome<br>• 2-4% false positive rate |

REPRODUCTIVE

| Test | Purpose/ Indication | Measurements | Accuracy |
|------|---------------------|--------------|----------|
| Enhanced FTS (11-13 wks GA) | Estimates risk of Down Syndrome and indicates high risk for Trisomy 18. More sensitive and specific than FTS. | • Nuchal Translucency (U/S)<br>• PAPP-A<br>• β-hCG<br>• Placental growth factor (PlGF)<br>• Alpha fetoprotein (AFP) | • 85-90% sensitivity for Down Syndrome<br>• 3-6% false positive rate |
| Non Invasive Prenatal Testing (NIPT). Offered as early as 9wks. | To test for trisomies 21, 18, 13. Option for women at increased risk, or those with abnormal serum screen. | Uses parallel sequencing of cell-free fetal DNA in maternal blood.<br><br>*note: funding of this test differs depending on provincial criteria and funding model. | • 99.5% sensitivity for Down Syndrome<br>• <0.1% false positive rate |

### Genetic Diagnostic Tests
Offered to women at higher risk as determined by genetic screening, family history or personal medical history
- Chorionic Villus Sampling: 10-14 weeks GA
  - Placental biopsy (transabdominal or transcervical)
  - Additional miscarriage risk <1%
  - Indications: high risk population for chromosomal abnormalities: » Ashkenazi Jewish
    - Increased maternal age
    - FHx of abnormality
- Amniocentesis: After 15 weeks GA
  - Aspirate of amniotic fluid (U/S guided transabdominal)
  - Additional miscarriage risk <0.5%
  - Indications: high risk population for chromosomal abnormalities, gold standard test used to verify positive genetic screening test

### Antenatal Monitoring
- Non-Stress Test (NST):
  - Assess fetal heart rate patterns
  - Indications: suspected uteroplacental insufficiency or fetal distress
- Doppler ultrasound of umbilical/fetal vessels:
  - Altered blood flow through these vessels due to vascular maldevelopment may indicate underlying fetal/maternal pathology (i.e. fetal growth restriction, preeclampsia)
  - Indications: pregnancies at increased risk of complications
- Biophysical Profile (BPP)[4]:
  - U/S assessment of fetus
  - Indications: nonreassuring NST, fetal distress, postterm pregnancy o Goal: to detect fetal hypoxia early enough to allow for delivery
  - Scores: (Total /8)
    - Amniotic fluid volume (most important parameter) /2
    - Fetal tone /2
    - Fetal movement /2
    - Fetal breaths /2
    - Fetal heart rate

**Table 11.** Components and Scoring of the Biophysical Profile[4]

| BPP Variable | Normal Score= 2 | Abnormal Score= 0 |
|---|---|---|
| Amniotic fluid volume | Pocket of at least 1 cm in 2 perpendicular planes | Pockets absent or pocket <1 cm in 2 perpendicular planes |
| Fetal Tone | 1 episode of motion of limb from flexion to extension and rapid return to flexion | Fetus in semi or full limb extension with no return or slow return to flexion |
| Fetal Gross Bosy Movement | 3 or more in 30 minutes, simultaneous limb and trunk movements | 2 or less movements in 30 minutes |
| Fetal Breathing Movements | At least 30 seconds of sustained breathing in 30 minutes of observation | Absent |
| Fetal Heart Rate | >2 episodes of accelerations (>15 beats/min) in 20 min, each lasting >15 sec and associated with fetal movement | Less than 2 accelerations or no acceleration >15 beats/min in 20 minutes |

| Score | Interpretation | Management |
|---|---|---|
| 8-10 | No fetal hypoxia | Repeat testing at weekly interval or more |
| 6 | Suspect chronic asphyxia | If >36 weeks, deliver |
| 4 | Suspect chronic asphyxia | If >36 weeks, deliver |
| | | If <32 weeks, repeat testing in 4-6 hours |
| 0-2 | Strongly suspect asphyxia | Test for 120 min. Persistent score <4, immediate delivery regardless of GA |

### 4.3 Labour

Labour = regular uterine contractions leading to cervical dilatation and effacement and resulting in the expulsion of the products of conception (fetus, membranes, and placenta)
- Preterm labour: 20-37 wk GA
- Term labour: 37-42 wk GA
- Postterm labour: >42 wk GA

Braxton-Hicks contractions ("false labour") = irregular, occur throughout pregnancy and do not result in cervical dilatation, effacement or fetal descent (see **Table 12**)

# History

**Table 12.** True vs. False Labour

| | True Labour | False Labour |
|---|---|---|
| **Contraction Intervals** | Regular | Irregular |
| **Duration of Time Between Contractions** | Gradually shortens | Remains long |
| **Intensity of Contractions** | Gradually increases | Remains unchanged |
| **Discomfort** | Back and abdomen | Lower abdomen |
| **Relief by Sedation** | Not relieved by sedation | Often relieved by sedation |
| **Cervix** | Effacement and dilatation | No effacement and no dilatation |

## Physical Exam and Investigations

*On Admission*
- Vital signs and fluid status
- Abdominal examination
    - Determine fetal lie, position, and station of presenting part
- Urine for protein, glucose, and ketone bodies
- If placenta previa known/suspected, do not attempt vaginal exam

*Bimanual Vaginal Exam*
- Repeat every 2-3 h or as indicated
- To assess for:

*A) Cervical changes (see Figure 3):*

- *Effacement:*
    - Thinning of cervical walls caused by pressure of fetal head o Expressed as % of total effacement
        - 0%: none, 100%: complete thinning
    - May result in release of mucus plug within cervical canal ("bloody show")
- *Dilatation:*
    - Opening of cervical canal
    - Expressed in cm:
        - 0 cm: no dilatation, 10 cm: full dilatation

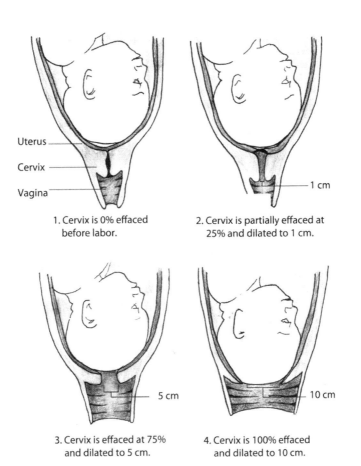

1. Cervix is 0% effaced before labor.

2. Cervix is partially effaced at 25% and dilated to 1 cm.

Uterus

Cervix

Vagina

1 cm

3. Cervix is effaced at 75% and dilated to 5 cm.

5 cm

4. Cervix is 100% effaced and dilated to 10 cm.

10 cm

Jan Cyril Fundano

**Figure 3.** Stages of Cervical Effacement and Dilatation

**How to perform:** separate vulva and labia with left hand and use right index and middle fingers to examine
* Assess position of cervix: anterior vs. posterior
* Assess degree of dilatation and effacement of cervix

*B) Position of the Presenting Part*

**How to perform:**
  **i. Station**
    ◆ Using index and middle fingers, palpate the ischial spines; locate most inferior aspect of presenting part, determine whether it is above, at or below level of ischial spines. (**Figure 4**)
    ◆ 0= level of ischial spines
    ◆ Estimate level in cm above (+) or below (-) ischial spines
  **ii. Position**
    ◆ Palpate suture lines and fontanelles in relation to pelvic diameters to determine whether the fetus is presenting occiput-posterior (OP) or occiput anterior (OA).

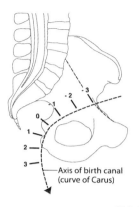

Krista Shapton 2010

**Figure 4.** Level of Head in Thirds Above or Below Ischial Spines

Occiput posterior

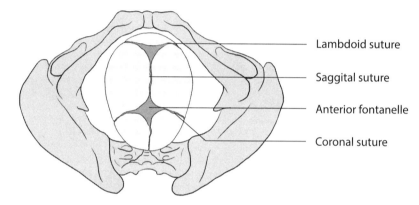

Lambdoid suture

Saggital suture

Anterior fontanelle

Coronal suture

Occiput anterior

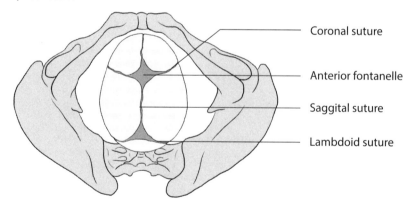

Coronal suture

Anterior fontanelle

Saggital suture

Lambdoid suture

Wendy Gu 2017

**Figure 5.** Fetal Head Position: Occiput Posterior and Occiput Anterior

**Table 13.** Assessing Latent Phase of Labor: Bishop Score for Assessing Cervical Ripeness

|  | 0 | 1 | 2 | 3 |
|---|---|---|---|---|
| **Effacement** (%) | 0-30 | 31-50 | 51-80 | >80 |
| **Cervical Dilatation** (cm) | 0 | 1 - 2 | 3 - 4 | ≥5 |
| **Cervical Consistency** | Firm | Medium | Soft | NA |
| **Position of Cervix** | Posterior | Central | Anterior | NA |
| **Fetal Head** (position in cm relative to ischial spine) | -3 | -2 | -1 or 0 | +1 or more |

### Speculum Exam

**How to perform:** See **Gynecological Exam**
- Assess if membranes have ruptured
    - Pooling of fluid in posterior fornix
    - pH of vaginal fluid (nitrazine paper colour change yellow to blue)
    - Ferning of fluid under light microscopy
- After membranes have ruptured, examine the amniotic fluid, noting any meconium (green or brown tinge of the amniotic fluid)
- Assessment of preterm labour
    - Fetal fibronectin swab (from 22 weeks to 35 weeks)
    - If negative, 99% certainty that patient will not go into labour in next 2 weeks
    - If positive, no assessment can be made
    - Test only valid if nothing has been in the vagina for past 24hrs

### Electronic Fetal Heart Rate Monitoring

- Assess baseline FHR, variability, and periodicity (decelerations and accelerations)

**Table 14.** Intrapartum FHR Monitoring (see also **Figure 6**)

|  | Normal | Atypical | Abnormal |
|---|---|---|---|
| **Baseline FHR** (bpm) | • 110-160 | • Slow 100-110<br>• Fast >160 for 30-80 min<br>• Rising baseline | • Slow <100<br>• Fast >160 for >80 min<br>• Erratic baseline |
| **Variability** (bmp) | • 6-25<br>• <5 for <40 min | • <5 for 40-80 min | • <5 for >80 min<br>• >25 for >10 min<br>• Sinusoidal |
| **Decelerations** | • None or occasional<br>• Early or variable decels | • Repetitive (>3) variable decels<br>• Occasional late decels<br>• Single prolonged decel for 2-3 min | • Repetitive (>3) variable decels<br>• Late decels >50% of contractions<br>• Single prolonged decel for 3-10 min<br>• Slow to return to baseline |
| **Acceleration** | • Spontaneous<br>• Occurs with fetal scalp stimulation | • Absence of accel with fetal scalp stimulation | • Absent |
| **Management** | • Routine intrapartum monitoring | • Frequent reassessment and further management as indicated clinically | • Confirm fetal wellbeing<br>• Fetal scalp blood sample<br>• Consider operative delivery<br>• Intrauterine resuscitation |

REPRODUCTIVE

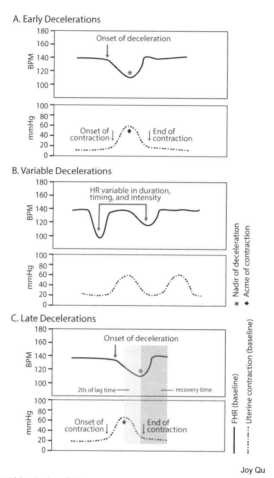

A. Early Decelerations

Onset of deceleration

Onset of contraction — End of contraction

B. Variable Decelerations

HR variable in duration, timing, and intensity

C. Late Decelerations

Onset of deceleration

20s of lag time —— recovery time

Onset of contraction — End of contraction

* Nadir of deceleration
♦ Acme of contraction

—— FHR (baseline)
⋯⋯ Uterine contraction (baseline)

Joy Qu

**Figure 6.** Fetal Heart Monitoring Strips

## Stages of Labour

*First Stage of Labour:* Onset of true labour to full dilatation of the cervix
- Latent phase: from the onset of labour to the onset of the active phase
- Active phase: accelerated cervical dilation generally beginning at 5 cm for multiparous and approximately 6 cm for nulliparous

*Second Stage of Labour:* Full dilatation of cervix to delivery of baby

Cardinal movements of fetus during delivery (see **Figure 7**)
1. Descent
   - Begins before onset of labor or during first stage
   - Continues until fetus is delivered
2. Flexion
   - Fetal head flexes chin to chest
   - Reduces diameter of presenting part
3. Internal Rotation
   - Fetal head rotates laterally during descent through the pelvis
4. Extension
   - Fetal neck extends to negotiate under the symphysis pubis
   - Crowning: largest diameter of fetal head is encircled by vulvar ring (station +3 or +5 if measuring station by thirds or fifths respectively)

5. Restitution/External Rotation
- Fetal head returns to the position at the time of engagement o Fetal back and shoulders align
6. Expulsion
- Delivery of anterior shoulder, posterior shoulder, then the rest of the body

REPRODUCTIVE

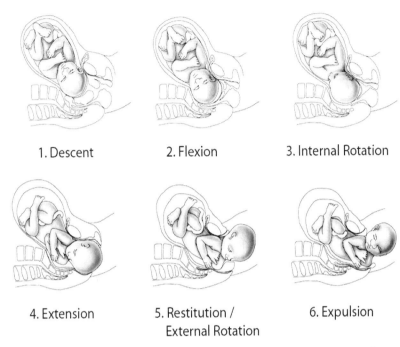

1. Descent    2. Flexion    3. Internal Rotation

4. Extension    5. Restitution / External Rotation    6. Expulsion

Joy Qu 2012 after Krista Shapton

**Figure 7.** Cardinal Movements of the Fetus During Delivery

Delivery of the fetus
- Mother is positioned left lateral decubitus or supine
- Episiotomy (incision in perineum) only if necessary
    - Midline: better healing but increased risk of deep tear
    - Mediolateral: reduced risk of extensive tear but poorer healing and more pain

i. Delivery of fetal head
    - Ritgen maneuver: exert forward pressure on the chin of the fetus
    - through the perineum just in front of coccyx with left hand while exerting pressure superiorly against occiput with right hand
ii. Check for nuchal cord
iii. Consider clear fetal airway using suction bulb: oral cavity first, then nares
iv. Delivery of anterior shoulder
    - Hold sides of the head with two hands and apply gentle downward pressure
v. Delivery of posterior shoulder
    - Gently elevate the head and apply upward pressure
vi. Delivery of rest of body

Check fetal Apgar scores (**Table 15**) 1 and 5 min after birth

### Examination of the Newborn
- Full neonatal examination within 24 h of delivery (see **The Pediatrics** chapter)

**Table 15.** Apgar Scores

| Sign | 0 | 1 | 2 |
|---|---|---|---|
| Appearance | Blue, pale | Body pink, extremities blue | Completely pink |
| Pulse | Absent | <100 bpm | >100 bpm |
| Reflexes: stimulation with NG tube | No response | Grimace | Sneeze or cough |
| Activity: muscle tone | Flaccid | Some flexion of extremities | Good flexion |
| Respiratory Effort | Absent | Weak, irregular | Good, crying |

*Third Stage of Labour:* Delivery of placenta
- Signs of placental separation:
  - Uterus becomes firm and globular
  - Gush of blood
  - Umbilical cord visibly lengthens
  - Uterine fundus rises in abdomen
- Patient is positioned supine
- Place left hand on abdomen over the uterine fundus
- Exert gentle pressure on uterine fundus while keeping the umbilical cord slightly taut with right hand
- Do NOT pull on umbilical cord!
- While applying fundal pressure, also apply upward pressure at the symphysis pubis to prevent uterine involution
- Monitor vital signs and ensure patient is stabilized
- Inspect placenta for completeness (i.e. no retained products) and blood vessels (2 arteries and 1 vein)
- Send cord blood gas samples of umbilical artery and umbilical vein cord to lab after every delivery
- Palpate to ensure uterine contraction and check for uterine bleeding
- Repair episiotomies or tears
- Administer oxytocic agent

*Fourth Stage of Labour:* Delivery of placenta until patient is stable

**Table 16.** Duration of Normal Labour[5]

| Stage | Nulliparous | Multiparous |
|---|---|---|
| First | 6-18 h | 2-10 h |
| Second | 30 min-3 h | 5-30 min |
| Third | 5-30 min | 5-30 min |
| Fourth | Until postpartum condition of patient has stabilized (usually 1 h) | |

## Operative Delivery
- Use of forceps, vacuum extraction or surgery to deliver the fetus

**Table 17.** Common indications for Cesarean section (C/S)[6]

| Maternal | Maternal-Fetal | Fetal |
|---|---|---|
| *Obstruction of birth canal | *Failure to progress in first stage | *Malpresentation: breech (3-4% of deliveries), transverse lie (0.3-0.4% of deliveries) |
| *Active herpetic lesions on vulva | *Placenta previa | |
| *Underlying severe maternal illness (eclampsia, HELLP syndrome [hemolysis, elevated liver enzymes, low platelet count]) requiring immediate delivery | *Abruptio placentae | Malposition (e.g. occiput posterior) |
| | *Prolapsed cord | Fetal distress, nonreassuring fetal heart rate (1-2% of cases) |
| | Cephalopelvic disproportion | |
| | Failure to progress in second stage | |
| *Elective | | Low birth weight infant |
| Previous C/S | Multiple gestations | Macrosomic infant (>4kg) |
| Poor obstetrical history | | |

*Absolute indications

Maternal risks associated with Vaginal Delivery:
- Deep vein thrombosis
- Pulmonary embolism
- Post partum hemorrhage
- Perineal tear
- Perineal and uterine infection
- Urinary incontinence
- Bowel problems, anal incontinence

Maternal risks associated with Cesarean Section:
- Uterine hemorrhage (due to atony, extension of incision, uterine rupture, presence of leiomyomata)
- Deep vein thrombosis
- Pulmonary embolism
- Postoperative infection (determined by length of labor, rupture of membranes, number of vaginal examinations)
- Risk of placenta previa or placenta accreta in future deliveries

### 4.4 Puerperium and Postpartum Period
- Postpartum period extends from 1 h after delivery of placenta to 6-week period after pregnancy when pregnancy-related anatomic and physiologic changes are reversed

### Physiological Changes in the Postpartum Period
- **Uterus**
  - Uterus decreases in size and cervix regains firmness
  - Uterus should involute 1 cm below umbilicus per day for first 4-5d o Uterine spasms can cause pain 4-7 d postpartum
  - Returns to non-pregnant state in 4-6 wk
- **Resumption of ovarian function**
  - Ovulation resumes in 45 d in non-lactating patients, and 3-6 mo in lactating women
  - Breastfeeding is NOT a method of contraception: unless patient wishes to conceive, use a barrier method
- **Lochia: normal vaginal discharge postpartum**
  - Decreases and changes color from red (lochia rubra) to yellow (lochia serosa) to white (lochia alba)
- **Breast changes**
  - Engorgement in late pregnancy
  - Colostrum expression can occur in late pregnancy up to 72 h postpartum
  - Full milk production by 3-7 d
  - Mature milk by 15-45 d

# 5. COMMON CLINICAL SCENARIOS

## 5.1 Pregnancy-Induced Conditions

**Table 18.** Medical Conditions Induced by Pregnancy

| Disorder | Definition | Signs/Symptoms | Physical Exam/ Investigations | Management |
|---|---|---|---|---|
| **Hypertensive Disorders:** | | | **\*For all hypertension in pregnancy** | |
| Preexisting Hypertension | Increased BP (>140/90) mmHg that precedes pregnancy or develops before 20 wks GA | Increased BP (>140/90) mmHg that precedes pregnancy or develops before 20 wks GA | Physical Exam HEENT: facial edema, scotomas, loss of peripheral vision | Consider pharmacologic antihypertensive therapy |
| Gestational Hypertension | Increased BP (>140/90) mmHg that develops after 20 wks GA | Increased BP (>140/90) mmHg that develops after 20 wks GA | Resp: crackles (pulmonary edema) CV: S3, S4, murmurs (CHF) Abdo: RUQ pain, ascites | Consider pharmacologic antihypertensive therapy |
| Preeclampsia | Clinical triad of HTN, proteinuria, edema | Clinical triad of HTN, proteinuria, edema | Neuro: hyperreflexia, clonus<br><br>Fetal evaluation: FHR, NST, BPP | Deliver. Antihypertensive therapy (labetalol, hydralazine, nifedipine) considered if premature fetus. Use of ASA 81mg from 16 weeks onwards to prevent this condition in high risk pregnancies (i.e. previous preeclampsia, pre-existing kidney disease, hypertension). |
| Eclampsia | Preeclampsia with seizure or coma | Preeclampsia with seizure or coma | | Magnesium sulfate therapy. Delivery. |

REPRODUCTIVE

| Disorder | Definition | Signs/Symptoms | Physical Exam/ Investigations | Management |
|---|---|---|---|---|
| **Gestational Diabetes Mellitus**[7] | Glucose intolerance present only in pregnancy | Asymptomatic | Screening at 24-28 wk GA<br>• Oral glucose challenge test (OGCT); 50g oral glucose<br>• Oral glucose tolerance test (OGTT) if OGCT abnormal; 75g oral glucose | Management<br>• Treated nutritionally (modify carbohydrate and kcal intake)<br>• Addition of insulin or oral antidiabetic agents if maternal glucose and/or fetal size parameters indicate risk |
| **Rhesus Discrepancies** | Sensitization of Rh- mother to Rh+ blood from fetus | No symptoms in pregnancy. Baby may exhibit signs of hemolytic anemia following birth. | Blood typing (Rh, ABO) | Administer Rh immune globulin (RhIg [©Rhogam]) |

## 5.2 Obstetrical Complications

**Table 19.** Antenatal, Intrapartum, Postpartum Complications

| Disorder | Signs/Symptoms | Physical Exam | Investigations | Management |
|---|---|---|---|---|
| **Antenatal Complications**[1,8] | | | | |
| **Miscarriage (Spontaneous abortion)**<br><br>**Definition:**<br>Pregnancy loss before 20 wk GA | • Vaginal bleeding<br>• Crampy pelvic pain<br>• Eventual expulsion of tissues | • Abdominal exam<br>• Leopold's maneuvers if GA appropriate<br>• Speculum exam to assess for expulsed tissue | • β-hCG<br>• U/S | • RhIg (©Rhogam) if Rh negative<br>• Follow up U/S to confirm expulsion of all tissues (retained products of conception may result in sepsis [pain, fever, bleeding]). |
| **Ectopic Pregnancy**<br><br>**Definition:**<br>Pregnancy occurring in location outside of the uterus (most often in fallopian tube, especially ampulla [80%]) | • Vague lower abdominal pain (95%)<br>• Minimal vaginal bleeding (50-80%)<br>• Adnexal mass/ tenderness<br>• Cervical motion tenderness<br>• Shock | • Abdominal exam (peritoneal signs may indicate rupture)<br>• Bimanual exam (to detect mass, cervical motion tenderness) | • β-hCG<br>• Pelvic U/S<br>• Laparoscopy in some cases | • RhIg (©Rhogam) if Rh negative<br>• Medical (methotrexate)<br>• Surgical resection |

REPRODUCTIVE

| Disorder | Signs/Symptoms | Physical Exam | Investigations | Management |
|---|---|---|---|---|
| **Abruptio Placentae**<br><br>**Definition:** Premature separation of normally implanted placenta. Hemorrhage from decidual spiral arteries. | • Pain<br>• Dark red vaginal bleeding in 80% of cases<br>• Internal/concealed (no visible vaginal bleeding) in 20% of cases<br>• Uterus firm, tender<br>• Onset of symptoms after 20 wk GA | • None | • Largely a clinical diagnosis<br>• Ultrasound (may identify retroplacental or subchorionicbleeding/ clot) | • RhIg (©Rhogam) if Rh negative<br>• Continuous FHR monitoring<br>• Rescusitation as necessary<br>• Vaginal delivery or C-section depending on fetal/ maternal stability |
| **Placenta Previa**<br><br>**Definition:** Abnormal location of placenta at or near the cervical os. May be marginal, partial or total. 1/150-250 births in T3. More than 90% resolve by T3. | • Bright red painless bleeding<br>• Uterus soft, nontender<br>• Onset of symptoms:<br>• 2/3 at 30 wk GA<br>• 1/3 before 30 wk GA | • Do NOT perform vaginal exams | • Diagnosis by Ultrasound | • RhIg (©Rhogam) if Rh negative<br>• Delivery by<br>• C-section |
| **Premature Rupture of Membranes (PROM)**[9]<br><br>**Definition:** Rupture of fetal membranes prior to onset of labour | • History indicating gush or trickling of fluid<br>• Pooling of fluid in vaginal vault<br>• Valsalva fluid leakage from cervical os | • Speculum exam | • Nitrazine paper indicator (turns blue with amniotic fluid but also with blood, urine, semen)<br>• Ferning of amniotic fluid on light microscopy (gold standard test) | • Delivery (induction of labour with oxytocin) |

| Disorder | Signs/Symptoms | Physical Exam | Investigations | Management |
|---|---|---|---|---|

**Intrapartum Complications[1]**

| Disorder | Signs/Symptoms | Physical Exam | Investigations | Management |
|---|---|---|---|---|
| **Breech Presentation**<br><br>**Definition:** Presentation of fetal buttocks or lower extremities into the maternal pelvis. Occurs in 3-4% of term pregnancies vs. 30% at 30 wks | Asymptomatic<br><br>3 types:<br>**1. Complete** (5-10%). Thighs and knees flexed, feet above buttocks<br>**2. Frank** (50-75%). Thighs flexed, knees extended<br>**3. Footling** (20%). Single: one thigh extended; foot is presenting part. Double: both thighs extended | • Leopold maneuvers | • Ultrasound | • External cephalic version (attempted after 34 wk)<br>• Delivery by C-section<br>• Vaginal breech delivery is an option |

**4.3 Postpartum Complications[1]**

| Disorder | Signs/Symptoms | Physical Exam | Investigations | Management |
|---|---|---|---|---|
| **Postpartum Hemorrhage**<br><br>**Definition:** Loss of >500 mL of blood at time of vaginal delivery or >1000 mL in C/S. Early (within 24 h of delivery) or delayed (24 h-6 wk post-delivery). Incidence 5-15%. | • Vaginal bleeding that is greater than expected<br>• Generally caused by one of the 4 Ts:<br>1. Tone (uterine atony)<br>2. Tissue (retained products i.e. placenta)<br>3. Trauma (tears)<br>4. Thrombosis (coagulopathy i.e. DIC) | • Inspection of vaginal tissue for tear or retained products<br>• Abdominal exam to assess for uterine tone | • Clinical diagnosis | • Manage according to likely cause<br>• Oxytocin, prostaglandin agents (Misoprostol, Carboprost, Ergot), and bimanual massage in context of uterine atony |
| **Endometritis**<br><br>**Definition:** Entry of normal GI or gyneco-logical bacteria into the usually sterile uterus. Occurring in 1-3% of vaginal deliveries. Increased risk in C-section deliveries, cho-rioamnionitis, PROM | • Postpartum fever<br>• Tachycardia<br>• Midline lower abdominal pain<br>• Uterine tenderness<br>• Foul smelling lochia | • Abdominal exam | • Largely clinical diagnosis (postpartum fever that cannot be attributed to another etiology) | • Intravenous antibiotics (clindamycin + gentamicin first line) |

| Disorder | Signs/Symptoms | Physical Exam | Investigations | Management |
|---|---|---|---|---|
| **Postpartum Depression**[10] <br><br> **Definition:** Major depression occurring within 4 wk postpartum. Incidence: 10-20%, 50% recurrence | • Despondent mood <br> • Feelings of inadequacy as a parent, thoughts of harming infant <br> • Impaired concentration <br> • Changes in appetite and sleep | • Diagnosis based on history | • Clinical Diagnosis | • Psychiatric referral <br> • Pharmacotherapy (SSRIs) <br> • Cognitive Behavioural Therapy |

## REFERENCES

1. Hacker NF, Gambone JC, Moore JG. Essentials of Obstetrics and Gynecology. Philadelphia: Saunders; 2009.
2. Chalmers I, Erkin M, Keirse MJNC (Editors). A Guide to Effective Care in Pregnancy and Childbirth. Oxford: Oxford University Press; 2000.
3. Screening Choices. Prenatal Screening Ontario web site. www.prenatalscreeningontario.ca/for-parents/screening-choices. Published 2016, Accessed Dec 2016.
4. Manning FA, Platt LD, Sipos I, Antepartum fetal evaluation development of a fetal biophysical profile. Am J Obstet Gynecol. 1980 136(5):787-795.
5. Steer P, Flint C. ABC of labour care: Physiology and management of normal labour. BMJ 1999; 31 8(71 86):793-796.
6. Chamberlain G, Steer P. ABC of labour care: Operative delivery. BMJ 1999; 318(7193):1260- 1264.
7. Buchanan TA, Xiang AH, Page KA. Gestational diabetes mellitus: Risks and management during and after pregnancy. Nat Rev Endocrinol 2012; 8(11 ):639-649.
8. Crochet, J. R., Bastian, L. A., & Chireau, M. V. Does this woman have an ectopic pregnancy?: the rational clinical examination systematic review.JAMA, 2013; 309(16), 1722-1729.
9. Erickson, H. (2010). Management of Premature Rupture of Membranes at Term.
10. O'Hara MW, McCabe JE. Postpartum depression: Current status and future directions. Annu Rev Clin Psychol 2013; 9:379-407.

REPRODUCTIVE

# CHAPTER 9D:

# The Urological Exam

**Editors:**
Matthew Da Silva, BMSc
Thomas Ying, BSc
Rushi Gandhi, BMSc

**Resident Reviewer:**
Jenny Li, MD, BMSc
Tristan Juvet, MD, BSc

**Faculty Reviewers:**
Michael Jewett, MD, FRCSC

## TABLE OF CONTENTS

# 1. ESSENTIAL ANATOMY

## Essential Male Anatomy

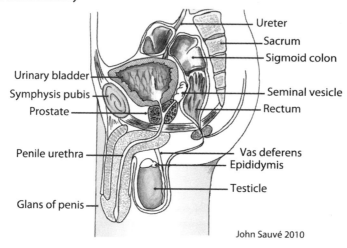

**Figure 1.** Anatomy of the Male Genitourinary Tract and Organs

## Essential Female Anatomy

- See the **Gynecological Exam** for a depiction of the external female genital anatomy

# 2. COMMON CHIEF COMPLAINTS

**Table 1.** Common urological chief complaints and differential diagnoses

| Chief Complaint | Differential Diagnosis | Distinguishing Features |
|---|---|---|
| **Hematuria** | Urothelial carcinoma | History of smoking, industrial occupational exposures, constitutional symptoms, chemotherapy |
| | Renal cell carcinoma | Incidental finding usually, rarely flank pain, flank bulge, paraneoplastic symptoms, obesity, history of smoking |
| | Urinary tract infection (UTI) | Dysuria, frequency, urgency |
| | Benign Prostatic Hyperplasia (BPH) | Older men, lower urinary tract symptoms (LUTS) |
| | Stone disease | Renal colic, previous stone former |
| | Coagulopathy | Anti-coagulants |
| | Medical renal disease | Proteinuria, urine casts (red cell, white cell, granular/epithelial) |

| Chief Complaint | Differential Diagnosis | Distinguishing Features |
|---|---|---|
| **Dysuria** | Urinary Tract Infections | Frequency, urgency, prior history of UTIs |
| | Sexually transmitted infections | Discharge, high risk sexual activity |
| | Anatomical variations: BPH, urethral strictures | Weak flow, incomplete emptying, instrumentation, urethral trauma |
| **Lower Urinary Tract Symptoms (LUTS)** | **Prostatic** BPH | Prostate is smooth, firm, and enlarged on DRE |
| | Prostatitis | Pain in the perineal area. Extreme tenderness on DRE if acute. |
| | Prostate Cancer | Most are asymptomatic, although may present with LUTS. May have bone pain from metastases. Potential hard nodule(s) found on DRE. |
| | **Urethral** Urethritis | Itching or irritation around the penile meatus. May have yellowish discharge from the urethra. |
| | Urethral Stricture | Straining on urination, weakened urinary stream, previous urethral instrumentation or trauma (catheter or cystoscope). |
| | Urethral Calculi | History of kidney stones. |
| | **Bladder** Cystitis | Prior history of UTI's. Any process that causes urine to be retained in the bladder. |
| | Bladder Cancer | History of smoking. |
| | Neurogenic Bladder | Result of nerve damage to the bladder. Includes conditions such as Diabetes, Parkinson's, Multiple Sclerosis, Cerebral Palsy, and stroke. |

REPRODUCTIVE

| Chief Complaint | Differential Diagnosis | Distinguishing Features |
|---|---|---|
| **Testicular Mass and Testicular Cancer** | Epididymitis | Scrotal pain and swelling, often one testicle affected. Fever is a common symptom, and patients will usually have recent history of dysuria or urethral discharge. Pain may be relieved by elevating the scrotum (Prehn's sign). |
| | Orchitis | Recent epididymitis, which can progress to orchitis. |
| | Testicular Torsion | Sudden, severe scrotal/testicular pain, often associated with nausea and vomiting. Testicle may sit higher than its normal position and be transverse. Anatomical defect "bell-clapper" deformity usually present |
| | Hematocele | Previous testicular operation, trauma. No transillumination. |
| | Hydrocele | Painless. Occasional history of trauma to the scrotum. Transillumination present. |
| | Spermatocele | Often an incidental finding. Can be confirmed with ultrasound. Transillumination present. |
| | Varicocele | Feeling of heaviness and tenderness in the scrotum. Presents as a feeling of a "bag of worms" which can be increased in size with Valsalva. Can lead to infertility. |
| | Hematoma | Previous scrotal operation. No transillumination. Can lead to an extremely enlarged and tender scrotum. |
| | Hemorrhagic testicular cancer | Testicular cancer can present as a painful mass in up to one fifth of cases. Low back pain may also occur with metastases to the retroperitoneum. |

| Chief Complaint | Differential Diagnosis | Distinguishing Features |
|---|---|---|
| **Incontinence** | Overactive bladder | Urgency incontinence: Sudden urge to urinate. Urine loss precedes urgency to urinate |
| | Cauda equina syndrome | Other neurological symptoms: Bowel and sexual dysfunction, sciatica, saddle numbness. Usually overflow and no sensation. |
| | Loss of anterior support of bladder (e.g. male: post-prostatectomy, female: postpartum) | Stress incontinence: Urine loss with increased intra-abdominal pressure |
| | Neurogenic bladder | Symptoms of urinary urgency following stroke, dementia or trauma |
| | Weak detrusor muscle | Overflow incontinence: Outflow obstruction causes build-up of urine in bladder. Eventually, the overfilled bladder begins to leak, and one can present with overflow incontinence. |
| | Pharmacologic | Urine loss secondary to medications such as anticholinergics, sedatives, sympathetic blockers |
| | Cystitis | Prior history of UTI's |
| | Prostatitis | Pain in perineal region. Severe pain on DRE. |
| **Pain** | Renal colic | Acute onset flank pain radiating to groin, nausea and vomiting |
| | Pyelonephritis | Costovertebral angle (CVA) tenderness, fever, nausea/vomiting, dysuria |
| | Bladder cancer | Hematuria and pain localized to suprapubic region |
| | Cystitis | History of UTIs or urinary obstruction |
| | Prostatitis | Pain in perineal region. Severe pain on DRE. Can radiate to rectum and penis. |
| | Epididymitis | Pain and swelling on one testicle, which usually hangs lower. Fever and recent history of dysuria or urethral discharge. Positive Prehn's sign. |
| | Testicular torsion | Sudden, severe testicular pain, often associated with nausea and vomiting. Testicle may sit higher than its normal position. |
| | Priapism | Inability of erect penis to detumesce to flaccid state. Painful. |
| | Peyronie's disease | Angulation of penile shaft on erection |

REPRODUCTIVE

# 3. FOCUSED HISTORY

### Lower Urinary Tract Symptoms (LUTS)

*Storage Symptoms*
- Frequency: How frequently do you urinate during the day?
- Nocturia: Do you wake up at night to urinate? If so, how many times?
- Urgency: Do you ever have a strong, sudden urge to urinate? Do you ever have such a strong urge to urinate that you fear not being able to make it to the toilet in time or actually leak?
- Dysuria: Do you ever have pain or burning during urination? At which point in the stream do you feel pain: beginning, middle, end or throughout?
- Incontinence (see **Table 2**)

*Voiding Symptoms*
- Straining: Do you ever have to strain to fully empty your bladder?
- Hesitancy: Do you ever have difficulty starting urination?
- Intermittency: Is your stream continuous, or are there times when the flow stops and restarts?
- Postvoid dribbling: Do you ever notice a continued release of drops of urine after voiding?
- Decreased force of urination: Have you noticed a weaker stream?
- Incomplete emptying (sensation that urine retained): Do you ever feel as though there is residual urine remaining in your bladder after you urinate? Do you have to urinate again a second time ("double voiding")?

### Genitourinary Pain (see **Table 3**)
- Onset, provoking/alleviating factors, quality, radiation, severity, duration, and location

### Discharge (from urethra)
- Continuous vs. intermittent discharge
- Bloody (urethral carcinoma) vs. purulent (infection)
- Gonococcal pus: thick, profuse, and yellow to gray (see **Infectious Diseases** chapter) vs watery with non-gonococal STD
- Sexual history: ask about multiple partners, previous STIs, and UTI history

### Gross Hematuria (see **Common Clinical Scenarios,** p.321)
- Timing: Is blood present at the beginning, middle, end or throughout the stream?
- Gross vs microscopic: Can you see blood or just lab test? Have you noticed any blood clots?
- Painful vs. painless: pattern suggests cause

### Past Medical History
- Previous urological problems
- Previous surgeries
- Ask about TB, DM, renal disease, malignancies

### Family History
- FHx of urological issues (stones, cancer, polycystic kidney disease, congenital abnormalities)

### Travel History
- Urological sequelae of schistosomiasis

### Social History
- Smoking (bladder cancer, erectile dysfunction [ED]) and alcohol use (testicular atrophy)
- Occupational exposures

**Table 2.** Classification of Incontinence

| Type of Incontinence | Definition | Possible Cause |
|---|---|---|
| Stress | Urine loss with increased intra-abdominal pressure (e.g. cough, sneeze, laugh) and not associated with the urgency to urinate | Postpartum, postmenopausal, or surgical loss of anterior vaginal support of bladder and proximal urethra, postoperative (e.g. prostatectomy) in men |
| Urgency | Urine loss due to uninhibited bladder contractions – precedes urgency to urinate | Overactive bladder, cystitis, neurogenic bladder (following stroke, dementia, cord lesion above sacral level) |
| Overflow | Urine loss due to chronically distended bladder – even after effort to void | Bladder outlet obstruction, weak detrusor muscle, impaired sensation (e.g. diabetic neuropathy) |
| Pharmacologic | Urine loss secondary to medication | Sedatives, tranquilizers, anticholinergics*, sympathetic blockers, potent diuretics |

*Note: anticholinergics lead to incontinence secondary to urinary retention

**Table 3.** Approach to Genitourinary Pain by Region

| Type of Pain | Location | Cause |
|---|---|---|
| Renal Capsule | Ipsilateral costovertebral angle (CVA). May radiate to upper abdomen/umbilicus | Distention of renal capsule (inflammation or obstruction) with flank ache |
| Ureteral | Mid-ureter: referred to ipsilateral lower quadrant of abdomen<br><br>Lower-ureter: referred to suprapubic area and genitals | Obstruction of ureter leading to distension and spastic peristalsis with colic - often severe |
| Vesical | Suprapubic region | Cystitis, interstitial cystitis/ bladder pain syndrome (IC/BPS), carcinoma, over-distension of bladder due to urinary retention |
| Prostatic | Referred to perineum, lower back, inguinal region or testes | Inflammation |
| Penile | Glans and shaft of penis | Flaccid: cystitis/urethritis, paraphimosis, trauma<br>Erect: Peyronie's disease (usually painless), priapism, trauma |
| Testicular | Scrotum | Epididymitis, torsion, tumour(rare), trauma |

## 3.1 Male-Focused Topics

### Scrotal Swelling
- Painful vs painless, onset, duration, provoking/alleviating factors, change over time, associated urinary, sexual or traumatic events

**Table 4.** Differential Diagnosis for Scrotal Swelling

| Painful | Painless |
|---|---|
| Epididymitis | Hydrocele |
| Orchitis | Spermatocele, epididymal cyst |
| Testicular torsion | Varicocele |
| Tumor (infarct/hemorrhage) | Tumor (non-hemorrhagic) |
| Hematocele (after trauma) | Scrotal hematoma |
| Strangulated inguinal hernia | Non-strangulated inguinal hernia |

### Erectile Dysfunction (Impotence)
- Inability to achieve and/or maintain an erection adequate for intercourse
- Onset, alleviation/aggravation (constant problem vs. situational)
- Psychogenic vs. organic (presence or loss of morning erections)
- Can be further classified: vasculogenic, neurogenic, anatomic, endocrinologic
- Differentiate from other male sexual disorders (loss of libido, failure to ejaculate, anorgasmia, premature ejaculation)

## 4. FOCUSED PHYSICAL EXAM[1]
### General Inspection
- Inspect the patient at rest
- Look for signs of distress or restlessness (e.g. renal colic)
- Inspect for supraclavicular lymphadenopathy (metastases from GU malignancy)

### Abdominal Exam
- Inspect for masses, scars, suprapubic distension suggesting urinary retention (palpable bladder) (see **The Gastrointestinal System** chapter)

### Kidneys (see **The Gastrointestinal System** chapter)
- Ballotment: place one hand under the patient's back and apply upward pressure near the 12th rib; attempt to 'catch' the kidney between your hands by placing the opposite hand firmly and deeply in the ipsilateral upper quadrant of the abdomen
- Costovertebral angle (CVA) tenderness: with a closed fist, percuss at the costovertebral angle (junction of the inferior margin of 12th rib and vertebral column)
- Tenderness: capsular distension

### Bladder
- Normal adult bladder (lies below pubic symphysis) cannot be palpated/ percussed unless filled with at least 150 mL of urine
- Palpation: deeply palpate the midline of the suprapubic abdomen
- Percussion: percuss immediately above the symphysis pubis and move cephalad until there is a change in pitch from dull to resonant (over the bladder should be dull)

### Femoral Hernias
- Inspect the femoral canal for bulging or mass
- Palpate on the anterior thigh in the femoral canal; attempt to reduce mass if present

### Inguinal Lymph Nodes (see **The Lymphatic System** chapter)
- Inspect for inguinal lymphadenopathy
- Only the superficial inguinal lymph nodes can be palpated on physical exam (indicates infection or tumor at distal 1/3 of urethra, scrotum or vulva)
- Drainage of the testes and internal female genitalia is to the abdomen, pelvic and paraaortic nodes (not palpable on exam)

## Genital Exam
- See Male-Specific Exam Maneuvers and Female-Specific Exam Maneuvers below

## Additional Exams
- ♂ Digital Rectal Exam
- ♀ Urinary Stress Test

## 4.1 Male-Specific Exam Maneuvers

### Penis
- Inspect prepuce (circumcised vs. uncircumcised), glans, shaft, and base for lesions, discoloration, masses, tumescence
- Inspect meatus: location (epispadias, hypospadias), blood, discharge, stricture/stenosis
- Open the urethral meatus by compressing the glans between the index finger and thumb; examine the inside for discoloration, inflammation, discharge, or lesions
- Ask patient to retract foreskin; if problematic: phimosis
- Ask patient to reduce foreskin; if problematic: paraphimosis (usually painful and edematous)
- Palpate the penis along the shaft from glans to base to assess for masses, nodularity, tenderness

### Scrotum and Contents
- While supine, have the patient flex his leg on the side of the scrotum being examined
- Examine each side separately
- Inspect for size, shape, symmetry, swelling, erythema, skin changes, presence of normal folds or rugae
- Lift the scrotum to examine the posterior surface
- Examine the scrotal sac by rolling the skin between the index finger and thumb
- Testicular exam
  - Palpate each testicle separately using both hands (left hand holding superior/inferior poles, right hand palpates and squeezes the anterior/posterior surfaces)
  - Note size, shape, and consistency (normal testicle: firm, rubbery consistency, smooth surface)
  - Abnormally small testicles suggests hypogonadism
  - Hard area or nodularity is malignant until proven otherwise
- Epididymis
  - Palpable mass attached to posterior surface of each testicle with prominent tail, head and body usually less obvious
  - Palpate for tenderness, nodularity or masses
  - Epididymitis: epididymis is very tender or painful with orchitis, indistinguishable from testis on palpation (E. coli, C. trachomatis, N. gonorrhoeae)
- Spermatic cord
  - Palpate both cords simultaneously with thumbs and index fingers
  - Note size, tenderness or beading
  - Cords should be firm from epididymis to superficial inguinal ring
  - Varicocele confirmed by pulsation when patient is asked to cough (Valsalva maneuver)
  - Transilluminate scrotal masses to differentiate between solid and cystic
  - Darken room, apply light source to side of scrotal enlargement
  - Cystic masses (hydrocele, spermatocele) transilluminate
  - Solid masses (tumor, varicocele, hernia) do not transmit light
- Inguinal area (hernias)
  - With the patient standing, invaginate the scrotal skin with the index finger of one hand
  - Palpate the external inguinal ring by following the spermatic cord toward the inguinal canal using the finger
  - Place the fingertips of the other hand over the abdomen in the area of the ipsilateral internal inguinal ring and ask the patient to turn his head and cough (Valsalva)
  - Hernia is felt as a bulge that descends against index finger at the external inguinal ring

## Digital Rectal Exam

- **Note:** if urinalysis is required, collect specimen before performing DRE
- Position
  - ◆ Explain why and how examination is done, allow time for patient to prepare, relax, and be draped appropriately
  - ◆ Patient should either be in left lateral decubitus (if the examiner is right-handed), right lateral decubitus (if the examiner is left-handed) or standing bent over the examination table
  - ◆ Put on glove and lubricate the index finger thoroughly
- Inspection (anus)
  - ◆ Inflammation, excoriation
  - ◆ Anal carcinoma or melanoma
  - ◆ Hemorrhoids: ask patient to bear down while inspecting
- Palpation (see **Figure 2**)
  - ◆ Relax sphincter with pressure from palmar surface of gloved, lubricated finger
  - ◆ Gently and slowly insert index finger into anus by rotating finger
  - ◆ Estimate sphincter tone
    - ▪ Flaccid or spastic sphincter suggests similar changes in urinary sphincter and may be suggestive of neurogenic disease
  - ◆ Assess for the presence of any rectal masses
  - ◆ Palpation of the prostate:
    - ▪ Do not massage prostate in patients with acute prostatitis
    - ▪ Assess size, consistency, sensitivity, and shape (see **Table 5**)
  - ◆ Withdraw index finger gently and slowly
  - ◆ Note color of stool on glove and test for occult blood
  - ◆ Wipe the anal area of lubricant with a tissue and provide patient tissues to clean himself

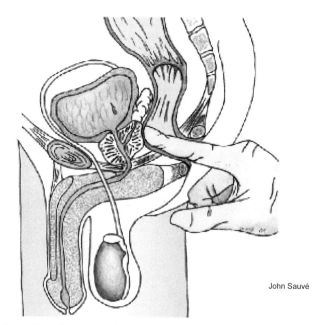

John Sauvé

**Figure 2.** Digital Rectal Examination and Palpation of the Prostate

**Table 5.** Features of the Prostate on DRE

| Feature | Normal | Pathologic |
|---|---|---|
| Size | Approximately 4 cm in length and width (chestnut size) | Enlarged (BPH, advanced prostate cancer) |
| Consistency | Rubbery | Firm/nodular (prostate cancer) |
| Mobility | Variable | Fixed |
| Sensitivity | Painless | Painful (prostatitis) Painless (prostate cancer) |

### 4.2 Female-Specific Exam Maneuvers

**Vagina**
- Inspect the vulva/vagina for swelling, erythema, atrophy (degree of estrogenization), and lesions
- Pelvic exam (see **The Gynecology Exam** chapter)
    - Examine for cystocele: bulge in anterior vaginal wall
    - Examine for rectocele: bulge in posterior vaginal wall
    - Assess anterior wall mobility by having patient perform Valsalva
- Urethral orifice
    - Examine for caruncle: small, red, benign tumor in urethral opening (posterior portion)
    - Examine for urethral prolapse: swollen red ring of urethral mucosa protruding from urethral opening

**Hernias**
- Occurrences in females are less common than in males; when occurring: indirect inguinal > femoral > direct inguinal
- Examination for inguinal hernias: palpate within the labia majora and move finger upward, ending just lateral to the pubic tubercle
- If a hernia is present, a bulge will be felt against finger tip when patient performs Valsalva

**Urinary Stress Test**
- Have patient assume the lithotomy position on the examining table with a full bladder; legs are spread and perineal area is relaxed
- Ask the patient to cough vigorously: if urine is lost, beginning and ending with the cough, the test is confirmatory for stress incontinence

## 5. COMMON INVESTIGATIONS

**Urinalysis**
- Should be performed in all urologic patients (see **Appendix 2**, p.651 (Urinalysis section))
- A complete urinalysis includes both chemical and microscopic analyses (R&M)

**Gram Stain and Culture**
- Include susceptibility testing if urethritis is suspected

**Cytology**
- Urine should be screened for tumor cells in:
    - High risk individuals (e.g. environmental exposures)
    - Presence of painless hematuria after ruling out other causes
    - Evaluation for recurrence after bladder tumor resection

**Cystoscopy**
- Visualization of the bladder via insertion of fiberoptic instrument (rigid or flexible) through the urethra

REPRODUCTIVE

- Aids in diagnosis of bladder tumors and calculi, management of urethral stricture or accessing bladder for visualization of ureters (with X-ray) and stent placement
- Caution should be exercised when performing in patients with an active UTI

## Ultrasound
- Often used to determine postvoid residual volume, total bladder capacity, and bladder proprioception in the setting of incontinence
- Scrotal ultrasound excellent to investigate scrotal masses
- Abdominal or pelvic ultrasound for hydronephrosis, renal masses, and lymph nodes

## Urodynamic Testing
- Uroflowmetry: patient urinates into device for catching and measuring urine and a computer calculates the flow rate
- Postvoid residual volume: the volume of urine remaining in the bladder after voiding; it can be measured via ultrasound or directly by inserting a catheter and measuring the output
- Cystometrogram: test to measure the response of the bladder filling
- Pressure/flow studies: can be used to test for outlet obstruction
- Video-urodynamics: use of X-ray contrast to obtain fluoroscopic images during urodynamic testing
- Catheter monitoring can be used to measure pressure during bladder filling and emptying

# 6. COMMON DISORDERS

## Kidneys
- Renal colic (stones)
- Renal mass (benign or malignant)
- Pyelonephritis

## Bladder
- Carcinoma
- Cystitis
- Interstitial cystitis/bladder pain syndrome (IC/BPS)

## Prostate ♂
- Prostatitis
- Carcinoma
- Benign prostatic hyperplasia (BPH)

## Penis ♂
- Erectile Dysfunction
- Phimosis (inability to retract foreskin over glans)
- Paraphimosis (inability to reduce foreskin: emergency)
- Priapism (low flow vs. high flow)
- Anterior urethral stricture
- Peyronie's disease (fibrous plaque in tunica albuginea)

## Vagina ♀
- Cystocele (bladder prolapse into vagina)
- Urethrocele (urethral prolapse into vagina)

## 7. COMMON CLINICAL SCENARIOS

**Table 6.** Common clinical scenarios in urology

| KEY SYMPTOMS & MANAGEMENT | PHYSICAL EXAM | INVESTIGATIONS |
|---|---|---|
| **Renal colic** | | |
| • Intense, sudden onset, unilateral pain in flank (or lower abdomen), restlessness, and vomiting<br>• Blood may be seen or detected in urine<br>• May be associated with infection (fever, chills, sweats) | • Complete abdominal and urological exam (including DRE)<br>• Rule out aortic aneurysm by checking for pulsating mass<br>• Rule out gallbladder pathology by assessing for Murphy's sign | • Urinalysis (R&M and C&S)<br>• Non-contrast helical CT abdomen is diagnostic test of choice<br>• Plain abdominal X-rays can assess already detected stone<br><br>**Management:**<br>• Non-interventional<br>• Medical: a-blocker<br>• Surgical: stenting, shockwave therapy, ureteroscopy, percutaneous lithotripsy |
| **BPH** | | |
| Storage/voiding LUTS | • DRE: note size and consistency (average prostate ~20 g)<br>• With BPH, prostate should be smooth, firm, elastic, and enlarged<br>• Induration found with DRE indicates further investigation for cancer<br>• Note: BPH is not a risk factor for prostate cancer | • Urinalysis (to exclude infection/ hematuria)<br>• Creatinine<br>• PSA (to exclude prostate cancer but controversial, see table 5)<br>• Transrectal ultrasound (TRUS) to assess size<br><br>**Management:**<br>• Medical: a-blocker, 5-alpha-reductase inhibitor<br>• Surgical: TURP |
| **Varicocele** | | |
| • Most are asymptomatic<br>• May present as infertile patient<br>• May report scrotal heaviness | • Careful inspection, may appear as "bag of worms" in scrotum<br>• Valsalva while palpating | • If unclear, then do high resolution Doppler ultrasonography<br>• Semen analysis to determine if surgery needed<br><br>**Management:**<br>• Surgery or interventional radiology embolization of vessels ONLY if symptomatic and affecting quality of life or fertility |
| **Testicular Torsion** | | |
| • Sudden onset of severe testicular pain followed by inguinal and/or scrotal swelling<br>• Testicle retracted upward<br>• 1/3 have GI upset<br>• May be preceded by trauma | • Swollen, tender, high-riding, transverse testis<br>• Lifting the testicle will increase pain (whereas in epididymitis, it will relieve pain Prehn's sign)<br>• Absence of cremasteric reflex supports diagnosis | • If physical exam suggests testicular torsion, refer patient to OR for immediate scrotal exploration<br>• Surgical emergency<br><br>**Management:**<br>• Surgery: detorsion and bilateral orchidopexy |

REPRODUCTIVE

**REPRODUCTIVE**

### Hematuria

| | | |
|---|---|---|
| Refer to Section 2: **Common Chief Complaints** | Refer to Section 4: **Focused Physical Exam** | • Refer to hematuria algorithm below (**Figure 3**)<br><br>**Management:**<br>• Microscopic: Renal U/S or CT Urogram +/- cystoscopy<br>• Gross: CT Urogram or MRI + cystoscopy<br>• Urinalysis, culture/sensitivity, cytology for both |

### Prostate Cancer

| | | |
|---|---|---|
| • Most are asymptomatic<br>• Storing or voiding LUTS may suggest advanced or metastatic disease<br>• Bone pain may be suggestive of metastases<br>• Paresthesias, weakness of lower extremities, and urinary or fecal incontinence may be observed in advanced disease with cord compression | • Today's cases often have normal DRE<br>• Induration found with DRE indicates further investigation to rule out cancer (i.e. PSA screen/ TRUS/biopsy) | • PSA Screening (**Table 5**)<br>• Percent free PSA (fPSA)<br>• PSA velocity<br>• TRUS (if appropriate)<br>• Biopsy (if appropriate)<br><br>**Management:**<br>• Watchful waiting<br>• Active surveillance<br>• Surgery<br>• Radiation<br>• Androgen Deprivation Therapy |

### Prolapse (Female specific)

| | | |
|---|---|---|
| • Often asymptomatic<br>• Vaginal bleeding (from exposed/ ulcerated mucous membrane)<br>• Sensation of vaginal fullness/pressure<br>• History of coital difficulties<br>• History of voiding or defecation difficulty<br>• Sacral back pain<br>• Bulge protruding into vagina or through vaginal introitus | • Examine the patient in lithotomy position as well as standing, both while relaxed and during maximal straining<br>• Urethral prolapse: swollen, red, ring around urethral meatus<br>• Cystocele if bulge in anterior vaginal wall<br>  • 1st Degree: protrusion to upper vagina<br>  • 2nd Degree: protrusion to the introitus<br>  • 3rd Degree: protrusion external to the introitus<br>• Rectocele if bulge in posterior vaginal wall<br>• Uterine (or vault) prolapse (may be associated with cystocele and/ or rectocele): progressive retroversion of uterus and descent into vagina with lowering of cervix:<br>  • 1st Degree: cervix remains within vagina<br>  • 2nd Degree: cervix is at the introitus<br>  • 3rd Degree: cervix and vagina are outside the introitus | • Assess for urinary retention: postvoid residual volume (ultrasound)<br>• Assess strength of pelvic floor musculature<br>• If patient is asymptomatic and there is no urinary retention, may do nothing<br><br>**Management:**<br>• Pelvic floor exercises<br>• Pessary<br>• Slings<br>• Surgery |

## Urinary Tract Infection

- Storage/voiding LUTS
- Hematuria
- Cloudy/malodorous urine
- Pain/tenderness (costovertebral angle, suprapubic, back)

- Pain suprapubic: cystitis
- Pain costovertebral angle: pyelonephritis

- Urinalysis
- Urine culture/sensitivity
- Organisms (KEEPS)
  - Klebsiella spp.
  - E coli
  - Enterococcus spp.
  - Proteus & Pseudomonas spp.
  - S. saprophyticus

### Management
- **Asymptomatic bacteriuria**: no treatment unless in pregnant women and before urological procedures
- **Acute cystitis**: Nitrofurantoin (100 mg PO BID x 5 days) or Septra (160/800 mg PO BID x 3 days, as sensitivity dictates)
- **Acute pyelonephritis**:
- *Inpatient*: Fluoroquinolone IV, ampicillin + gentamicin or 3rd generation cephalosporin IV x 14 days
- *Outpatient*: Ciprofloxacin (500 mg PO BID x 7 days) or Septra (160/800 mg PO BID x 14 days)

**Clinical Pearl: Clinical Suspicion of Hematuria**
Hematuria of any degree should never be ignored and, in adults, should be regarded as a symptom of urologic malignancy until proven otherwise.

REPRODUCTIVE

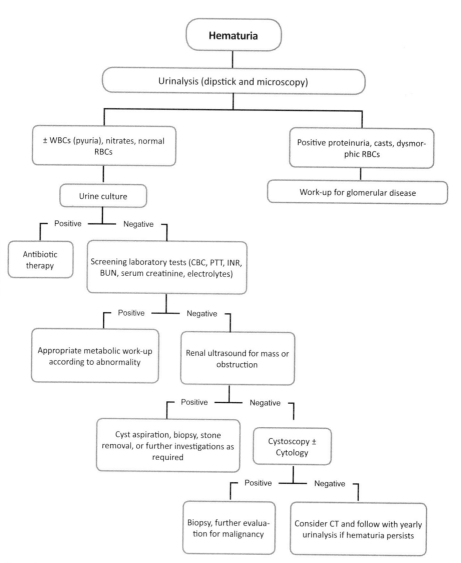

**Figure 3.** Investigations for Hematuria

**Clinical Pearl: PSA Measurements After Treatment of Prostate Cancer**
PSA measurements become an integral part of follow-up visits post-treatment. The frequency and parameters of these measurements will depend on the modality of treatment and the physician's or hospital's protocol.

**Table 7.** Screening for Prostate Cancer

Males 50-75 yr with life expectancy of >10 yr should be informed of the risks/benefits of PSA testing
- Men over 75 yr should not be tested

Men at a higher risk for prostate cancer:
- African-American descent
- 1st generation relative with prostate cancer
- High fat diet
- Prostatic nodule found on DRE
- Abnormal-feeling prostate
- Discrete change either in texture, fullness or symmetry

PSA has limited specificity because elevations also occur in men with benign disease (e.g. prostatic hyperplasia, prostatitis)

PSA levels vary according to age and degree of hyperplasia, but cancer produces excess levels

Consider tests such as PSA velocity or percent free PSA (fPSA) to supplement investigation

### Hernias (See **Figure 4**)
- Signs and Symptoms
  - Lump or swelling in groin or scrotum
  - Sudden pain in scrotum
  - Pain in scrotum while standing or moving
  - Heavy feeling in groin
- Physical Exam
  - Observe inguinal canal for bulge and size increased with cough
  - In male patients, the exam is best performed seated with patient standing; invaginate scrotum with finger, ask patient to cough and feel for impulse
  - In female patients, palpate within the labia majora and move finger superiorly, feel for bulge on Valsalva
  - Investigations are often not necessary to make diagnosis
  - Indicative of hernias if: masses return to the abdomen upon lying down, have bowel sounds on auscultation, and do not transmit light when transilluminated

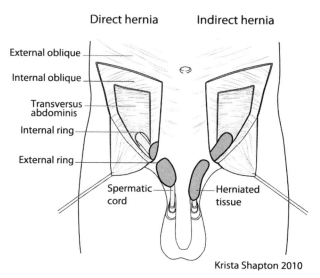

Direct hernia    Indirect hernia

External oblique
Internal oblique
Transversus abdominis
Internal ring
External ring

Spermatic cord

Herniated tissue

Krista Shapton 2010

**Figure 4.** Direct vs. Indirect Hernias

### 7.1 Pediatric Male-Specific Scenarios

**Table 8.** Common pediatric scenarios in urology

| KEY SYMPTOMS | PHYSICAL EXAM | INVESTIGATIONS & MANAGEMENT |
|---|---|---|
| **Hypospadias** | | |
| • Asymptomatic, signs present at newborn exam<br>• Foreskin has dorsal hooded prepuce<br>• Two apparent urethral openings, with blind meatus in normal location and displaced true meatus ventrally<br>• Abnormal penile curvature: chordee | • Meatal location<br>• Glans configuration<br>• Penile curvature<br>• Penile length assessment<br>• Scrotal exam | • Investigations not needed<br>• Surgery necessary to correct meatal opening and foreskin<br><br>**Management**<br>• Surgery: primary tubularization, onlay island flap, two-stage repairs |
| **Cryptorchidism** | | |
| • Testicle not found within scrotum<br>• Scrotum may be small and minimally rugated | • Genital exam to assess for other abnormalities<br>• Two-handed exam is needed; one soapy or lubricated hand making sweeping movements along anterior inguinal canal and the other over the scrotum assessing for a retractile or ectopic testis<br>• The child should be in a squatting position<br>• Testicular position: inguinal canal vs. scrotum vs. typical ectopic sites<br>• Testicular consistency<br>• Size of testicle in relation to opposite testis<br>• Evaluation for a non-palpable testis | • Radiologic examination not warranted, aside from cases in which the presence of a uterus needs to be excluded or in assessment of obese boys<br><br>**Management**<br>• Surgery: orchidopexy depending on viability of testis<br>• inguinal, scrotal or laparoscopic approach |

REPRODUCTIVE

## REFERENCES

1. Wein AJ, Kavoussi LR, Partin AW, Peters CA (Editors). Campbell-Walsh Urology, 10th ed. Philadelphia: Saunders Elsevier; 2016.
2. Andriole GL, Crawford ED, Grubb RL 3rd, Buys SS, Chia D, Church TR, et al. 2009. N Engl J Med 360(13):1310-1319.
3. Hugosson J, Carlsson S, Aus G, Bergdahl S, Khatami A, Lodding P, et al. 2010. Lancet Oncol 11(8):725-732.
4. Schröder FH, Hugosson J, Roobol MJ, Tammela TL, Ciatto S, Nelen V, etal. 2009. N Engl J Med 360(13):1320-1328.
5. University of Michigan Health System. Urinary Tract Infection. Ann Arbor: University of Michigan; 2011.

REPRODUCTIVE

RESPIRATORY

CHAPTER 10:

# The Respiratory System

**Editors:**
Arnav Agarwal, BHSc
Marie Yan, BHSc, MD

**Resident Reviewer:**
Benny Dua, MD, PhD

**Faculty Reviewers:**
Meyer Balter, MD, FRCPC
David Hall, MD, PhD, FRCPC

## TABLE OF CONTENTS

# 1. ESSENTIAL ANATOMY

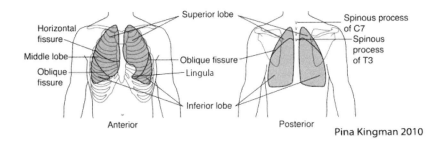

**Figure 1.** Locations of Lobes and Landmarks

## Landmarks
- **Apex:** 2-4 cm above medial third of clavicle
- **Oblique fissure** (both lungs): line from T3 spinous process, through 5th rib in the mid-axillary line, ending at the 6th rib in the mid-clavicular line
  - Right oblique fissure: separates the lower lobe from the upper and middle lobes
  - Left oblique fissure: separates the upper and lower lobes
- **Horizontal fissure** (right lung): separates the upper and middle lobes; extends from the 5th rib in the right mid-axillary line to the 4th rib at the sternal border
- **Inferior margins** (both lungs): extend from T10 posteriorly, through the 8th rib in the mid-axillary line to the 6th rib in the mid-clavicular line
- **Carina:** located at the level of the angle of Louis (T4)
- **Right hemidiaphragm:** at the level of the 5th rib anteriorly and T9 posteriorly at the end of respiration (higher than left due to liver)

# 2. COMMON CHIEF COMPLAINTS

**Table 1.** Common Respiratory Complaints

| Chief Complaint | Differential Diagnosis | Distinguishing Features |
|---|---|---|
| Chronic cough* (>3 months) | • Asthma | • Diffuse wheezing, dyspnea, chest tightness, history of atopy |
| *with normal CXR | • GERD | • Burning chest pain, acid taste in mouth, association with meals |
| | • Post-nasal drip | • Throat clearing, sensation of dripping in back of throat |
| Shortness of breath (dyspnea) | | |
| • **Acute SOB** | • URTI | • Rhinitis, sneezing, sore throat |
| | • Pneumonia | • Fever, cough |
| | • Anaphylaxis | • Rash/hives, angioedema, GI symptoms |

| Chief Complaint | Differential Diagnosis | Distinguishing Features |
|---|---|---|
| • **Chronic SOB** | • COPD | • Chronic productive cough, chest tightness, history of smoking |
| | • Cardiac (e.g. angina, heart failure) | • Retrosternal chest pain, bilateral leg swelling, orthopnea, PND |
| **Coughing up blood (hemoptysis)\*** | • COPD/Chronic bronchitis | • See above |
| *all conditions listed here can also present with dyspnea, therefore should be considered in DDx | • Pulmonary embolism | • Pleuritic chest pain, symptoms of DVT, PE risk factors |
| | • Lung cancer | • Constitutional symptoms, history of smoking |
| | • Tuberculosis | • Fever, travel to/born in TB endemic areas |
| | • Vasculitis/connective tissue disease | • Rash, joint pain, constitutional symptoms, hematuria/AKI |
| **Wheezing** | • Asthma/COPD | • See above |
| | | • See above |
| | • Anaphylaxis | |
| | | • Focal wheezing, history of choking with food |
| | • Aspiration/foreign body | |
| | | • Focal wheezing, constitutional symptoms, history of smoking |
| | • Tumour | |

Other Common Chief Complaints:
- Phlegm production (sputum)
- Chest pain
- Chest radiographic abnormalities (as reason for referral)

# 3. APPROACH TO THE RESPIRATORY HISTORY AND PHYSICAL EXAM

## 3.1 Overview of the History

In addition to general history taking, important aspects of the respiratory history include:

**Associated Symptoms:**
- Cough ± sputum production, hemoptysis
- Wheezing/stridor, dyspnea
- Pleuritic chest pain
- Cyanosis
- Edema

**Risk Factors:**
- Past history of respiratory infections
- Atopy
- Smoking
- Previous abnormalities on CXR or pulmonary function testing
- Animal exposure, allergies
- Environmental/occupational exposures
- Travel history/birthplace (TB endemic)

- Sexual history

## 3.2 Overview of the Physical Exam
- **Inspection**
    - Rate and pattern of respiration
    - Signs of respiratory effort and distress (accessory muscle use, paradoxical breathing)
    - Cyanosis (central, peripheral)
    - Chest configuration (kyphosis, scoliosis, barrel chest)
    - Clubbing
    - Pursed-lip breathing
    - Presence of supportive care measures and monitors
- **Palpation**
    - General tenderness and deformities
    - Position of trachea
    - Chest expansion
    - Tactile fremitus
- **Percussion**
    - General percussion (resonance, dullness)
    - Diaphragmatic excursion
- **Auscultation**
    - Type of breath sounds (vesicular, bronchovesicular, bronchial, tracheal)
    - Symmetry of breath sounds
    - Presence of adventitious sounds (crackles, wheezes, stridor, pleural rub)

# 4. KEY COMPONENTS OF RESPIRATORY HISTORY

### Cough
- OPQRST: onset/duration - acute/chronic, time of day; palliating/provoking factors - body position, season, different environments; quality (see **Table 2**)
- Associated Symptoms: sputum, constitutional symptoms (fever, chills, night sweats, weight loss), post-nasal drip, runny nose, hoarseness, wheezing, heartburn
- Risk Factors: smoking, sick contacts, travel history, pets, occupational history

**Table 2.** Cough Descriptors and Possible Etiologies to Consider

| Cough Descriptors | Possible Etiologies |
| --- | --- |
| Dry, hacking | Viral pneumonia, interstitial lung disease, tumor, laryngitis, allergies, anxiety |
| Chronic, productive | Bronchiectasis, chronic bronchitis, abscess, pneumonia, TB |
| Barking | Epiglottal disease (e.g. croup) |
| Morning | Smoking |
| Nocturnal | Post-nasal drip, CHF, asthma |
| Upon eating/ drinking | Neuromuscular disease of the upper esophagus |

Note: While the descriptions of a cough obtained by history may be helpful when considering the differential diagnosis of cough, these descriptions alone cannot determine the etiology of cough. A clinical anatomic-pathologic diagnostic approach and supportive tests, such as spirometry, pulmonary function tests, imaging, and 24-h esophageal pH monitoring, are crucial steps in diagnosis after taking a history

### Sputum
- OPQRST: onset/duration, frequency, progression, quantity, color, consistency, odor
- Associated Symptoms: hemoptysis, mucoid sputum (odorless, transparent, and whitish-gray), purulent sputum (infected; yellow-green in bronchiectasis and COPD; yellow or green in asthma, more often due to eosinophilia than infection), foul-smelling sputum (suggestive of a lung abscess)

### Wheezing/Stridor
- CC: High-pitched sound caused by partially obstructed airway (wheezing due to

intrathoracic obstruction on expiration; stridor due to extra thoracic upper airway obstruction on inspiration)
- OPQRST: onset, duration of episodes, frequency, progression, palliating factors, provoking factors (food, odors, emotions, animals, allergens (e.g. dust, pollen))
- Risk Factors: history of nasal polyps, cardiac disease (e.g. CHF), smoking

## Dyspnea
- OPQRST: onset (gradual vs. sudden), palliating/provoking factors, duration, progression (e.g., current symptoms vs. 6 months prior), on exertion (quantify with exercise tolerance e.g., number of blocks walked or flights of stairs climbed before onset; **Table 3**), timing (paroxysmal nocturnal dyspnea - sudden onset of dyspnea that awakens an individual from sleep; patient classically describes needing to go to an open window for air), body position (see Table 3)
- Associated Symptoms: constitutional symptoms (fever, chills, night sweats, weight loss), cough, hemoptysis, sputum, fatigue, chest pain, palpitations, peripheral edema
- Risk Factors: sick contacts, industrial exposure (e.g. asbestos, sandblasting), travel history

**Table 3.** Medical Research Council (MRC) Dyspnea Scale

| Grade | Description |
|---|---|
| 1 | Not troubled by breathlessness except with strenuous exercise |
| 2 | Troubled by shortness of breath when hurrying on the level or walking up a slight hill |
| 3 | Walks slower than people of the same age on the level because of breathlessness or has to stop for breath when walking at own pace on the level |
| 4 | Stops for breath after walking about 100 yards (90 m) or after a few minutes on the level |
| 5 | Too breathless to leave the house or breathless when dressing or undressing |

**Table 4.** Types and Etiologies of Positional Dyspnea

| Type | Etiology |
|---|---|
| **Orthopnea** (dyspnea when lying horizontally) | CHF Mitral valve disease Severe asthma (rare) COPD (rare) Neurological diseases (rare) |
| **Trepopnea** (dyspnea when lying on one side) | CHF |
| **Platypnea** (dyspnea when seated) | Status post-pneumonectomy Neurological diseases Cirrhosis (intrapulmonary shunts) Hypovolemia |

## Hemoptysis
- OPQRST: onset, number of episodes, quantity, quality (clots or blood-tinged sputum), precipitating factors (cough, nausea/vomiting)
- Associated Symptoms: fever, chills, night sweats, weight loss, pleuritic chest pain, leg pain, leg edema, persistent cough, dyspnea, palpitations, arrhythmias
- Risk Factors: recent surgery (DVT/PE), smoking, anticoagulants, clotting disorders, oral contraceptives, bronchiectasis, cystic fibrosis, TB exposure
- Notes: Important to distinguish hemoptysis and hematemesis. Hemoptysis: associated with coughing and dyspnea; red, frothy, mixed with sputum, alkaline. Hematemesis: associated with nausea/vomiting; red/brown, not frothy, may be mixed with food, acidic (unless on antacids/proton pump inhibitors)

## Pleuritic Chest Pain

- CC: localized "knife-like" pain associated with inspiration or coughing; suggests involvement of parietal pleura
- Risk Factors: domestic exposures (pets, hobbies, pollution), occupational exposures (see **Table 5**), recent travel and immigration history
- Etiologies: primary diseases of the pleura: mesothelioma, pleuritic; pulmonary diseases that can extend to the pleura: pneumonia, pulmonary embolism

**Table 5.** Occupational Exposures

| Type | Etiology |
|---|---|
| **Grain dust, wood dust, tobacco, pollens etc.** | Occupational asthma |
| **Asbestos** | Pleural mesothelioma<br>Pulmonary fibrosis |
| **Coal** | Pneumoconiosis |
| **Sandblasting and quarries** | Silicosis |
| **Industrial dusts** | Chronic bronchitis |

## 5. FOCUSED PHYSICAL EXAM

### Inspection
- **Signs of Respiratory Distress**
  - General difficulty breathing (stridor or wheezing, pursed-lip breathing on expiration)
  - Use of accessory muscles (trapezius, sternocleidomastoids, retraction of intercostal muscles, nasal flaring)
  - Orthopnea: dyspnea that occurs when lying down and improves upon sitting up
  - Tripoding: sitting upright and leaning forward on outstretched arms
  - Paradoxical Breathing: inward movement of abdomen on inspiration
  - Use of $O_2$ therapy/respiratory equipment (e.g. nasal prongs, mask, transtracheal $O_2$, endotracheal/tracheostomy tube with ventilator, oximeter)
- **Cyanosis (Central or Peripheral)**
  - Signs of peripheral cyanosis include coolness and bluish color of extremities (fingers, toes, nose, ears)
  - Signs of central cyanosis include bluish mucous membranes (lips, frenulum, buccal mucosa)
  - Central cyanosis occurs when oxygen saturation falls below 85% (and patient is not anemic)
- **RR and Pattern** (assessed immediately after measuring pulse so patient is unaware of it being done)
  - Normal adults: RR = 14-20 breaths/min
  - Apnea: a period without breathing
  - Bradypnea: abnormally slow rate of respiration (RR <14)
  - Tachypnea: abnormally fast rate of respiration (RR >20)
  - Hyperpnea (Kussmaul's breathing): increased depth and rate of breathing
  - Cheyne-Stokes Breathing: periods of deep breathing alternating with periods of apnea
- **Chest Configuration (AP and Lateral)**
  - Masses, scars, lesions, lacerations
  - Normal: AP diameter < lateral diameter
  - Barrel chest: AP diameter equal to lateral diameter
  - Pectus excavatum (funnel chest): a depression of the sternum; associated with mitral valve disease
  - Pectus carinatum (pigeon chest): an anterior protrusion of the sternum
  - Kyphosis: abnormal AP curvature of spine
  - Scoliosis: abnormal lateral curvature and torsion of spine
- **Clubbing**
  - Nail-fold/hyponychial angle: abnormal if angle > ~180 degrees
  - Phalangeal depth ratio: abnormal if ratio > 1.0 (i.e. distal phalangeal finger depth is greater than interphalangeal finger depth)

- Look for Schamroth sign: loss of diamond-shaped window when dorsal surfaces of terminal phalanges on opposite fingers are opposed
- Sponginess of nail bed
- Refer to **Dermatology** Chapter for more details

## Palpation

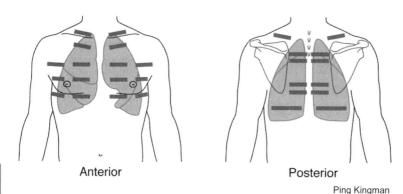

Anterior

Posterior

Ping Kingman

**Figure 2.** Sites of Lung Percussion, Palpation, and Auscultation

- **Chest Wall Tenderness**
  - Gently palpate all areas of chest for tenderness and deformities; check for MSK pain (beware of rib fractures)
- **Tactile Fremitus**
  - Place ulnar side of the hand against chest wall and ask patient to say "ninety-nine" or "boy-oh-boy"
  - The hand must be moved from side-to-side to compare left to right sides and from the top downward (see **Figure 2**)
  - Each lung field should be palpated both posteriorly and anteriorly (including the supraclavicular fossae, mid-axillary line, and anterior intercostal spaces beginning at the clavicle)

**Table 6.** Interpretation of Tactile Fremitus[1]

| Transmission | Pathologies |
| --- | --- |
| **Increased** | Consolidation (e.g. pneumonia) |
| **Decreased: Unilateral** | Atelectasis, bronchial obstruction, pleural effusion, pneumothorax, pleural thickening |
| **Decreased: Bilateral** | Chest wall thickening (muscle, fat), COPD, bilateral pleural effusion |

- **Evaluation of Position of Trachea**
  - Palpate the trachea in the suprasternal notch to determine if it is midline
  - Trachea is deviated to ipsilateral side in atelectasis, fibrosis, lung collapse
  - Trachea is deviated to contralateral side in pleural effusion, hemothorax, tension pneumothorax
  - Non-pulmonary causes: lateral tracheal deviation can be caused by neck mass or retrosternal goiter
- **Evaluation of Trachea Mobility**
  - A tracheal tug may be used to assess if the trachea is fixed in the mediastinum
  - With the patient's neck slightly flexed, support the back of the patient's head and position the middle fingers of the opposite hand into the cricothyroid space
  - Push the larynx upward
  - Normally, the trachea and larynx will move up 1-2 cm
  - Slowly lower the larynx before removing fingers

- A fixed trachea may be due to mediastinal fixation (neoplasm or TB)
- **Chest Expansion**
    - Place hands flat on back with thumbs parallel to the midline at the level of the 10th rib and fingers gripping the flanks
    - Ask patient to exhale completely and then inhale deeply: look for symmetry in outward movement of hands
    - Asymmetrical with pleural effusion, lobar pneumonia, pulmonary fibrosis, bronchial obstruction, pleuritic pain with splinting, pneumothorax

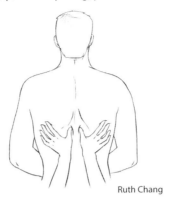

Ruth Chang

**Figure 3.** Technique for Examining Chest Expansion

## Percussion
- Percussion is performed in the same areas as tactile fremitus (see **Figure 2**)
- Normally, chest is resonant everywhere except in the left 3rd-5th intercostal spaces anteriorly (cardiac dullness); loss of dullness suggests hyperinflation (e.g. emphysema) (see **Table 7**)

**Table 7.** Interpretation of Percussion Notes[2]

| Percussion Note | Pathologies |
| --- | --- |
| **Dull** | Lobar pneumonia, hemothorax, empyema, atelectasis, tumor, pleural effusion (can be flat/"stony dull") |
| **Hyperresonant** | Emphysema, asthma, pneumothorax (can be tympanic) |

**Clinical Pearl: Pleural Effusions[3]**
Dullness to percussion is the most useful clinical finding to suggest the presence of a pleural effusion (positive likelihood ratio: 8.7, 95% CI 2.2 – 33.8), but diagnosis requires radiographic confirmation.

## Diaphragmatic Excursion
- Locate level of diaphragm during quiet respiration by percussing in an inferior direction for a change from resonant to dull
- The level of the diaphragm may be stated in reference to the vertebral level by counting down the vertebrae starting with the vertebral prominence (C7)
- Have the patient hold as full an inhalation as possible and locate the new (inferior) level of the diaphragm
- Have the patient hold as full an exhalation as possible and relocate the level of the diaphragm (now superior)
- Measure the change in diaphragm level from inspiration to expiration; normal diaphragmatic excursion is 4-5 cm
- Consider percussing bilaterally to compare excursion (i.e. check for hemiparalysis)

## Auscultation

- Instruct patient to breath deeply through an open mouth and listen to breath sounds using the stethoscope's diaphragm in the same areas as for tactile fremitus (see **Figure 2**)
- Note intensity, pitch, and ratio of duration of inspiration to expiration (see **Table 8**)
- Bronchial breath sounds can be heard over the trachea, are louder than vesicular breath sounds, and have a gap between inspiration and expiration
- Vesicular breath sounds are heard best at the bases of lungs and have no gap between inspiration and expiration
- Compare breath sounds on both sides
- Over peripheral lung fields:
  - Bronchial breath sounds usually indicate consolidation
  - Bronchovesicular breath sounds may indicate bronchospasm or interstitial fibrosis

**Table 8.** Interpretation of Breath Sounds[1]

| Characteristic | Tracheal | Bronchial | Bronchovesicular | Vesicular |
|---|---|---|---|---|
| **Description** | Harsh | Air rushing through tube | Rustling but tubular | Gentle rustling |
| **Normal Location** | Extrathoracic trachea | Manubrium | Mainstem bronchi | Peripheral lung fields |
| **Pitch** | Very high | High | Moderate | Low |
| **Inspiration: Expiration** | 1:1 | 1:3 | 1:1 | 3:1 |

**Adventitious Sounds**
- Listen for sounds that are superimposed upon the usual breath sounds (see **Table 9**)

**Table 9.** Adventitious Sounds

| Sound | Description | Mechanism | Causes |
|---|---|---|---|
| **Crackles** | Short, discontinuous, nonmusical sounds heard mostly during inspiration Fine: high-pitched Coarse: low-pitched | Often excess airway secretions (exception is pulmonary fibrosis) | Timing in inspiratory cycle can be important: atelectasis (early), pneumonia (mid), fibrosis (late), CHF (late), pulmonary edema (late) |
| **Wheezes** | Continuous, musical, high-pitched sounds; usually heard on expiration | Rapid airflow through obstructed airway | Asthma, secretions, pulmonary edema, bronchitis, CHF, bronchiectasis, foreign body, tumor |
| **Stridor** | Inspiratory musical sounds best heard over trachea during inspiration | Upper airway extrathoracic obstruction | Partial obstruction of larynx or trachea |
| **Pleural Rub** | Grating or creaking sounds best heard at end of inspiration and beginning of expiration | Inflammation of the pleura | Pneumonia, pulmonary infarction |

**Consolidation**
- Higher-pitched sounds are better transmitted through consolidated lung than air-filled lung (sound travels faster in solids than gases)
- **Egophony:** when patient utters "E-E-E", sounds like "A-A-A" over area of consolidation
- **Whispered pectoriloquy:** whispered words (e.g. "one-two-three") by patient are auscultated more clearly over area of consolidation

## 6. COMMON INVESTIGATIONS

### Pulse Oximetry
- LED device on finger, toe, or earlobe measures oxygen saturation of hemoglobin
- Does not measure the oxygen tension ($P_aO_2$); interpret $O_2$ saturation with the oxyhemoglobin dissociation curve in mind
- Reads incorrectly high in certain conditions (e.g. carbon monoxide poisoning)
- Reads incorrectly low if there is movement, highly calloused skin, nail polish, or hypoperfusion to extremity being used for monitoring (cold, use of vasopressor)

### Arterial Blood Gases (ABGs)
- Arterial oxygen tension ($P_aO_2$), carbon dioxide tension ($P_aCO_2$) and pH are measured; bicarbonate concentration is calculated using Henderson-Hasselbalch equation
- Useful for assessing acid/base disturbances (see **Fluids, Electrolytes, and Acid/Base Disturbances** Chapter)
- Alveolar air equation used to determine theoretical alveolar oxygen tension ($P_AO_2$), where RQ = Respiratory quotient
    - $P_AO_2 = FiO2 (P_{ATM}-P_{H2O}) - (P_aCO_2/RQ)$
    - $= 150 - (P_aCO_2/0.8)$
- The alveolar-arterial oxygen gradient (A-a $D_{O2}$) is the difference between the calculated $P_AO_2$ and the measured $P_aO_2$
    - Normally <15 mmHg in healthy patients breathing room air
    - A-a $D_{O2}$ increases with normal aging. Expected A-a $D_{O2}$ = 2.5 + (0.21 x age)
    - Elevated A-a $D_{O2}$ occurs with ventilation-perfusion (V/Q) mismatch or shunting, or increasing FiO2

### Ventilation Perfusion Scan
- Radioactive gas is respired; radiolabeled albumin is injected intravenously and deposits in the pulmonary capillaries
- Radiation from both sources is measured simultaneously to visualize the distribution of both ventilation and perfusion

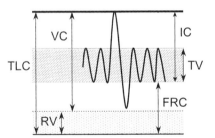

**Figure 4.** Lung Volumes
FRC = functional residual capacity, IC = inspiratory capacity, RV = residual volume, TLC = total lung capacity, TV = tidal volume, VC = vital capacity

### Pulmonary Function Tests (PFTs)
- Patient exhales into a spirometer from TLC down to RV with max effort; the max expiratory flow-volume envelope is plotted
    - $FEV_1$ = forced expired volume in one second
    - FVC = forced vital capacity
    - $V_{50}$ = forced expired flow at 50% of vital capacity
    - $V_{25}$ = forced expired flow at 25% of vital capacity

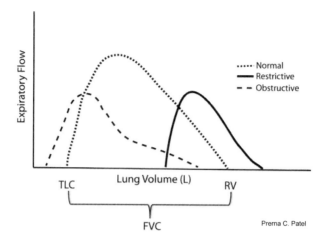

Prerna C. Patel

**Figure 5.** Flow-Volume Curves for Normal, Obstructed, and Restricted Lungs

- Response to bronchodilator and/or methacholine can be used to test for asthma
  - Obstructive lung diseases have characteristic "scooped-out" expiratory flow-volume curves
  - Restrictive lung diseases show generally decreased lung volumes
- A plethysmograph measures TLC, FRC and RV; panting against a closed shutter allows total airway resistance (Raw) to be measured
- Carbon monoxide is used to measure diffusion capacity ($D_{CO}$)

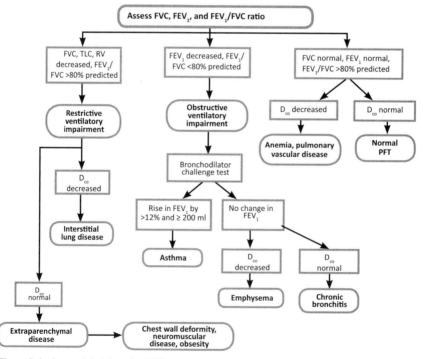

**Figure 6.** An Approach to Intepreting PFTs

## Chest X-ray
- See **Medical Imaging** Chapter

RESPIRATORY

**Table 10.** Characteristic Results of Pulmonary Function Tests in Obstructive and Restrictive Lung Disease

| | | Obstructive | Restrictive |
|---|---|---|---|
| **Lung Volumes** | VC | ↓ or N | ↓ |
| | FRC | ↑ | ↓ |
| | RV | ↑ | ↓ |
| | TLC | ↑ or N | ↓ |
| **Flow Rates** | $FEV_1$ | ↓ | ↓ or N |
| | $FEV_1/FVC$ | ↓ | ↑ or N |
| | $V_{50}$ | ↓ | ↑, ↓ or N |
| | $V_{25}$ | ↓ | ↑, ↓ or N |
| **Airway Resistance** | Raw | ↑ | N |

N = normal

## 7. COMMON DISORDERS

Disorders marked with (✓) are discussed in **Common Clinical Scenarios**
✓ Asthma
✓ COPD (chronic bronchitis, emphysema)
✓ Infections (TB and pneumonia)
✓ Pulmonary embolism
✓ Obstructive lung diseases
  • Asthma
  • COPD (chronic bronchitis, emphysema)
  • Bronchiectasis
✓ Restrictive lung diseases
  • Interstitial lung disease
  • Obstructive sleep apnea
  • Pneumothorax
  • Bronchogenic carcinoma
  • Acute respiratory distress syndrome
  • Occupational lung disease

## 8. COMMON CLINICAL SCENARIOS

**Table 11.** Features of Common Clinical Scenarios[4-10]

| Key Symptoms | Physical Exam Findings | Investigations | Management |
|---|---|---|---|
| **Asthma:** chronic inflammatory disorder of the airways | | | |
| • Dyspnea<br>• Wheezing<br>• Chest tightness<br>• Cough (especially nocturnal) | • Respiratory distress (accessory muscle use, nasal flaring)<br>• Pulsus paradoxus<br>• Expiratory wheezes on auscultation (silent chest if severe) | • Peak expiratory flow rate (PEFR) meter to monitor response to therapy<br>• Spirometry with bronchodilator reversibility assessment<br>• Methacholine challenge<br>• Consider CXR if no response to therapy<br>• Consider ABG if hypoxemic or no response to therapy | Acute management:<br>• Manage ABCs, $O_2$<br>• SABA and SAAC<br>• Systemic corticosteroids (PO or IV)<br>• If severe (e.g. decreased LOC, exhaustion, silent chest), consider $MgSO_4$, ICU<br><br>Long-term management:<br>• Asthma education<br>• Control of triggers<br>• Inhaled corticosteroids (first-line) +/- adjuncts (LABA, LTRA, etc)<br>• SABA PRN |

RESPIRATORY

**COPD:** progressive, partially reversible airway obstruction; clinical subtypes include chronic bronchitis ("blue bloaters") and emphysema ("pink puffers")

| Key Symptoms | Physical Exam Findings | Investigations | Management |
|---|---|---|---|
| • Dyspnea<br>• Productive cough<br>• Increased sputum | **Chronic bronchitis:**<br>• Crackles and wheezes on auscultation<br>• Cyanosis<br><br>**Emphysema**<br>• Tachypnea<br>• Pursed-lip breathing<br>• Accessory muscle use<br>• Hyperresonance on percussion<br>• Decreased breath sounds on auscultation<br>• Decreased diaphragmatic excursion | • CXR may show hyperinflation, flat hemidiaphragm, increased AP diameter and retrosternal airspace<br>• CBC<br>• Sputum cultures<br>• ABG to assess acid-base, hypoxemia, hypercapnia | Acute management:<br>• ABC, $O_2$ (target 88-92% if $CO2$ retainer)<br>• SABA and SAAC<br>• Systemic corticosteroids (PO or IV)<br>• Consider antibiotics if moderate/severe exacerbation or presents with at least 2 of increased sputum purulence, volume, or dyspnea<br>• If severe, consider noninvasive positive pressure ventilation, ICU<br><br>Long-term management:<br>• LAAC +/- LABA<br>• SABA/SAAC PRN<br>• Smoking cessation<br>• Vaccinations*<br>• Home oxygen<br>• Pulmonary rehabilitation |

**Pneumonia**: infection of lung parenchyma

| Key Symptoms | Physical Exam Findings | Investigations | Management |
|---|---|---|---|
| • Cough<br>• Dyspnea<br>• Fever<br>• Pleuritic chest pain | • Tachycardia<br>• Tachypnea<br>• Dullness to percussion<br>• Increased tactile fremitus<br>• Bronchial breath sounds on auscultation | • CXR may show consolidation<br>• CBC<br>• Sputum culture<br>• Blood cultures +/- tests for *Legionella*, TB | • Manage ABCs, $O_2$<br>• Determine need for hospitalization using CURB-65 score<br>• Empiric antibiotics (Table 12)<br>• Prevention through vaccinations* |

RESPIRATORY

**Pulmonary embolism:** blockage of an artery in the lung by a blood clot (most common), air, fat, or another substance that has travelled into the lungs

| Key Symptoms | Physical Exam Findings | Investigations | Management |
|---|---|---|---|
| • Dyspnea<br>• Chest pain (classically pleuritic)<br>• Hemoptysis<br>• Syncope<br>• Fever | • Tachycardia<br>• Tachypnea<br>• Signs of venous thrombosis (see peripheral vascular exam) | • Use PERC and Wells criteria to determine pretest probability and guide investigations<br>• Pulmonary angiogram (gold standard)<br>• Ventilation/ perfusion (V/Q) scan<br>• ECG to rule out ACS; commonly shows sinus tachycardia +/- S1Q3T3 (rare)<br>• CXR to rule out other lung diseases and help interpret V/Q scan<br>• Venous thrombosis studies (i.e. Doppler U/S) | • ABC, $O_2$<br>• Anticoagulation<br>• Duration of anticoagulation depends on cause of PE and thrombosis and bleeding risk<br>• Thrombolytic therapy for cases of massive unstable PE<br>• Consider inferior vena cava filter for patients with contraindications to anticoagulation |

SABA = short-acting β2-agonist; LABA = long-acting β2-agonist; SAAC = short-acting anticholinergic; LAAC = long-acting anticholinergic; LTRA = leukotriene receptor antagonist
* Pneumovax for high-risk patients (including all COPD patients) and annual influenza vaccination

**Table 12.** Common Organisms in Community-Acquired and Hospital-Acquired Pneumonias and their Empiric Antibiotic Treatment

| Sites of Pathogen Acquisition | Organism | Empiric Antibiotic Coverage |
|---|---|---|
| **Community** | S. pneumoniae<br>M. pneumoniae<br>C. pneumoniae<br>H. influenzae<br>Respiratory viruses: influenzas A and B, adenoviruses | **Outpatient:** Macrolide (no risk factors for MDR), respiratory fluoroquinolone (if comorbidities)<br><br>**Inpatient:** Respiratory fluoroquinolone or beta-lactam + macrolide (such as ceftriaxone + azithromycin) |
| **Hospital** | Think about patient's risk of MDR pathogens<br><br>S. pneumoniae<br>S. aureus<br>C. pneumoniae<br>Legionella spp.<br>H. influenzae<br>Gram-negative bacilli<br>Pseudomonas (common MDR pathogen) | **No Risk Factors for MDR Infection:**<br>Respiratory fluoroquinolone or ceftriaxone or ampicillin or ertapenem<br><br>**Risk Factors for MDR Infection*:**<br>Antipseudomonal cephalosporin (cefepime, ceftazidime) or antipseudomonal carbapenem or piperacillin-tazobactam PLUS respiratory fluoroquinolone or aminoglycoside PLUS vancomycin (for MRSA) |

*Risk factors for multiple drug resistant (MDR) pathogen causing HAP, HCAP or VAP include: hospitalization >5 d, antimicrobial therapy in preceding 90 d, immunosuppressive disease/

RESPIRATORY

therapy, residence in nursing home, dialysis, home wound care, hospitalization >2 d in
preceding 90 d
MRSA = methicillin-resistant Staphylococcus aureus

## 8.1 Obstructive Lung Disease
- Asthma
- COPD (emphysema, chronic bronchitis)
- Bronchiectasis

### Clinical Pearl: Obstructive Airway Disease (OAD)[11]
Four elements of history and physical exam are significantly associated with the diagnosis of OAD:

| Finding | Likelihood Ratio |
| --- | --- |
| Smoking history >40 pack yr | 8.3 |
| Self-reported history of chronic OAD | 7.3 |
| Maximum laryngeal height of ≤4 cm | 2.8 |
| Age at least 45 yr | 1.3 |

Patients with all 4 findings had LR+ of 220. Those with none had LR- of 0.13.

## 8.2 Restrictive Lung Disease
- Interstitial lung disease (e.g. idiopathic pulmonary fibrosis [IPF], pneumoconiosis, hypersensitivity pneumonitis, iatrogenic)
- Neuromuscular disease (e.g. polio, myasthenia gravis)
- Chest wall disease (e.g. kyphoscoliosis)
- Space-occupying lesions (e.g. tumors, cysts)
- Pleural disease (e.g. effusions, pneumothorax)
- Extrathoracic conditions (e.g. obesity, ascites, pregnancy)

### Clinical Pearl: Community-Acquired Pneumonia (CAP)[12]

Recommendations for diagnostic testing remain controversial. The overall low yield and infrequent positive effect on clinical care argue against the routine use of common tests such as blood and sputum cultures. However, these cultures may have a major impact on the care of individual patients and are important for epidemiologic reasons. The most definite indication for extensive diagnostic testing is in the critically ill CAP patient. "Such patients should at least have blood drawn for culture and an endotracheal aspirate obtained if they are intubated."

RESPIRATORY

# REFERENCES

1. Swartz M. *Textbook of Physical Diagnosis*, 6th ed. Philadelphia: Elsevier; 2010.
2. Bickley LS, Szilagyi PG, Bates B. *Bates' Guide to Physical Examination and History Taking*, 10th ed. Philadelphia: Lippincott Williams & Wilkins; 2009.
3. Wong CL, Holroyd-Leduc J, Straus SE. Does this patient have a pleural effusion? *JAMA*. 2009; 301(3): 309–317.
4. Lemière C, Bai T, Balter M, et al. Adult asthma consensus guidelines update. *Can Respir J*. 2003; 11(Suppl A): 9A-18A.
5. Lougheed M, Lemière C, Dell S, et al. Canadian thoracic society asthma management continuum – 2010 consensus summary for children six years of age and over, and adults. *Can Respir J*. 2010; 17(1): 15-24.
6. Sin DD, Man J, Sharpe H, Gan WQ, Man SF. Pharmacological management to reduce exacerbations in adults with asthma: A systematic review and meta-analysis. *JAMA*. 2004; 292(3): 367-376.
7. O'Donnell DE, Aaron S, Bourbeau J, et al. Canadian thoracic society recommendations for management of chronic obstructive pulmonary disease. *Can Respir J*. 2003; 10(SupplA): 11A-65A.
8. O'Donnell DE, Hernandez P, Kaplan A, et al. Canadian thoracic society recommendations for management of chronic obstructive pulmonary disease – Highlights for primary care. *Can Respir J*. 2008; 15(Suppl A): 1A-8A.
9. Mandell LA, Marrie TJ, Grossman RF, Chow AW, Hyland RH. Canadian guidelines for the initial management of community-acquired pneumonia: An evidence-based update by the Canadian infectious diseases society and the Canadian thoracic society. *Clin Infect Dis*. 2000; 31(2): 383-421.
10. Metlay JP, Kapoor WN, Fine MJ. Does this patient have community-acquired pneumonia? Diagnosing pneumonia by history and physical examination. *JAMA*. 1997; 278(17):1440-1445.
11. Straus SE, McAlister FA, Sackett DL, Deeks JJ. The accuracy of patient history, wheezing, and laryngeal measurements in diagnosing obstructive airway disease. *JAMA*. 2000; 283(14): 1853-1857.
12. Mandell LA, Wunderink RG, Anzueto A, et al. Infectious diseases society of America/American thoracic society consensus guidelines on the management of community-acquired pneumonia in adults. *Clin Infect Dis*. 2007; 44(Suppl 2): S27-S72.
13. Kalil AC, Metersky ML, Klompas M, et al. Management of adults with hospital-acquired and ventilator-associated pneumonia: 2016 clinical practice guidelines by the infectious diseases society of America and the American thoracic society. *Clin Infect Dis*. 2016; 63(5): e61-e111.

# CHAPTER 11:

# Anesthesiology and Pain Management

**Editors:**
Sangwoo Leem
Gary Tran, MSc
Stephanie Zhou, HBSc

**Faculty Reviewer:**
Natalie Clavel, MD, FRCPC
Doreen Yee, MD, FRCPC

## TABLE OF CONTENTS

# 1. PAIN BASICS

- Pain is an unpleasant sensory and emotional response associated with actual or potential tissue damage, or described in terms of such damage, subjectively modified by a patient's past experiences and expectations[1].
- The ascending pathways that mediate pain consist of three different tracts: (1) neospinothalamic tract, (2) paleospinothalamic tract, and (3) archispinothalamic tract. Each pain tract originates in different spinal cord regions and ascends to terminate in different areas in the CNS.

# 2. FOCUSED PAIN HISTORY

- See Physical Exam for a detailed approach (p. 347)
- OPQRSTUVW questions regarding each complaint

## Associated Symptoms
### Common Pain Patterns and Symptoms

- **Acute Pain**: Lasts min to week; concordant with degree of tissue damage and resolves spontaneously with tissue healing (e.g. dental extraction, surgery, renal calculi, trauma, acute illness)[2]
- **Chronic Pain**: Lasts >3-6 mo; can be associated with no underlying pathology identified to explain the pain, may be intermittent or persistent, may be associated with depression (e.g. chronic lower back pain, osteoarthritis, diabetic polyneuropathy, migraines, fibromyalgia)[2]
  - Can be further divided into nociceptive and neuropathic pain (see **Table 1**)
- **Localized Pain**: pain confined to site of tissue injury (e.g. cutaneous pain, some visceral pain, arthritis, tendonitis)
- **Referred Pain**: pain that is referred to a distant structure (e.g. pain produced by a MI may feel as if it is in the arm, diaphragmatic irritation causing shoulder tip pain) (i.e. referred diaphragmatic pain after laparoscopic surgery)
- **Projected (transmitted) Pain**: pain transferred along the course of a nerve with a segmental distribution (e.g. herpes zoster) or a peripheral distribution (e.g. trigeminal neuralgia)
- **Dermatomal Pattern**: peripheral neuropathic pain (due to distinct spinal cord lesion / nerve root compression)
- **Non-dermatomal Pattern**: central neuropathic pain (i.e. after stroke), fibromyalgia
- **Hyperalgesia**: increased sensitivity to pain that is abnormally out of proportion to the painful stimuli; occurs from damage to nociceptors or peripheral nerves (often a feature of chronic pain)
- **Allodynia**: pain from a stimulus which does not normally cause pain; associated with neuropathic and chronic pain syndromes
- **Paresthesia**: a subjective skin sensation with no apparent physical cause that may be described as numbness, tingling, burning, prickling, pin pricks, pins and needles, etc.

**Table 1.** Peripheral Pain Classification

| Classification | Description | Example |
|---|---|---|
| Nociceptive | Pain from normal activation of peripheral nociceptors by a noxious stimulant (e.g. heat, cold, pressure) Involves actual tissue damage Well-localized (can be diffuse if involve viscera or deep structures) | Soft tissue injuries (e.g. burn, laceration) Fracture Arthritis Abscess Ischemia |
| Neuropathic | Pain from direct injury to neural tissue Causes altered function of CNS or PNS Bypasses nociceptive pathways May or may not have tissue damage Commonly described as burning, tingling, or lancinating | Peripheral Syndromes Peripheral neuropathy Phantom limb Central Syndromes Post-stroke MS Spinal cord injury Trigeminal neuralgia |

Progression of symptoms over time and response to treatment; can use validated tools to assess severity and change:

**Visual Analog Scale**: 100 mm line on which patient indicates his/her level of pain; a reduction of 30 mm or more is clinically significant

**Numeric Rating Scale:** patient rates pain on a scale of 0-10; a reduction of 3 digits or more is significant

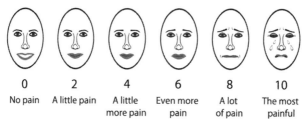

| 0 | 2 | 4 | 6 | 8 | 10 |
|---|---|---|---|---|---|
| No pain | A little pain | A little more pain | Even more pain | A lot of pain | The most painful |

Zaria Chowdhury

**Figure 1.** Numeric Rating Scale

- Pain is the 6th vital sign. Should always ask patient how pain is. Acceptable pain scores are ≤4/10

**Risk Factors**
- Pain medication history (prescription, non-prescription (i.e. OTC), naturopathic, recreational)
- Previous experience with opioid therapy (including precise medication history: drug, dose, frequency, route)
- Effectiveness on pain and function
- Compliance
- Side effects of opioid therapy: N/V, constipation, pruritus, sedation/respiratory depression, tolerance, addiction
- Use of opioids for non-prescribed purposes (e.g. insomnia, stress, mood)
- The Opioid Risk Tool (**Table 2**) is used for safe prescribing of opioids for non-cancer pain.

**Table 2.** ORT Opioid Risk Tool from Canadian Guidelines for Safe Prescribing of Opioids for Non-Cancer Pain

| Item | Score if Female | Score if Male |
|---|---|---|
| Family History of Substance Abuse | | |
| • Alcohol | 1 | 3 |
| • Illegal Drugs | 2 | 3 |
| • Prescription Drugs | 4 | 4 |
| Personal History of Substance Abuse | | |
| • Alcohol | 3 | 3 |
| • Illegal Drugs | 4 | 4 |
| • Prescription Drugs | 5 | 5 |
| Age (mark box if 16-45) | 1 | 1 |
| History of Preadolescent Sexual Abuse | 3 | 0 |
| Psychological Disease | | |
| • Attention Deficit Disorder, Obsessive-Compulsive disorder, or Bipolar, Schizophrenia | 2 | 2 |
| • Depression | 1 | 1 |
| Total | | |

**Total Score Risk Category:**
Low Risk: 0-3
Moderate Risk: 4-7
High Risk: 8+

## 3. FOCUSED PHYSICAL EXAM

### General Inspection
- Observe posture, gait, pain behaviors (e.g. favoring a limb or extremity, dyspnea/respiratory splinting)
- Document any physical stigmata of a substance use disorder (e.g. skin tracks, skin abscesses, stigmata of liver disease, edema, venous insufficiency, lymphadenopathy)

### Peripheral Pain Assessment
- Consider performing MSK and neurological exams of the painful body locations (look for tenderness, trigger points)
- Look specifically for signs of neuropathic pain (hyperalgesia, allodynia, paresthesia)
- Look for secondary consequences of chronic pain (e.g. stiffness, disuse muscle atrophy, weakness)
- Assess the patient's pretreatment mental status and changes in mental status following treatment (e.g. Glasgow coma scale [GCS])

## 4. GENERAL APPROACH TO PAIN MANAGEMENT
- Treat the underlying cause where possible (e.g. steroids for polymyalgia rheumatica, appendectomy for appendicitis)
- Use a multimodal approach where possible for additive effects of analgesics with fewer side effects
- Pain control should be continuous with regularly scheduled dosing and "PRN" dosing for intermittent breakthrough pain
- Manage pain preemptively (e.g. give pain control before painful procedures: i.e. before dressing changes, before physiotherapy)
  - Oral medications can take up to 20-40 minutes to take effect.
  - Intramuscular medications can take 10-20 minutes to take effect.
  - Intravenous medications take 30 sec – 5 min to work
- Multidisciplinary approach and non-pharmacological management also beneficial (see **Complementary and Alternative Therapies**, p. 353)
- Ask the patient to rate the pain as mild, moderate or severe and treat according to the WHO approach to pain management (see **Figure 2**)
- If patient is experiencing neuropathic pain, consider using practice guidelines from the Canadian Pain Society (See neuropathic pain management)
- Choice of analgesic and delivery method depend on:
  - Type of pain
  - Underlying medical condition
  - Patient restrictions: i.e. nil per os (NPO), swallowing problems, etc.
- ***Note:*** it may be necessary to switch therapies as clinical course changes

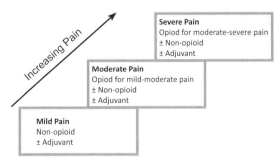

**Figure 2.** WHO Pain Ladder
http://www.who.int/cancer/palliative/painladder/en/

**Table 3.** Common Pain Management Medications

| | Acetaminophen | NSAIDS | Opioids |
|---|---|---|---|
| **Doses** | Acetaminophen 500 mg-1 g q6h PO | Naproxen 250-500 mg q12h PO<br><br>Ibuprofen 200-400 mg q6h PO<br><br>Celecoxib 50-200 mg q12h PO | See dosing in Opioids Management Principles, p. 348 |
| **Indications** | first-line for mild acute pain | Mild to moderate acute pain | Chronic pain refractory to other treatments<br><br>Codeine, Tramadol: Mild to moderate acute pain Morphine, Hydromorphone, Oxycodone: Moderate to severe pain |
| **Cautions** | Liver disease<br>Elderly | Asthma<br>Coagulopathy<br>GI ulcers<br>Renal disease<br>CAD<br><br>Do not take if have sulfa allergy | History of substance abuse<br>Drug-seeking<br>Liver disease<br>Renal disease<br>COPD<br>Sleep apnea |
| **Side Effects** | Liver failure (rare) | Bleeding, pruritus, rash, worsen preexisting renal disease | Constipation or decreased GI motility, nausea, sedation, pruritus, respiratory depression, delirium |
| **Comments** | Analgesia and antipyretic but no anti-inflammatory properties | Analgesia<br>Anti-inflammatory therefore good for tissue damage and inflammation | Caution with concurrent sedating medications (e.g. benzodiazepines)<br><br>Switch from intravenous to oral administration when able to tolerate and taper dose as acute pain resolves |

## 4.1 Medications
### Opioids Management Principles
- When introducing opioids in patients with chronic non-cancer pain, consider a trial period with a defined deadline and outcome
- Mild to moderate acute pain
  - Start with oral immediate release (IR)/short-acting (SA) opioids compounded with acetaminophen (e.g. Tylenol® #3 or Tramacet™) dosed 1-2 tablets, q4-6h PRN
    - Tylenol #3 = acetaminophen 300 mg, codeine 30 mg and caffeine 15 mg
    - Tramacet = acetaminophen 325 mg and tramadol 37.5 mg

---

**Clinical Pearl: Opiod Therapy**
Codeine is a PRODRUG. It is converted to MORPHINE in the body. Codeine is ineffective in ~30% of population.

---

  - If insufficient pain control and acetaminophen dose exceeds 3-4 g/day, switch to stronger compound (e.g. Percocet®) dosed 1-2 tablets, q4-6h PRN
    - Chronic use of Tylenol can cause renal and liver impairment and toxicity

ANESTHESIOLOGY

- Percocet = acetaminophen 325 mg + oxycodone 5 mg, no caffeine
  - Ensure acetaminophen dose from all sources does not exceed 4g/day
- Moderate to severe pain
  - Start with the maximum allowable dose of acetaminophen and add in an NSAID if appropriate. Consider an opioid for moderate to severe pain such as morphine, hydromorphone, or oxycodone either standing or as a PRN medication.
- Severe acute pain
  - Maximize acetaminophen and NSAID (if appropriate) and then titrate IV opioids to effect so pain becomes controlled. Switch as soon as appropriate to oral opioids as effect is longer lasting and easier to administer
  - Note: avoid IM opioid injections for acute, severe pain as absorption is slow and erratic – peak effect in 15-20 mins
  - Taper dose as acute pain resolves
  - Pay attention to and treat side effects: constipation, sedation, nausea
  - Be wary of sedating medication: especially benzodiazepines – for patients on opioids
  - Breakthrough doses of analgesia should be prescribed to manage sudden outbursts of pain. Two methods:
  1. Half the q4h standing dose of an opioid. For example, if someone is taking 10 mg of morphine PO every four hours and requires breakthrough pain medicine, a breakthrough dose of 2.5 mg IV morphine or 5 mg PO morphine every 2 h PRN is given
  2. 10% of the daily dose
- NOTE: morphine not routinely used in hospital because of accumulation of active metabolite during renal failure and in elderly
- In palliative and end-of-life care: dose of morphine is titrated to patient's pain control requirements (no maximum dose)

## Indications for/Contraindications to Opioids
- See **Table 3**

**Clinical Pearl: Opioid Therapy**
For opioid therapy in older patients or those with severe renal/liver disease: Start LOW, go SLOW.
*Initial dose should be half the usual starting dose

- In screening for opioid medication misuse or abuse, verified tools such as the Screener and Opioid Assessment for Patients with Pain (SOAPP) questionnaire (www.painedu.org/soapp.asp) can be used

## Opioid Analgesic Equivalencies
- When converting from one opioid to another, use 50-75% of the equivalent dose to allow for incomplete cross-tolerance
- Rapid titration and PRN use may be required to ensure effective analgesia for the first 24 h
- Dose equivalencies provided in **Table 3** are approximate; individual patients vary

**Table 4.** Approximate Equivalent Doses

| General Name | PO (mg) | IV/IM/SC (mg, unless specified otherwise) | Comments |
|---|---|---|---|
| **Morphine** | 30 | 10 (IV) | Parenteral 10 mg morphine is standard for comparison |
| **Hydromorphone** | 7.5 | 1.5 (IV) | |
| **Oxycodone** | 20 | X | Often formulated in combination with acetaminophen/Aspirin® (Percocet®/Percodan®) Use with caution if administering additional acetaminophen or Aspirin® |

| General Name | PO (mg) | IV/IM/SC (mg, unless specified otherwise) | Comments |
|---|---|---|---|
| Codeine | 180-200 | 130 (IV) | Morphine is more commonly administered orally; Morphine IV is used less frequently. |
| Fentanyl (transdermal) | 25 mcg/h transdermal patch (equiv. to 50 mg PO morphine) | 167 mcg | Usually for stable chronic pain, especially in patients with GI dysfunction<br>Refer to CPS for additional help<br>Not used as first-line treatment for acute pain |
| Methadone | Dosing is not directly proportional; depends largely on starting dose of PO morphine | Equivalent dosing not reliably established | Long, variable half-life, which may complicate titration<br>Variable conversion rates occur |
| Hydrocodone | 30 | Not available | Often combined with other analgesics<br>Use with caution if administering additional acetaminophen or Aspirin® |
| Meperidine | 300 | 75 (IV) | Not first-line opioid/rarely used<br>May cause seizures due to metabolite accumulation |

Stanford University. Opioid Equivalent Dosing. 2016. http://web.stanford.edu/~jonc101/tools/OpioidEquivalentDosing.htm

*For all sustained release drugs: do not crush, break or chew oral controlled release medications

## Neuropathic Pain Management
- Consider using the stepwise approach proposed by the Canadian Pain Society for neuropathic pain management (**Figure 3**)
- Neuropathic pain (e.g. post-herpetic neuralgia, diabetic neuropathy) not usually relieved by typical analgesics (e.g. acetaminophen, NSAIDs)
- 4 main classes of treatment for neuropathic pain:
  - Anticonvulsants
    - Most common class of medication for treatment of neuropathic pain
    - e.g. Gabapentin 300 mg TID PO
      - Titrate up starting from 100 mg TID PO to avoid excessive drowsiness
      - Usual effective dose: 300-1200 mg TID PO
      - Decrease dose in patients with impaired renal clearance
    - Others: Pregabalin, Carbamazepine
  - Tricyclic Antidepressants (TCAs)
    - e.g. Amitriptyline
      - Starting dose: 10 mg qhs PO, then titrate up by 10 mg qwk
      - Max daily dose: 150 mg/d
    - Others: Nortriptyline, Desipramine
    - Contraindications: cardiac arrhythmias, recent MI, MAOI use, hyperthyroidism, narrow angle glaucoma
  - Opioid Analgesics
    - Can be effective, usually in conjunction with adjuvant medications
  - Topical Agents
    - e.g. Lidocaine patch, Capsaicin cream (substance P inhibitor)
- Fourth Line Agents
  - e.g. SSRIs, other anticonvulsants (e.g. lamotrigine, lacosamide, topiramate, valproate acid), methadone, topical lidocaine/ capsaicin, and tapentadol

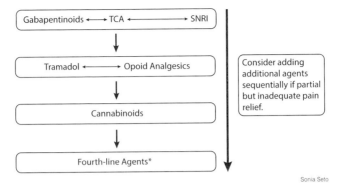

Sonia Seto

**Figure 3:** Stepwise approach from the Canadian Pain Society[15]
*Topical lidocaine (second line for postherpetic neuralgia), methadone, lamotrigine, lacosamide, tapentadol, botulinum toxin; Note: Limited randomized controlled trial evidence to support add-on combination therapy. TCA Tricyclic antidepressants; SNRI Serotonin noradrenaline reuptake inhibitors

## 4.2 Routes of Delivery
- **Oral (immediate vs. Extended release)**
- **Intramuscular**
- **Subcuticular**
- **Intravenous**
- **Systemic Analgesic Delivery**
    - Patient-Controlled Analgesia (PCA)
        - Use of computerized (usually parenteral) pumps that can deliver a predetermined dose of medication when requested by a patient, within set parameters, allowing the patient to reach his/her own minimum effective analgesic concentration
        - PCA parameters: bolus dose, lockout interval, continuous infusion (optional), maximum 4 h limit
        - Most commonly used agents for PCA are morphine and hydromorphone
        - Shown to lessen postoperative pain, decrease complications, lead to earlier discharge, and lessen the overall opiate level consumed[3]

---

**Clinical Pearl: Analgesic Therapy**
Use of multimodal anesthesia approach (various systemic medications ± regional anesthesia techniques) can improve pain management, reduce doses of individual medications, and thus reduce side effects.

---

- **Rectal**
- **Transdermal (fentanyl patch)**

## Local Nerve Block (infiltration by surgeon OR by regional anesthesia)
- Definition: blockade of nerve fibers that transmit pain and sensation from the region of interest by local anesthetics; prevents conduction of electrical impulses by the nerve
- Uses:
    - Diagnostic procedures
    - Minor surgical procedures
    - Peri-operative analgesia
    - Post-operative analgesia
    - Management of chronic pain
- Benefits:
    - Better pain control during the peri-operative period
    - Avoids adverse effects of general anesthesia: myocardial and respiratory depression

- Side effects:
  - Block failure or excessive duration of anesthetic
  - Dizziness (rare) and hypotension
- Contraindications:
  - Infection at the block site/systemic infection
  - Allergy to anesthetics/analgesics
  - Anticoagulation
  - Patient refusal
  - Pre-existing nerve injury
  - Lack of skill
  - Lack of resuscitation equipment
- Complications:
  - Local Anesthetic Systemic Toxicity (LAST)
    - Low concentrations: drowsiness, lightheadedness, visual/auditory disturbances, restlessness, circumoral and tongue numbness, metallic taste
    - High concentrations: nystagmus, muscular twitching, tonic-clonic convulsions/seizures, arrhythmia
    - Treatment: Intralipid® 20%: 1.5 mL/kg bolus, followed by 0.25 mL/kg/min
  - Injury of targeted nerve or nerve plexus
  - Inadvertent injection of agent intravascularly or around non-targeted neurological tissues
  - Damage to other tissues around injection site (e.g. pneumothorax for blocks near thorax)
  - Infection
  - Perineural hematoma could result, especially in patients with an underlying bleeding disorder, or those on anticoagulation/antiplatelet therapy

**Table 5.** Regional Anesthesia Techniques

| Regional Anesthesia Technique | Main Uses |
| --- | --- |
| **Local Anesthesia** | Small incisions, sutures, and excisions of small lesions |
| **Infiltration Anesthesia** | Small dermal surgeries/procedures |
| **Bier Block (IV regional anesthesia)** | Short procedures in the distal limbs (<60 min) |
| **Tumescent Anesthesia** | Liposuction procedures |
| **Peripheral nerve blocks:** | |
| **Brachial Plexus Block** | Shoulder and upper limb procedures |
| **Paravertebral Sympathetic Ganglion Block** | Treatment of reflex sympathetic dystrophy |
| **Lumbar Plexus Block** | Pelvic girdle, knee, and proximal tibia procedures |
| **Femoral Nerve Block** | Open knee procedures (total knee replacement) |
| **Fascia Iliaca Block** | Hip procedures (total hip replacement) |
| **Sciatic Nerve Block** | Foot and distal lower limb procedures |
| **Neuroaxial Blocks:** | |
| **Spinal (subarachnoid anesthesia)** | Procedures on anatomical structures below upper abdomen |
| **Thoracic Epidural** | Abdominal and chest wall procedures |
| **Lumbar Epidural** | Gynecological procedures, orthopedic surgery, general surgery, vascular surgery (for structures innervated by lumbar spine and below) |

# 5. COMPLEMENTARY AND ALTERNATIVE THERAPIES

## Transcutaneous Electric Nerve Stimulation (TENS)
- Definition: application of electrical current through the skin for pain control
- Effect:
  - Activation of opioid reception in CNS[4]
  - Reduces excitation of CNS nociceptive neurons
- Meta-analyses have shown effectiveness in treating chronic and acute pain[5,6]

## Physiotherapy
- Effects[4]:
  - Inhibits pain perception by stimulation of sensory afferents (gate-control theory)
  - Avoid painful movements by improvement in the quality of movement (muscle strength and coordination)
- Indicated in all pain syndromes where motor dysfunction is involved and in chronic pain (to reduce depression)
- Active therapy should start early, discourage long-term immobilization
- Apply in combination with other treatments such as analgesic drugs

## Acupuncture
- Definition: the technique of inserting and manipulating fine filiform needles into specific points on the body
- Effects: excites receptors and nerve fibers (mechanical activation of somatic afferents)[4]
- "Ashi points"
  - Near the source of pain (local points)
  - On the forearms and lower legs (distal points)
- Meta-analyses have yet to consistently show effectiveness for pain management[7]

## Massage
- Synonyms: effleurage, petrissage, friction, tapotement, vibration
- Effects[8]:
  - Stimulation of large diameter nerve fibers (gate-control theory)
  - Blood flow, temperature, and histamine release are all increased by dilatation of superficial blood vessels
  - Physical and mental relaxation
- The most consistently proven effect is decreased anxiety and perception of tension
- Contraindications: any area of acute inflammation, skin infection, nonconsolidated fracture, DVT, burns, active cancer tumors, advanced osteoporosis

## Cognitive Behavioural Therapy (CBT) / Psychotherapy
- Addresses underlying mental health components
- Stress reduction and mindfulness

# 6. GENERAL ANESTHESIA & PREOPERATIVE ANESTHESIA ASSESSMENT

## General Anesthesia
- Definition: a reversible state of amnesia, analgesia, loss of consciousness, immobility, and inhibition of sensory and autonomic reflexes
- Typical approach: induced with IV anesthetic agents and maintained with inhalational and/or IV anesthetics and/or regional anesthesia; may be used in combination with muscle relaxants and/or intubation with mechanical ventilation.
- Risks associated with general anesthesia are: dental injury, corneal injury, aspiration, nerve injury, anaphylaxis, death, postoperative nausea vomiting, postoperative delirium.
- Patient perioperative risk can be predicted using the ASA score or NSQUIP Risk Calculators ASA score (see Essentials of General Surgery).

## Preoperative Assessment / Consult
The goal of preoperative assessment by the anesthesiologist is to:
1. Optimize the patient's medical condition for the proposed surgery such that perioperative risk and morbidity are as low as possible (May not be possible for emergency surgery).

2. Inform the choice of an appropriate perioperative and anesthetic care plan that minimizes the patient's risk of complications. Routine preoperative testing is not required for patients having low-risk surgery.[11-13] Some higher risk patients with cardiac risk factors may benefit from non-invasive cardiac stress testing.[14]

History:

- Identifying data (age, sex), proposed surgery and diagnosis
- Previous anesthetics and adverse outcomes, previous post-operative N/V, history of difficult intubation, family history of anaesthetic problems (e.g. malignant hyperthermia, cholinesterase deficiency)
- Drug allergies
- Current medications (including dose and frequency)
- PMHx/Review of systems (cardiovascular – hypertension, coronary artery disease, CHF, arrhythmias, valvular disease; respiratory – asthma, bronchitis, COPD, smoking history, OSA; renal; neurology; MSK; GI; hematology; endocrinology – diabetes mellitus)

Physical Exam:

- Vitals (HR, RR, BP, temp, O2 saturation)
- Airway
    - Neck range of motion: flexion and extension (sniffing position)
    - 3-2-1 rule (3 fingers between thyroid cartilage and mandible, 2 fingers between upper and lower teeth with mouth open, 1 finger behind condylar process of mandible during anterior subluxation)
    - Dental anatomy (dentures/cap/crown, chipped/cracked/loose teeth)
    - Mallampati score (see **Figure 4**)
- Cardiovascular exam - 4 Metabolic Equivalents (METS), pacemakers, defibrillators, heart murmurs, rhythm
- Respiratory exam - airway anatomy, features of difficult airway, presence of wheezes, rhonchi
- Spine exam if considering neuraxial technique: scoliosis, tattoos over insertion sites
- Other exams pertinent to surgery or medical conditions
- Investigations:
    - Consider investigations relevant to the surgical procedure and medical history of the patient11-13 (e.g. CBC, electrolytes, coagulation profile, blood group and screen or cross-match, ECG, CXR, etc.)
    - Review medical records: i.e. anesthesia records (adverse events, ease of intubation), previous testing (echocardiogram, pulmonary function testing, etc.)
- Preparation for Anesthesia and Surgery:
    - NPO Guidelines (Canadian Anesthesiologists' Society)
        - ≥2 h clear fluids
        - ≥4 h breast milk
        - ≥6 h light meal (i.e. toast and clear fluids)
        - ≥8 h regular meal
        - Medications are often ok, with sips of water
    - Medications
        - Anticoagulants may need to be discontinued several days prior, depending on surgery and patient risk (5 days for warfarin, 1-2 days for the new oral anticoagulant drugs)
        - Ensure patient takes usual pain medication (± NSAIDs) day of surgery
        - Many essential medications should be continued the day of surgery:
        - Blood pressure medication (i.e. steroids, anti-seizure; not diuretics, ACE inhibitors or angiotensin II receptor blockers)
        - Respiratory medications (i.e. puffers)
        - Reflux/heartburn medications
        - Diabetic medications are often held the day of surgery because patient is NPO and the concern is regarding perioperative hypoglycemia
        - Glucose should be measured by patient in morning and on arrival to hospital
- Optimization
    - Does the patient require further consultations, investigations, treatments prior to surgery?
- Types of Anesthesia
    - Local anesthesia only
    - Local + light sedation (neurolept)

ANESTHESIOLOGY

- General anesthesia
- Regional anesthesia
- General anesthesia + regional anesthesia (for post-operative pain control)
  - Disposition
    - Does the patient require special care/monitoring in the post-operative phase (i.e. step-down unit, intensive care unit)?

### Mallampati Scores

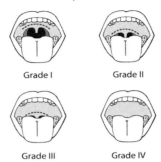

Grade I     Grade II

Grade III     Grade IV

Zaria Chowdhury

**Figure 4.** Mallampati Score

~~Opioid Overdose Management~~

**Clinical Pearl: Opioid Overdose Management**

Opioid toxidrome: respiratory depression, pinpoint pupils, altered mental states (incl. unresponsive)

Naloxone (opioid antagonist) for opioid reversal
- Half-life of 40 mins – requires ICU admission or infusion when overdose suspected (half-life shorter than most opioids; re-narcotization may recur)
- MUST be diluted x10 before use (0.04mg/mL)
- 0.04-0.08mg (IV q3-5 min)

Differential Diagnosis: seizure, stroke, other medications, hyper/hypoglycemia, hyper/hyponatremia, hypoxia, HTN, MI, sepsis

* overdose of naloxone may cause symptoms of opioid withdrawal

## REFERENCES

1. Schmidt RF, Willis WD (Editors). Encyclopedia of Pain. Berlin: Springer-Verlag; 2007.
2. Barash PG, Cullen BF, Stoelting RK, Cahalan MK, Stock MC. Clinical Anesthesia. 6th ed. New York: Lippincott Williams & Wilkins; 2009.
3. Ballantyne JC, Carr DB, Chalmers TC, Dear KB, Angelillo IF, Mosteller, F. Postoperative patient-controlled analgesia: Meta-analyses of initial randomized control trials. J Clin Anesth. 1993; 5(3):182-193.
4. Belgrade MJ, Schamber CD. Evaluation of Complementary and Alternative Therapies. In: Wilson PR, Jensen TS, Watson PJ, Haythornthwaite JA (Editors). Clinical Pain Management: Chronic Pain. 2nd ed. Oxford: Oxford University Press; 2008.
5. Johnson M, Martinson M. Efficacy of electrical nerve stimulation for chronic musculoskeletal pain: A meta-analysis of randomized controlled trials. Pain. 2007; 130(2):157-165.
6. DeSantana J, Walsh DM, Vance C, Rakel BA, Sluka KA. Effectiveness of transcutaneous electrical nerve stimulation for treatment of hyperalgesia and pain. Curr Rheumatol Rep. 2008; 10(6):492-499.
7. Hopton A, MacPherson H. Acupuncture for chronic pain: Is acupuncture more than an effective placebo? A systematic review of pooled data from meta-analyses. Pain Pract. 2010; 10(2):94- 102.
8. Paley CA, Johnson MI, Tashani QA, Bagnall AM. Acupuncture for cancer pain in adults. Cochrane Database of Syst Rev. 2010; 1; CD 007753.
9. Swartz MH. Textbook of Physical Diagnosis: History and Examination. 6th ed. Philadelphia: Saunders Elsevier; 2010.
10. Wilson PR, Jensen TS, Watson PJ, Haythornthwaite JA (Editors). Clinical Pain Management: Chronic Pain, 2nd ed. Oxford: Oxford University Press; 2008.
11. Schein, OD, Katz, J et al. The Value of Routine Preoperative Testing before Cataract Surgery. NEJM. 2000; 342:168-175
12. Choosing Wisely: Anesthesiology – Five Things Physicians and Patients Should Question http://www.choosingwiselycanada.org/recommendations/anesthesiology
13. Kirkham, KR, Wijeysundera, DN, et al. Pre-operative Testing before low-risk surgical procedures. CMAJ. 2015; 187(11):E349-E358.
14. Wijeysundera, DN, Beattie WS et al. Non-invasive cardiac stress testing before elective major non-cardiac surgery: population based cohort study. BMJ. 2010; 340:b5526
15. Moulin D, Boulanger A, Clark AJ, et al. Pharmacological management of chronic neuropathic pain: revised consensus statement from the Canadian Pain Society. Pain Res Manag. 2014; 19(6):328-35

# CHAPTER 12:

# **Dermatology**

**Editors:**
Andrea Copeland, BSc
Danny Mansour, HBSc

**Resident Reviewer:**
Emily Moon, MD, CCFP

**Faculty Reviewers:**
David N. Adam, MD, FRCPC
Jensen Yeung, MD, FRCPC

## TABLE OF CONTENTS

# 1. COMMON CHIEF COMPLAINTS

**Table 1.** Common Chief Complaints[1]

| Chief Complaint | Differential Diagnosis |
|---|---|
| **Red Scale** | Inflammatory: dermatitis, psoriasis, lichen planus |
| | Infectious: pityriasis rosea |
| | Other: mycosis fungoides, gold toxin |
| **Red Facial Rash** | Inflammatory: acne vulgaris, perioral dermatitis, rosacea, seborrheic dermatitis |
| | Infectious: impetigo |
| **Red Papule** | Inflammatory: acne vulgaris, lichen planus, rosacea, psoriasis, urticaria |
| | Infectious: folliculitis, scabies |
| | Other: arthropod bite, dermatofibroma, miliaria rubra |
| **Brown Macule** | Inflammatory: Post-inflammatory hyperpigmentation |
| | Other: congenital café-au-lait spots, congenital nevus, junctional nevus, pigmented BCC, lentigo maligna melanoma |
| **Pustule** | Inflammatory: acne vulgaris, rosacea, pustular psoriasis, dyshidrotic dermatitis |
| | Infectious: candida, dermatophyte, impetigo |
| | Other: acute generalized exanthematous pustulosis |
| **Vesicle** | Inflammatory: acute contact dermatitis, dyshidrotic dermatitis |
| | Infectious: impetigo, viral (HSV, HZV, VZV, molluscum, coxsackie), scabies |
| | Other: dermatitis herpetiformis |
| **Bulla** | Inflammatory: acute contact dermatitis, erythema multiforme, Stevens-Johnson syndrome, toxic epidermal necrolysis |
| | Infectious: bullous impetigo |
| | Other: pemphigus vulgaris, bullous pemphigoid, dermatitis herpetiformis |

DERMATOLOGY

# 2. FOCUSED HISTORY

In contrast to most areas of medicine, it can be helpful in dermatology to do a physical exam before taking a detailed history; this allows for interpretation of the lesion without predetermined ideas and for a more objective interpretation of the history.

### History of Presenting Illness: OPQRST

- **O**nset
- **P**alliating/**P**rovoking:
  - Provoking Factors: are there any things that make/have made it worse (e.g. sunlight, temperature)
  - Palliating Factors: have any treatments been tried? Has anything helped?
- **Q**uality: are there any symptoms such as pruritus (itch), pain, or numbness?
- **R**elevant exposures & **R**adiation:
  - Exposures: sun, tanning beds, swimming pools, plants, contact allergens, chemicals, contact with people with similar lesions, travel, animals/pets
  - Radiation: where is the lesion and has it been spreading?
- **S**ystems review: fever, joint pain, weight loss, malaise
- **T**iming (course): is this eruption/lesion recurrent or persistent?
  - Emphasis on change over time
- **Associated Symptoms**
  - Hair loss
    - Symmetric/asymmetric
    - Focal/diffuse
    - Rash/no nails
  - Nails
    - Recent illnesses or stressors
    - Exposure (e.g. toxins, commercial nail products, chemicals)

### Past Medical History

- History of skin disease or skin cancer (e.g. non-melanoma skin cancer, melanoma)
- Inflammatory skin disorders (e.g. psoriasis, atopic dermatitis)
- Chronic disease (e.g. DM, rheumatologic, thyroid, collagen vascular)

### Medications and Allergies

- Complete list of medications and allergies with resulting symptoms

### Family History

- Atopy, autoimmunity, skin cancer, etc.

## 3. FOCUSED PHYSICAL EXAM

The focused physical exam includes:
1. A general examination of the skin
2. Inspection of skin lesion(s); confirm location, distribution, and characteristics of the lesion
3. Palpation of lesion
4. Examination of secondary sites such as the nails, hair, and mucosal sites
Ensure appropriate lighting for this exam

> **Clinical Pearl: Lesion Interpretation**
> Some skin eruptions are so characteristic that they do not require an initial history; seeing the lesion first can allow for more objective interpretation of the complaint.

### General Skin Inspection

- General inspection: Does the patient look sick or not sick?
- Skin color: erythema (red), cyanosis (blue), pale (white), jaundice (yellow), pigmentary abnormalities
- State of skin: dry, normal, moist

## Inspection of Skin Lesions
- The ability to correctly characterize the lesion is half the challenge in dermatology; when characterizing the lesion, avoid the word "rash" and apply this mnemonic: SCALDA
  - **S**ize/Surface area
  - **C**olor
  - **A**rrangement (see **Table 3** and **Figure 2**)
  - **L**esion morphology (see **Table 2** and **Figure 1**)
  - **D**istribution
  - **A**lways check hair, nails, mucous membranes, and intertriginous areas

## Primary Skin Lesion Morphology

**Clinical Pearl: Scaling and Crusting**
Scaling and crusting may obscure diagnostic features; careful physical removal of surface crusts may be helpful (use appropriate sterile techniques such as wiping the lesion with rubbing alcohol prior to inspection).

**Table 2.** Primary Lesion Morphology

| Classification | General Size | |
| --- | --- | --- |
| | <1 cm Diameter | >1 cm Diameter |
| **Flat, Smooth** | Macule (e.g. freckle) | Patch (e.g. vitiligo) |
| **Raised, Superficial** | Papule (e.g. wart) | Plaque (e.g. psoriasis) |
| • *If edematous* | Wheal (e.g.urticaria) | |
| **Raised, Fluid-Filled** | Vesicle (e.g. HSV) | Bulla (e.g. bullous pemphigoid) |
| • *If purulent* | Pustule | |
| **Palpable Deep** (dermal) | Nodule (e.g. dermatofibroma) | Tumor (e.g. lipoma) |
| • *If Semi-Solid or Fluid-Filled* | Cyst | |

DERMATOLOGY

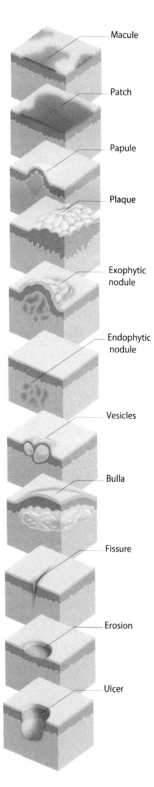

Macule

Patch

Papule

Plaque

Exophytic
nodule

Endophytic
nodule

Vesicles

Bulla

Fissure

Erosion

Ulcer

Miguel Luis Reyes

**Figure 1.** Primary Lesion Morphology[2]

DERMATOLOGY

**Table 3.** Arrangements and Patterns of Skin Lesions[3]

| Shape/Pattern | Examples |
|---|---|
| **Annular** | Granuloma annulare (non-scaling), tinea corporis (scaling) |
| **Arcuate** | SLE, urticaria |
| **Confluent** | Psoriasis plaques, scaly macules of pityriasis versicolor (yeast), serious drug or viral reaction |
| **Cribriform** | Pyoderma gangrenosum heals with this pattern |
| **Dermatomal** | Shingles (herpes zoster) |
| **Digitate** | Digitate dermatosis |
| **Discoid/Nummular** | Discoid eczema, psoriasis |
| **Exanthematous** | Viral infections, drug eruptions |
| **Grouped** | Insect bites, herpes simplex |
| **Linear** | Striae, scabetic burrows, insect bites, excoriations |
| **Livedo** | Cutis marmorata, erythema ab igne, vasculitis |
| **Oval** | Pityriasis rosea |
| **Polycyclic** | Psoriasis, tinea corporis |
| **Reticulate** | Wickham's striae in lichen planus |
| **Serpiginous** | Track left by hookworm in cutaneous larva migrans |
| **Satellite** | Local malignant spread, candida diaper dermatitis |
| **Scattered and Disseminated** | Varicella, disseminated metastases, cutaneous lymphoma, benign nevi |
| **Stellate (rare)** | Meningococcemia |
| **Target/Iris** | Erythema multiforme |

DERMATOLOGY

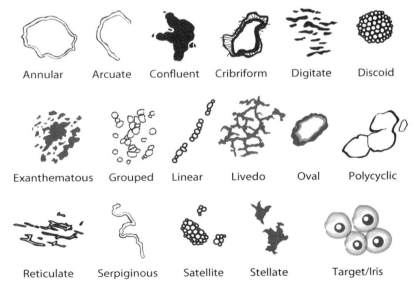

Tess Peters

**Figure 2.** Common Arrangements and Patterns of Skin Lesions[3]

## Secondary Skin Lesion Morphology
- **Scaling:** increase in keratin, dead cells on surface of skin (e.g. dermatitis, psoriasis)
- **Crust:** dried fluid (pus, blood, serum) originating from lesion (e.g. impetigo)
- **Lichenification:** thickening of skin with accentuated skin markings (e.g. chronic atopic dermatitis, lichen simplex chronicus)

## Other Morphology
- **Purpura:** bleeding into dermis
  - Petechiae <3 mm diameter
  - Ecchymoses (bruises) >3 mm diameter
- **Telangiectasia:** dilated superficial blood vessels; blanchable
- **Excoriation:** a scratch mark
- **Erosion:** disruption of skin involving epidermis alone; heals without scarring
- **Ulcer:** disruption of skin into the dermis or beyond; heals with scarring
  - Can form dark colored crust called eschar

## Palpation
- It is recommended to wear gloves when palpating a lesion; however, many clinicians do not wear gloves as it is more difficult to assess (most only wear gloves if there is a concern of infection)
- Assess for texture, consistency, fluid, adjacent edema, tenderness, blanching
- Texture:
  - Superficial (largely epidermal) or deep (more likely in dermis)
  - Soft (e.g. lipoma) or doughy (e.g. hypothyroidism) vs. hard (e.g. scleroderma, calcification), firm (e.g. lichen planus, sarcoid, amyloid) or indurated (e.g. pretibial myxedema)
  - Dry (e.g. hypothyroidism) vs. wet
  - Velvety (acanthosis nigricans, Ehlers-Danlos syndrome)
  - Leathery and "bark-like" (lichenification): epidermal hypertrophy from prolonged rubbing/scratching, pruritic cutaneous disorder (e.g. lichen simplex chronicus, neurodermatitis)

## Hair
- Texture should be examined (e.g. coarse: hypothyroidism, fine: hyperthyroidism)
- Alopecia (loss of hair) (see **Alopecia**, p.373)
- Hirsutism (abnormally exuberant hair growth) should be examined (e.g. polycystic ovarian disease, neoplasm of the adrenals and gonads)

## Nails
- Shape, size, color, and brittleness should be noted
- Hemorrhages under the nail (e.g. splinter hemorrhages in bacterial endocarditis)
- Grooves in the nail (e.g. trauma, Beau's lines)
- Increased white area under the nail bed (e.g. renal disease, liver disease)

DERMATOLOGY

**Table 4.** Typical Nail Changes Associated with Medical Conditions

| Abnormality | Characteristics | Common Associations |
|---|---|---|
| Clubbing | **Nail-Fold Angles:** nail projects from nail bed (hyponychial angle) ~160° (normal), approaches 180° in clubbing<br>**Phalangeal Depth Ratio:** distal phalangeal depth smaller than interphalangeal depth (normal), reversed in clubbing<br>**Schamroth Sign:** diamond-shaped window when dorsal surfaces of terminal phalanges of similar fingers are opposed (normal), no diamond-shaped window in clubbing<br>**Palpation:** clubbed nails perceived as "floating" within soft tissues, in advanced cases may be able to feel proximal edge of the nail, elicited by rocking the nail | **Lungs:** bronchial cancer, bronchiectasis, lung abscess, CF, idiopathic pulmonary fibrosis, asbestosis<br>**Heart:** congenital cyanotic heart disease, infective endocarditis<br>**GI:** cirrhosis (especially primary biliary cirrhosis), IBD, celiac disease<br>**Others:** hyperthyroidism, subclavian artery stenosis, familial, idiopathic |
| Splinter Hemorrhages | Longitudinal red-brown flecks on nail bed | <1 mm, in nail itself (i.e. will grow out): trauma (e.g. manual work)<br>>1 mm, in nail bed: infections (e.g. endocarditis, septicemia) |
| Leukonychia | White marks across nail bed | Fungal infections<br>TB<br>Chemotherapy<br>Cirrhosis |
| Koilonychia | Spoon-shaped nails | Iron deficiency anemia |
| Onycholysis | Separation of nail from nail bed | Fungal infection<br>Thyrotoxicosis<br>Psoriasis<br>Drugs |
| Pitting | Slight depression (<1 mm diameter) in nail bed | Psoriasis<br>Psoriatic arthritis |
| Beau's Lines | Single transverse, non-pigmented ridge | Past debilitating illness: distance from cuticle corresponds to time since recovery from illness |
| Mees' Band | White lines across pink nail bed | Arsenic poisoning |
| Lindsay's Nails | "1/2 and 1/2 nails", pink-white proximally and brown distally | Chronic liver disease<br>Azotemia |
| Terry's Nails | White nail beds with 1-2 mm of distal border of the nail | Cirrhosis<br>Hypoalbuminemia |

CF = cystic fibrosis

DERMATOLOGY

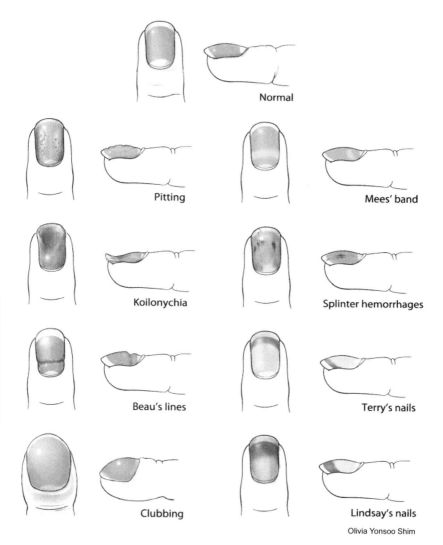

Normal

Pitting

Mees' band

Koilonychia

Splinter hemorrhages

Beau's lines

Terry's nails

Clubbing

Lindsay's nails

Olivia Yonsoo Shim

**Figure 3.** Common Nail Changes Associated with Systemic Disease

**Table 5.** Hand Abnormalities and Possible Causes

| Signs and Symptoms | Possible Causes |
|---|---|
| **Asterixis (Flapping Tremor)** | Metabolic Encephalopathy |
| **Blue** | Peripheral Cyanosis |
| **Bouchard's (PIP) and Heberden's (DIP) Nodes** | Arthritis |
| **Enlarged** | Acromegaly |
| **Pallor of Palmar Creases** | Anemia |
| **Pigmented** | Jaundice |
| **Tremor or Muscle Wasting** | Neurological Disease |

# 4. COMMON CLINICAL SCENARIOS

- The type, prevalence, and incidence of many skin diseases varies with age, gender, race, geographic location, culture, and socioeconomic status
- Appropriate management includes psychosocial interventions as skin diseases can have a major impact on the quality of life of the patient

**Table 6.** Common Clinical Scenarios

| | Morphology | Risk Factors | Investigations | Management |
|---|---|---|---|---|
| **Acne** | • Discrete papules, pustules, nodules, open and closed comedones <br> • Common sites include the face, chest, and back | • Systemic medications – steroids, lithium, androgens, etc. <br> • Mechanical pressure and emotional stress <br> • Topical agents – steroids, tars, ointments, oily cosmetics | • Clinical diagnosis <br> • May perform the following to R/O other conditions: testosterone, DHEAS, Sex-hormone binding globulin, prolactin, FSH/LH | • First line – behavioural changes, topical agents (benzoyl peroxide, antibiotics, retinoids, etc.) <br> • Second line – anti-inflammatory oral antibiotics <br> • Third line – systemic isotretinoin |
| **Eczema** | • Papular lesions with erythema, scale, severe pruritus <br> • Chronic lesions may be dull, red, and lichenified <br> • Distribution varies with age but may involve cheeks, ears, extensor surface of feet and elbows and flexural involvement | • Personal or family history of atopy | • Clinical diagnosis <br> • May consider: skin biopsy, immunoglobulin serum levels (elevated IgE level), patch testing and skin prick tests | • Avoid triggers <br> • Moisturizers <br> • Topical corticosteroids and calcineurin inhibitors |
| **Psoriasis** | • Plaque: well-demarcated erythematous papules/plaques with silvery-white scales <br> • Guttate: discrete salmon-pink small papules: "drop-like" lesions <br> • Erythrodermic: generalized erythema <br> • Inverse: erythematous plaques on flexural surfaces which may be macerated <br> • Pustular: erythematous macules and papules which can evolve into painful pustules | • Polygenic inheritance <br> • Infection – streptococcal pharyngitis <br> • Triggers include physical trauma, stress, smoking, heavy alcohol consumption also rebound exacerbation from stopping systemic corticosteroids, lithium, antimalarials, B-blockers, and interferon <br> • Associated with psoriatic arthritis, DM, obesity, depression | • Biopsy if atypical presentation (rare) | • Depends on severity of disease as well as classification but may include: avoiding triggers, topical steroids, topical vitamin D3 analogues, or a combination of the two (eg. Dovobet - combination betamethasone and calcipotriol), phototherapy, methotrexate, cyclosporine, acitretin, biologics |

| | Morphology | Risk Factors | Investigations | Management |
|---|---|---|---|---|
| **Cellulitis** | • Unilateral, poorly demarcated, erythematous patch<br>• Pits on pressure<br>• Tender<br>• Sites: commonly on legs | • Intravenous drug use<br>• Obesity<br>• Immunodeficiency<br>• Diabetes | • Blood culture, skin biopsy, or aspirate of advancing edge for C&S should be obtained | • IV penicillin or first generation cephalosporins |
| **Skin Malignancies** | • Several variants, see **Common Skin Malignancies** p.376 | • Personal or FHx of skin cancer<br>• Immunosuppression<br>• Sun exposure, tanning bed use<br>• Nevi<br>  • 1+ giant congenital nevi (>20 cm)<br>  • >5 atypical nevi<br>  • >50 normal nevi<br>• Skin phenotype: Fitzpatrick Skin Type I or II | • If shallow, may do shave biopsy; otherwise an excisional or punch biopsy may be more appropriate | • Depends on malignancy but may involve: topical imiquimod, surgical excision, Mohs surgery |

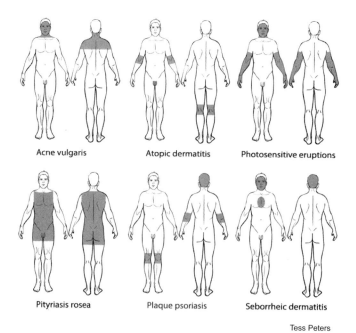

Acne vulgaris     Atopic dermatitis     Photosensitive eruptions

Pityriasis rosea     Plaque psoriasis     Seborrheic dermatitis

Tess Peters

**Figure 4.** Distribution Patterns of Skin Lesions

## 4.1 Acne

- A common disease of the pilosebaceous unit
- Epidemiology[2]: age of onset 10-17 yr in females, 14-19 yr in males; however, can continue into 40s and beyond

### Types of Lesions

- Inflammatory: discrete papules, pustules, nodules
- Non-inflammatory (comedones):
    - Open comedones (blackheads)
    - Closed comedones (whiteheads)

Closed comedone (whitehead)  vs.  Open comedone (blackhead)

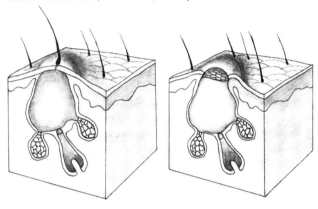

Jan Cyril Fundano

**Figure 5.** Closed vs. Open Comedones

### Pathogenesis

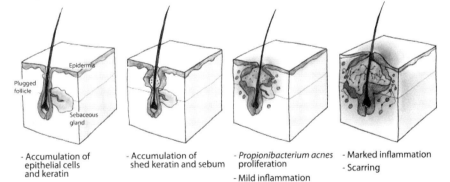

- Accumulation of epithelial cells and keratin
- Accumulation of shed keratin and sebum
- *Propionibacterium acnes* proliferation
- Mild inflammation
- Marked inflammation
- Scarring

Jan Cyril Fundano

**Figure 6.** Pathogenesis of Acne Vulgaris[4]

**Clinical Pearl: Acne**
Emotional stress and mechanical pressure can exacerbate acne; contrary to popular belief, chocolate and fatty foods do not.

**Clinical Pearl: Acne Treatment**
The use of benzoyl peroxide and a topical antibiotic in combination is recommended in order to make bacterial resistance to the antibiotic alone negligible.

## Treatment

### First Line
- Behavioral changes
  - Cleanse face daily, but not aggressively
  - Use non-comedogenic sunblocks and facial products
- Topical agents
  - Benzoyl peroxide: 2.5-10%
  - Antibiotic: clindamycin, erythromycin
  - Topical retinoids (Vitamin A acid derivatives; unplugs sebaceous gland)

### Second Line
- Anti-inflammatory oral antibiotics: tetracycline, doxycycline, minocycline, erythromycin

### Third Line
- Systemic isotretinoin (Accutane®)
  - Teratogenic; female patients must use two forms of contraception
  - Monitor monthly: CBC, triglycerides, liver function tests
  - Especially important to monitor β-hCG monthly

## Variants of Acne
- **Hormonal Acne**
  - Women in high-androgen state
  - Acne along jaw line
  - Associated with: hirsutism, polycystic ovarian syndrome, irregular periods, metabolic syndrome, infertility
- **Neonatal Acne**
  - 20% of newborns
  - Appears at 2 wk, clear by 3 mo
- **Infantile Acne**
  - Appears at 3 mo, clear by 6 mo
- **Acne Conglobata**
  - Acne with systemic symptoms: fever, myalgias, arthralgias
  - Severe, explosive, inflammatory, and nodular acne

> **Clinical Pearl: Psychosocial Effects of Acne[5]**
> The social, psychological, and emotional impairment that can result from acne has been reported to be similar to that associated with epilepsy, asthma, diabetes, and arthritis.

## 4.2 Rosacea[7]
- A chronic condition characterized by facial erythema, typically beginning across the cheeks, nose, and forehead. It can also affect the ears, scalp, or neck. In most cases it is a medically harmless condition, although it may greatly affect quality of life

> **Clinical Pearl: Acne vs. Rosacea[6]**
> Compared to acne, rosacea usually occurs in older patients and lacks comedones, nodules, cysts, or scarring. Patients may have both rosacea and acne. The presence of facial flushing, which is provoked by heat, alcohol, or spicy food helps distinguish rosacea from acne.

- Epidemiology: found in all skin types, but most common in those with fair skin; female > male, usual age of onset is 30-50 yr, with peak incidence between 40-50 yr
- Exacerbating Factors: hot food/drink, spices, alcohol (especially red wine), sun exposure
- Lesion:
  - Vascular component: erythema, flushing, blushing, and telangiectasia (visible dilatation of dermal venules)
  - Eruptive component: papules and pustules
- Distribution: eruptions on the forehead, cheeks, nose, chin

DERMATOLOGY

- Associated Symptoms: mild conjunctivitis with soreness, grittiness, and lacrimation; chronic, deep inflammation of the nose leading to irreversible hypertrophy in men (known as rhinophyma)
- Clinical Diagnosis: bacterial culture to rule out folliculitis, KOH test to rule out tinea, biopsy to rule out SLE if not responsive to standard therapy

**Clinical Pearl: Rosacea and Ocular Changes[6]**
Ocular changes are present in more than 50% of patients.

## 4.3 Dermatitis/Eczema
- Noninfectious inflammation of the skin accompanied by edema and blistering

## Contact Dermatitis
- Generic term for acute or chronic inflammatory reaction to substances which contact the skin (endogenous and exogenous agents)
- Irritant Contact Dermatitis: caused by exposure to chemical irritant; given enough exposure, all individuals react to irritants
- Allergic Contact Dermatitis: caused by antigen with type IV (cell mediated/delayed-type) hypersensitivity reaction (e.g. reaction to poison ivy)
- Common Allergens: nickel, chromate, cobalt, rubber additives in gloves and shoes, preservatives in water-based cosmetics, fragrances, dyes
- Lesion:
  - Vesicles, edema, erythema, extreme pruritus, papules, scale
  - Bullae may be present
- Distribution (for both irritant and allergic contact dermatitis):
  - Appearance at a specific site suggests contact with certain objects
  - Hands, forearms, and face
  - Usually first confined to the area of exposure
  - Distributed in linear streaks if caused by plants
    - May be patchy and asymmetric if caused by topical products
    - In chronic exposure, may spread beyond the area of contact

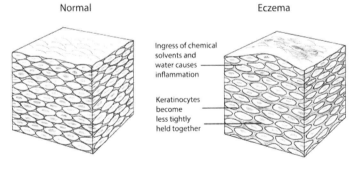

Normal

Eczema

Ingress of chemical solvents and water causes inflammation

Keratinocytes become less tightly held together

Jan Cyril

**Figure 7.** Skin Changes in Eczematous Skin

## Atopic Dermatitis/Eczema
- A skin disorder defined by the presence of four of the following major diagnostic criteria:
  - Pruritus
  - Young age of onset
  - Typical morphology and distribution (see below)
  - Chronic and relapsing course
  - Personal or family history of atopy: asthma, allergic rhinoconjunctivitis
- Aggravated by contact irritants, allergens, perspiration, excessive heat, and stress

- Lesion:
  - Papular lesions with erythema, scale, and severe pruritus
  - Acute lesions may be oozing and vesicular
  - Subacute lesions: scaly and crusted
  - Chronic lesions: dull red and lichenified
- Distribution (varies with age):
  - **Infantile** (2 mo-2 yr): often exudative lesions: cheeks, perioral area, scalp, around ears, and extensor surfaces of feet and elbows; spares the diaper area if present on the body
  - **Childhood** (2-12 yr): flexural involvement: antecubital and popliteal fossae, neck, wrists, and ankles
  - **Adult:** flexural involvement, hands, and face

## 4.4 Psoriasis
- Chronic, noninfectious, inflammatory condition with increased epidermal cell proliferation (epidermal turnover reduced to 4 days)
- Recurrent exacerbations and remissions; may be associated with arthritis
- Epidemiology[4]: equal sex incidence; onset at any age but has bimodal peaks in 20s/30s and 50s/60s
- Etiology: recognized familial genetic component (FHx is important)

### Plaque Psoriasis (most common)
- Lesion:
  - Well-demarcated, erythematous (red or salmon-pink) plaques topped with silvery scales; redness is constant
  - May bleed when scales detached (Auspitz's sign)
  - Symmetrical distribution
  - Classical presentation involves elbows, knees, sacrum, and scalp
- Margins:
  - Extensor > flexor surfaces
  - Scalp: scaling is very dense and may be very thick
  - Nails (matrix or nail bed involvement): pitting, onycholysis (separation of nail from nail bed), discoloration (oily or salmon-pink)
  - Nail changes support diagnosis if skin changes are questionable or absent

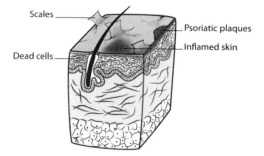

Bonnie Tang

**Figure 8.** Skin Changes in Psoriasis

### Eruptive/Guttate Psoriasis (Youths and Adolescents)
- Acute symmetrical appearance of small, bright red, well-demarcated "drop-like" lesions on trunk and limbs
- Streptococcal pharyngitis may stimulate first episode: confirm presence of streptococci; may be widespread
- May develop rapidly; may disappear spontaneously in 2-3 mo
- DDx: secondary syphilis (malaise, lymphadenopathy, or may see lesions on palms and soles), pityriasis rosea (light pink, scaling only around the edge of plaques)

DERMATOLOGY

## Flexural Psoriasis (Elderly)
- Located in the axillae, submammary flexures, or other intertriginous areas
- Scales may only be present on the edge

## Pustular Psoriasis
- In contrast to regular psoriasis, pustules, not papules are predominant in two subtypes:
  - Localized pustular psoriasis (pustulosis palmaris et plantaris)
    - Palmoplantar pustules: chronic, relapsing eruption on palms and soles
    - Pustules can be white, yellow, orange, or brown; do not rupture – turn brown and scaly as they reach the surface
  - Generalized pustular psoriasis (Von Zumbusch)
    - Life threatening, rare, and serious: requires immediate hospitalization
    - Small, sterile, yellow pustules on bright red, burning erythematous background
    - Rapid spread
    - Accompanied by acute fever, malaise, leukocytosis, "toxic" appearance

> **Clinical Pearl: Psoriasis**
> In psoriasis, pustules on the palms and soles vary in color; this can help distinguish localized psoriasis from both tinea and eczema (which have uniform color).

## 4.5 Fungal Infections
### Cutaneous Fungal "Ringworm" Infections
- Due to dermatophytes (Trichophyton, Microsporum, Epidermophyton)

**Table 7.** Forms of Cutaneous Fungal Infections[4]

| Infection | Lesion Description | Lesion Location |
|---|---|---|
| **Tinea Capitis** | Annular patches of alopecia with surface scaling | Invasion of stratum corneum and hair shaft |
| **Tinea Corporis** | Annular lesions in a classic ringworm pattern; begin as flat scaly spots; develop a raised advancing border extending in all directions with central clearing; lesions can coalesce | Trunk and limbs, face (Tinea faciei), beard (Tinea barbae) |
| **Tinea Cruris** (Jock Itch) | Often bilateral beginning in the crural fold; half-moon red plaque with a well-defined scaling border advancing onto thigh | Groin: moist environment with excessive sweating/itching |
| **Tinea Pedis** (Athlete's Foot) | Classic ringworm pattern: scaly advancing border, may present with an acute vesicular eruption | Plantar surface/dorsum of foot, soles of feet, interdigital: toe webs between 4th and 5th digits |

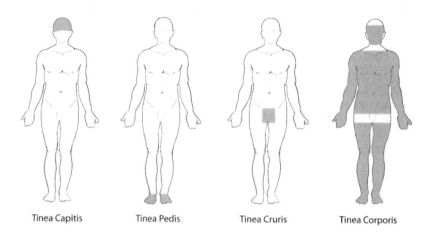

Tinea Capitis     Tinea Pedis     Tinea Cruris     Tinea Corporis

Bonnie Tang

**Figure 9.** Distribution of Tinea Infections

## Tinea Versicolor
- Common infection caused by the yeast Malassezia spp. (commensal flora)
- Epidemiology: adolescents and young adults, often first noticed after sun exposure
- Characteristics: usually asymptomatic, occasionally pruritic
- Risk Factors: adrenalectomy, Cushing's disease, pregnancy, malnutrition, burns, corticosteroid therapy, immunosuppression, oral contraceptives
- Lesion:
  - Multiple, small, circular macules with superficial, subtle scale
  - Hypopigmented or hyperpigmented, minimally scaly papules
- Distribution: upper trunk, upper arms, neck, abdomen
- Clinical Diagnosis: scale scrapings for culture; Wood's light: irregular, pale, yellow-to-white fluorescence which in some cases fades with improvement

## 4.6 Bacterial and Viral Infections
See **The Infectious Disease** Chapter

## 4.7 Cysts
- Cysts can contain air, fluid, or semi-solid material; if pus is present it is then considered an abscess
- Most cysts in body are benign; however, a few have potential to become malignant (e.g. dermoid cysts)

> **Clinical Pearl: Scraping vs. Biopsy**
> If it scales, scrape it. Biopsy *thick* skin.

**Table 8.** Differentiating Cysts[4]

| Type | Description | Signs and Symptoms |
|---|---|---|
| **Epidermal/ Epidermoid/ Sebaceous** | Cyst from follicular origin; keratin-containing cyst lined by squamous epithelium; most common cutaneous cyst; youth to middle age | Present on parts of body with little hair; round, flesh-colored and slow growing, firm and mobile nodule; punctum often visible |
| **Pilar** | Keratin-containing cysts that form in hair follicles; second most common | Present most often on scalp; smooth, hard and mobile, can be tender; do not have central punctum |

DERMATOLOGY

| Type | Description | Signs and Symptoms |
|------|-------------|--------------------|
| **Dermoid** | Cystic lesion often filled with skin and/ or skin appendages and other mature tissue | Most common location is at the lateral third of eyebrow or midline under nose (along embryonal cleft closure lines); grow slowly and non-tender |
| **Ganglion/ Synovial** | Cyst filled with clear, gelatinous fluid that originated from joint or tendon sheath; female > male; usually found in older patients | Around joints and tendons; solitary, rubbery, and translucent |

## 4.8 Scars

- Scars are a natural part of the healing process (**Figure 10** illustrates a simple scar that is flat and pale)
- Two additional types of scars can result from the overproduction of collagen (see **Table 9**)
- Can be caused by surgery, trauma, or body piercing
- Most common locations: back, shoulders, sternum

**Table 9.** Hypertrophic vs. Keloid Scars[4]

| Scar Type | Description | Distinguishing Features |
|-----------|-------------|-------------------------|
| **Hypertrophic** | Erythematous, pruritic, raised lesion | Does not grow beyond boundaries of original wound |
| **Keloid** | Dense, thick nodules, can be single or multiple, familial tendency, common in black and Asian populations | Grows beyond boundaries of original wound |

DERMATOLOGY

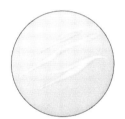 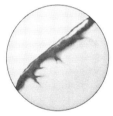 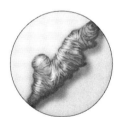

Flat, Pale Scar     Hypertrophic Scar     Keloid Scar

Miguel Luis Paler Reyes

**Figure 10.** Type of Scar[4]

## 4.9 Alopecia

- Definition: hair loss
- Investigations: CBC, thyroid function tests, ferritin, consider SLE, VDRL
- Hair Pull Test: Pull gently on a group of hairs (40-60) from proximal to distal end. Normally less than 3 hairs come out with each pull. If more than 10% come out, the pull test is positive

**Clinical Pearl: Telogen Hair Loss[8]**
The scalp loses approximately 100 telogen hairs per day.

## Nonscarring Alopecias

- Usually no scalp symptoms
- Follicular openings can all be seen

## Androgenic Alopecia
- Epidemiology: males may begin any time after puberty, females later (40% of cases occur in 60s)[4]
- Pull test: negative
- With dermatoscope: progressive miniaturization (thinning) of hair shafts
- Males: androgens have essential role
  - Hair loss starts in temples and/or vertex
- Women: androgens do not have same defined role
  - Slow thinning over frontal and mid-scalp (front hair line usually not lost)
- Treatment:
  - Males:
    - Minoxidil 2-5%
    - Oral finasteride
    - Hair transplantation
  - Females:
    - Minoxidil 2-5%
    - Androgen-blocking medication (spironolactone, oral contraceptive)
    - Hair transplantation

## Alopecia Areata
- Epidemiology: young onset (<25 yr), equal in both sexes
- Relatively common; about 1% of population has at least one episode by age 50 yr
- Circular areas of scalp hair loss for >5 mo
- Pull test: positive early on
- Etiology: autoimmune attack at level of hair
  - Can be associated with other autoimmune diseases (thyroid disease, vitiligo)
- Treatment: none (can resolve on its own), topical steroids, intralesional steroid injections

## Telogen Effluvium
- Diffuse loss all over scalp for many months
- Pull test: positive
- Etiology:
  - Hair follicles shifted into telogen/shedding stage
  - Three months after some trigger (e.g. surgery, pregnancy, endocrine, nutritional deficiency, drugs)
- Treatment: treat underlying cause, reassure patient that hair will grow back

# Scarring Alopecias
- Usually has scalp symptoms (itching, burning, pain)
- Follicular openings cannot be seen

## Central Centrifugal Cicatricial Alopecia
- Almost always occurring in African-American patients
- No scalp symptoms
- Central hair loss, starting at vertex and moving outward
- Possible contributing factors are styling techniques such as tight braids, extensions, and relaxing chemicals
- Treatment: steroids (topical and injections), immunomodulators

## Lichen Planopilaris
- Diffuse hair loss, especially centrally
- Loss of follicular openings with perifollicular redness and scale
- Associated with lichen planus in other areas
- Etiology thought to be autoimmune
- Treatment: steroids (topical and injections), immunomodulators

## Folliculitis Decalvans
- Discharge of blood and pus
- Pustules, crusting, and tufting (multiple hairs from a single follicle)
- Scalp swabs often grow *S. aureus*
- Treatment: antibiotics

## 4.10 Common Pediatric Dermatologic Skin Conditions

- See **The Pediatric Exam** Chapter

## 4.11 Nevi

- Epidemiology: nevi (which are often referred to as moles) are very common (most people have 10-40 nevi)
- Lesion:
  - ◆ Color: pink, tan, brown, or flesh-colored; may darken with sun exposure
  - ◆ Shape: flat or raised
  - ◆ Can change over time
- Distribution: over entire body
- Classification (see **Figure 11**):
  - ◆ **Junctional Nevi:** usually flat with dark brown color; appear in childhood and adolescence; nevus cells are found at the dermal-epidermal junction
  - ◆ **Compound Nevi:** slightly raised with less intense color than junctional nevi; the nevus cells are migrating into the dermis
  - ◆ **Intradermal Nevi:** dome-shaped papules with even less pigmentation; nevus cells are completely within the dermis
  - ◆ **Melanocytic Nevi:** usually appear in adolescence and have dysplastic features

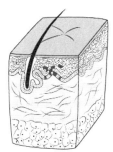

A. Junctional

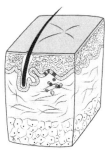

B. Compound

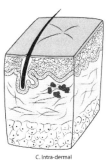

C. Intra-dermal

Bonnie Tang

**Figure 11.** Types of Nevi

DERMATOLOGY

## 4.12 Common Skin Malignancies

### Basal Cell Carcinoma (BCC)
- Most common primary skin malignancy (>75% of skin malignancies)[2]
- Increased prevalence in patients >40 yr, male > female
- Clinical variants: sclerosing, noduloulcerative, superficial, and pigmented
- Characterized by local destruction and slow growth
- Risk Factors: chronic sun exposure, ionizing radiation
- Rarely metastatic but local tissue destruction can be debilitating
- Distribution: face (80%), scalp, ears, neck; less often on sun-exposed areas of the trunk and extremities; rarely on the dorsum of the hand

### Squamous Cell Carcinoma (SCC)
- Second most common primary skin malignancy
- Primarily in elderly, male > female
- Clinical variants: keratoacanthoma (low-grade SCC), SCC *in situ* (Bowen's disease)
- Risk Factors: chronic sun exposure, immunosuppression, HPV
- More rapid enlargement and more likely to metastasize than BCC
- Clinically looks like crusted nodule with erythematous base

> **Clinical Pearl: Squamous Cell Carcinoma**
> In the case of immunosuppressed patients (transplant patients, patients on immunosuppressive medications, etc.), the incidence of squamous cell carcinoma becomes greater than basal cell carcinoma.

### Malignant Melanoma (MM)
- Most serious cutaneous malignancy
- Potentially curable, thus early diagnosis is important
- All pigmented lesions should be examined periodically: 30% of melanomas develop from a pre-existing nevus, 70% develop de novo[8]
- Early signs (see **Table 10** and **Figure 12**)
- Early symptom: nonspecific pruritus
- Later symptoms: tenderness, bleeding, ulceration
- Associated Symptom: regional lymphadenopathy; sentinel node biopsy is an important factor in determining prognosis

**Table 10.** Two Scales for Assessing Signs of Melanoma and When to Refer[9,10]

| Checklist | ABCD(E) | 7-Point |
|---|---|---|
| Criteria | Asymmetry: Overall shape is asymmetrical<br>Border: Uneven edges<br>Color: Heterogenous color, two or more shades<br>Diameter: >6 mm<br>Evolution: Changes or grows over time | Major (2 points each):<br>• Irregular color<br>• Irregular shape<br>• Change in size<br><br>Minor (1 point each):<br>• Diameter >7 mm<br>• Inflammation<br>• Crusting/bleeding<br>• Sensory changes |
| Refer | When one or more of the above is present | Point score of 3 or more |
| Sensitivity | 92-100% | 79-100% |
| Specificity | 98% | 30-37% |

### Superficial Spreading Melanoma (>50%)
- Most common form of melanoma
- Affects mainly caucasians
- Distribution on trunk and extremities; spreads laterally
- Lesions >6 mm, flat, asymmetric with varying coloration: ulcerate and bleed with growth

DERMATOLOGY

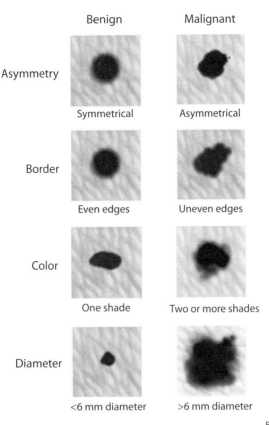

|  | Benign | Malignant |
|---|---|---|
| Asymmetry | Symmetrical | Asymmetrical |
| Border | Even edges | Uneven edges |
| Color | One shade | Two or more shades |
| Diameter | <6 mm diameter | >6 mm diameter |

Bonnie Tang

**Figure 12.** Visual Depiction of ABCD Checklist[10]

## Nodular Melanoma (30%)
- Extremities; extends vertically: rapidly fatal
- Lesions are elevated, appear rapidly, and develop papules
- May be accompanied by local hemorrhage

## Lentigo Maligna Melanomas (15%)
- Affects older Caucasian patients with a history of chronic sun exposure
- Distribution: face, neck, dorsal arms
- Lesions: flat and irregular in shape, brown in color but mottled; nodules and ulceration may indicate local invasion

## Acral Lentiginous Melanoma (5%)
- Occurs mainly on the extremities
- Most common type of melanoma in darker skinned individuals

**Clinical Pearl: Melanoma[8]**
Not all black-blue pigmentation is due to melanoma (e.g. benign blue nevus).

## Premalignant Skin Tumors
- May transform into malignancies and should be carefully monitored

DERMATOLOGY

**Table 11.** Precursors to Malignant Tumors

| Malignant Tumor | Precursors |
|---|---|
| Basal Cell Carcinoma | Actinic keratosis, rarely nevus sebaceous |
| Squamous Cell Carcinoma | Actinic keratosis, oral leukoplakia |
| Melanoma | Multiple "dysplastic" nevi or giant/congenital hairy nevi (>20 cm in diameter) <br> Lentigo maligna |

## Skin Cancer Risk Factors
1. Personal or FHx of skin cancer
2. Immunosuppression
3. Sun exposure, tanning bed use
4. Nevi[7]
   - 1+ giant congenital nevi (>20 cm)
   - >5 atypical nevi
   - >50 normal nevi
5. Skin phenotype: Fitzpatrick Skin Type I or II

**Table 12.** Fitzpatrick Skin Phenotypes[11]

| Skin Type | Skin Color | Characteristics |
|---|---|---|
| I | White, very fair; red/blond hair; blue eyes | Always burns, never tans |
| II | White, fair; red/blond hair; blue/hazel/green eyes | Usually burns, tans with difficulty |
| III | Cream white; fair with any eye or hair color | Sometimes mild burn, gradually tans |
| IV | Brown | Rarely burns, tans with ease |
| V | Dark brown | Very rarely burns, tans very easily |
| VI | Black | Never burns, tans very easily |

## 4.13 Sun Safety
### UVA vs. UVB
- Mnemonic: UVA = aging, UVB = burning
- UVA
   - Penetrates deep into the dermis
   - Rays go through windows
   - Leads to premature skin aging (lentigines, wrinkles, leathery skin)
   - Lentigines are commonly known as sunspots, age spots, or liver spots
   - Suppresses immune system
   - Indirectly leads to skin cancer
- UVB
   - Burns the superficial layers of the epidermis, leading to traditional erythematous sunburn
   - Intensity of rays vary by season, location, and time of day
   - Directly leads to skin cancer

### Sunscreen
- Broad-spectrum sunscreen (both UVA and UVB protection) of SPF (Sun Protection Factor) 30 or higher[11]
- SPF measures protection from UVB only (not UVA)
- Moisturizers and cosmetics with SPF protect from UVB only
- Sunscreen application:
   - Best applied liberally (1 teaspoon for face, 1 shot glass full for body)
   - Best reapplied every 2 h

**Clinical Pearl: Skin Cancer and Tanning Beds**[13]
Skin cancer risk increases over 75% when tanning bed use occurs before age 30.

## 4.14 Dermatologic Emergencies

**Table 13.** Dermatologic Emergencies and Key Features

| Condition | Morphology | Key Signs and Symptoms | Management |
|---|---|---|---|
| Angioedema | Well-circumscribed areas of edema[9-11] | Acute swelling usually of the face, extremities, or genitalia | Airway patency; cool, moist compresses; antihistamines |
| Exfoliative Erythroderma | Erythematous skin eruption involving more than 90% of the cutaneous surface[9-11] | Fluid and protein loss through the skin can lead to life-threatening hypotension, electrolyte imbalance, CHF, and enteropathy | Supportive therapy, skin care involves emollients and compresses as well as topical corticosteroid therapy and antihistamines for pruritus |
| Meningococcemia | Abrupt onset of morbiliform (maculopapular) or petechial rash on the extremities and trunk (50-60% of cases) | "Flu-like" symptoms (fever, chills, malaise, and disorientation)[9-11]<br><br>Altered mental state, neck stiffness, URTI | Obtain blood cultures; supportive management and therapy with third generation cephalosporin or intravenous penicillin G therapy (chloramphenicol if patient allergic to penicillin) |
| Necrotizing Fasciitis | Poorly demarcated and rapidly spreading erythema, purplish discolouration<br><br>Late findings: dusky blue/black, bullae, eschars | Non-pitting edema; pain out of proportion to findings; diabetic or immunocompromised patient<br><br>Subcutaneous emphysema (crepitus), systemic symptoms | Aggressive management of sepsis and surgical debridement of necrotic tissue |
| Rocky Mountain Spotted Fever | Petechial lesions that start on ankles and wrists, and then spread centrally to trunk and face | 60% of patients present with fever, headache, and rash following tick bite<br><br>Abdominal pain (mainly children), fever, headache (almost all adults) | Symptomatic support and antibiotic treatment (doxycycline); tick should be removed if embedded in the skin |

DERMATOLOGY

| Condition | Morphology | Key Signs and Symptoms | Management |
|---|---|---|---|
| **Stevens-Johnson Syndrome** (<10% Body Surface Area) and **Toxic Epidermal Necrolysis** (>30% Body Surface Area) | Erythema, epidermal necrosis, and desquamation[12-14] | Fever, malaise, headache, cough, and conjunctivitis 3d before rash | Identification and withdrawal of culprit drug, transfer of patient to appropriate unit (burn unit, intensive care unit), supportive care, medical management (systemic corticosteroids, cyclosporine, TNF inhibitors), mucous membrane management[15] |
| | Atypical targets with central dusky purpura | Positive Nikolsky sign (exfoliation of skin when rubbed) | |
| | Bullae and blister formation | Erythroderma and hypotension | |
| **Toxic Shock Syndrome** | Rapid onset of generalized erythema with desquamation[12-14] | Prodrome: 2-3 d of malaise and patient presents usually with fever, chills, nausea, and abdominal pain | Supportive management and obtain culture specimens; treat with B-lactamase-resistant anti-staphlococcal antibiotic |
| | | Strawberry tongue (inflamed red papillae) | |

**Clinical Pearl: Necrotizing Fasciitis**
Draw a line around erythematous area on admission to determine if rash is spreading.

**Clinical Pearl: Disseminated Varicella**
Disseminated varicella presents as widespread, discrete vesicles or papulovesicles. Early treatment with IV acyclovir is life-saving.

## Conditions that Mimic Dermatologic Emergencies

*Red Skin*
- More itchy than painful: allergic contact dermatitis
- Itchy, lower extremities: stasis dermatitis
- Sun-exposed area: sunburn
- Emergencies: necrotizing fasciitis; Stevens-Johnson syndrome and toxic epidermal necrolysis; toxic shock syndrome[12-14]

*Desquamation*
- Localized with no systemic manifestations: bullous impetigo
- Emergencies: Stevens-Johnson syndrome and toxic epidermal necrolysis; toxic shock syndrome[12-14]

*Petechiae and Purpura*
- Trauma
- Healthy appearance: pigmented purpuric dermatosis; viral exanthema
- Emergencies: meningococcemia; Rocky Mountain spotted fever[9-11]

DERMATOLOGY

*Generalized Pruritus*
- In the absence of rash and dry skin may be due to a systemic cause[12]:
  - **Hematologic Disorders:** iron deficiency anemia, myeloproliferative disorders, monoclonal gammopathy, and multiple myeloma and lymphoma
  - **Renal Disorders:** uremia
  - **Liver Disorders:** cholestasis
  - **Endocrine Disorders:** hyperthyroidism or hypothyroidism

**Clinical Pearl: Scabies and Pruritus[8]**
Always suspect scabies in any patient with severe pruritus.

*Erythema Nodosum*
- Symmetric, tender, hot, erythematous nodules over the extensor legs
- Commonly affects young women
- Potential causes: think NODOSUMM[12-14]
  - **N**O cause in 50%
  - **D**rugs (bromides, iodides, sulfur drugs)
  - **O**CP (most common drug)
  - **S**arcoidosis
  - **U**lcerative Colitis and Crohn's Disease
  - Many **I**nfections (e.g. TB)
  - **M**alignancies (leukemia)
  - Other: pregnancy, Beçhet's disease

**Clinical Pearl: Sarcoidosis and Erythema Nodosum[8]**
Consider and exclude sarcoidosis in all cases.

*Systemic Diseases*

**Table 14.** Dermatological Manifestations of Systemic Diseases[4]

| Systemic Disease | Skin Manifestations |
| --- | --- |
| **Addison's Disease** | Generalized hyperpigmentation |
| **Paget's Disease (Breast)** | Persistent unilateral dermatitic-looking lesion on the breast |
| **Cushing's Syndrome** | Moon facies, purple striae, acne, hyperpigmentation, hirsutism, atrophic skin with telangiectasias |
| **Hepatitis C Infection** | Cutaneous vasculitis, polyarteritis nodosa, porphyria cutanea tarda, lichen planus, necrolytic acral erythema |
| **HIV** | Kaposi's sarcoma, seborrheic dermatitis, psoriasis |
| **Hyperthyroidism** | Moist warm skin, seborrheic dermatitis, acne, hirsutism, nail atrophy, onycholysis |
| **Hypothyroidism** | Cool dry scaly thickened skin, toxic alopecia, coarse hair, brittle nails |
| **Liver Disease** | Spider nevi, palmar erythema, alopecia |
| **Rheumatic Fever** | Nodules over bony prominences, erythema marginatum |
| **SLE** | Malar erythema, discoid rash, patchy/diffuse alopecia, photosensitivity |
| **Thyroid Carcinoma** | Sipple's syndrome: multiple mucosal neuromas |
| **Inflammatory Bowel Disease** | Pyoderma gangrenosum, erythema nodosum |

DERMATOLOGY

## 4.15 Drug-Induced Skin Reactions
**Stevens-Johnson Syndrome and Toxic Epidermal Necrolysis** (see **Dermatologic Emergencies,** p.379)

**Exanthematous Reactions:** bright red rash and skin may feel hot, burning or itchy
- Erythema, or morbilliform (maculopapular) lesions
- Location: often start on the trunk and also often involve extremities and intertriginous areas; face may be spared
- Common Causative Drugs: allopurinol, antimicrobials, barbiturates, captopril, carbamazepine, furosemide, gold salts, lithium, phenothiazines, phenylbutazone, phenytoin, thiazides

**Urticaria:** hives present as raised, itchy, red blotches or wheals that are pale in the center and red around the outside
- Common Causative Drugs: NSAIDs including Aspirin® and pharmaceutical excipients
- Urticaria has many causes that do not include medications

**Erythroderma and Exfoliative Dermatitis:** widespread confluent erythematous rash often associated with desquamation
- Systemic symptoms may be present such as fever, lymphadenopathy, and anorexia
- Common Causative Drugs: chloroquine, isoniazid, penicillin, phenytoin, sulfonamides

**Fixed Drug Eruption:** erythematous round or oval lesions of a reddish, dusky purple or brown color, sometimes featuring blisters, either bullae or vesicles
- Location: within hours at the same site; frequently hands, feet, tongue, penis, or perianal areas
- Common Causative Drugs: ACEIs, allopurinol, antimicrobials, barbiturates, benzodiazepines, calcium channel blockers, carbamazepine, dextromethorphan, diltiazem, fluconazole, lamotrigine, NSAIDs, proton pump inhibitors

**Acne:** papulopustular but comedones are often absent
- Common Causative Drugs: think "B PIMPLES"
  - ◆ Bromides (halides, iodides)
  - ◆ Phenytoin
  - ◆ Isoniazid
  - ◆ Moisturizers
  - ◆ Prednisone
  - ◆ Lithium
  - ◆ EGFR inhibitors
  - ◆ Systemic hormones (androgens, OCPs)

**Psoriasis:** erythematous plaques with large dry silvery scales
- Common Causative Drugs: ACEIs, β-blockers, chloroquine and hydroxychloroquine, digoxin, lithium, NSAIDs, tetracyclines, TNF-α antagonists

## Management of Drug-Induced Reactions
- Accurate medication history including all recent medications and OTC medicines, herbal and homeopathic preparations
- Note the times when medications taken and if patient has taken medications before
- Note proprietary and generic name in order to have a record of pharmaceutical excipients
- Record any known or suspect adverse drug reactions with details of cause; advise that future exposure can be avoided and report to relevant regulatory authority

# REFERENCES

1. Jiang M, Stewart E. Dermatology. In: *Toronto Notes*. 32nd Ed. Toronto, ON: Toronto Notes for Medical Students, Inc; 2016
2. Chiang N. Verbov J. *Dermatology: A handbook for medical students and junior doctors*. Liverpool: British Association of Dermatologists; 2009.
3. Burns DA. *Rook's textbook of dermatology*. 8th ed. New York: Blackwell Publishing; 2009.
4. Fitzpatrick T, Johnson RA, Wolff K, Suurmond R. In: *Color atlas & synopsis of clinical dermatology: Common and serious conditions*. New York: McGraw-Hill; 2001.
5. Mallon E, Newton JN, Klassen A, Stewart-Brown SL, Ryan TJ, Finlay AY. *The quality of life in acne: A comparison with general medical conditions using generic questionnaires*. Br J Dermatol. 1999; 140(4): 672-676.
6. Powell FC. *Clinical practice – Rosacea*. N Engl J Med. 2005; 352(8): 793-803.
7. Shapiro J. *Clinical practice – Hair loss in women*. N Engl J Med. 2007; 357(16): 1620-1630.
8. Goldstein BG, Goldstein AO. *Diagnosis and management of malignant melanoma*. Am Fam Physician. 2001; 63(7): 1359-1368.
9. Whited JD, Grichnik JM. *JAMA*. 1998; 279(9): 696-701.
10. Erian A. *Advanced surgical facial rejuvenation: Art and clinical practice*. New York: Springer; 2012.
11. Moyal DD, Fourtanier AM. *Broad spectrum sunscreens provide better protection from solar ultraviolet-simulated radiation and natural sunlight-induced immunosuppression in human beings*. J Am Acad Dermatol. 2008; 58(5 Suppl 2): S149-154.
12. Freiman A, Borsuk D, Sasseville D. *Dermatologic emergencies*. CMAJ. 2005; 173(11): 1317-1319.
13. Usatine RP, Sandy N. *Dermatologic emergencies*. Am Fam Physician. 2010; 82(7): 773-780.
14. McQueen A, Martin SA, Lio PA. *Derm emergencies: Detecting early signs of trouble*. J Fam Pract. 2012; 61(2): 71-78.
15. Dodiuk-Gad RP, Chung WH, Valeyrie-Allanore L, Shear NH. *Stevens-Johnson syndrome and toxic epidermal necrolysis: An update*. Am J Clin Dermatol. 2015; 16(6): 475-493.

**DERMATOLOGY**

# CHAPTER 13:

# Emergency Medicine

**Editors:**
Devon Alton, HBSc
Graham Mazereeuw, PhD
Daniel Tae Oh Yoo, BHSc

**Resident Reviewers:**
Andrew Prine, MD

**Faculty Reviewers:**
Jacques S Lee, MD, MSc, FRCPC
Catherine Varner, MD, MSc, CCFP(EM)

EMERGENCY

## TABLE OF CONTENTS

# 1. RAPID PRIMARY SURVEY (RPS) OF TRAUMA

In order of priority, **ABCDE**:

<u>A</u>irway
- Assume cervical spine injury for trauma patient and use collar for immobilization
- Assessment:
    - Patent: patient speaking normally
    - Compromised: altered voice, moaning, stridor, absence of sounds, decreased LOC (GCS < 8)
- Differential Diagnosis
    - Foreign body (i.e. tooth), soft tissue swelling from direct trauma or inhalational injury, neck hematoma, facial or neck fracture, obstructive substance (i.e. emesis, blood, saliva), tongue obstruction
- Management: Basic Airway
    - To open airway, use chin lift or jaw thrust. AVOID head tilt; C-Spine precautions to be maintained on ALL patients
    - To remove foreign material, sweep and suction
    - To maintain airway
        - Nasopharyngeal airway (contraindicated if suspected basal skull fracture or severe facial trauma)
        - Oropharyngeal airway (contraindicated if gag reflex present)
        - Bag-mask ventilation
        - Laryngeal mask airway (supraglottic airway device)
- Management: Definitive Airway
    - Indications for intubation (**4 Ps**):
        - **P**atency: obstructed or impending obstruction (burns, inhalational injury, neck hematoma, tongue if decreased LOC)
        - **P**ositive-pressure ventilation: to correct deficient oxygenation and/or ventilation (decreased O2 sat, cyanotic)
        - **P**rotection: decreased LOC (GCS < 8), apnea (resp failure)
        - **P**redicted deterioration
    - Intubation must be confirmed with end-tidal $CO_2$ detector, perspiration in the tube, symmetrical chest rising, and auscultation of air entry bilaterally
    - If intubation unsuccessful, return to bag valve mask ventilation, and consider advanced airway techniques including: bougie (tracheal tube introducer), video laryngoscopy (Glidescope)
    - If intubation still unsuccessful, consider surgical airway with cricothyroidotomy or tracheostomy
    - Once airway is secured, move on to assess breathing

<u>B</u>reathing
- Assessment:
    - Inspect: RR, symmetric rising of the chest, decreased LOC, anxiety, cyanosis, nasal flaring, pursed-lip breathing, tracheal tug, intercostal indrawing, distended neck veins
    - Auscultate: equal/absent breath sounds, wheezes, crackles
    - Palpate: tracheal shift, chest tenderness, flail segments, sucking chest wound, subcutaneous emphysema
- Differential Diagnosis:
    - Life-threatening: respiratory (tension pneumothorax, hemothorax, flail chest, diaphragmatic rupture, pulmonary embolus, pleural effusion), cardiac (tamponade, ACS)
- Investigations:
    - Many of the above diagnoses should be made clinically, but chest x-ray may help to confirm
- Management:
    - General: nasal prongs, face mask, non-rebreather mask, bag-mask ventilation
    - Tension pneumothorax: needle thoracostomy for immediate stabilization followed by tube thoracostomy (chest tube)
    - Hemothorax: tube thoracostomy (note: if high output from chest tube, consider opening chest to control bleeding source)
- Move on to assess circulation once airway is secure and/or breathing (oxygenation and ventilation) is appropriate

EMERGENCY

#### Circulation
- Shock: an abnormality of the circulatory system causing insufficient perfusion of tissue and organs with oxygenated blood which, if uncorrected, will result in cell death
- Assessment:
  - Weak peripheral pulses, tachycardia, tachypnea, hypotension, widened pulse pressure, delayed capillary refill time, decreased urine output, mental status changes (anxiety, confusion, lethargy)
  - Note: hypotension is an insensitive marker of tissue perfusion as it does not occur until there has been a blood loss > 30% total blood volume
  - Skin – cool & pale (cardiogenic/hypovolemic cause) vs. warm & flushed (distributive cause), signs of external/internal hemorrhage
  - JVP – low (hypovolemia/distributive cause) vs high (obstructive cause)
- Differential Diagnosis: SSHOCK mnemonic
  - **S**eptic – vasogenic and distributive
  - **S**pinal/neurogenic – vasogenic and distributive
    - Features warm extremities
    - Suspect if hypotensive and bradycardic
  - **H**ypovolemic – most common cause is hemorrhage
  - **O**bstructive – tension pneumothorax, massive PE, severe asthma, cardiac tamponade
  - **C**ardiogenic – MI, LV failure, arrhythmia
  - Anaphyla**K**tic – vasogenic and distributive
- Investigations:
  - Bedside Ultrasound – FAST U/S (Focused Assessment with Sonography in Trauma Ultrasound) can detect intraabdominal hemorrhage, IVC filling (marker of hypovolemia), and pericardial tamponade
  - X-ray – chest +/- pelvis
  - Head CT (if trauma suspected)
  - Order blood work – CBC, low bicarbonate/high anion gap (metabolic acidosis), elevated serum lactate, group and screen
- Management:
  - General: cardiac monitors, oxygen and O2 sat monitor, IV access (2 large bore IVs – 14G or 16G, or central line), control external bleeding by direct pressure, Foley catheter to monitor urine output
  - Specific
    - Hemorrhage – aggressive IV infusion of warmed crystalloid (NS or RL) – 1-2 L bolus (or 20mg/kg in children), pRBCs (O- for women < 50; O+ for rest) if Class III/IV shock or no response to fluids, tranexamic acid, platelets and FFP
    - Anaphylactic – epinephrine IM, IV crystalloid, antihistamines (H1, H2 blockers), corticosteroids
    - Septic – IV crystalloid, broad-spectrum antibiotic, early goal directed therapy
    - Cardiogenic – inotropes, intra-aortic balloon pump, angioplasty
    - Cardiac tamponade – IV crystalloid, pericardiocentesis or pericardial window
    - Tension pneumothorax – needle thoracostomy followed by chest tube
    - Massive PE – IV crystalloid, inotropes, thrombolysis
- For details on fluid replacement (see **Fluids, Electrolytes, and Acid/Base Disturbances Chapter**)

**Table 1.** Classes of Shock

| Class | I | II | III | IV |
|---|---|---|---|---|
| Respiratory Rate | 20 | 30 | 35 | >45 |
| Pulse | <100 | 100-120 | >120 | >140 |
| Blood Pressure | Normal | Normal | ↓ | ↓ |
| Capillary Refill | Normal | ↓ | ↓ | ↓ |
| % Blood Volume | <15% | 15-30% | 30-40% | >40% |
| Fluid Replacement | Crystalloid | Crystalloid | Crystalloid and blood | Crystalloid and blood |

- **D**isability
  - ◆ Assess LOC using Glasgow Coma Scale (GCS) or **AVPU** (**A**lert, responds to **V**oice, responds to **P**ain, **U**nresponsive) (see **Table 2**)
  - ◆ GCS score: "numbers go low to high with head-to-toe" – eyes (1-4), verbal (1-5), motor (1-6)
    - ▪ Mild disability (13-15)
    - ▪ Moderate disability (9-12)
    - ▪ Severe disability (≤8): "GCS less than 8, intubate"

- **E**xposure/**E**nvironment
  - ◆ Expose entire body and assess for injuries
  - ◆ Must log-roll patient to assess the back
  - ◆ Avoid hypothermia with warm blankets, warm IV blood/fluids

**Table 2.** Glasgow Coma Scale

| Eye Opening | | Verbal Response | | Motor Response | |
|---|---|---|---|---|---|
| Spontaneous | 4 | Oriented | 5 | Obeys commands | 6 |
| To verbal command | 3 | Confused | 4 | Localizes to pain | 5 |
| To pain | 2 | Inappropriate words | 3 | Withdraws from pain | 4 |
| None | 1 | Incomprehensible sounds | 2 | Flexion (decorticate) | 3 |
| | | No verbal response | 1 | Extension (decerebrate) | 2 |
| | | | | No response | 1 |

## 2. SECONDARY SURVEY
A more detailed head-to-toe exam to identify significant injuries and concerns.

### 2.1 Sample History
- • **S**igns and symptoms
- • **A**llergies
- • **M**edications
- • **P**ast medical history
- • **L**ast meal
- • **E**vents surrounding episode

### 2.2 Focused Physical Exam
**Neurological and Head & Neck**
- • Evaluate GCS or AVPU
- • Evaluate for spinal cord injury: sensory level and motor exam
- • Cranial nerve exams
  - ◆ Pupillary reactivity and reflex
    - ▪ Reactive pupils (symmetrical) + decreased LOC: metabolic/structural cause
    - ▪ Nonreactive pupils (or asymmetrical) + decreased LOC: structural cause
  - ◆ Extraocular movements, nystagmus
- • Fundoscopy
- • Assess tympanic membrane for CSF leakage/hemotympanum
- • Evaluate for facial trauma
  - ◆ Signs of basal skull fracture:
    - ▪ Hemotympanum, CSF rhinorrhea, CSF otorrhea
    - ▪ Battle's sign (retroauricular hematoma), raccoon eyes (periorbital ecchymosis) (see **Figure 1**)

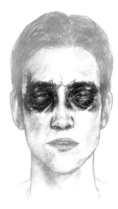
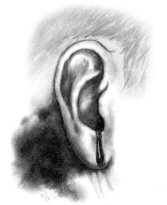

Periorbital ecchymosis        Periauricular ecchymosis        Jan Cyril Fundano

**Figure 1.** Common Signs of a Basal Skull Fracture

### Chest
- Inspection: contusions, flail segments, symmetrical chest expansion, paradoxical breathing (seesaw respiration in children)
- Palpation: subcutaneous emphysema
- Auscultation: all lung fields

### Abdomen/Pelvis
- Assess for intraperitoneal bleeding, acute abdomen (consider acute abdomen if abdominal wall does not move with breathing)
- DRE (look for gross blood, sphincter tone, high-riding or mobile prostate), blood at urethral meatus, bimanual exam

### MSK
- Log-roll and palpate cervical, thoracic, and lumbar spines for fractures
- Palpate pelvic girdle, pubic symphysis for instability indicating "open-book" fracture
- Extremity exam for fracture and neurovascular status

### Investigations
- X-rays: C-, T-, and L-spine, chest, pelvis
- CT scans: head, chest, abdomen, pelvis

> **Clinical Pearl: Canadian CT Head Rules[1]**
> Risk criteria where CT head required
> - High Risk: GCS <15 two hours after injury, suspected open/depressed skull fracture, signs of basilar skull fracture, vomiting >2 episodes, age >65 yr
> - Medium Risk: amnesia >30 min, dangerous mechanism (e.g. pedestrian struck by motor vehicle, occupant ejected, fall >3 ft (0.9 m) or 5 stairs)

## 3. COMMON CLINICAL SCENARIOS

### 3.1 Anaphylaxis/Anaphylactoid Reaction
Immune response mediated by massive release of histamine, leukotrienes, prostaglandins and tryptase resulting in severe systemic reaction occurring within minutes

EMERGENCY

**Table 3.** Overview of Anaphylaxis

| Key Symptoms | Physical Exam Findings | Investigations | Management |
|---|---|---|---|
| **Anaphylaxis (general)** | | | |
| • Respiratory distress: bronchospasm, upper airway obstruction or laryngeal edema<br><br>• Swelling, hives<br><br>• Syncope, presyncope<br><br>• GI pain, vomiting | • Hypotension<br><br>• Skin/mucosal involvement: pruritis, urticaria or angioedema | • Dx based on clinical presentation and history at time of acute event<br><br>• Can be supported by elevated tryptase or histamine | • Prehospital care: Epi-pen, oral antihistamines<br>• IV normal saline<br>• Epinephrine<br>• If bronchospasm, β-agonist aerosol (salbutamol) via nebulizer<br>• Antihistamines (diphenhydramine)<br>• Glucocorticoids |
| **Mild to Moderate Anaphylaxis** | | | |
| • Minimal airway edema<br><br>• Mild bronchospasm<br><br>• Mild cutaneous reactions | • See above | • See above | • Diphenhydramine only:<br>  • Adults: 50mg IM or IV q4-6h<br>  • Children: 1mg/kg IM or IV q4-6h |
| **Moderate to Severe Anaphylaxis** | | | |
| • Laryngeal edema<br><br>• Severe bronchospasm<br><br>• Respiratory distress/arrest<br><br>• Shock<br><br>• MI<br><br>• Arrhythmia | • See above | • See above | • Diphenhydramine<br>• IM/SC epinephrine: 0.3-0.5mL of 1:1000 (adults); 0.01-0.4mL of 1:1000 (children)<br>• Antihistamine (ranitidine)<br>• IV epinephrine if severe: 1 mL of 1:10000 (adult); 0.01 mL/kg (child); repeat every 5-10 min until symptoms resolve<br>• Glucocorticoids as adjunct to epinephrine |

IM = intramuscular, SC = subcutaneous

**Clinical Pearl: Rule of 5s for Adult Dosing**
- Epinephrine: 0.5 mg, 1:1000 IM
- H1 Histamine blockers (diphenhydramine): 50 mg IV
- H2 Histamine blockers (ranitidine): 50 mg IV
- Glucocorticoids (methylprednisolone): 125 mg IV
- β-agonist aerosol (salbutamol): 5 mg in 3 cc normal saline IH

**Focused History**

**OPQRST** (especially time of exposure to anaphylactic agent)

**Past Medical History**: allergic/systemic reactions, previous ICU admissions, check for allergy-identifying jewelry items and wallet

Focused Physical Exam
- **General:** marked anxiety, tremor, weakness, cold sensation
- **CNS:** weakness, syncope, dizziness, seizures
- **Head & Neck:** facial edema, lip/tongue swelling, lacrimation, ocular pruritus, conjunctival injection, mydriasis
- **Respiratory:** tachypnea, accessory muscle use, cyanosis, laryngeal edema (lump in throat, hoarseness, stridor), bronchospasm (cough, wheezing, chest tightness, respiratory distress)
- **CVS:** tachycardia, hypotension, chest pain
- **GI:** N/V, crampy abdominal pain, bloody diarrhea
- **Derm:** pruritic urticaria, edema, erythema

Management
- ABCDE
- Identify and treat responsible agent as soon as anaphylaxis is suspected
  - ♦ Should stop all IV meds until responsible agent identified
- IV normal saline
- Medications
  - ♦ If administered epinephrine, must also be given steroids and remain 4 hours for observation

### 3.2 Hypothermia
Decline in core temperature below 35°C due to increased heat loss (convection, radiation, conduction, evaporation) or decreased heat production (metabolic, toxic, catatonic state)[2,3]
- Primary hypothermia from environmental exposure
- Secondary hypothermia from underlying medical condition which disrupts thermoregulatory mechanism (e.g. bacterial infection, thyroid disease, malnutrition, stroke, DM, spinal cord injury, use of medication or substance which affects CNS)

**Table 4.** Clinical Features of Hypothermia

| | Key Symptoms | Physical Exam Findings | Investigations | Management |
|---|---|---|---|---|
| **Hypother-mia** (general) | • Shivering <br><br> • Altered mental status <br><br> • Tachypnea, tachycardia | • Core temperature using rectal or esophageal probes <br> • Neurological exam: lowered GCS, hyporeflexia, dilated pupils <br> • Cardiac exam for arrhythmias | • ECG <br><br> • Blood work: hypoglycemia, hypomagnese-mia, hypophos-phatemia | • Monitor core temperature <br><br> • Rewarming |
| **Mild** (32-34.9°C) | • Lethargy, shivering, tachypnea, tachycardia, altered judgment, ataxia | • See above | • See above | • Passive rewarming (since thermoregulatory mechanism intact) |
| **Moderate** (28-31.9°C) | • Stupor, attention/ memory deficits, loss of shiver, dilated pupils, arrhythmias, slowed reflexes, muscle rigidity | • See above | • See above | • Active external rewarming: blanket, heating lamp |
| **Severe** (<28°C) | • Unresponsive, coma, hypotension, fixed pupils, ventricular fibrillation, apnea, areflexia | • See above | • See above | • Active core rewarming: warmed humidified O2, IV fluids, peritoneal dialysis, irrigation of cavities |

**Focused History**
- **OPQRST** (especially duration of exposure)
- **Risk factors:** age (extremes of age at greatest risk), drug or alcohol overdose, toxins, cold water immersion, trauma, outdoor sports, impaired CNS-mediated thermoregulation (hypothalamus, spinal cord injury or surgery), malnutrition, endocrine failure

**Focused Physical Exam**
- **General:** decreased core temperature (use rectal or esophageal probes), lethargy, shivering
- **CNS:** altered judgement, decreased level of consciousness
- **Respiratory:** tachypnea, apnea
- **CVS:** tachycardia, arrhythmias
- **Neuro:** hyporeflexia/areflexia, ataxia, muscle rigidity, dilated/fixed pupils

**Investigations**
- **ECG:** wide QRS, prolonged QT, atrial fibrillation, J or Osborne wave (positive deflection at the J point)
- **Blood work:** hypoglycemia, hypomagnesemia, hypophosphatemia

**Management**
- ABCDE
- Secondary survey
- Monitor core temperature: rectal or esophageal temperature probes are most accurate
- Rewarming:
  - Passive
  - Active external (forced air blankets/"bear hugger", heated blanket, heating lamp, warm baths)
  - Active core (warmed humidified oxygen, IV fluids, peritoneal dialysis, irrigation of cavities, cardiopulmonary bypass: most effective and rapid, but not readily available)

## 3.3 Hyperthermia

Increase in core temperature >37.5°C without a change in the body's temperature set-point[2]. This may lead to:
- Dilation of peripheral venous system, increased blood flow to skin, stimulation of sweat glands
- Severe hyperthermia: dehydration with electrolyte abnormalities → dysfunction of thermoregulatory mechanism → multi-system organ failure

Caused by:
- Increased heat production
  - Muscular activity, metabolism, drugs, severe infection
- Decreased heat loss
  - ↓ sweating, ↓ CNS response, ↓ cardiovascular reserve, drugs

**Table 5.** Overview of hyperthermia

| Key Symptoms | Physical Exam Findings | Investigations | Management |
|---|---|---|---|
| • Fatigue, dizziness, irritability, weakness, headache, N/V<br><br>• Myalgias, muscle cramps | • Elevated core temperature > 38.5°C (or severe heatstroke > 40°C)<br>• Neuro: mental status changes, ataxia<br>• Resp: tachypnea, dyspnea<br>• CVS: tachyarrhythmias<br>Signs of dehydration: hypotension, hot/dry skin, etc. | • ECG<br>• Arterial/venous blood gas;<br>• Liver enzymes, PT/PTT, creatinine, creatine kinase<br>• Toxicology screening if appropriate | • Rest and cooling<br>• Fluid and salt replacement<br>• Cooling measures: fan, spray bottle, ice packs to groin and axillae, gastric lavage, iced peritoneal lavage, cooling blanket |

Focused History
- **OPQRST** (including peak ambient temperature)
- **Associated symptoms:** fatigue, dizziness, irritability, weakness, headache, N/V, myalgias, muscle cramps
- **Risk factors:**
  - **Excessive heat load:** fever, environment, lack of acclimatization, exertion
  - **Circulatory insufficiency:** extremes of age, obesity, dehydration, CHF, diuretics, laxatives
  - **Medications:** sympathomimetics (e.g. cocaine, ecstasy), lysergic acid diethylamide (LSD), anticholinergics, antihistamines, MAOIs, phencyclidine (PCP), drug or alcohol withdrawal, β-blockers, sympatholytics, anesthetic gases (i.e. malignant hyperthermia)

**Table 6**. Clinical Features of Heat Disorders[2]

| Heat Disorder | Clinical Features | Management |
|---|---|---|
| **Heat Edema** | Vasodilation and venous stasis → swelling of feet and ankles | Elevation of limbs |
| **Heat Syncope** | Peripheral pooling of intravascular volume → ↓ preload → orthostatic hypotension → syncope | Rest, cooling, and rehydration |
| **Heat Cramps** | Dehydration → salt depletion (Na$^+$/K$^+$ shifts) → spasms of voluntary muscles of abdomen and extremities | Fluid and salt replacement |
| **Heat Exhaustion** | Prolonged heat exposure → primary water loss or primary sodium loss → dehydration signs; no CNS symptoms | Rehydration and cooling |
| **Heat Stroke** | Extremely high body temperature (>40.5°C) → multiorgan dysfunction (e.g. rhabdomyolysis and hepatic damage) including CNS symptoms → altered mental status, confusion, bizarre behavior, hallucinations, disorientation, coma | Rapid reduction in body temperature |

Focused Physical Exam (for Heat Exhaustion and Heat Stroke)
- **General:** fatigue, malaise, sweating (anhidrosis when severe), fever
- **CNS:** confusion/lethargy, weakness, headache, agitation, delirium, seizure, ataxia, coma
- **H&N:** fixed dilated pupils (heat stroke), subconjunctival hemorrhage
- **CVS:** tachycardia, hypotension, dehydration
- **Respiratory:** tachypnea, alkalosis, hemoptysis
- **GI:** N/V, diarrhea ± bright red blood or melena
- **GU:** oliguria or anuria (acute renal failure), hematuria
- **Derm:** dry, warm, diaphoretic, piloerection

Management
- **ABCDE**
- **Cooling measures:** convection (fan), evaporation (spray bottle), conduction (ice packs to groin and axillae, gastric lavage, iced peritoneal lavage), cooling blanket

## 3.4 Burns

**Table 7.** Overview of Burns

| Key Symptoms | Physical Exam Findings | Investigations | Management |
|---|---|---|---|
| • Skin: local erythema, pain, blisters, swelling, loss of sensation, charring<br><br>• Respiratory distress, cardiac irritability | • Assess degree of burn and affected body surface area using rule of nines<br><br>• Assess for circumferential burns<br><br>• Assess mental status<br><br>• Ensure intact respiratory, cardiac and neurological function | • ECG<br><br>• Routine bloods and arterial blood gas/CO levels<br><br>• Creatine kinase, lactate | • ABC<br><br>• Correct hyponatremia and hyperkalemia<br><br>• Sedatives/narcotics as needed, tetanus<br><br>• Dress wounds, evaluate for other associated injuries (e.g. fractures) |

**Focused History**
- **OPQRST**
  - ◆ Type of exposure: thermal, chemical, electrical, inhalation, UV
  - ◆ Environment: e.g., enclosed space
  - ◆ Materials involved: e.g., smoke, fire, CO, cyanide poisoning
- **Associated symptoms:** respiratory illness (persistent cough, wheeze, hoarseness from respiratory burns, soot-stained sputum), related injuries (eg. electrical/blast injury)
- **Risk factors:** immunodeficiency, DM, respiratory illness, renal disease

**Focused Physical Exam**
- Degree of burn assessed by:
  - ◆ Burn size: rule of nines for percentage of affected body surface area (BSA) in 2° and 3° burns (see **Figure 2**)
    - ▪ Add up all the burned areas of the body that have blisters or worse
  - ◆ Burn site: serious injuries if hands/feet, face, eyes, ears, perineum affected
- **H&N:** corneal damage, singed nasal hair, facial charring, mucosal burns
- **Respiratory:** hypoxic, stridor, wheezing, respiratory obstruction (due to inhalational injury), circumferential burns (i.e. eschar)
- **CVS:** cardiac irritability (electrical burns)
- **CNS:** neurologic dysfunction (electrical burns)
- **GU:** genital or perineal burns in children (suspect child abuse)
- **MSK:** reduced joint movement due to scarring over joints, mobility
- **Derm:** minimal surface wounds with extensive deep damage (electrical burns)

**Table 8.** Classification of Burns

| Burn Depth | Layers Involved | Signs and Symptoms |
|---|---|---|
| **First Degree** | Epidermis | Local erythema, pain |
| **Second Degree** | A: Superficial partial thickness<br>B: Deep partial thickness | Blisters and bullae-covered skin that is erythematous, moist, and swollen (intact sensation); hair follicles are preserved |
| **Third Degree** | All layers of skin | No sensation, charring if severe/eschar formation |
| **Fourth Degree** | Fat, muscle, bone | As above |

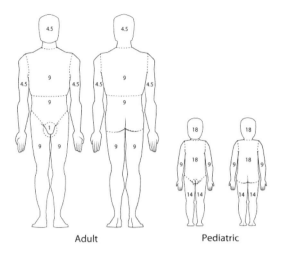

Adult        Pediatric

Caitlin O'Connell

**Figure 2.** Rule of Nines

**Management**
- **ABCDE** with attention to
- **Airway:** Control early with endotracheal tube (ETT) if:
  - ◆ Signs of upper airway and laryngeal edema (severe burns to lower face and neck, inhalation of superheated air in confined space, carbonaceous sputum, associated chemical inhalation)
  - ◆ Full thickness circumferential chest wall or abdomen involvement: emergency escharotomy if circumferential burns constrict chest movements
- **Circulation:** if hemodynamically unstable, initial fluid resuscitation with NS, then:
  - ◆ IV Ringer's lactate using **Parkland** formula
    - ▪ Fluid for first 24 h = Total body surface area burn (%) × Weight (kg) × 4 (mL); give ½ over first 8 h, ½ over next 16 h
    - ▪ Target urine output of 0.5-1.0 mL/kg/h
  - ◆ Correct hyponatremia and hyperkalemia (check ECG for peaked T waves)
- **Disposition/drugs/draw bloods/drains:** routine bloods and arterial blood gas (ABG)/ CO levels, CK if concern for tissue damage/rhabdomyolysis, lactate if concern for cyanide toxicity, sedatives/narcotics as needed, tetanus, Foley catheter, nasogastric (NG) tube
- **Exposure and secondary survey:** dress wounds (irrigation with sterile saline ± dressing to prevent heat loss and infection)

### 3.5 Wound Care
- Establishment of absolute hemostasis before wound care through indirect and direct methods (to prevent further blood loss and formation of hematoma)
  - ◆ **Indirect:** elevation of injured part above level of heart, direct pressure over wound or tourniquets for complex injuries, epinephrine-containing solutions (contraindicated in wounds on penis, digits, tip of nose)
  - ◆ **Direct:** ligation, electrocautery, chemical cautery

**Table 9.** Overview of Wound Care

| Key Symptoms | Physical Exam Findings | Investigations | Management |
|---|---|---|---|
| • Bleeding<br>• Pain | • MSK: assess for any loss of function of injured part<br>• Neuro: two-point discrimination on each side of digits<br>• Vascular: assess pulses | • X-ray if suspect open fracture | • Anesthetic agents (lidocaine ± epinephrine) via local infiltration<br>• Cleansing: irrigation (normal saline), cleaning agent (e.g. iodine, chlorhexidine), mechanical scrubbing<br>• Debridement<br>• Wound closure |

**Focused History**
- **OPQRST**
  - Time of injury (increased risk of infection if sutured >6 h after time of injury)
  - Site of injury, contact with contaminants
    - Less infectious: face, hands
    - More infectious: back, buttocks
  - Mechanism of injury, especially crush injuries
  - Tetanus immunization status
- **Past Medical History**
  - Tetanus immunization status (up to date in last 10 years)

**Focused Physical Exam**
- **MSK:** loss of function in injured part, involvement of underlying structures (e.g. nerves, major blood vessels, ligaments, bones), degree of contamination, foreign body
- **Neuro:** use two-point discrimination on the finger to document nerve status (<4 mm is normal) on each side of the digits
- **Vascular:** assess pulses

**Management**
- Assess neurovascular status before using anesthetic agents (lidocaine ± epinephrine) via local infiltration
- Cleansing: irrigation (normal saline), cleaning agent (e.g. iodine, chlorhexidine), mechanical scrubbing
- Debridement
- Wound closure (absorbable or nonabsorbable sutures, steri-strips, steel and metallic clips or staples, wound tapes, wound staples, tissue adhesives)

## 3.6 Abdominal Pain

**Table 10.** Selected Causes of Abdominal Pain

| Key Symptoms | Physical Exam Findings | Investigations | Management |
|---|---|---|---|
| **Appendicitis** | | | |
| • Initial vague, colicky central abdominal pain; progresses to localized RLQ pain over McBurney's point | • Peritoneal signs (guarding, rebound tenderness esp. over McBurney's point), Rovsing's sign, psoas sign, obturator sign | • Contrast-enhanced CT if diagnosis uncertain; U/S in females of reproductive age; can consider MRI | • Morphine<br>• Antibiotics (either perioperative or as primary treatment for uncomplicated cases) |
| • Anorexia; N/V; fever (50% of patients) | | • Leukocytosis (50% of patients) | • Appendectomy (laparoscopic, open) |
| **Abdominal Aortic Aneurysm (AAA)** | | | |
| • Majority asymptomatic | • Pulsatile abdominal mass; if ruptured, shock, hypotension and mottled abdominal wall | • CT if symptomatic and diagnosis uncertain; U/S in females of reproductive age | • Emergency repair (open vs endovascular) |
| • Consider rupture if symptomatic with sudden acute abdominal, back, or flank pain | | | |

| Key Symptoms | Physical Exam Findings | Investigations | Management |
|---|---|---|---|
| **Acute Ischemic Bowel** | | | |
| • Abdominal pain out of proportion with physical exam<br><br>• N/V, fever, bloody diarrhea | • Peritoneal signs<br><br>• Abdominal distension<br><br>• Absent bowel sounds<br><br>• Occult blood in stool<br><br>• Shock (tachycardia; hypotension) | • Leukocytosis, lactic acidosis<br><br>• Contrast CT: thickened bowel wall loops (thumbprinting); abdominal angiography: may show embolus or thrombus | • Fluid resuscitation<br><br>• Broad-spectrum antibiotics<br><br>• Anticoagulation<br><br>• Arterial occlusion: surgical/endovascular revascularization<br><br>• Venous occlusion: thrombolysis<br><br>• Non-occlusive: vasodilators |
| **Cholecystitis** | | | |
| • Steady, severe RUQ or epigastric pain (may radiate to right shoulder or back), fever, anorexia, N/V | • Abdominal guarding<br><br>• Positive Murphy's sign<br><br>• Tachycardia | • Leukocytosis<br><br>• U/S: gallstones, sonographic Murphy's sign, gallbladder wall thickening, pericholecystic fluid | • IV fluid, correct electrolytes, analgesia<br><br>• Antibiotics<br><br>• Cholecystectomy |
| **Obstruction** | | | |
| • Cramping abdominal pain, often periumbilical<br><br>• N/V, decreased oral intake, minimal passage of gas or stool | • Abdominal distension<br><br>• Abnormal bowel sounds<br><br>• Dehydration (tachycardia, hypotension) | • Abdominal X-ray: dilated bowel, air fluid levels | • IV fluid, correct electrolytes<br><br>• Antibiotics if perforation/ischemia<br><br>• GI decompression with NG tube<br><br>• Water soluble contrast<br><br>• Surgery |
| **Splenic Rupture** | | | |
| • LUQ pain, left shoulder tip pain when supine (Kehr's sign), or diffuse abdominal pain | • Hypotension<br><br>• Peritoneal signs | • CT (only in a stable patient): rupture seen, blood detected; U/S: free fluid around spleen | • Splenectomy<br><br>• Angiography and embolization |
| **Ectopic Pregnancy** | | | |
| • Abdominal pain and vaginal bleeding following a missed period | • Adnexal mass<br><br>• Hypotension if ruptured | • Transvaginal U/S: blood or mass in adnexa, ectopic cardiac activity or gestational sac; β-hCG >1500 and no intrauterine pregnancy | • Methotrexate<br><br>• Salpingectomy/salpingostomy |

Note: Although atypical, one should consider myocardial infarction in the differential for

EMERGENCY

abdominal pain as well (See **The Precordial Exam** Chapter)

> **Clinical Pearl: Abdominal Pain**
> • Abrupt, severe onset is suggestive of a vascular cause or viscus rupture
> • Gradual onset is more suggestive of inflammatory or infectious causes
> • Crampy, cyclic pain occurring in crescendo-decrescendo cycles may indicate small bowel obstruction
> • Despite its name, "renal colic" pain is typically constant, however it may present as colicky as well

**Focused History**
- **OPQRST**
  - Location and radiation of pain vital for differential (see **Figure 3**)
  - Consider referred pain (e.g. cholecystitis causing subscapular pain)
- **Associated symptoms:** Anorexia, N/V, constipation, diarrhea, hematochezia, melena, fever, rigors

**Focused Physical Exam**
- See **The Gastrointestinal System** Chapter

**Investigations**
- Vitals (temperature, HR, RR)
- CBC w/ differential, electrolytes
- Serum creatinine/BUN, lactate, LFTs, lipase
- Urinalysis
- β-hCG in <u>all</u> women of reproductive age
- ECG (especially if >40 yr)
- Abdominal X-ray (AXR), CXR, CT, U/S as needed

**Management**
- NPO, NG tube, IV fluids
- Treat shock
- Analgesia: judicious use of IV narcotics has been shown to aid the diagnostic process by making the physical exam more reliable
- Antiemetics and NG suction if necessary
- Consider holding back antibiotics unless sepsis/infection is obvious or until diagnosis is established
- Immediate surgical consult if hemodynamically unstable, acute abdomen, pulsatile abdominal mass

> **Clinical Pearl: Screening for Abdominal Aortic Aneurysm**
> • Abdominal palpation is useful for detecting large aneurysms, warranting surgery, but it cannot exclude the diagnosis
> • Investigate with imaging (U/S or CT) whenever AAA is suspected, regardless of physical exam findings

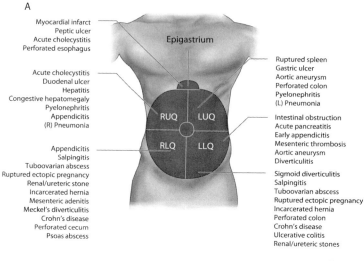

A

Myocardial infarct
Peptic ulcer
Acute cholecystitis
Perforated esophagus

Epigastrium

Ruptured spleen
Gastric ulcer
Aortic aneurysm
Perforated colon
Pyelonephritis
(L) Pneumonia

Acute cholecystitis
Duodenal ulcer
Hepatitis
Congestive hepatomegaly
Pyelonephritis
Appendicitis
(R) Pneumonia

Intestinal obstruction
Acute pancreatitis
Early appendicitis
Mesenteric thrombosis
Aortic aneurysm
Diverticulitis

RUQ    LUQ

RLQ    LLQ

Appendicitis
Salpingitis
Tuboovarian abscess
Ruptured ectopic pregnancy
Renal/ureteric stone
Incarcerated hernia
Mesenteric adenitis
Meckel's diverticulitis
Crohn's disease
Perforated cecum
Psoas abscess

Sigmoid diverticulitis
Salpingitis
Tuboovarian abscess
Ruptured ectopic pregnancy
Incarcerated hernia
Perforated colon
Crohn's disease
Ulcerative colitis
Renal/ureteric stones

Ahmed Aly

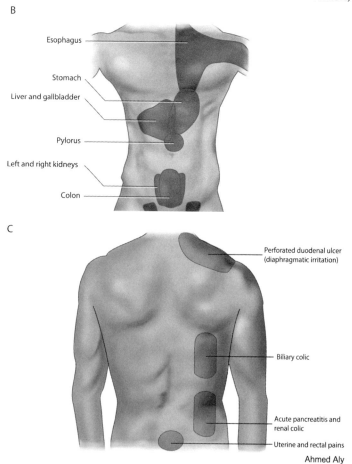

B

Esophagus

Stomach

Liver and gallbladder

Pylorus

Left and right kidneys

Colon

C

Perforated duodenal ulcer
(diaphragmatic irritation)

Biliary colic

Acute pancreatitis and
renal colic

Uterine and rectal pains

Ahmed Aly

**Figure 3.** (A) Differential Diagnoses for Pain in Abdominal Quadrants; (B) Localizations of Pain for Common Abdominal Pathologies, Anteriorly and (C) Posteriorly

EMERGENCY

## 3.7 Chest Pain

**Table 11.** Differential Diagnosis of Chest Pain

| Differential Diagnosis of Chest Pain | |
|---|---|
| **Cardiovascular**<br>• **Aortic dissection**<br>• **Cardiac tamponade**<br>• **ACS (STEMI, NSTEMI, unstable angina)**<br>• Pericarditis, myocarditis<br>• Stable angina<br>• Aortic stenosis, aortic insufficiency, mitral prolapse<br>• Sickle cell crisis<br>• Cocaine use | **Gastrointestinal**<br>• **Boerhaave's syndrome/esophageal rupture**<br>• Cholecystitis<br>• Esophagitis<br>• GERD<br>• Gastritis<br>• Peptic ulcer disease<br>• Pancreatitis |
| **Respiratory**<br>• **Pulmonary embolism**<br>• (Tension) pneumothorax<br>• Pleurisy<br>• Pneumonia | **Musculoskeletal**<br>• Costochondritis<br>• Intercostal muscle strain<br>• Rib fractures<br>• Thoracic outlet syndrome |
| **Neurological & Psychogenic**<br>• Spinal nerve root compression<br>• Anxiety | **Dermatological**<br>• Herpes zoster |

*Note:* life-threatening conditions that always need to be ruled out are in **bold**
**ACS** = acute coronary syndrome, **NSTEMI** = non-ST segment elevation myocardial infarction, **STEMI** = ST segment elevation myocardial infarction

> **Clinical Pearl: Postemesis Chest Pain**
> • Onset of postemesis chest pain is suggestive of Boerhaave's syndrome
> • Consider drug use, especially cocaine and other sympathomimetics

**Focused History**
- OPQRST
- N/V, diaphoresis
- Dyspnea, palpitations, syncope
- Cardiac or other risk factors (e.g. travel, oral contraceptive, DVT/PE)
- Trauma
- Sense of doom

**Focused Physical Exam**
- See **The Precordial Exam** Chapter

**Investigations**
- Vitals (temperature, HR, RR)
- CBC, electrolytes, serum glucose
- Serum creatinine, BUN
- Lipase (preferred) or amylase
- Cardiac enzymes: creatine kinase isoform (CK-MB), troponins I/T, brain natriuretic peptide (BNP)
- Consider D-dimer to rule out PE
- ECG
- CXR, EDE

**Management**
- Supplemental oxygen by facemask, nasal prongs
- Establish IV access (saline lock)
- Continuous cardiac monitoring or serial ECGs
- Evaluate for hypotension/shock
  - If hypovolemic: IV crystalloids, type and crossmatch 6-8 units pRBCs
- IV analgesia
- Correct arrhythmias if present

**Table 12.** Selected Causes of Chest Pain

| Key Symptoms | Physical Exam Findings | Investigations | Management |
|---|---|---|---|
| **ACS (STEMI, NSTEMI, unstable angina)** | | | |
| • Pain: retrosternal pressure +/- radiation to arms, neck, epigastrium N/V<br>• Dyspnea<br>• Palpitations | • Diaphoresis<br>• Restlessness<br>• Shock | • **CK-MB**<br>• **Troponin:** elevated in STEMI/NSTEMI, not in UA. Note: may also take a few hours to rise<br>• **ECG:** ST elevation in STEMI, no changes in NSTEMI or UA | • Oxygen (SpO2 > 90%)<br>• Anti-platelet (ASA and ticagrelor or clopidogrel)<br>• Anti-coagulants (heparin or enoxaparin)<br>• Anti-ischemics (nitroglycerin + beta blocker)<br>• Statin<br>• ACE inhibitor<br>• Reperfusion (PCI vs thrombolysis) |
| **Cardiac Tamponade** | | | |
| • Chest pain following trauma, MI, or post-op heart surgery | • <u>Beck's triad</u>: hypotension, increased JVP, muffled heart sounds<br>• Pulsus paradoxus | • **ECG:** low voltage QRS complexes, or electrical alternans (QRS amplitude ↑ then ↓ on alternating beats)<br>• **Echo** | • Pericardiocentesis<br>• Pericardial window |
| **Aortic Stenosis** | | | |
| • Triad: heart failure, angina, syncope | • Crescendo-de-crescendo systolic ejection murmur | • **ECG:** LVH<br>• **Echo:** ↓ aortic valve area and ↑ pressure gradient across valve | • If symptomatic: diuretics, ACEi, digoxin<br>• Surgery is gold-standard |
| **Pericarditis** | | | |
| • Pain: retrosternal sharp and pleuritic chest pain<br>• Worse with cough, inspiration, lying flat<br>• Improved with leaning forward | • Pericardial friction rub | • **ECG:** diffuse ST elevation across all leads (with exception of aVR and V1); T wave inversion | • NSAIDs (1st line) for short period<br>• Colchicine can be added<br>• PPI for gastric protection |

EMERGENCY

| Key Symptoms | Physical Exam Findings | Investigations | Management |
|---|---|---|---|

### Aortic Dissection

| | | | |
|---|---|---|---|
| • Pain: abrupt onset, retrosternal tearing-sensation radiating to back<br><br>• May lead to MI or CVA symptoms<br><br>• Syncope | • Usually ↑ BP but may be ↓ (worse prognosis)<br><br>• BP/pulse differences between right & left<br><br>• Aortic insufficiency murmur<br><br>• Neuro deficits | • **CXR:** widened aortic silhouette (>80% but ~16% will be normal)[5]<br><br>• **ECG:** MI (~1-2%)<br><br>• **CT angio:** gold-standard for diagnosis | • Urgent BP reduction with IV anti-hypertensive<br><br>• STAT consult cardiac surgery (Type A) or vascular surgery (Type B) |

### Pulmonary Embolism

| | | | |
|---|---|---|---|
| • Pain: abrupt onset, sharp and pleuritic<br><br>• Dyspnea<br><br>• Tachypnea<br><br>• Unilateral leg pain and swelling | • Friction rub (rare)<br><br>• Hypoxia | • **ECG:** sinus tachycardia, inverted T waves in precordial leads, new RBBB, S1Q3T3<br><br>• **CT pulmonary angiography**<br><br>• **V/Q scan:** if pregnant<br><br>• **D-dimer:** can R/O PE if negative and low risk | • Anti-coagulation (LMWH or unfractionated heparin) |

### Pneumothorax

| | | | |
|---|---|---|---|
| • Dyspnea<br><br>• Tachycardia | • Absent breath sounds unilaterally<br><br>• Tracheal deviation<br><br>• Shock + ↑ JVP = tension PTX | • **CXR:** absence of peripheral lung markings; mediastinal shift if tension PTX<br><br>• **EDE:** absence of comet tails or lung sliding | • Needle decompression in 2nd interspace midclavicular line<br><br>• Tube thoracostomy |

### Esophgeal Rupture

| | | | |
|---|---|---|---|
| • Pain: sudden onset, retrosternal pain following frequent emesis | • Subcutaneous emphysema<br><br>• Hamman's sign – raspy, crunchy sound on auscultation of precordium | • **CXR:** pneumomediastinum, pleural effusion<br><br>• **Contrast esophagogram** is diagnostic | • Protect airway<br><br>• IV antibiotics and analgesia<br><br>• NG tube<br><br>• Surgical consult |

ACS = acute coronary syndrome, EDE = emergency department echocardiogram, NSTEMI = non-ST segment elevation myocardial infarction, PCI = percutaneous coronary intervention, STEMI = ST segment elevation myocardial infarction, V/Q = ventilation-perfusion

EMERGENCY

## 3.8 Headache

**Table 13.** Selected Causes of Headache

| Key Symptoms | Physical Exam Findings | Investigations | Management |
|---|---|---|---|
| **Increased intracranial pressure** | | | |
| • Pain is worse in morning, with coughing/sneezing | • Papilledema, loss of venous pulsations | • CT or MRI | • Urgent neurosurgery consult |
| **Meningitis** | | | |
| • Fever, N/V | • Meningismus, purpuric rash, decreased LOC | • Lumbar puncture for CSF profile, gram stain, C&S, PCR | • IV antibiotics (do not delay for LP) |
| **Subarachnoid hemorrhage** | | | |
| • Sudden onset 10/10 pain, N/V | • Meningismus, focal neurological deficits, decreased LOC | • CT (90-95% sensitivity), lumbar puncture if CT negative | • Urgent neurosurgery consult |
| **Temporal arteritis (typically age > 50)** | | | |
| • Scalp tenderness, jaw claudication, fever, malaise, myalgia, visual loss/disturbance | • Weight loss | • ESR (elevated >50 mm/h), temporal artery biopsy (definitive) | • High-dose steroids |

**Focused History** (refer to **The Nervous System** Chapter for greating detail)
- **Onset:** acute onset or sudden change in pattern is serious
- **Quality:**
  - ◆ Shooting pain in V1, V2 distribution indicative of trigeminal neuralgia
  - ◆ Steady, band-like pain indicative of tension headaches
- **Timing:** headaches secondary to raised intracranial pressure (ICP) are often worst on awakening (prolonged supine position)
- Nausea and vomiting, myalgia, jaw claudication, scalp tenderness
- Photophobia, phonophobia, aura, vision changes
- Meningeal signs
- History of recent head trauma

**Focused Physical Exam**
- **General:**
  - ◆ Establish stability of patient: evaluate appearance, LOC and responsiveness, vital signs (especially BP and temperature)
  - ◆ Inspection: neurofibromas, café-au-lait spots, cutaneous hemangiomas, purpuric rash
- **Neurologic:**
  - ◆ Neurological exam and fundoscopy: neurological deficits or papilledema are suggestive of intracranial lesion
  - ◆ Meningeal signs
  - ◆ Palpate for scalp tenderness (temporal arteritis) and nuchal line tenderness (occipital neuralgia)
  - ◆ Measure intraocular pressure to rule out glaucoma

## 3.9 Toxicology/Acute Poisonings

Toxidrome: a set of physiologically-based abnormalities (signs and symptoms) that typically occur due to a specific class of substances

**Table 14.** Common Toxidromes

| Toxidrome | Signs and Symptoms |
|---|---|
| **Anticholinergics**<br><br>Antihistamines, antiemetics, antispasmotics, atropine, belladonna, Jimson weed, tricyclic antidepressants | **"Mad as a hatter"**: agitation/hallucinations<br>**"Blind as a bat"**: dilated pupils<br>**"Dry as a bone"**: dry skin<br>**"Hot as a hare"**: fever<br>**"Red as a beet"**: vasodilation<br>**"The bowel and bladder lose their tone and the heart goes on alone"**: ileus, urinary retention, tachycardia |
| **Cholinergics**<br><br>Carbamates<br>Nerve gas<br>Organophosphates (i.e. pesticides) | **DUMBELS**<br>Decreased blood pressure/diaphoresis/defecation<br>Urination<br>Miosis<br>Bradycardia/bronchorrhea/bronchospasm<br>Emesis<br>Lacrimation<br>Salivation/seizures |
| **Sympathomimetics**<br><br>Amphetamines<br>ASA<br>Cocaine<br>LSD<br>PCP<br>Theophyllines<br>Sedative/alcohol withdrawal | CNS excitation<br>Diaphoresis<br>Dilated pupils<br>HTN<br>Increased temperature<br>Nausea/vomiting<br>Tachycardia |
| **Narcotics & Sedatives**<br><br>Opioids<br>GHB<br>Barbiturates<br>Benzodiazepines<br>Ethanol | CNS depression<br>Respiratory depression<br>Hypotension<br>Miosis (narcotics) |

*Note:* other common toxidromes include hallucinogens, and heart-blocking agents (β-blockers, calcium channel blockers, digoxin)

### Focused History
- Time of exposure
- Type of exposure
- Amount/dose of exposure
- Route of exposure: inhalation, ingestion, mucous membrane exposure, cutaneous exposure, or injection
- Intent of poisoning (e.g. suicide)
- History of suicide attempts, suicidal ideation or other psychiatric illness
- In children, focus on potential environmental/household substances

### Focused Physical Exam
- **Vitals:** BP, pulse, RR, $O_2$ saturation, temperature, capillary glucose
- **General:** fever, agitation, confusion, obtundation, somnolence, level of consciousness, sweating, hypothermia, hyperthermia
- **CNS:** seizures, LOC, altered deep tendon reflexes, coordination, cognition, tremor, fasciculations, cranial nerve assessment, slurred speech, psychosis, hallucinations
- **H&N:** eyes (nystagmus, constricted/dilated pupils, pupil reactivity, dysconjugate gaze, excessive lacrimation); oropharynx (hypersalivation, burning in the mouth, excessive dryness)
- **CVS:** assess rhythm, rate, regularity (e.g. arrhythmias, tachycardia, bradycardia)

- **Respiratory:** bronchorrhea, wheezing, pulmonary edema, bronchoconstriction, apnea, pneumothorax, alveolar hemorrhage, hypoventilation, tachypnea
- **GI:** N/V, diarrhea, abdominal tenderness/rigidity, bowel sounds, cramps
- **Derm:** flushing, diaphoresis, dryness, signs of injury/injection, ulcers, bullae, staining, bruising
- **GU:** discolored urine, urinary retention

Management
- Stabilize vital functions: ABCs, appropriate monitoring
- If mental status depressed, administer universal antidotes (**DON'T** mnemonic - **D**extrose, **O**xygen, **N**aloxone, **T**hiamine)
- Obtain history and perform physical exam
- Identify agent(s) and/or toxidromes
- Apply methods to decrease absorption of toxin: decontamination (see **Pharmacology and Toxicology** Chapter)
- Obtain general labs and specific drug identification or levels as indicated, use ancillary tests as needed
- Continuous reevaluation, administer symptomatic and supportive care, correct fluid/electrolyte imbalances
- Perform enhanced metabolism and elimination
- Administer sodium bicarbonate to facilitate elimination of weak acids (i.e. ASA and barbiturates): drug in anionic form becomes "ion trapped" in lumen
- Call poison control in overdose situations as they can often provide invaluable information and suggestions for management
- Tylenol (Acetaminophen) Overdose
    - Most common overdose in the ED
    - Draw plasma acetaminophen levels at least 4 hours after time of ingestion
    - Use the Rumack-Matthew Nomogram (**Figure 4**) to plot acetaminophen plasma level vs. time to determine whether treatment with N-acetyl cysteine (Mucomyst) is warranted
- Hemodialysis to remove chemical (not possible with digoxin)
- Use physiological antagonist or antidotes/chelators (see **Pharmacology and Toxicology** Chapter)

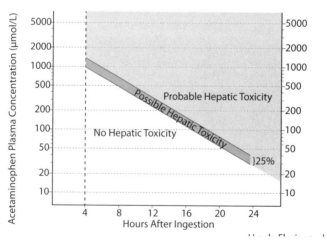

**Figure 4.** Rumack-Matthew Nomogram

REFERENCES
1. Stiell IG, Wells GA, Vandemheen K, et al. The Canadian CT Head Rule for patients with minor head injury. Lancet. 2001; 357(9266): 1391-1396.
2. Becker JA, Stewart LK. Heat-related illness. Am Fam Physician. 2011; 83(11): 1325-1330.
3. Petrone P, Asensio JA, Marini CP. Management of accidental hypothermia and cold injury. Curr Probl Surg. 2014; 51(10): 417-431
4. Cartotto RC, Innes M, Musgrave MA, Gomez M, Cooper AB. How well does the Parkland formula estimate actual fluid resuscitation volumes? J Burn Care Rehabil. 2002; 23(4): 258-265.
5. Hagan PG, Nienaber CA, Isselbacher EM, et al. The international registry of acute aortic dissection (IRAD): New insights into an old disease. JAMA. 2000; 283(7): 897-903.

# CHAPTER 14:

# Fluids, Electrolytes, and Acid/Base Disturbances

**Editors:**
Waleed S. Ahmed, BHSc
Taraneh Tofighi, BHSc

**Faculty Reviewers:**
Martin Schreiber, MD, MMedEd, FRCPC
Gemini Tanna, MD, FRCPC

## TABLE OF CONTENTS

FLUIDS

# 1. VOLUME STATUS

## 1.1 Clinical Features of Volume Overload
- Symptoms
  - Pulmonary edema: shortness of breath on exertion, paroxysmal nocturnal dyspnea, orthopnea
  - Peripheral edema: swelling of ankles (especially at the end of the day), hands (rings feel tight), and around the eyes; recent weight gain
- Signs
  - Vital Signs: hypertension
  - Pulmonary: edema (bibasilar crackles on auscultation) or pleural effusion
  - Peripheral: ankle edema (in ambulatory patients), sacral edema (in bed-ridden patients); evidence of ascites; elevated JVP with abdominojugular reflex

## 1.2 Clinical Features of Volume Depletion
- History
  - Excessive fluid loss
  - GI: vomiting, diarrhea
  - Renal: diuretics, polyuria
  - Skin: excessive sweating (fever, exercise, hyperthermia), burns
  - Hematologic: blood loss
  - Neurologic: altered mental status leading to reduced intake
- Symptoms
  - Recent weight loss
  - Excessive thirst
  - Postural dizziness
  - Fatigue
  - Weakness
  - Cramps
- Signs
  - Vital Signs:
    - Resting supine tachycardia and hypotension
    - Orthostatic tachycardia (rise in HR >30 from supine to standing)
    - Orthostatic hypotension (fall in systolic BP >20 on standing, or any fall in diastolic BP). This has been summarized as the 30-20-10 rule: rise in HR >30, fall in sBP >20, and fall in dBP >10
  - Low JVP
  - Dry mucous membranes
  - Dry axilla
  - Oliguria or anuria
  - In infants: Soft fontanelles, reduced skin turgor, dry cry, dry diaper (in newborns)

**Clinical Pearl: Hypovolemia[1]**
The finding of dry axilla has a LR+ of 2.8 and a LR- of 0.6 while the finding of orthostatic tachycardia has a LR+ of 1.7 and a LR- of 0.8.

## 2. DISORDERS OF SODIUM CONCENTRATION

**Table 1.** Overview of hyponatremia and hypernatremia

| Key Signs and Symptoms | Physical Exam Maneuvers | Investigations | Management |
|---|---|---|---|
| **Hyponatremia - Serum sodium < 135 mM**<br>Details in Section 2.1 | | | |
| Slow onset:<br>• Often asymptomatic<br>• Nausea<br>• Anorexia<br>• Malaise<br><br>Rapid onset:<br>• Headache<br>• Lethargy<br>• Decreased LOC<br>• Seizures<br>• Can be fatal | Vital Signs<br>• HR, BP<br>• Orthostatic signs<br><br>Volume status<br>• Signs of edema<br>• Volume depletion | • Serum Na$^+$<br>• Serum osmolality<br>• Urine Na$^+$<br>• Urine osmolality | • Treat underlying cause<br>• Water restrict<br>• IV NaCl 3% (if patient has severe symptoms)<br>• Correct Na levels slowly to avoid complications |
| **Hypernatremia - Serum sodium > 145 mM**<br>Details in Section 2.2 | | | |
| • Mild symptoms<br>• Weakness<br>• Lethargy<br>• Irritability<br>• Confusion<br>• Intracerebral hemorrhage<br>• Seizures<br>• Coma<br>• Can be fatal | • ECF volume status<br>• JVP | • Serum electrolytes<br>• Creatinine<br>• Urea<br>• Glucose<br><br>If hypovolemic:<br>• Urine Na$^+$<br>• Urine osmolality<br><br>If euvolemic:<br>• Urine osmolality | Hypovolemic<br>• IV normal saline<br>• Free water by mouth or hypotonic fluid<br><br>Hypervolemic<br>• Loop diuretic<br>Dialysis |

### 2.1 Hyponatremia

### Clinical Features
- Symptoms: vary depending on severity and speed of onset
  - Mild hyponatremia manifests with slow, gradual onset:
    - Often asymptomatic (due to compensation)
    - Nausea, anorexia, malaise
  - Severe hyponatremia may present acutely
    - More likely symptomatic as water enters cells, and there is no time for compensation
    - Headache, lethargy, decreased LOC
    - Seizures and death may occur due to cerebral edema

FLUIDS

## Classification and Causes

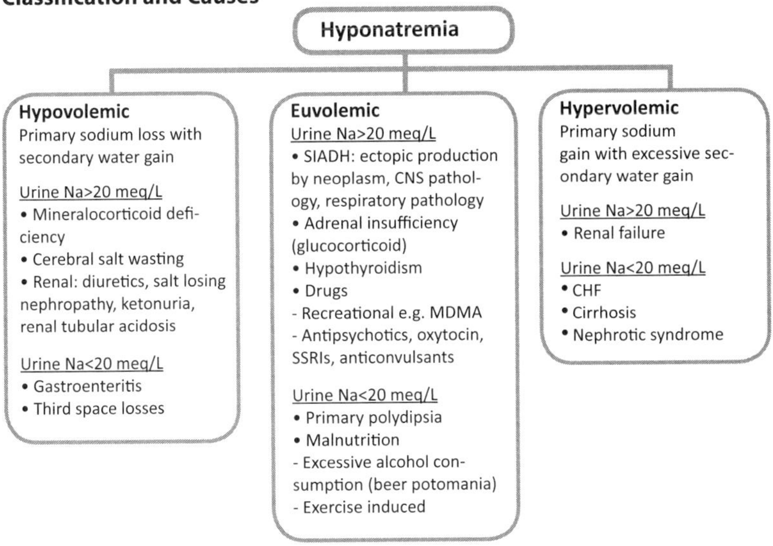

**Figure 1.** Classification and Causes of Hyponatremia
SIADH = syndrome of inappropriate antidiuretic hormone secretion

## Other Classifications
- Pseudohyponatremia: Serum [Na+] appears falsely lowered
  - Normal osmolality: An increase in lipids or proteins falsely lowers [Na+]
    - Hyperlipidemia
    - Hyperproteinemia
  - Increased plasma osmolality: Excess water in plasma dilutes [Na+]
    - Hyperglycemia
    - Hypermannitolemia

## Investigations
- Assess volume status (HR, BP, signs of edema or volume depletion)
- Measure serum sodium, osmolality
- Measure urine sodium, osmolality

## Management
- Warning: Monitor serum sodium and urine osmolality to ensure that chronic hyponatremia is not corrected too rapidly (serum [Na+] should never increase more than 8 mM/d in patients with chronic hyponatremia)
- For <u>acute, symptomatic hyponatremia</u> (seizures, coma) treat with intravenous 3% NaCl until symptoms stop. Aim to correct [Na+] by 3-5% in the first few hours
- For <u>chronic, symptomatic hyponatremia</u>, aim to correct [Na+] by 4-6 mM in first several h and not more than 8 mM in the first 24 h

## 2.2 Hypernatremia
- Symptoms: mild unless thirst mechanism is defective or water access is restricted
  - Weakness, lethargy, irritability, confusion
  - Intracerebral hemorrhage, seizures, coma, and death if severe

## Classification and Causes

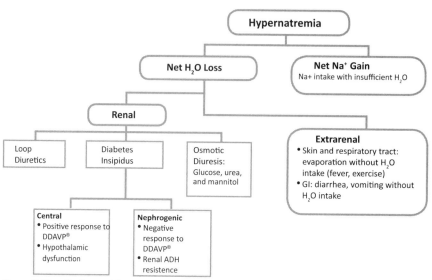

**Figure 2.** Classification and Causes of Hypernatremia
ADH = antidiuretic hormone, DDAVP = desmopressin

## Investigations
- If hypovolemic:
  - Check urine osmolality (UOsm) and sodium (UNa)
    - Renal loss: UOsm 300-600 and UNa >20
    - Nonrenal loss: UOsm >600 and UNa <20
- If euvolemic:
  - Check UOsm
    - UOsm <300 suggests diabetes insipidus

## Management
- **Hypovolemic Hypernatremia**
  - If evidence of hemodynamic instability, correct with bolus of NS:
    - Calculate free water deficit and replace with water PO/NG or IV hypotonic infusates (maximum 12 mM decrease of [Na$^+$] over 24 h)
    - Free H$_2$O deficit = [Total body water (TBW) x (serum [Na$^+$] -140)] / 140
- **Hypervolemic Hypernatremia**
  - Loop diuretic (or dialysis if renal failure):
    - Replace water deficit with 5% dextrose in water (D5W)

FLUIDS

# 3. DISORDERS OF POTASSIUM CONCENTRATION

**Table 2.** Overview of hypokalemia and hyperkalemia

| Key Signs and Symptoms | Physical Exam Maneuvers | Investigations | Management |
|---|---|---|---|
| **Hypokalemia - Serum potassium < 3.5 mM** <br> Details in Section 3.1 | | | |
| Skeletal muscle: <br> • Fatigue <br> • Myalgia <br> • Cramps <br> • Weakness <br><br> Heart: <br> • Arrhythmia <br> (tachycardias) | • Vital Signs <br> • Muscle power <br> • Cardiac exam <br><br> • May be within normal ranges | • Serum $K^+$ <br> • ECG <br> • Blood glucose <br> • 24 h urine $K^+$ excretion (UK) <br> • Urine $[K^+]$ <br> • Urine $[Cr]$ <br> • ABGs <br> • Plasma renin, aldosterone, $Mg^{2+}$ | • Treat underlying cause <br><br> • KCl <br><br> • Avoid dextrose-containing fluids and insulin |
| **Hyperkalemia - Serum potassium > 5 mM** <br> Life threatening when serum potassium > 7 mM <br> Details in Section 3.2 | | | |
| • Asymptomatic when mild <br><br> Skeletal muscle: <br> • Weakness <br> • Stiffness <br><br> Cardiac <br> • Arrhythmias <br> (bradycardias) | • Vital Signs <br> • Muscle power <br> • Cardiac exam <br><br> • May be within normal ranges | • Serum $K^+$ <br> • ECG <br> • Estimate GFR <br> • Urine $[K^+]$ <br> • Urine $[Cr]$ | <u>3 Principles:</u> <br> • Protect the heart (Ca gluconate) <br><br> • Shift $K^+$ into cells (insulin, $\beta_2$ agonists e.g. salbutamol) <br><br> • Promote excretion (diuretics, cation exchange resins, dialysis) |

## 3.1 Hypokalemia

## Clinical Features
- Symptoms
  - Skeletal muscle: fatigue, myalgia, cramps, weakness
- Signs
  - Metabolic alkalosis
  - Cardiac: arrhythmia (ventricular premature beats [VPBs], ventricular tachycardia)
  - ECG changes: flattened T waves, premature ventricular beats, prolonged QT interval, U waves

## Classification and Causes

```
                          ┌─────────────────────┐
                          │     Hypokalemia     │
                          └─────────────────────┘
```

**Redistribution Into Cells**
- Insulin, metabolic alkalosis, exogenous catecholamines (salbutamol at very high doses), thyrotoxic periodic paralysis, vitamin B12 treatment of pernicious anemia

**Increased Losses**
- GI: diarrhea, bowel obstruction, ileus
- Skin: sweating
- Renal: increased distal flow (non-K+ sparing diuretics, osmotic diuresis), increased potassium secretion (vomiting with bicarbonate), increased mineralocorticoid activity, diabetic ketoacidosis, hypomagnesemia

**Decreased Potassium Intake**
(contributory rather than causative)

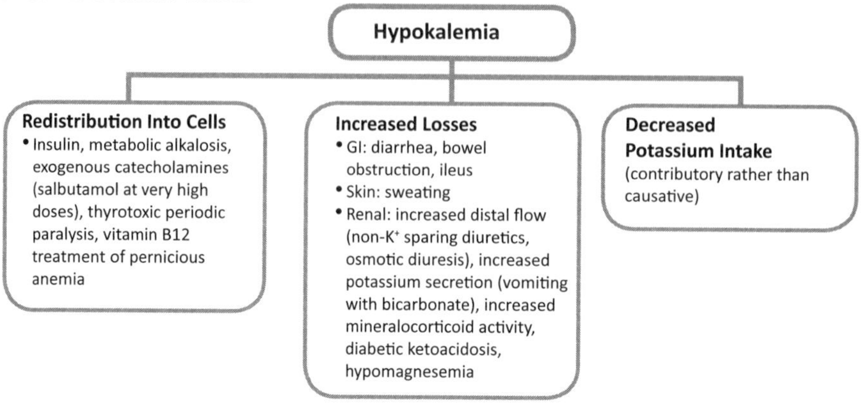

**Figure 3.** Classification and Causes of Hypokalemia

### Investigations
- Rule out shift into cells (check blood glucose to see if insulin is low)
- 24 h urine K+ excretion (UK)
    - UK <20 mEq/d suggests extrarenal loss
    - UK >40 mEq/d suggests renal loss
- Urine [K+] / Urine [Cr]
    - Ratio > 1.5 suggests a renal problem is contributing to hypokalemia
- Assess serum renin, aldosterone, and [$Mg^{2+}$]

### Management
- ECG should be checked if potassium level <3.0 mM
- Treat underlying cause (if fluid repletion needed, avoid dextrose-containing solutions since dextrose raises insulin and drives an intracellular potassium shift)
- Mild-moderate hypokalemia:
    - KCl (40 mEq) PO BID for 2 days and then repeat K+
- Severe hypokalemia or patient not able to take oral therapy:
    - Maximum IV [KCl] is 40 mEq/L in peripheral veins or 60 mEq/L in central lines

## 3.2 Hyperkalemia

### Clinical Features
- Symptoms: none if mild
    - Skeletal muscle: weakness, stiffness
- Signs
    - Cardiac: arrhythmia (sinus bradycardia, heart block, asystole, junctional rhythms, etc.)
    - ECG changes (if severe): peaked T waves, widened QRS, small/absent P waves, "sine wave", asystole

## Classification and Causes

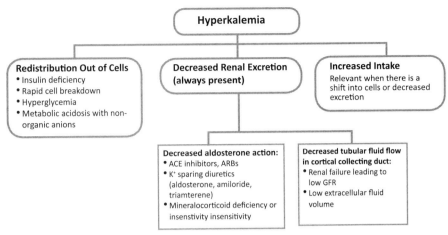

**Figure 4.** Classification and Causes of Hyperkalemia
ARBs = angiotensin receptor blockers, GFR = glomerular filtration rate

### Specific Physical Findings Depending on Cause of Hyperkalemia
- If patient is hypovolemic or euvolemic consider these possibilities:
    - Decreased renal function and decreased potassium secretion
    - Decreased mineralocorticoid level
        - Addison's Disease
        - Mineralocorticoid resistance
        - Aldosterone blockers (spironolactone), blockage of Na+ channel in cortical collecting duct (amiloride, trimethoprim, triamterene), other medications (ACE inhibitors, ARBs, direct renin inhibitor [DRI])
- If patient is hypervolemic, consider these possibilities:
    - Due to enhanced chloride absorption in cortical collecting duct (and therefore reduced intraluminal negative charge to attract potassium secretion)
    - Gordon's syndrome (rare)
    - Calcineurin toxicity (i.e. cyclosporine, tacrolimus)
    - Hyporeninemic hypoaldosteronism of diabetes

### Investigations
- Rule out factitious hyperkalemia (e.g. hemolysis during venipuncture)
- Check to make sure that if receiving IVF, there is no KCl in fluid
    - Rule out shift of $K^+$ out of cells
    - Estimate glomerular filtration rate (GFR)
    - Measure urine $[K^+]$ and urine [creatinine]; if ratio of urine $[K^+]$/[Creatinine] is <3-4, impaired renal excretion of $K^+$ may be contributing to hyperkalemia

### Management
- Emergent reaction if symptoms, ECG changes, or serum $[K^+]$ >6.5 mEq
- Tailor response to severity of increase in $K^+$ and ECG changes

**Table 3.** Treatment of Hyperkalemia

| Principle | Intervention | Onset | Dose |
|---|---|---|---|
| **Protect heart** | Calcium Gluconate | mins | 1-2 amps (10 mL of 10% solution) IV |

| Principle | Intervention | Onset | Dose |
|-----------|-------------|-------|------|
| **Shift K+ into cells** | Insulin | 15-30 min | 1 amp D50W IV then 10-20 units insulin R IV |
| | Bicarbonate | 15-30 min | 1-3 amps IV |
| | β2-agonists | 30-90 min | Salbutamol: 10 mg inhaled |
| **Promote excretion** | Diuretics (urinary excretion) | 30 min | ≥40 mg furosemide IV ± IV NS to prevent hypovolemia |
| | Cation-Exchange Resins (gut excretion) | 1-2 h, not for acute cases | Sodium polystyrene sulfonate 15-30 g; needs to be given with laxative – avoid sorbitol due to risk of intestinal necrosis; likely limited benefit |
| | Dialysis | | |

## 4. DISORDERS OF CALCIUM CONCENTRATION

**Table 4.** Overview of hypocalcemia and hypercalcemia[2]

| Key Signs and Symptoms | Physical Exam Maneuvers | Investigations | Management |
|---|---|---|---|
| **Hypocalcemia - Total serum Ca$^{2+}$ <2.2 mM** Details in Section 4.1 | | | |
| Acute: • Paresthesias • Hyperreflexia • Tetany • Seizures  Chronic: • Parkinsonism • Dementia | • Neurological Exam » Sensory » Reflexes • Other Signs » Chvostek's » Trousseau | • Serum ionized Ca$^{2+}$ • PO$_4^{3-}$ • Mg$^{2+}$ • Creatinine • PTH | Treat underlying cause  • Acute: » Oral Ca » IV Ca gluconate  • Chronic: » Calcium and Vitamin D PO |
| **Hypercalcemia - Total serum Ca$^{2+}$ >2.6 mM** Details in Section 4.2 | | | |
| • "Bones, stones, abdominal groans, mental overtones" » Bone pain, renal colic, abdominal pain, altered LOC | • Vital Signs (HTN) • Neurological exam » Tone • Volume status | • PTH, PTHrP • PO$_4^{3-}$, HCO$_3^-$ • Albumin, ALP • Globulin, serum free light chains • Radiographic imaging | Treat underlying cause  • Saline to restore ECFV • Bisphosphonates • Calcitonin SC |

- Calcium (Ca$^{2+}$) Measurement
  - Total serum calcium includes calcium bound to albumin and free calcium (aka ionized calcium)
  - Ionized calcium is the most physiologically relevant, but measurement is difficult and can be compromised by exposure to air and the presence of anticoagulants in the tube
  - Adjusting the total serum Ca$^{2+}$ for the albumin level is the intermediate choice

> **Clinical Pearl: Correcting Calcium in a patient with hypoalbuminemia[3]**
> Rule of thumb: add 0.2 mM $Ca^{2+}$ for every 10 g/L albumin drop.

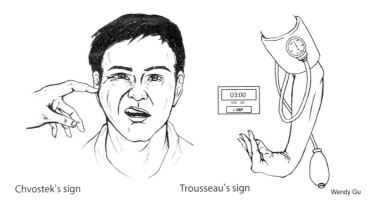

Chvostek's sign       Trousseau's sign

Wendy Gu

**Figure 5.** Chvostek's and Trousseau's Signs

## 4.1 Hypocalcemia

### Clinical Features
- Symptoms
    - Acute, mild hypocalcemia: paresthesias, hyperreflexia
    - Acute, severe hypocalcemia: tetany, confusion, seizures, laryngospasm, bronchospasm
    - Chronic hypocalcemia: parkinsonism, dementia, cataracts, abnormal dentition, dry skin
- Signs
    - Chvostek's sign
        - Facial spasm when facial nerve or branch is tapped
    - Trousseau's sign
        - Carpal spasm induced with arterial occlusion using a BP cuff (1-3 min above systolic on the forearm)
    - Papilledema
    - ECG: prolonged QT interval

### Classification and Causes
*Associated with Low PTH Levels (Hypoparathyroidism)*
- Genetic disorders
- Surgical removal of parathyroid glands
- Autoimmune hypoparathyroidism
- Hypomagnesemia

*Associated with Elevated PTH Levels (Secondary Hyperparathyroidism)*
- Deficiency of vitamin D
- Renal failure (low calcitriol levels)
- Malabsorption syndromes
- Drugs: phosphate, calcitonin, aminoglycosides
- Shift out of circulation: sepsis, osteoblastic metastases, pancreatitis, post-parathyroidectomy (hungry bone syndrome)
- Respiratory alkalosis (total calcium level is normal, but a greater fraction is bound to albumin, so ionized fraction falls)
- Hyperphosphatemia
- Hypoalbuminemia (ionized calcium will be normal)

FLUIDS

## Investigations
- Measure serum ionized calcium, phosphate, magnesium, creatinine, and PTH
- Serum phosphorus usually elevated except in hypocalcemia from vitamin D deficiency
- Serum PTH usually elevated except in hypoparathyroidism and magnesium deficiency

## Management
- Treat underlying cause
- Do not treat hypocalcemia if suspected to be transient response
- Mild/asymptomatic
  - Oral $Ca^{2+}$ 1000-2000 mg/d (of elemental $Ca^{2+}$)
- Acute/symptomatic
  - Calcium gluconate: 1 g IV over 10 min ± slow infusion (10 g in 1000 mL D5W over 10 h)
  - Check serum $Ca^{2+}$ q4-6h
  - If hypomagnesemia present, must be treated to correct hypocalcemia
- If parathyroid hormone (PTH) recovery not expected (e.g. hypoparathyroidism), treat with vitamin D and calcium long-term (use calcitriol for vitamin D replacement if patients have hypoparathyroidism or renal failure)

## 4.2 Hypercalcemia

### Clinical Features
- Symptoms
  - "Bones, stones, abdominal groans with mental overtones"
    - Skeleton "bones": bone pain/myalgia
    - Renal "stones": renal colic, polyuria, polydipsia
    - "Abdominal groans": N/V, anorexia, constipation, pancreatitis, peptic ulcer disease
    - "Mental overtones": cognitive changes, decreased level of consciousness
- Signs
  - Hypotonia, HTN
  - Evidence of dehydration, may lead to acute kidney injury (AKI)
  - ECG: shortened QT interval

### Classification and Causes
- Parathyroid hormone
  - Primary hyperparathyroidism
  - Tertiary hyperparathyroidism of renal failure
- Malignancy
  - Humoral hypercalcemia of malignancy (paraneoplastic parathyroid hormone related peptide [PTHrP])
  - Squamous cell carcinoma (lung), renal carcinoma, bladder carcinoma, breast cancer, leukemia
  - Solid tumors causing local bone resorption
  - Hematologic malignancy (e.g. multiple myeloma)
- Vitamin D elevation (sarcoidosis, TB or exogenous)
- Drugs: thiazides, lithium, calcium carbonate (milk alkali syndrome)
- Familial hypocalciuric hypercalcemia, Addison's disease, hyperthyroidism

### Investigations
- Intact PTH is first step in work-up
- Further investigations: phosphate, bicarbonate, PTHrP, albumin, globulin, ALP, serum free light chains, radiographic imaging

**Clinical Pearl: Causes of Hypercalcemia[2]**
90% of cases of hypercalcemia are caused by primary hyperparathyroidism or malignancy.

FLUIDS

## Management
- Treat underlying cause
- Normal saline to restore extracellular fluid volume
- Use furosemide if, and only if, extracellular fluid volume overload develops
- Bisphosphonates (e.g. pamidronate) for hypercalcemia of malignancy
- If emergency situation, can use calcitonin subcutaneously
- In primary hyperparathyroidism, symptomatic patients and some asymptomatic ones should be referred for parathyroidectomy or cinacalcet management (if not surgical candidates)

# 5. DISORDERS OF PHOSPHATE CONCENTRATION

**Table 5.** Overview of hypophosphatemia and hyperphosphatemia[3]

| Key Signs and Symptoms | Physical Exam Maneuvers | Investigations | Management |
|---|---|---|---|
| **Hypophosphatemia - Serum phosphate <0.84 mM**<br>Details in Section 5.1 | | | |
| • Typically asymptomatic<br>• Proximal muscle weakness<br>• CNS<br>&raquo; Paresthesia<br>&raquo; Seizures<br>&raquo; Delirium<br>&raquo; Coma | • Vital Signs<br>• Muscle power<br>• Cardiac exam<br>• Respiratory exam<br>• Neurological exam<br>• May be within normal ranges | • Serum phosphate<br>• Serum PTH<br>• Urine phosphate | Treat underlying cause<br><br>Chronic cases:<br>• Oral phosphate supplement for chronic cases<br><br>Acute/symptomatic cases:<br>• IV potassium phosphate or sodium phosphate |
| **Hyperphosphatemia - Serum phosphate >1.8 mM**<br>Details in Section 5.2 | | | |
| • Ectopic soft tissue calcification<br>• Clinical features of hypocalcemia | • Clinical features of hypocalcemia | • Serum phosphate<br>• Serum PTH<br>• Urine phosphate | Treat underlying cause, restrict diet phosphate<br><br>• Oral phosphate binders in Stage 3-4 chronic kidney disease (CKD): calcium carbonate, calcium acetate, lanthanum, or sevelamer given with meals |

## 5.1 Hypophosphatemia

### Classification and Causes
- Decreased intestinal absorption
  - Poor intake
  - Aluminum- or magnesium-containing antacids
  - Fat malabsorption
  - Vitamin D deficit
- Excessive renal excretion of phosphate (tends to be chronic)
  - Hyperparathyroidism
  - Fanconi syndrome
- Rapid shift of phosphate from extracellular fluid to bone or soft tissue
  - Insulin (either exogenous [treatment of diabetic ketoacidosis] or endogenous

[refeeding in patients with severe malnutrition])
- ◆ Acute respiratory alkalosis
- ◆ Hungry bone syndrome

## 5.2 Hyperphosphatemia

### Classification and Causes
- • Increased intake
  - ◆ Phosphate-containing laxatives
- • Decreased output
  - ◆ Renal failure
  - ◆ Hypoparathyroidism
- • Shift of phosphate out of cells
  - ◆ Massive cell death (rhabdomyolysis, tumor lysis, hemolysis)
  - ◆ Respiratory acidosis

# 6. DISORDERS OF MAGNESIUM CONCENTRATION

**Table 6.** Overview of hypomagnesemia and hypermagnesemia[3]

| Key Signs and Symptoms | Physical Exam Maneuvers | Investigations | Management |
|---|---|---|---|
| **Hypomagnesaemia - Serum Mg$^{2+}$ <0.7 mM** Details in section 6.1 | | | |
| • Muscle cramps<br>• CNS<br>  » Apathy<br>  » Depression<br>  » Delirium<br>  » Paresthesias<br>• Seizure<br>• Arrhythmias | • Vital signs<br>• Muscle power<br>• Cardiac exam<br>• Neuro exam<br>  » Reflexes | • Measure 24 h urine Mg$^{2+}$ excretion (>2 meq/d indicates excessive renal loss)<br>• Normal serum Mg$^{2+}$ does not exclude total body Mg$^{2+}$ deficiency | Mild/chronic<br>• Oral magnesium oxide or magnesium lactate<br><br>Severe symptomatic<br>• 1-2 g magnesium sulphate IV over 15 min followed by infusion of 6 g in ≥1 L over 24 h, repeated over 7 d to replete Mg$^{2+}$ stores |
| **Hypermagnesaemia - Serum Mg$^{2+}$ >1.2 mM** Details in section 6.2 | | | |
| • Mild:<br>  » N/V<br>  » Skin flushing<br>  » Bradycardia<br>• Moderate:<br>  » Weakness<br>  » Somnolence<br>• Severe:<br>  » Muscle paralysis<br>  » Coma | • Vital signs<br>• Muscle power<br>• Cardiac exam<br>• Respiratory exam<br>• Neuro exam<br>  » Reflexes | • Measure serum Mg$^{2+}$<br>• Assess kidney function (creatinine, urea) | Asymptomatic<br>• Stop magnesium-containing products<br><br>Severe symptomatic:<br>• 1-2 g calcium gluconate IV over 10 min (plus dialysis in severe renal failure) |

## 6.1 Hypomagnesemia

### Classification and Causes
- • Decreased intake
  - ◆ Malabsorption/malnutrition
- • Increased losses
  - ◆ Renal
    - ▪ Diuretics (thiazide, furosemide)
    - ▪ Alcohol

- Nephrotoxic drugs (amphotericin, cisplatin, cyclosporine)
- Rare inherited renal tubular disorders (Bartter syndrome, Gitelman syndrome)
- Diarrhea

### 6.2 Hypermagnesemia

#### Classification and Causes
- Increased intake
  - Iatrogenic (most commonly in setting of treatment of preeclampsia)
- Decreased output
  - Renal failure (most common cause)

## 7. DISORDERS OF ACID-BASE BALANCE
Information required to evaluate the status of a patient with an acid-base disturbance:
- Arterial blood gases (for ABG see **The Respiratory System** Chapter)
- Plasma anion gap (see below)
- Clinical evaluation of respiration

Table 7. Normal ABG Values

| Normal ABG Values | |
|---|---|
| **pH** | 7.35-7.45 |
| **pCO$_2$** | 35-45 mmHg |
| **pO$_2$** | 80-100 mmHg |
| **HCO$_3$-** | 22-28 mM |

### 7.1 Respiratory Acidosis
- Pathophysiology: hypoventilation leads to accumulation of $CO_2$ from metabolism, which lowers the pH of body fluids

#### Common Causes
- COPD or any severe lung disease associated with excessive work of breathing can eventually lead to respiratory muscle fatigue and hypoventilation
- Drugs (excess amounts of opioids, benzodiazepines, sedating antihistamines, tricyclic antidepressants, barbiturates, anesthetics) or other causes of decreased LOC, hypothyroidism
- Problem with respiratory muscles or chest wall (e.g. nerve problem such as Guillain-Barré syndrome; neuromuscular junction disorder such as myasthenia gravis; severe chest wall abnormality such as kyphoscoliosis)

#### Normal Compensation
- Increased levels of bicarbonate raises the pH and buffers against respiratory acidosis
- Acute: bicarbonate increases 1 mM for every 10 mmHg increase in pCO$_2$
- Chronic (after 2-3 d): the kidney increases rate of production of new bicarbonate, resulting in a rise of 3 mM for every 10 mmHg increase in pCO$_2$

Table 8. Compensation in respiratory acidosis

| Condition | Primary Change | Expected Compensation |
|---|---|---|
| **Acute respiratory acidosis** | Increased P$_{CO2}$ | Increased HCO$_3$- = 0.1 x Δ P$_{CO2}$ |
| **Chronic respiratory acidosis** | Increased P$_{CO2}$ | Increased HCO$_3$- = 0.3 x Δ P$_{CO2}$ |

### 7.2 Respiratory Alkalosis
- Pathophysiology: hyperventilation lowers pCO$_2$ and thereby raises pH of body fluids

FLUIDS

## Common Causes

- Any lung disease tends to cause hyperventilation and therefore respiratory alkalosis, provided work of breathing not so great that patient develops respiratory muscle fatigue (e.g. pneumonia, pulmonary embolism, asthma, pulmonary fibrosis, pulmonary edema)
- Sepsis
- Pregnancy
- Liver failure
- ASA overdose

## Normal Compensation

- Decreased levels of bicarbonate lowers the pH and buffers against respiratory alkalosis
- Acute: bicarbonate decreases 2 mM for every 10 mmHg decrease in $pCO_2$
- Chronic: the kidney reduces bicarbonate production, resulting in a drop of 5 mM for every 10 mmHg decrease in $pCO_2$

**Table 9.** Compensation in respiratory alkalosis

| Condition | Primary Change | Expected Compensation |
|---|---|---|
| **Acute respiratory alkalosis** | Decreased $P_{CO2}$ | Decreased $HCO_3^- = 0.2 \times \Delta P_{CO2}$ |
| **Chronic respiratory alkalosis** | Decreased $P_{CO2}$ | Decreased $HCO_3^- = 0.5 \times \Delta P_{CO2}$ |

## 7.3 Metabolic Acidosis

- Pathophysiology: reduction in ECF bicarbonate concentration results in a lower pH
  - This can be caused directly by the addition of $H^+$ (which binds to bicarbonate to reduce the concentration), loss of bicarbonate from the body, or the failure of the kidneys to produce bicarbonate at the usual rate
  - Use plasma anion gap to help determine etiology

## Plasma Anion Gap (PAG)

- $PAG = Na^+ - (HCO_3^- + Cl^-)$, normal value is 12 (range 10-14)
- Proportional to albumin concentration
- If the compound that caused the acidosis contributes an anion, this will be reflected in an increased PAG because the newly ingested substance dissociates into H+ and an anion in the body; this new $H^+$ is buffered by $HCO_3^-$ and is now reflected in the above formula as a lower amount of $HCO_3^-$, thus elevating the PAG
- In a pure increased anion gap acidosis, the drop in bicarbonate closely matches the increase in PAG
- If the drop in bicarbonate is significantly greater than the increase in PAG, then there is both an increased anion gap type of metabolic acidosis and also a normal anion gap type of acidosis
- If the drop in bicarbonate is significantly less than the increase in PAG, then there is both an increased anion gap type of metabolic acidosis and also a metabolic alkalosis

## Common Causes of Increased PAG Metabolic Acidosis: MUDPILES

- **M**ethanol
- **U**remia
- **D**iabetic ketoacidosis
- **P**araldehyde or Propylene glycol (in car radiator fluid)
- **I**soniazid
- **L**actic acidosis
- **E**thylene glycol
- **S**alicylates

## Common Causes of Non-Anion Gap Metabolic Acidosis

- Diarrhea
- Mild to moderate renal failure
- Renal tubular acidosis
- Mineralocorticoid deficiency

FLUIDS

## Normal Compensation
- Hyperventilation should decrease the $pCO_2$ (in mmHg) by the same amount as the decrease in bicarbonate (in mM)
- Kussmaul's breathing: respiratory compensation (i.e. hyperventilation) for metabolic acidosis may be clinically detectable in terms of deep and perhaps rapid breathing

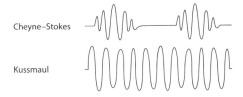

Cheyne–Stokes

Kussmaul

**Figure 6.** Cheyne-Stokes and Kussmaul Respirations

## 7.4 Metabolic Alkalosis
- Pathophysiology: a rise in pH due to an increase in ECF bicarbonate secondary to:
  - Exogenous source
  - Stomach production from emesis
  - Renal overproduction, most commonly caused by hypokalemia
- Under normal conditions, the kidneys excrete the extra bicarbonate, which corrects the elevated bicarbonate levels, thus preventing metabolic alkalosis
  - During volume and/or potassium depletion, the kidneys retain the extra bicarbonate and thus cause metabolic alkalosis

## Common Causes
- Diuretics
- Vomiting
- Excess mineralocorticoid activity

## Normal Compensation
- Hypoventilation with a variable increase in $pCO_2$ (range is 3-8 mmHg for each 10 mM rise in bicarbonate level)

## Summary: Approach to Evaluating Acid-Base Disorders[5]
1. Assess pH – is it acidemic or alkalemic?
2. Determine primary acid-base disorder
   - If pH is acidemic, then there is either metabolic acidosis (reflected by low $HCO_3^-$ level) or respiratory acidosis (reflected by high $pCO_2$)
   - If pH is alkalemic, then there is either metabolic alkalosis (reflected by high $HCO_3^-$ level) or respiratory alkalosis (reflected by low $pCO_2$)
   - If pH is normal, then the patient either has no abnormalities, or has two abnormalities that happen to balance each other (e.g. metabolic acidosis and respiratory alkalosis)
3. Determine compensation
   - If primary disorder is metabolic acidosis, then for compensation expect to observe hyperventilation leading to a fall in $pCO_2$
   - If primary disorder is respiratory acidosis, then for compensation expect to observe increase in $HCO_3^-$ level
   - If primary disorder is metabolic alkalosis, then for compensation expect to observe hypoventilation leading to rise in $pCO_2$
   - If primary disorder is respiratory alkalosis, then for compensation expect to observe decrease in $HCO_3^-$ level
4. Always calculate PAG
   - $PAG = Na^+ - (HCO_3^- + Cl^-)$
   - Any changes in PAG should be compared to $HCO_3^-$ changes to evaluate any additional acid/base disturbances at play
5. Calculate osmolar gap (OG) to detect toxic alcohol
   - OG = Osmolarity(measured) – Osmolarity(calculated)

FLUIDS

**Figure 7.** Algorithm for Evaluation of Acid-Base Status

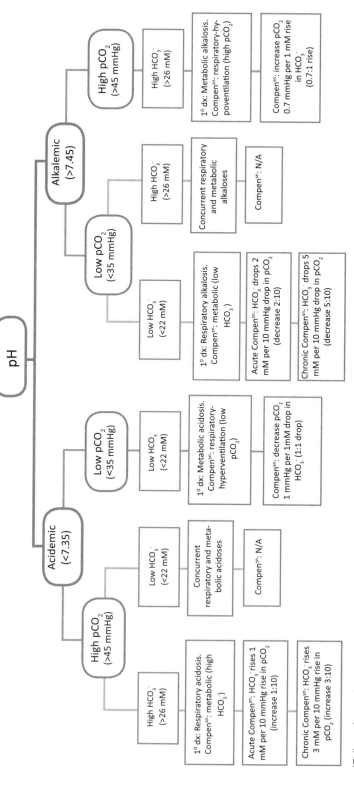

*Failure of normal compensation or overcompensation indicates the presence of a second acid-base disturbance. For example, a patient with a bicarbonate of 10 mM (i.e. a drop of 15) with a $pCO_2$ of 35 (i.e. a drop of only 5) would represent a combined metabolic and respiratory acidosis – manifested by a failure to reach normal compensation for the metabolic acidosis. When comparing changes in $pCO_2$ and $HCO_3^-$ levels, use middle values of normal ranges: for $pCO_2$, 40 mmHg; for $HCO_3^-$ level, 24 mM.

> **Clinical Pearl: Acidosis vs Acidemia (or alkalosis vs alkalemia)**
>
> Acidemia/alkalemia refer to whether the pH of the plasma is low/high. In contrast, acidosis/alkalosis refer to the kind of process which leads to changes in pH.
>
> For example, an acidosis is a process which leads to a rise in [H+], i.e., a fall in pH, i.e., an acidemia. An alkalosis is a process which leads to a fall in [H+], i.e., a rise in pH, i.e., an alkalemia.

## 8. INTRAVENOUS FLUIDS AND DIURETICS

Table 10. Commonly Used IV Solutions (Crystalloids)

| Fluid | Components | Tonicity | Indications |
|---|---|---|---|
| **D5W (5% dextrose in water)** | 50 g/L Dextrose | Hypotonic (100% free water) | • Hypernatremia |
| **0.9% NaCl (Normal Saline [NS])** | 154 mM Na<br>154 mM Cl | Isotonic | • Fluid resuscitation<br>• Fluid maintenance<br>• Large volumes can cause hyperchloremic non-anion gap metabolic acidosis |
| **0.45% NaCl (½ NS)** | 77 mM Na<br>77 mM Cl | Hypotonic (50% free water) | • Avoid in elevated ICP |
| **Ringer's Lactate** | 130 mM Na<br>109 mM Cl<br>4 mM K<br>3 mM Ca<br>28 mM Lactate | (nearly) Isotonic | • Avoid in hyperkalemia<br>• Useful in large volume resuscitation (lactate metabolized by liver to bicarbonate)<br>• Avoid in elevated ICP |
| **2/3rds and 1/3rd** | 33 g/L Dextrose<br>51 mM Na<br>51 mM Cl | Hypotonic (66% free water) | • Avoid in elevated ICP |
| **3% NaCl** | 513 mM Na<br>513 mM Cl | Hypertonic | • Cerebral edema due to hyponatremia |

### Fluid Balance
- TBW = 60% total body weight = 2/3 ICF + 1/3 ECF
(where ICF = intracellular fluid and ECF = 3/4 interstitial + 1/4 intravascular)

### Maintenance Fluids
- To calculate maintenance fluids (4/2/1 Rule):
  - 4 mL/kg/h for 1st 10 kg of patient's body weight
  - 2 mL/kg/h for 2nd 10 kg
  - 1 mL/kg/h for the patient's remaining weight
- To calculate maintenance electrolytes:
  - Na+: 2 mEq/kg/d
  - K+: 1 mEq/kg/d

FLUIDS

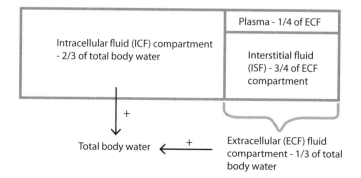

Plasma compartment changes manifest as changes in blood pressure and JVP. IV fluids are added to this compartment initially. The fluid will then equilibrate over the other body fluid compartments as per its tonicity.

For example, if isotonic saline is given it will equilibrate ¼ to plasma and ¾ to ISF. If hypotonic saline is given, the free water component will distribute 2/3 into ICF and 1/3 into ECF (of this amount, ¾ will go to ISF, and ¼ will stay in the plasma). If hypertonic saline is given, it will cause water to move out of the ICF and into the ECF (distributing in proportion), causing cells to shrink.

Increases in ISF will manifest as edematous states.

ICF changes will determine swelling or shrinkage of cells (i.e. especially affects brain cells and cognition).

**Figure 8.** Concept of Total Body Water[6]

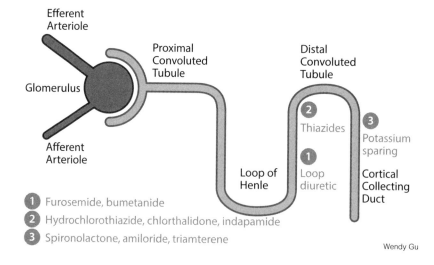

Wendy Gu

**Figure 9.** Commonly used diuretics and their sites of action[7]

## REFERENCES

1. McGee S, Abernethy WB, Simel DL. Is this patient hypovolemic? *JAMA*. 1999; 281: 1022-1029.
2. Moe SM. Disorders involving calcium, phosphorous and magnesium. *Prim Care*. 2008; 35(2): 215-237.
3. Baird GS. Ionized calcium. *Clinica Chimica Acta*. 2011; 412: 696-701.
4. Bilezikian JP, Khan AA, Potts JT. Guidelines for the management of asymptomatic primary hyperparathyroidism: Summary statement from the third international workshop. J *Clin Endocrinol Metab*. 2009; 94: 2335-2339.
5. Tanna, G. Metabolic acidosis. Course Lecture for *Metabolism and Nutrition*. Toronto: University of Toronto; 2014.
6. Schreiber, M. Intravenous fluids: Why and how? Course Lecture for *Mechanisms, Manifestations, and Management of Disease*. Toronto: University of Toronto; 2015.
7. Schreiber, M. Hypertension. Course Lecture for M*echanisms, Manifestations, and Management of Disease*. Toronto: University of Toronto; 2015.

FLUIDS

# CHAPTER 15:

# General Surgery

**Editors:**
Maya Deeb, HBSc
Mark Shafarenko

**Faculty Reviewers:**
Peter K. Stotland, HBSc, MSc, MD, FRCSC
Tulin Cil, MEd, MD, FRCSC

## TABLE OF CONTENTS

# 1. SURGICAL HISTORY AND PHYSICAL EXAM[1-2]

In addition to general history taking and physical exam, important aspects of assessing a surgical patient include:
- Cardiac, respiratory, and abdominal H&P (see **Table 1**)
- Assessing risk of cardiac complication in a noncardiac surgical setting using the Revised Cardiac Risk Index (see **Table 2**)
- Assessing risk of pulmonary complication using the Canet Risk Index (see **Table 3**)
- Assessing overall surgical risk using the American Society of Anesthesiologists Physical Status Classification (see **Table 4**)
- The American College of Surgery Risk calculator is also frequently used (http://riskcalculator.facs.org/RiskCalculator/)

**Table 1.** Cardiac, Pulmonary, and Abdominal Evaluation[3]

| | History | Physical Exam |
|---|---|---|
| **CV** | • Symptoms: SOB, angina, syncope, palpitations<br>• Diagnoses: DM, MI, valvular heart disease, CHF<br>• Procedures: CABG, angioplasty, prosthetic heart valve | See the **Circulatory System** chapter |
| **Resp** | • Habitus: smoking, occupational exposure, obesity<br>• Symptoms: sputum production, exertional dyspnea, functional status (e.g. walk up a flight of stairs), wheezing<br>• Diagnoses: COPD, asthma | See the **Respiratory System** chapter |
| **Abdo** | • Symptoms: pain, changes in bowel habits, vomiting, bleeding (hematemesis, melena, hematochezia). Check groin for hernia. | See the **Gastrointestinal System** chapter |

CABG = coronary artery bypass grafting, SOB = shortness of breath

**Table 2.** Assessing Cardiac Risk: Revised Cardiac Risk Index[4]

| Factors | Points |
|---|---|
| **History of CHF** | 1 |
| **History of Ischemic Heart Disease** | 1 |
| **History of Cerebrovascular Disease** | 1 |
| **Preoperative Treatment with Insulin** | 1 |
| **Preoperative Serum Creatinine Level >177 µM** | 1 |
| **High-Risk Surgical Procedure** | 1 |
| **Probability of Major Cardiac Complication:** 0 points, 0.4 - 0.5%; 1 point, 0.9 - 1.3%; 2 points, 4.0 - 7.0%; 3+ points, 9.0 - 11.0% | |

**Table 3.** Assessing Pulmonary Risk: Canet Risk Index[4]

| Factors | Points |
|---|---|
| **Age** | |
| • ≤50 yr | 0 |
| • 51-80 yr | 3 |
| • >80 yr | 16 |
| **Preoperative O$_2$ Saturation** | |
| • ≥96% | 0 |
| • 91-95% | 8 |
| • ≤90% | 24 |
| **Respiratory Infection in the Last Month** | 17 |

| Factors | Points |
|---|---|
| **Preoperative Anemia: Hemoglobin ≤100 g/L** | 11 |
| **Surgical Incision**<br>• Upper abdominal<br>• Intrathoracic | <br>15<br>24 |
| • **Duration of Surgery**<br>• ≤2 h<br>• 2-3 h<br>• >3 h | <br>0<br>16<br>23 |
| **Emergency Surgery** | 8 |

**Probability of Pulmonary Complication:** <26 points, low risk (1.6%); 26-44 points, intermediate risk (13.3%); ≥45 points, high risk (42.1%)

**Table 4.** Assessing Surgical Risk: American Society of Anesthesiologists (ASA) Physical Status Classification[5]

| Class | Patient Status |
|---|---|
| I | Healthy patient (non-smoking, no or minimal alcohol use). |
| II | Patient with mild systemic disease (eg. patient with well-controlled DM, normal HbA1C, mild lung disease). |
| III | Patient with severe but not incapacitating systemic disease (eg. patient with symptomatic cardiac disease, on medication, implanted pacemaker) |
| IV | Patient with severe systemic disease that poses constant threat to life (e.g. recent (<3 months) MI, CVA, TIA; ongoing cardiac ischemia or severe valve dysfunction) |
| V | Moribund patient who is not expected to survive without surgery (e.g. ruptured abdominal/thoracic aneurysm, massive trauma, intracranial bleed) |
| VI | Patient who has been declared brain-dead and whose organs are being removed for donor purposes |

ASA classes I and II correspond to low risk; class III corresponds to moderate risk; and classes IV and V correspond to high risk.

## 2. PREOPERATIVE MANAGEMENT

### Preoperative Admission[1]
*Investigations*
- CXR for patients with cardiopulmonary disease, or >50 yr undergoing major surgery
- ECG for patients >50 yr
- Anaesthesiology consult and ASA classification (see **Table 4** above)

See **Table 5** for indications for other investigations (note: tests mentioned in Table 5 are generally done on all patients having emergency surgery). For patients with low preoperative risk and low risk elective procedures, the preoperative investigations below may not be necessary.

*Laboratory Tests*
- CBC, Hb, electrolytes, creatinine, sickle test in high risk groups☐
- Type and Screen for ABO and Rh status; if expected blood loss, want minimum 2 units packed RBCs
- Check INR if patient on anticoagulation therapy or at risk for bleeding
- Classic anticoagulants: should be discontinued prior to surgery (ASA, 7-10 d prior; Plavix, 5 d prior; Warfarin, 3-5 d prior)

- Novel anticoagulant (NOAC) drugs: usually need to be held for 48-72 hours prior

*Forms*
- Informed consent (refer to Ethics section)
- Code status: discuss advance directives

*Calls and Contacts*
- Book the operating room (OR) and indicate case acuity (A-D)
- Consult with anesthesia and OR nurses
- Be proactive and try to anticipate potential issues impacting post-operative discharge planning

**Table 5.** Indications for Preoperative Laboratory Investigations[6]

| Investigations | Indications |
|---|---|
| Hb | Procedure associated with significant blood loss |
| WBC | Infection symptoms, myeloproliferative disease, myelotoxic medications |
| Platelets | Bleeding disorder, myeloproliferative disease, myelotoxic medications |
| PTT and INR | Bleeding disorder, chronic liver disease, malnutrition, long term antibiotic or anticoagulant use |
| Electrolytes | Renal insufficiency, CHF, diuretic, digoxin, ACE inhibitors |
| Creatinine | Age >50 yr, DM, HTN, cardiac disease, medications that influence renal function (ACE inhibitors, NSAIDs), major surgery |
| Glucose | Obesity, known DM or symptoms thereof, infection or suspected infection |
| Albumin | Liver disease, serious chronic illness, recent major illness, malnutrition |
| Urinalysis | No indication |
| Chest X-ray | Age >50 yr, known cardiopulmonary disease or symptoms thereof |
| ECG | Males >40 yr, females >50 yr, CAD, HTN, DM |

Smetana GW, Macpherson DS. 2003. Med Clin North Am 87(1):7-40.

# 3. OPERATIVE MANAGEMENT

**Operative Note**
- Date and time of procedure
- Preoperative diagnosis
- Postoperative diagnosis
- Procedure(s)
- Surgeon, assistants, anesthetist
- Anesthesia type (e.g. general, regional, local)
- Operative findings
- Complications
- Estimated blood loss (EBL)
- Crystalloid replaced (type and volume)
- Blood products administered
- Drains and tubes (e.g. nasogastric [NG], Foley, Jackson-Pratt [JP])
- Urine output
- Specimens collected: cultures, blood, pathology
- Intraoperative X-rays
- Patient status on transfer to post-anesthesia care unit (PACU)
- Disposition after PACU
- Signature

There are many different memory aids to help remember components of the OR note. For example, **PPP SAFE SCDD:**

**P** – Preoperative diagnosis
**P** – Postoperative diagnosis
**P** – Procedure(s)

**S** – Surgeon, assistants, anesthetist
**A** – Anesthesia type
**F** – Fluids
**E** – Estimated blood loss (EBL)

**S** – Specimens
**C** – Complications
**D** – Drains
**D** – Disposition

Please refer to **Appendix 3, Basics of Suturing & Needles**

## 4. POSTOPERATIVE MANAGEMENT

### 4.1 Postoperative Orders: ADDAVID
**Admit** to ward/service, under the care of Dr._____

### Diagnosis Pre/Postoperatively

### Diet
- Preoperative: NPO (nil per os = nothing by mouth), must have IV, see below
- Postoperative: NPO, sips/clear fluids (CF), diet as tolerated (DAT), etc.
- Total parenteral nutrition nutrition (TPN) requires Interventional Radiology consult to insert peripherally inserted central catheter (PICC) line

### Activity
- Activities as tolerated (AAT)
- Bed rest/elevate head of bed/other special positions

### Vital Signs
- Vital signs routine (VSR, as per floor)
- Vitals q4h (vitals every 4 h)
- Notify MD if: systolic BP <90 mmHg, HR >120 bpm, temperature >38.5°C or O2 saturation <92%

### IV, Ins/Outs, Investigations
*IV*
- Normal saline (NS) at 125 cc/h (+10-20 mEq/L KCl)
  - Note: avoid K+ if oliguric
  - Remember to change to maintenance IV (with K+ and glucose) after 48 hours
- If dehydrated, bolus with NS or Ringer's lactate (typically preferred)
- If patient drinking well postoperatively, common orders include:
  - IV TKVO WDW (IV to keep vein open when drinking well; means IV running at 5 cc/h)
  - IV to SL (saline lock)
  - D/C (discontinue) IV

*Ins/Outs*
- NG tube (to low intermittent suction "low gomco"/straight drain) – especially upper GI obstruction
  - If excessive losses via NG, then replace losses 1:1 with NS + 20 mEq/L KCl

- JP drains to bulb suction
- Foley catheter to straight drain/urometer
- Measure IV/PO in and all fluids out
- Maintain O2 saturation >92%

## Investigations
- Routine blood work (b/w): CBC, electrolytes, BUN, creatinine
- Assess for coagulopathy: partial thromboplastin time (PTT), INR, platelet count (in CBC differential)
- Imaging/tests (as indicated):
  - CXR, X-ray of extremity
  - ECG
- Consults (as indicated):
  - Internal Medicine
  - Anesthesia, Acute Pain Service
  - Discharge Planning – send referrals to out-patient community services as appropriate; arrange follow-up appointments in clinic as indicated

## Drugs (6 A's)
- **Analgesics**
  - Morphine 5-10 mg SC q3h PRN for pain
  - Tylenol® #3 1-2 tabs PO q4h PRN for pain
    - **Note:** maximum acetaminophen from all sources is 4 g/24 h
  - NSAID often used to reduce opioid need:
    - Choice of ketorolac (Toradol) parenteral, indomethacin suppository, or oral ibuprofen
    - Keep course short to avoid risk of GI bleed, coagulopathy, other complications in elderly
    - There is some evidence that links perioperative NSAID use and anastomotic leaks in patients having a colorectal resection. However, this evidence is inconclusive
    - For patients having a colorectal resection WITH anastomosis, NSAIDs should only be prescribed with the agreement of the surgeon, and following discussion between the surgeon and the pain team/anesthesiologist
    - **Note:** unless fresh GI anastomosis, may order stool softener with opioid pain medications (constipating)

- **Antiembolics**: Standard anticoagulation for prophylaxis is LMWH like Fragmin 5000 U OD or Enoxaparin 40 mg SC OD

- **Antecedents**
  - While NPO, may need to withhold oral medications taken prior to admission (e.g. antihypertensives, thyroid, hormone replacement, etc.) or replace with IV medications
  - Note potential contribution of medications to coagulopathy (see the **Pharmacology and Toxicology** chapter)
    - ASA (Aspirin®) = antiplatelet
    - Warfarin (Coumadin®) = anticoagulant
    - NSAIDs = reversible COX-1, 2 inhibitors
  - Postoperative: restart medications

- **Antibiotics**
  - Base empiric treatment on likely causative organisms until culture results are available[7]
  - Common intra-abdominal organisms acquired in hospital: hospital organisms (e.g. Pseudomonas aeruginosa, ESBL-producing Enterobacteriaceae, Acinetobacter, Methicillin-resistant Staphylococcus aureus) and fungi
    - Organisms in cellulitis: Group A streptococcus, gram positive (GP) cocci (includes GAS), gram negatives (GNs)
    - Organisms in pneumonia: GN rods and S. aureus (including anaerobes if

aspiration)

- Hospital resistance patterns should guide therapy once culture results obtained
- Refer to The Sanford Guide to Antimicrobial Therapy and/or Compendium of Pharmaceuticals and Specialties (CPS) for comprehensive and updated information

- **Antiemetics**
  - Dimenhydrinate (Gravol®) 25-50 mg IV/IM/PO q3-4h for nausea

- **Anxiolytics**
  - Benzodiazepines (e.g. diazepam, lorazepam)
    - Caution in elderly patients

- CAUTION: Do NOT order medications PO with concurrent NPO order. Other routes are needed in this case (IV, SC, PR).

## 4.2 Progress Note: SOAP
- Date/Time, Service, your Name and Designation
- One-line description including patient age, postoperative day (POD) #, surgical procedure, and pertinent medical history

## Subjective
- Changes in symptoms, pain, GI function, mobility, significant events, physical complaints in patient's own words

## Objective
- Vital signs
- Intake and output (urinary output [UO], NG, JP)
- Physical exam: Wound exam (take off dressing from 48 h onward), lines, chest, neurovascular status
- Investigations (if applicable): CBC, electrolytes, imaging, etc.

## Assessment and Plan
- Increase activity; may involve physiotherapist to help with ambulation
- Plan discharge in advance
- For each identified problem, devise an appropriate therapeutic regimen

## 4.3 Postoperative Complications

**Table 6.** Presentation and Management of Common Postoperative Complications[8]

| Complication | Presentation | Management |
|---|---|---|
| Fever | If caused by infection, tend to reach higher temperatures (>38.3°C) and associated with moderately elevated WBC on POD 3 or later | **Investigations:** WBC, respiratory exam (cough, sputum, respiratory effort), check lines, further work-up as indicated (CXR, sputum cultures, blood cultures, urinalysis, CT abdomen)<br>**Treatment:** discontinue any unnecessary Tx, treat underlying cause; think **4 W's: W**ind (atelectasis), **W**ater (UTI), **W**ound (SSI), **W**hat did we do (DVT/PE, hospital acquired infections, drug reaction) |
| Pneumonia | Fever, SOB, hypoxia, productive cough, and rales on lung auscultation | **Investigations:** CXR, sputum cultures<br>**Treatment:** see **Postoperative Note** (Drugs – Antibiotics), pg. 431 |

GENERAL SURGERY

| Complication | Presentation | Management |
|---|---|---|
| **Surgical Site Infection (SSI)** | Pain, erythema, swelling at the surgical site; usually after POD 5, but can occur within first 24-48 hours with very aggressive bacteria (e.g. clostridium) | **Investigations:** cultures of purulent material from SSI<br>**Treatment:** open and drain the wound, allow to heal by secondary intention, antibiotics depending on presence of cellulitis and for remote endoprosthesis |
| **Deep Vein Thrombosis (DVT)** | Lower extremity pain or one leg is noticeably more swollen than the other; physical exam unreliable | **Investigations:** venous duplex U/S<br>**Treatment:** heparin infusion or Fragmin SC, switch to warfarin when patient is stable |
| **Pulmonary Embolism (PE)** | Decreased O2 saturation or SOB, chest pain, tachycardia, diaphoresis | **Investigations:** spiral CT<br>**Treatment:** heparin infusion or Fragmin SC (may be appropriate to start before Dx is confirmed) |

POD = postoperative day, SOB = shortness of breath

**Clinical Pearls: Most Common Causes of Post-Op Fever**

12-24 h: atelectasis, wound cellulitis, UTI, indwelling catheter infection, transfusion reaction, thrombophlebitis, surgical complications

24-72 h: pneumonia, UTI, wound cellulitis, necrotizing fasciitis or clostridial myositis, thrombophlebitis, DVT, wound infection, pancreatitis

POD 3-7: UTI, pneumonia, intravascular infection, transfusion-related acute infection, drug fever

>POD 8: leaking anastomosis, deep wound infection, abscess, infected prosthetic material, occult bacteremia

## 4.4 Discharge Note

- Date and time
- Diagnoses
- Therapy and operations during hospital stay
- Investigations: ECG, CXR, CT
- Discharge medications
- Follow-up arrangements

**Clinical Pearls: Prevention of Surgical Site Infections (SSI)**

**Timing of prophylactic antibiotics**: Prophylactic antibiotics should be administered within 60 min of skin incision*.

**Maintenance of normothermia**: Patient's core temperature should be maintained intraoperatively†.

**Skin preparation**: Chlorhexidine-alcohol should be used for preoperative cleansing of the patient's skin instead of povidone-iodine‡.

**Hair removal**: Clipping or no hair removal**.

*Classen DC, et al. 1992. N Engl J Med 326(5):281-286.
†Kurz A, Sessler DI, Lenhardt R. 1996. N Engl J Med 334(1 9):1 209-1216.
‡Darouiche RO, et al. 2010. N Engl J Med 362(1):18-26.
**Cruse, PJ, Foord, R. 1973. Arch Surg 107:206-210.

## 4.5 Postoperative Pain Management

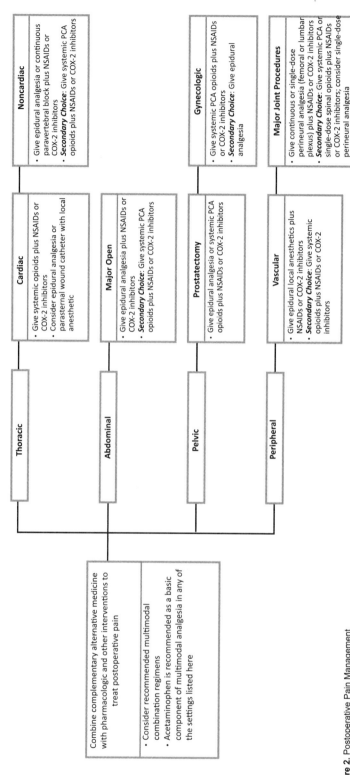

**Figure 2.** Postoperative Pain Management
Liu SS, Kehlet H. Postoperative Pain. In: Ashley SW (Editor). ACS Surgery: Principles and Practice.
Hamilton: BC Decker; 2012.

# 5. SPECIAL CIRCUMSTANCES

## Common Emergency Neonatal Surgical Problems[8]
- Congenital diaphragmatic hernia (CDH)
- Esophageal atresia
- Congenital lobar emphysema
- Intestinal obstruction
- Omphalocele, gastroschisis
- Exstrophy of the bladder
- Meningomyelocele

## Common Surgical Problems in Infants and Children[4]
- Pyloric stenosis
- Gastroesophageal reflux
- Neck and soft tissue masses (refer to the **Pediatrics** chapter for this presentation in infants and children)
- Inguinal hernia
- Undescended testes
- Acute appendicitis
- Intussusception
- Meckel's diverticulum and lower GI hemorrhage

## Approach to Acute Abdominal Pain in the Pregnant Patient[9]
- History, physical exam (3rd trimester: appendix is in right upper quadrant [RUQ])
- Place IV, start fluids as needed
- Insert NG tube if significant vomiting
- Perform routine labs
- Use fetal monitor after 24 wks
- Limit X-rays, avoid radionuclide scans, use abdominal and pelvic U/S

**Table 7.** General Surgical Approaches for the Pediatric, Pregnant, and Elderly Patient

| Pediatric Patient[8,10,11] | |
|---|---|
| **Preoperative Assessment** | • Assess for the following in the context of increasing postoperative risk of complications: not full term; ASA score >3; undergoing cardiovascular or neurosurgery; receiving intraoperative albumin transfusion<br>• Assess for the following in the context of increasing intraoperative complications: not full term; ASA score >3; Hx of CV disease; undergoing CV, neurological, orthopaedic surgery |
| **Postoperative Management** | • Infants in the first year experience highest rates of failure to rescue, infection, postoperative hemorrhage/hematoma, PE/DVT, and postoperative sepsis |
| **Pregnant Patient[8,9]** | |
| **Preoperative Assessment[9]** | • Assess for Hx of DVT/PE, thrombocytopenia, bleeding disorders<br>• Assess for Hx of CV disease, involve specialists as needed<br>• If asthmatic: assess severity, watch Sx in context of histamine-releasing opioids (will worsen Sx)<br>• Confirm antepartum HIV testing, on HAART if HIV+ |
| **Intraoperative Considerations** | • Watch for severe preeclampsia, fetal bradycardia, emergent C-section<br>• Remember to position pregnant patient appropriately - after 20 weeks, she needs to be in left lateral decubitus position to avoid compression of IVC. |
| **Postoperative Management[10]** | • Slightly higher rates of complications due to cholecystectomy: VTE; infection; return to OR<br>• 20% and 5% chance of fetal loss during surgery for perforated appendicitis and Sx of cholelithiasis, respectively (this varies with the time of surgery and trimester) |

| **Preoperative Assessment**[7] | • Comprehensive geriatric assessment (CGA), including: functional status, comorbidities, nutrition, cognition, depression, social support, polypharmacy<br>• DVT prophylaxis<br>• Anticipate potential need for blood transfusion (ensure group & screen is done) |
|---|---|
| **Intraoperative Considerations** | • Difficulties with sedation, intubation (as per anesthesia); prolonged operative time; coagulopathy complications |
| **Postoperative Management** | • Initiate respiratory therapy early<br>• Encourage early ambulation<br>• Pressure ulcer prevention (i.e. frequent turning, visual inspection)<br>• Monitor for delirium |

CV = cardiovascular, HAART = Highly Active Anti-Retroviral Therapy, Sx = symptom, VTE = venous thromboembolism

GENERAL SURGERY

# 6. COMMON CLINICAL SCENARIOS

**Table 8.** Common clinical scenarios in general surgery, summarized

| Signs and Symptoms | Physical Exam Findings | Investigations and Tests | Management |
|---|---|---|---|
| **Acute Appendicitis[8, 14]** | | | |
| Acute abdominal pain (<48 h), pain initially periumbilical/ epigastric then may localize to right lower quadrant (RLQ), ± N/V, anorexia, diarrhea, constipation, fever | Assess general appearance and positioning (i.e. pain), vitals; auscultate heart and lungs; perform abdominal exam, including DRE and groin inspection; perform pelvic exam; look for rigidity, a positive psoas sign, fever, or rebound tenderness (Refer to the **Gastrointestinal System** chapter) | • **Investigations:** abdominal CT scan if diagnosis not obvious; ECG in elderly with heart Hx <br> • **Laboratory Tests:** CBC, hematocrit, serum electrolytes, BUN, serum creatinine, urinalysis | Laparoscopy or laparotomy: immediately if spreading peritonitis, very sick or worsening clinically |
| **Acute Cholecystitis[8, 14]** | | | |
| Acute abdominal pain, localized to RUQ, ± referred pain (R subscapular area), ± N/V, anorexia, diarrhea, fever, fat intolerance | Assess general appearance and positioning (i.e. pain), vitals; auscultate heart and lungs; perform abdominal exam, including DRE and groin inspection; perform pelvic exam; look for Murphy's sign | • **Investigations:** abdominal U/S; ECG in elderly with heart Hx <br> • **Laboratory Tests**: CBC, hematocrit, serum electrolytes, LFTs and enzymes (serum bilirubin, ALP, albumin, INR, PTT, ALT/AST), amylase, urinalysis, lipase (> amylase for dx of pancreatitis) | 75% of patients improve with IV fluids, analgesics & antibiotics. If no improvement, laparoscopic cholecystectomy is indicated (may require conversion to laparotomy) |

GENERAL SURGERY

**Perforated Bowel[8]**

| Signs and Symptoms | Physical Exam Findings | Investigations and Tests | Management |
| --- | --- | --- | --- |
| On history, ask: Peptic ulcer disease? NSAID use? Diverticulitis? Vasculopathy?<br><br>**Phase 1 (<2 h)**: sudden onset severe abdominal pain, usually epigastric and generalized; tachycardia, weak pulse, low temperature;<br><br>**Phase 2 (2-12 h)**: lessened pain, abdominal rigidity, tender on DRE;<br><br>**Phase 3 (>12 h)**: increasing abdominal distention, elevated temperature, hypovolemia, signs of peritonitis | Assess general appearance and positioning (i.e. pain), vitals; auscultate heart and lungs; perform abdominal exam focusing on peritoneal signs, include DRE | · **Investigations:** CXR, abdominal X-ray<br>· **Laboratory Tests:** CBC, hematocrit, serum electrolytes, blood cultures if suspecting sepsis, LFTs and enzymes (serum bilirubin, ALP, albumin, INR, PTT, ALT/AST), amylase, urinalysis; rule out *C. difficile*, *Cytomegalovirus*, *E. coli* | Urgent laparotomy (may start with laparoscopic approach) |

**Bowel Obstruction (BO)[8]**

| Signs and Symptoms | Physical Exam Findings | Investigations and Tests | Management |
| --- | --- | --- | --- |
| On history, ask: previous episodes of BO? Previous abdominal/pelvic surgery? Hx of abdominal cancer? Hx of intra-abdominal inflammation, e.g. IBD, pelvic inflammatory disease (PID), pancreatitis, trauma? Recent change in bowel habits? Weight loss? Passage of flatus? Metabolic conditions? Radiation exposure? Current medications? (e.g. anticoagulants, anticholinergics)<br><br>Abdominal pain or distention, N/V, obstipation | Assess general appearance, vitals, hydration status, cardiopulmonary system; perform abdominal exam – special considerations: auscultate 1 min, thoroughly search for hernias, perform DRE | · **Investigations:** determine if small BO (surgery often initially unnecessary if not closed loop and/or there are no signs of peritonitis) or large BO (commonly cancer needing OR, cecum may burst if distended) with abdominal X-rays (supine, upright, lateral decubitus; usually CT and/or water-soluble contrast enema); alarmed if cecum >10 cm; sometimes GI endoscopy (rare unless subacute chronic partial obstruction)<br>· **Laboratory Tests:** serum electrolytes, hematocrit, serum creatinine, coagulation profile | Place NG tube to low intermittent suction, Foley catheter, IV; or colonic BO = immediate or urgent operation; partial and/or small BO = may try conservative management with NG suction, reassess hourly, then q4h; repeat X-rays, consider OR if not resolved within 48-72 hours |

GENERAL SURGERY

# REFERENCES

1. Blankstein U, Blankstein M. 2012. The 'perfect' pre-operative admission: A practical guide. UTMJ 89:170-171.
2. Ashley SW (Editor). ACS Surgery: Principles and Practice. Hamilton: BC Decker; 2012.
3. Lee TH, et al. 1999. Circulation 100(10):1043-1049.
4. Canet J, et al. 2010. Anesthesiology 113(6):1338-1350
5. Dripps RD, Lamont A, Eckenhoff JE. 1961. JAMA 178:261-266
6. National Institute for Clinical Excellence. Preoperative Tests: The Use of Routine Preoperative Tests for Elective Surgery. Clinical Guideline 3. 2003. Available from: http://www.nice.org.uk/ nicemedia/pdf/CG3NICEguideline.pdf.
7. Armstrong, C., 2010. Updated guideline on diagnosis and treatment of intra-abdominal infections. American Family Physician, 82(6), pp.694-709.
8. Ashley SW. ACS Surgery: Principles and Practice. Hamilton: BC Decker; 2012
9. Hinova A, Fernando R. 2010. The preoperative assessment of obstetric patients. Best Pract Res Clin Obstet Gynaecol 24(3):261-276.
10. Miller MR, Zhan C. 2004. Pediatric patient safety in hospitals: A national picture in 2000. Pediatrics 113(6):1741-1746.
11. Weinberg AC, Huang L, Jiang H, Tinloy B, Raskas MD, Penna FJ, et al. 2011. Perioperative risk factors for major complications in pediatric surgery: A study in surgical risk assessment for children. J Am Coll Surg 212(5):768-778.
12. Souba WW, Fink MP, Jurkovich GJ, Kaiser LR, Pearce WH, Pemberton JH, et al. ACS Surgery: Principles and Practice, 6th ed. Hamilton: BC Decker; 2007.
13. Kirshhtein B, Perry ZH, Mizrahi S, Lantsberg L. 2009. Value of laparoscopic appendectomy in the elderly patient. World J Surg 33(5):918-922.
14. Garner J. 2010. The Rational Clinical Examination: Evidence-Based Clinical Diagnosis, edited by David L. Simel, MD, MHS, and Drummond Rennie, MD.Proceedings (Baylor University Medical Center). 23(1):0087.

# FURTHER READING:

1. Sprung J, Gajic O, Warner DO. 2006. Age related alterations in respiratory function – Anesthetic considerations. Can J Anesth 53(12):1244-1257.
2. Egol KA, Strauss EJ. 2009. Perioperative considerations in geriatric patients with hip fracture: What is the evidence? J Orthop Trauma 23(6):386-394.
3. Corneille MG, Gallup TM, Bening T, Wolf SE, Brougher C, Myers JG, et al. 2010. The use of laparoscopic surgery in pregnancy: Evaluation of safety and efficacy. Am J Surg 200(3):363- 367.
4. Erekson EA, Brousseau EC, Dick-Biascoechea MA, Ciarleglio MM, Lockwood CJ, Pettker CM. 2012. Maternal postoperative complications after nonobstetric antenatal surgery. J Matern Fetal Neonatal Med 25(12):2639-2644.
5. Fagarasanu, A., Alotaibi, G., Hrimiuc, R., Lee, A. and Wu, C. (2016). Role of Extended Thromboprophylaxis After Abdominal and Pelvic Surgery in Cancer Patients: A Systematic Review and Meta-Analysis. Annals of Surgical Oncology, 23(5), pp.1422-1430.
6. Sawyer J, Morningstar B, Chung F, Siddiqui N, McCluskey S. Enhanced Recovery after Surgery Guideline: Perioperative Pain Management in Patients Having Elective Colorectal Surgery. Best Practice in General Surgery. 2013.

# CHAPTER 16:

# Geriatrics

**Editors:**
Saurabh Kalra, MD, BHSc
Reha Kumar, BHSc
Yasmin Nasirzadeh, BSc

**Resident Reviewer:**
Shixin Shen, MD, MSc

**Faculty Reviewers:**
Samir Sinha, MD, DPhil, FRCPC
Camilla Wong, MD, FRCPC

## TABLE OF CONTENTS

# 1. COMMON CHIEF COMPLAINTS

**Table 1.** Common chief complaints in the geriatric population and differential diagnoses

| Chief Complaint | Differential Diagnosis | Distinguishing Features |
|---|---|---|
| **Cognitive Concerns** | Dementia | Insidious onset, gradual cognitive decline (months-years). Normal level of consciousness. Poor memory without inattention. |
| | Delirium | Acute onset (days-weeks), fluctuating course (hypoactive and/or hyperactive), inattention, disorganized thinking |
| | Depression/Anxiety | Normal/reduced memory with inattention, normal level of consciousness, low self-esteem, may be reversible |
| **Urinary Incontinence (UI)**[1] | Stress UI | Voiding with coughing, sneezing, laughing |
| | Urge UI | Urgency with or without increased frequency |
| | Mixed UI | Combination of urge and stress UI symptoms |
| | Functional UI | Decreased cognitive/physical functioning, environmental factors |
| | Overflow UI | Dribbling, hesitancy, weak stream, intermittency |
| **Falls/Mobility Concerns**[2,3] | Cardiovascular | History of arrhythmias, CHF, coronary artery disease, claudication |
| | Psychiatric | History of sleep disorders, depression, substance abuse, delirium, dementia |
| | Musculoskeletal | History of osteoarthritis, osteoporosis, gout |
| | Metabolic | History of diabetes, B12 deficiency, hypo/hyperthyroidism, obesity |
| | Neurological | History of stroke, Parkinson's disease, cerebellar dysfunction, multiple sclerosis |
| | Sensory | Hearing or visual impairment, peripheral neuropathy |
| | Other | Acute illness, recent hospitalization/surgery, polypharmacy |
| | Common disorders: Parkinson disease | Bradykinesia, rigidity, tremor |
| | Arrhythmias, CHF | Chest pain or dyspnea on exertion, palpitations |
| | Deconditioning | Recent hospitalization, sedentary lifestyle |
| | Peripheral Neuropathy | Sensory loss, paresthesia |
| | Orthostatic Hypotension | Lightheadedness with sudden rise from sitting or supine position |
| | Osteoporosis | Kyphosis, decrease in height, history of fractures |
| | Osteoarthritis | Joint pain and deformities |

GERIATRICS

| Chief Complaint | Notes |
|---|---|
| **Poly-pharmacy**[4] | Common causes: multimorbidity, patient/prescriber expectations, communication gaps, clinical practice guidelines, prescribing cascade |
| **Functional Decline**[5] | Limitation in the ability to perform basic functional and self-care activities. <u>Multiple causes:</u><br>Medical conditions (examples stated above under mobility concerns)<br>Impairments: cognition, mood, pain, nutrition<br>Contextual Factors: lack of social support, limited finances, environmental factors, personality traits |

## 2. FOCUSED HISTORY

The geriatric history is similar to a complete, general medical history. However, there are a few specific issues that must be addressed when assessing a geriatric patient.

As early as possible during the interview, evaluate the patient's ability to hear, see, understand, and give an accurate historical account in the language you speak or understand. Consider encouraging the use of sensory aids to assist in history taking. It is important to obtain collateral history from the family doctor, family, and community agencies when needed.

### Identification Data
- Age, sex/gender, and handedness
- Marital status, past/current occupation, and current living status (i.e. living alone at home vs. retirement home)

### Chief Complaint
- Illness often presents as a change in function, a geriatric syndrome, or atypical symptoms
- To elicit a vague CC, use questions such as "What has changed recently?" and "What is your most concerning issue today?"

### History of Present Illness
- Patients may present with multiple issues and noanspecific symptoms (eg. fatigue, confusion) without clear involvement of a particular organ system.
- Creation of a comprehensive problem list is helpful for addressing all complaints in order of functional importance

### Past Medical, Surgical, and Psychiatric History
- Often long, complicated, and difficult to remember for many patients
  - The use of collateral history from family doctors, family members, caregivers, and prior patient records is often helpful
- Include hospitalizations, general state of health
- Asking more specific questions may be helpful: "Have you ever had a heart attack?" or "Have you ever had heart surgery?" instead of "Do you have any medical problems?"

### Medications
- Polypharmacy is prevalent in the elderly and you must ask, in detail, about drugs they are taking, drugs they may have recently stopped taking, route(s) of administration (e.g. blister pack, dosette, orally), OTC medications, herbal remedies/teas, supplements/vitamins
  - It may be useful to have the patient or caregiver bring in everything they are taking
- Note that polypharmacy is one of the risk factors of non-adherence: ask to see if they are taking all medications as directed
- The risk of drug-drug interactions and adverse drug reactions increases with the number of prescriptions
- Ask about pneumococcal, influenza, shingles, and tetanus vaccinations

### Social History
- Determine living arrangements, type of housing, mobility barriers and assistive devices (stairs, adaptive equipment etc.), marital status, family members, social/community support, and willingness to accept help

- Document existence of designated power of attorney for personal care and finances and a living will
- Ask if plans exist for times of illness or functional decline. Advanced care planning should be discussed
- Ask caregivers whether a back-up plan of care exists for the patient in case of caregiver misfortune or ill-health
- Do not forget that some elders are lesbian, gay, bisexual or transgender, queer etc; therefore, use of inclusive language such as 'partner' will help build better rapport
- Ask about the content of a typical day for the patient, extent of social relationships, suitability and safety of home, occupational/educational history, cultural background, religion/spirituality, interests/hobbies, sources of income, and veteran status
- Substance use/abuse (smoking, alcohol intake, recreational drug use, sleep aids, and daily caffeine consumption) is an important and often overlooked aspect of the geriatric history[6]
- Enquire about availability and attitude of caregivers and neighbors, as well as availability of emergency help. Pay attention to potential caregiver fatigue
- For hospitalized patients, enquire about their discharge plans

## Mental Status Examination
- The Folstein MMSE is a screen for assessing cognitive impairment (see **Psychiatry** Chapter)
- Some patients may be upset or offended by the nature of the questions. Avoid using the word "test" or "exam". One approach is to introduce the MMSE by saying, "I have a few questions and tasks that will allow me to see how your memory and concentration are functioning today." Also telling them in advance that a memory screen is a standard part of your exam would allow them to expect it and even choose when to do it.
  - Note that MMSE scores may also be low in patients with sensory impairments, dysphasia, depression, poor English skills or low education level[7]
- The MoCA (Montreal Cognitive Assessment) is a more sensitive tool for detecting mild cognitive impairment compared to the MMSE[8]
- The RUDAS (Rowland Universal Dementia Assessment Scale) is another cognitive assessment scale that is likely more neutral to culture, educational attainment, and language[9]

## The Functional Assessment
- Used as a screen to identify any impairments and dependence on others

*Activities of Daily Living (ADLs) (**DEATH: D**ressing, **E**ating, **A**mbulating, **T**oileting, **H**ygiene)*
- Are you able to dress yourself?
- Are you able to feed yourself?
- Are you able to get out of bed by yourself in the morning?
- Are you able to walk without any assistance (person, cane, walker)?
- Do you experience difficulty going up or down stairs?
- Can you use the bathroom on your own?
- Do you bathe yourself and do your own grooming?

**Hint: These are the things you do every morning!**

*Instrumental Activities of Daily Living (IADLs) (**SHAFT**: **S**hopping, **H**ousework, **A**ccounting, **F**ood preparation, **T**ransport, **T**elephoning, **T**aking medications)*
- Do you do the shopping, cleaning, or laundry?
- Are you able to take care of banking, paying the bills, and making financial decisions?
- Are you able to cook for yourself?
- Does anyone help you make or get to your appointments?
- Are you driving at the moment? If yes, are you experiencing any difficulties with your driving? (see Driving Competency and Safety, p. 449)
- Are you able to keep track of your own medications? Do you ever forget to take your medications?

## Geriatric Review of Systems
Remember to ask about these systems in particular:
- **General:** fatigue, sleep patterns, constitutional symptoms
- **H&N:** visual changes, hearing loss, denture use
- **GI:** incontinence, constipation
- **GU:** incontinence, frequency, nocturia, sexual function

GERIATRICS

- **Cognition:** memory, visuo-spatial, language or time/place orientation concerns, executive function
- **CNS/MSK:** gait, balance, falls, and other injuries
- **Psychiatric:** mood changes, isolation, recent loss of loved ones
- **Nutrition:** weight loss, appetite
- **Derm:** skin integrity, wounds, skin changes
- **Safety:** abuse, neglect

## Hints and Tips for the Geriatric History
When taking a geriatric history, remember to ask about the geriatric giants and the 5 I's:

| Geriatric Giants | 5 I's |
| --- | --- |
| Falls | Immobility |
| Confusion | Intellect |
| Incontinence | Incontinence |
| Polypharmacy | Iatrogenesis<br>Impaired homeostasis |

- Due to communication difficulties or potentially multiple comorbidities, history taking may be a lengthy process. If the patient is medically stable, the history need not be completed at once and can be broken down into several sessions. Setting priorities is important for efficient time management.

- Underreporting of symptoms is a common occurrence in the elderly population due to health beliefs, fear, depression, cognitive impairment, or cultural barriers. A thorough review of systems and asking specific questions may help uncover medical problems.

- Corroborative history, from a family member or caregiver, is often important.

# 3. FOCUSED PHYSICAL EXAM[10]

## Vital Signs (see **General History and Physical Exam** Chapter)
- **Weight**: unintentional weight loss (>5-10%) may be a sign of dehydration (if acute), lack of access to food, depression, or malignancy
- **Height**: reduction may indicate osteoporosis, vertebral compression fractures
- **Blood Pressure:** screen for hypertension, orthostatic hypotension
    - May be a normal consequence of aging, medication side effect, or a disease state
    - Do not miss auscultatory gap in elderly hypertensive patients

## Head and Neck
- **Eyes** (see **Ophthalmology** Chapter)
    - Test visual acuity, central and peripheral visual fields
    - Screen for cataracts, macular degeneration, glaucoma
    - *Note*: previous cataract surgery can cause unequal and less reactive pupils but not RAPD (RAPD is always due to optic neuropathy)
- **Ears** (see **The Head, Neck, and Throat** Chapter)
    - Hearing impairment can be caused by wax impaction (can result in a 30% conductive hearing loss)
    - High frequency hearing loss is common with aging
    - Assess for presbycusis and tinnitus
- **Dentition**
    - Ask patient to remove dentures when examining the mouth
    - Check for dryness, odor, signs of oral cancers
    - Lack of dental work and ill-fitting dentures may lead to difficulty eating, weight loss, and malnutrition
- **Neck** (see **The Head, Neck, and Throat** Chapter)
    - Auscultate for carotid bruits (which indicates diffuse vascular disease and should lead to detailed questioning about symptoms of CAD and past TIAs/strokes)
    - Thyroid exam (*Note:* patients can have subclinical hypothyroidism)
    - Assess for neck masses (malignancy, infection, inflammation)
- **Lymph Nodes** (see **The Lymphatic System** Chapter)
    - With advanced age, lymph nodes usually become smaller, decrease in number, and

GERIATRICS

become more fibrotic and fatty

## Chest (see **The Precordial Exam** Chapter)
- Examine for arrhythmias, murmurs, and extra heart sounds
  - Aortic stenosis, aortic sclerosis, and mitral regurgitation are common in the elderly
  - Examine for cyanosis, signs of pneumonia, COPD exacerbation, and airway pathology (see **The Respiratory System** Chapter)
- **Posterior Chest**: Dorsal kyphosis may indicate vertebral compression fractures and osteoporosis

## Peripheral Vascular System (see **The Peripheral Vascular Exam** Chapter)
- Examine for peripheral pulses, edema
- Auscultate for bruits
- Screen for arterial or venous insufficiency and its complications (clubbing, cyanosis, varicose veins, ulcerations, hair loss) - especially in diabetics

## Gastrointestinal
- Screen for abdominal pain, constipation, rectal bleeding, fecal incontinence
- Examine for abdominal aortic aneurysm, abdominal, and umbilical hernia

## Genitourinary (see **The Gynecological Exam** Chapter and **The Urological Exam** Chapter)
- Screen for urinary incontinence or retention, cystocele, rectocele, atrophic vaginitis, enlarged prostate
- Examine for inguinal or femoral hernia

## Dermatological
- Screen for premalignant/malignant lesions (esp. on face and hands)
- Look for any pressure sores, especially in immobile patients
- Examine for unexplained bruises (elder abuse), ulcerations/edema in the lower extremities (vascular or neuropathic impairments)

## Musculoskeletal
- Determine range of motion of all joints, especially hips and shoulders
- Impairment in extremities may interfere with ADLs
- Screen for deformity, joint pain, muscle weakness/wasting
- Check foot hygiene, footwear, assess need for chiropody

## Gait Assessment
- Observe gait for: use of arms and foot stance, gait initiation, velocity, trajectory, cadence, posture, ataxia
  - Parkinsonian patients: exhibit delayed gait initiation, reduced gait velocity, multi-step turn
  - Abnormal trajectory may be indicative of vestibular disease
  - Sway and/or use of walking aid may indicate cerebellar dysfunction
  - Step height and step length usually decrease in elderly
    - Asymmetry in step height or length may result from stroke
    - Parkinsonian shuffle: patient's feet never leave the ground, stance is narrow, and stride length is decreased
  - Observe turning (one-step turn vs. multi-step) and balance
    - Parkinsonian patients exhibit a multi-step turn
  - Assess balance using in-bed mobility, transfers and ambulation

## Neurological
- Examine: cognition, cranial nerves, peripheral strength, tone and sensation, deep tendon reflexes
  - Diminished vibration sense and absent ankle jerk reflex are common in elderly patients
- Cognitive Assessment include MMSE, RUDAS and MOCA for dementia, Confusion Assessment Method (CAM) for delirium and Geriatric Depression Scale (GDS) and PHQ-9 for depression
- Tests should be used in conjunction with history and information from the family/caregiver(s).
- Specifically ask about mood, memory, behavior, and functional status

GERIATRICS

# 4. COMMON CLINICAL SCENARIOS

**Table 2.** Common clinical scenarios in geriatric medicine

| History | Key Physical Exams | Risk Factors | Investi- gations | Treatment |
|---|---|---|---|---|
| **Delirium[4,11,12]** | | | | |
| • Acute change in mental status<br>• Fluctuating course<br>• Inattention<br>• Altered LOC<br>• Disorganized thinking | • Vitals<br>• Hydration status<br>• Infectious source<br>• Skin condition<br>• Neuro exam: focal neuro signs | <u>Predisposing:</u><br>Dementia<br>Visual/hearing impairment<br>Depression<br><br><u>Precipitating:</u><br>Restraints<br>Medications<br>Surgery<br>Infection or any concurrent illness | CBC<br>Electro-lytes<br>(Calcium, Magne-sium, Phos-phate)<br>Glucose<br>Creati-nine<br>LFT's<br>TSH | Prevention is very effective:*<br>• Cognitive stimulation<br>• Early mobilization<br>• Glasses/hearing aids<br>• Oral volume repletion<br>• Promote sleep<br>• Involve family |
| **Dementia[4,13,14]** | | | | |
| Symptoms: Amnesia, aphasia, apraxia, agnosia, executive dysfunction<br><br>Functional impact<br><br>Onset and progression<br><br>Presence of BPSDs (Behavioral and Psychological Symptoms)<br><br>Safety concerns<br><br>Review meds, especially those with anticholinergic properties<br><br>Comorbidities | • MMSE/ MoCA<br>• Neurologic exam<br>• Signs of parkinsonism (see 4.1 for expected find-ings) | • Age<br>• Genetic<br>• Vascular: hypertension, diabetes, smoking, heart disease<br>• Low physical activity<br>• Low education level | CBC<br>Eletro-lytes<br>BUN/Cr<br>Glucose<br>TSH<br>B12<br>LFT's<br>Calcium<br>Albumin | • Multidisciplinary approach<br>• Promote cognitive and physical activities<br>• Caregiver support<br>• Address vascular risk factors<br>• Pharmacologic: limited evidence for cholinesterase inhibitors & NMDA antagonists<br>• Safety: medication monitoring, OT home safety assessment, wandering registry, driving retirement, financial risk minimization strategies |

| History | Key Physical Exams | Risk Factors | Investi-gations | Treatment |
|---|---|---|---|---|

**Urine Incontinence[1,17] (Also see Section 1)**

| History | Key Physical Exams | Risk Factors | Investi-gations | Treatment |
|---|---|---|---|---|
| Voiding record: time and volume of each void | Volume status: CHF | Stress UI: age, vaginal deliveries, obesity, pelvic surgery | Urinalysis Post void residual | Stress UI: Kegel exercises, regular and prompted voiding, surgery |
| Onset, previous treatment | Neuro exam: sacral reflexes, perineal sensation | Urge UI: CNS disorders, local GU conditions | | Urge UI: antimuscarinic drugs, bladder training |
| Symptoms of overactive bladder, stress incontinence | | | | |
| Voiding difficulty: hesitancy, straining, dribbling etc. | Abdominal: suprapubic palpation for distended bladder | Overflow UI: enlarged prostate, acontractile bladder due to diabetes or spinal cord injury | | Overflow UI: bladder training, catherization, surgery |
| Pain, dysuria, hematuria | | | | Functional UI: |
| Precipitating factors (eg. cough) | Rectal: sphincter tone, impaction, prostate exam | Functional UI: severe dementia, depression, limited mobility | | environmental adjustment |
| Fluid intake | | Transient UI: DIAPPERS | | Common Strategies: manage constipation, address polypharmacy, weight loss, avoid caffeine, regular and prompted voiding, limiting fluids before bedtime, kegel exercises |
| Bowel habits | External genitalia | D: Delirium I: Infection (UTI) A: Atrophic P: Pharma-cological P: Psych-chologic E: Endocrine R: Reduced mobility S: Stool impaction | | |
| | Pelvic: atrophy, vaginitis, prolapse, mass | | | |

*Limited evidence for prevention and treatment with antipsychotics in hyperactive and mixed deliriums and none for patients with hypoactive delirium

## 4.1 Common dementias and distinguishing clinical features[18-20]

- Alzheimer's disease: predominant cognitive and functional impairment (slow progression); memory loss; aphasia and apraxia; +/- gait impairment

- Vascular: cognitive decline (step-wise progression); focal neurological symptoms; +/- vascular lesions on CT and/or MRI; often develops post-stroke

- Frontotemporal: young age of onset (40s-early60s); personality and behavioral changes; significant difficulty with language

- Parkinson's (dementia develops after motor disorder): resting tremor; bradykinesia; cogwheel rigidity; slow, narrow-based "shuffling" gait; stooped posture; hallucinations (late in disease)

- Lewy Body (dementia develops before/at same time as motor disorder): progressive; fluctuating cognition; visual hallucinations; REM sleep behavior disorder; parkinsonism motor symptoms

GERIATRICS

**Clinical Pearl: Tips for Management of Geriatric Patients**

1. Urinary retention: rule out fecal impaction
2. Driving: always consider assessment of fitness to drive in management of any condition in the elderly
3. Renal function: creatinine clearance is a more accurate way to assess renal function than serum creatinine level. This is due to the decline in renal clearance and lean muscle mass that may make serum creatinine normal in the elderly
4. Delirium prevention strategies: hydration, early mobilization, glasses/hearing aids, involve family, regular orientation
5. Advance care directives: make sure these are known to the team during routine visits. Such discussions are preferably held during normal outpatient visits rather than when an acute life-threatening event is imminent or occurring
6. For pain control, a good trial of acetaminophen should be attempted first. If a narcotic is needed, hydromorphone is generally better tolerated than codeine or morphine in the elderly

**Clinical Pearl: Adverse effects of medications in the elderly[21]**

| Common Medication | Adverse Effect |
| --- | --- |
| Sulfonylureas/Insulin | Hypoglycemia |
| Anticholinergics | Cognitive effects |
| Opioids | Constipation |
| Benzodiazepines/sedatives | Falls |
| Warfarin/NOAC's | GI, intracranial bleeding |

For further readings on medication management in elderly, please consult the Beers Criteria[22] and the STOPP/START[23] criteria

## 5. MANAGEMENT OF COMMON CONCERNS IN THE GERIATRICS POPULATION

### 5.1 Falls

**History (SPLATT)**
- **S**ymptoms: dizziness, palpitations, dyspnea, chest pain, weakness, loss of consciousness
- **P**revious falls (frequency, time of day)
- **L**ocation, witnesses
- **A**ctivity
- **T**ime of fall
- **T**rauma: physical, psychological (fear of falls)
- **O**ther: recent medication changes, availability of gait aids or Life Line

Risk Factors:
- Prior falls
- Balance impairment
- Decreased muscle strength
- Polypharmacy
- Vision concerns
- Cognitive impairment

### Physical Exam
- Complete physical exam with emphasis on:
  - **CVS:** orthostatic changes in blood pressure and pulse, arrhythmias
  - **MSK:** injury secondary to fall, lower extremity function, podiatric problems, poorly fitting shoes
  - **CNS:** vision, muscle power and symmetry, lower extremity peripheral nerve sensation, reflexes, gait (turning, getting in/out of a chair) and balance (Romberg test and sternal push), cognitive screen

### Overview of Management:
- Manage meds
  - Withdraw or minimize psychoactive medication
  - Optimize hypertensive medication to prevent postural hypotension
  - Withdraw or minimize sedatives and benzodiazepines
- Prescribe vitamin D
- Physical therapy & exercise
- OT home safety assessment
- Proper footwear
- Support patient and caregiver(s)

## 5.2 Driving Competency and Safety
Assessing an elderly patient's ability to operate a motor vehicle is a common task in many geriatric settings. In Ontario, the Ministry of Transportation requires everyone over 80 years of age to pass a vision test as well as a clock drawing and attention test.*

### Summary: Evaluate SAFE DRIVE
- **S**afety and record (from Ministry of Transportation)
- **A**ttention skills
- **F**amily report
- **E**thanol
- **D**rugs: analgesics, hypoglycemic, anticholinergics, anticonvulsants, antidepressants, antipsychotics, opiates, sedatives, stimulants
- **R**eaction time
- **I**ntellectual impairment
- **V**ision and visuospatial ability
- **E**xecutive functions

*Refer to the CMA Driver's Guide (https://www.cma.ca/En/Pages/drivers-guide.aspx) for more information.[24]

# 6. ELDER ABUSE

### Features suggestive on history
- Injuries inconsistent with explanation
- Discrepancies between patient and caregiver account of illness/injury
- Behavior: withdrawn, depressed, fearful, anxious
- Neglect and financial abuse should be considered.

### Physical Exam
- General: signs of neglect, malnourishment or physical abuse
- Dermatological: unexplained bruises, scars, welts, alopecia

### Risk Factors
- Family history of violence
- Caregiver stress
- Dementia
- Shared living environment
- Social isolation
- Female gender

### Assessment
- Elder Abuse Suspicion Index (EASI)
- Separate interviews with patient and caregiver

**Management**
- Treat physical/emotional manifestations of abuse
- Try to resolve or improve issue that may be triggering abuse
- Consult social worker
- If abuse occurred in the setting of retirement or nursing home, it is reportable (mandatory reporting is province/state specific)

GERIATRICS

# REFERENCES

1. Frank C, Szlanta A. Office management of urinary incontinence among older patients. Can Fam Physician. 2010; 56(11):1115-1120.
2. Ganz DA, Bao Y, Shekelle PG, Rubenstein LZ. Will my patient fall? JAMA. 2007; 297(1 ):77-86.
3. Salzman B. Gait and balance disorders in older adults. Am Fam Physician. 2010; 82(1), 61-68.
4. Ontario Geriatrics Learning Centre. http://geriatrics.otn.ca. Accessed June 20, 2016.
5. Colon-Emeric C, Whitson H, Pavon J, Hoenig H. Functional Decline in Older Adults. Am Fam Physician. 2013; 88(6): 388-394.
6. Blazer DG, Wu LT. The epidemiology of at-risk and binge drinking among middle-aged and elderly community adults: National Survey on Drug Use and Health. Am J Psychiatry. 2009; 166(10):1162- 1169.
7. Crum RM, Anthony JC, Bassett SS, Folstein MF. Population-based norms for the Mini- Mental State Examination by age and educational level. JAMA. 1993; 269(18):2386-2391.
8. Nasreddine ZS, Phillips NA, Bédirian V, et al. The Montreal Cognitive Assessment, MoCA: A brief screening tool for mild cognitive impairment. J Am Geriatr Soc. 2005; 53(4):695-699.
9. Rowland JT, Basic D, Storey JE, Conforti DA. The Rowland Universal Dementia Assessment Scale (RUDAS) and the Folstein MMSE in a multicultural cohort of elderly persons. Int Psychogeriatr. 2006; 18:111-120.
10. Bickley LS, Szilagyi PG, Bates B. Bates' Guide to Physical Examination and History Taking, 10th ed. Philadelphia: Lippincott Williams & Wilkins; 2009.
11. Hospital Elder Life Program. http://www.hospitalelderlifeprogram.org. Accessed July 2, 2016.
12. Inouye SK. Delirium in older persons. N Engl J Med. 2006; 354(11):1157–65.
13. Chen J, Lin K, Chen Y. Risk Factors for Dementia. J Formos Med Assoc. 2009; 108(10):754–764.
14. Scott KR, Barrett AM. Dementia syndromes: evaluation and treatment. Expert Rev Neurother. 2007; 7(4), 407-422.
15. Tideiksaar R. Preventing falls: How to identify risk factors and reduce complications. Geriatrics. 1996; 51 (2):43-53.
16. American Geriatrics Society. American Geriatrics Society/British Geriatrics Society Clinical Practice Guideline for Prevention of Falls in Older Persons. New York: American Geriatrics Society; 2010.
17. DeMaagd G,Davenport T. Management of Urinary Incontinence. P T. 2012; 37 (6), 345-361.
18. Karantzoulis S, Galvin, J. Distinguishing Alzheimer's disease from other major forms of dementia. Expert Rev Neurother, 2011; 11(11), 1579-1591.
19. McKeith I, Galasko D, Kosaka K, et al. Consensus guidelines for the clinical and pathologic diagnosis of dementia with Lewy bodies (DLB): Report of the consortium on DLB international workshop. Neurology, 1996; 47(5), 1113-1124.
20. Shaik S, Varma A. Differentiating the dementias: a neurological approach. Prog. Neurol. Psychiatry. 2012; 16(1), 11-18.
21. Steinman M, Hanlon J. Managing medications in clinically complex elders: "There's got to be a happy medium." JAMA. 2010; 304 (14): 1592-1601.
22. American Geriatrics Society. American geriatrics society 2015 updated beers criteria for potentially inappropriate medication use in older adults. Journal of the American Geriatrics Society. 2015; 63:2227–2246.
23. O'Mahony D, O'Sullivan D, Byrne S, O'Connor MN, Ryan C, & Gallagher P. STOPP/START criteria for potentially inappropriate prescribing in older people: version 2. Age Aging. 2014; 44 (2): 213-218.
24. Canadian Medical Association. Determining medical fitness to operate motor vehicles. CMA Driver's Guide, 7th ed. Ottawa: Canadian Medical Association; 2006.
25. Lachs MS, Pillemer K. Elder abuse. Lancet. 2004; 364(9441):1263-1272.
26. McDonald L, Collins A. Abuse and Neglect of Older Adults: A Discussion Paper. Ottawa: Family Violence Prevention Unit, Health Canada; 2000.
27. Imbody B, Vandsburger E. Elder Abuse and Neglect: Assessment Tools, Interventions, and Recommendations for Effective Service Provision. Educ Gerontol. 2011; 37(7), 634-650

GERIATRICS

# CHAPTER 17:

# Infectious Disease

**Editors:**
Claudia Frankfurter, BHSc
Stephanie Zhou, HBSc

**Resident Reviewer:**
Shixin Shen, MD, MSc

**Faculty Reviewers:**
Andrew Morris, MD, SM, FRCPC
Susan M. Poutanen, MD, MPH, FRCPC

## TABLE OF CONTENTS

# 1. RESPIRATORY TRACT INFECTIONS

- See **The Respiratory System** chapter for a general history and exam of the respiratory system
- **Red flag** signs and symptoms suggest a non-benign, infectious condition that require further investigation and medical management (see **Table 1**)

**Table 1.** Potentially dangerous respiratory conditions that require medical management

| Differential Diagnosis | Distinguishing Features |
| --- | --- |
| Pharyngitis[1] | Severe and sudden throat pain, absence of cough, odynophagia, painful lymphadenopathy, tonsillar exudates |
| Epiglottitis[1] | Fever, severe sore throat, stridor, hoarseness, dysphagia, drooling, dyspnea |
| Pneumonia | Fever, productive cough, dyspnea, chills |
| Tuberculosis | Long standing cough, hemoptysis, chest pain, constitutional symptoms (weight loss, fatigue, fever, chills, night sweats) |
| Influenza in vulnerable populations (elderly, children) | Fever, malaise, myalgia. May lead to complications such as pneumonia and may require hospitalization. |

## 1.1 Upper Respiratory Tract Infections

An infection of the upper respiratory tract can range from self-limiting to lethal presentations depending on the patient's age, immune status, and the infectious agent.

### Etiology
- Mostly viral, but can be bacterial, mycobacterial or fungal in origin

### Focused History
- Signs and symptoms to inquire when differentiating benign conditions from those that require treatment (see **Table 1** and **2**)
- Make sure to ask **OPQRSTUVW** questions in addition
- See **Respiratory History** p.330 for details

### Focused Physical Exam
- See **The Respiratory System** chapter
- See **The Head, Neck, and Throat** chapter
- If specific localization of symptoms is observed – such as sinus, ears, pharynx, lower airway – then specific examinations of those structures are required
- Ear and mastoid: pneumatic otoscopy, focused neurological exam of CN VIII (see **The Nervous System** chapter)
- Larynx: direct laryngoscopy

**Table 2.** Common Upper Respiratory Tract Infections[2]

| Diagnosis | Presenting Signs/ Symptoms | Investigations | Complications |
| --- | --- | --- | --- |
| **Common Cold** | Sneezing, nasal congestion and discharge (rhinorrhea), sore throat, cough, low grade fever, headache, and malaise | Clinical diagnosis; suspect alternative dx if >2 wk or high fever | Secondary bacterial rhinosinusitis, lower respiratory tract infections (LRTIs), otitis media |

| Diagnosis | Presenting Signs/ Symptoms | Investigations | Complications |
|---|---|---|---|
| **Acute Rhinosinusitis** | Nasal congestion, obstruction, discharge, maxillary tooth pain, facial pain, fever, cough, headache, hyposmia | Clinical diagnosis; suspect bacterial etiology if >10 d without improvement; severe symptoms at the onset of illness; worsening symptoms after initial improvement | Bacterial sinusitis, meningitis, orbital cellulitis |
| **Pharyngitis** | Sore throat, tonsillar edema/exudate, tender anterior cervical lymph nodes, splenomegaly; cough and significant rhinorrhea are usually absent | Swab for culture, rapid streptococcal antigen testing (RSAT) | Peritonsillar/ retropharyngeal abscess, post-strep glomerulonephritis (GN), rheumatic fever |

**Clinical Pearl:** Epiglottis on the Differential
Epiglottitis should always be considered on the differential diagnosis. May find drooling, respiratory distress, and dysphagia. This can lead to respiratory compromise and is a medical emergency.[1]

## Common Investigations
- The common cold is generally self-resolving with nonspecific laboratory examinations, and thus should not be routinely investigated.
- Pharynx and oral cavity: key investigation is to distinguish Group A streptococcal pharyngitis from viral pharyngitis.
  - Throat swab culture (takes 24-48 h)
  - Rapid antigen detection testing for Group A β-hemolytic streptococci (GABHS) (less sensitive)
- Epiglottitis: Fiber optic laryngoscopy in the OR for visualization, or "thumb-printing" on lateral neck x-ray[2] (direct visualization in the examination room with tongue blade and laryngoscope NOT recommended)

## Management
- Antibiotic therapy not indicated for uncomplicated common colds; symptomatic management includes over-the-counter nasal saline rinse, decongestants, NSAIDs, dextromethorphan (for cough), lozenges, etc.
- Pharyngitis: Refer to Centor Score for Strep Pharyngitis (**Figure 1**) for management criteria
- See **The Head, Neck, and Throat** chapter for treatment options for sinusitis

INFECTIOUS DISEASE

| Criteria | Points |
|---|---|
| Absence of cough | 1 |
| Swollen and tender anterior cervical nodes | 1 |
| Temp. > 100.4 °F (38 °C) | 1 |
| Tonsillar exudates or swelling | 1 |
| Age<br>3-14<br>15-44<br>>44 | 1<br>0<br>-1 |

**Antibiotic selection**

**First line treatment:**
Penicillin V PO x10 days
Amoxicillin PO x10 days
Penicillin G IM x1 dose

**Penicillin allergy:**
Erythromycin PO x10 days
Cefadroxil PO x10 days
Cephalexin PO x 10 days

Apply criteria

| Cumulative score | Risk of GABHS pharyngitis |
|---|---|
| ≤0 | 1-2.5% |
| 1 | 5-10% |
| 2 | 11-17% |
| 3 | 28-35% |
| ≥4 | 51-53% |

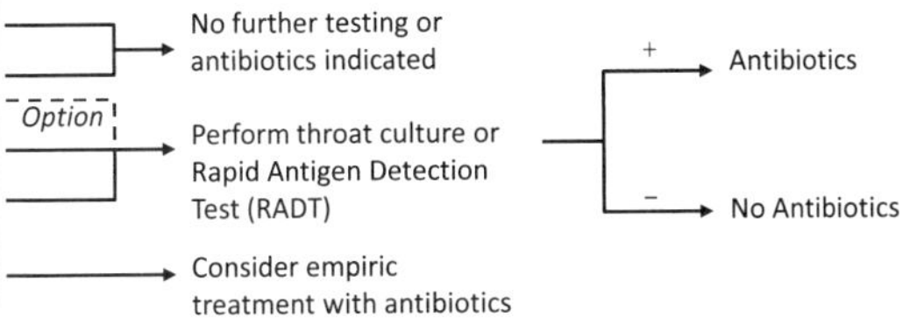

No further testing or antibiotics indicated

Option

Perform throat culture or Rapid Antigen Detection Test (RADT)

+ Antibiotics

− No Antibiotics

Consider empiric treatment with antibiotics

**Figure 1.** Modified Centor score and management options for sore throat.[3] *Adapted.*

## 1.2 Lower Respiratory Tract Infections
### Acute Bronchitis
- Etiology: primarily viral
- Focused history: similar to URTI with cough ± sputum >5 d
- Focused physical exam (see **The Respiratory System** chapter)
- Investigations: no cultures recommended; CXR if pneumonia is suspected
- Management: no antibiotics indicated

### Pneumonia
- Etiology: bacterial, viral, and less often, fungal in origin
- Focused history: fever, productive cough, pleuritic chest pain, dyspnea
- Focused physical exam (see **The Respiratory System** chapter)
- Investigations: CXR, sputum and blood cultures; consider nasopharyngeal swab for influenza during influenza season
- Management: empiric antibiotic therapy; during influenza season, consider empiric antivirals for influenza while awaiting influenza test results; refer to **CURB-65 Criteria** (**Table 3**) for admission criteria

**Table 3:** Criteria for admission in patients with pneumonia. [4]

| CURB-65 Criteria | | |
|---|---|---|
| C | Confusion | 1 |
| U | Blood urea nitrogen ≥ 20 mg/dL | 1 |
| R | Respiratory rate ≥ 30 breaths/min | 1 |
| B | Systolic BP < 90 mm Hg or Diastolic BP ≤ 60 mm Hg | 1 |
| 65 | Age ≥ 65 | 1 |
| Scoring, Risk Level, Suggested Site-of-Care | 0=Low risk, outpatient; 1=Low risk, outpatient; 2=Moderate risk, short inpatient/supervised outpatient; 3=Moderate-high risk, inpatient; 4=High risk, inpatient/ICU | |

INFECTIOUS DISEASE

# 2. TUBERCULOSIS

- Caused by the *Mycobacterium tuberculosis* complex, manifesting as pulmonary and extrapulmonary disease (see **Table 6**)
- Transmission via airborne droplets produced by coughing from individuals with active pulmonary TB

## 2.1 Pulmonary Tuberculosis
### Focused History
- **HPI**:
  - ◆ Pulmonary Symptoms
    - ▪ Cough: may be initially nonproductive and subsequently purulent
    - ▪ Sputum ± hemoptysis
    - ▪ Pleuritic chest pain
    - ▪ Dyspnea or acute respiratory distress syndrome (ARDS)
  - ◆ Nonspecific Symptoms:
    - ▪ fever that persists more than 2 wk, night sweats, weight loss, chills, general malaise, weakness
- **Past Medical History**: Immunosuppression (organ transplant, long-term corticosteroids, DM, chronic kidney disease [CKD])
- **Medications**: Antacids inhibit the absorption of certain TB drugs. Many drugs and foods interact with TB medications. A comprehensive medication and diet history is essential to ensure patient safety when they begin their treatment regimen.
- **Social History / Travel:**
  - ◆ HIV/AIDS
  - ◆ First Nations peoples
  - ◆ Homelessness, history of imprisonment, lack of social support, joblessness, and poverty
  - ◆ Substance abuse
  - ◆ Family members with TB
  - ◆ Actual exposure to known TB cases
  - ◆ Travel to endemic areas: Eastern Europe, Mediterranean, Russia, China, Southeast Asia, India, Pakistan, Africa, and South America (assume exposure regardless of whether the patient recognizes an exposure or not)

### Focused Physical Exam
- General inspection: age, degree of nutrition, emotional and anxiety states, cyanosis
- Tachypnea
- Fever
- Wasting
- Chest examination (see **The Respiratory System** chapter, p.333)
- Persistent rales in involved areas during inspiration, especially after coughing
- Rhonchi due to partial bronchial obstruction
- Whispered pectoriloquy may be helpful in finding small areas of local consolidation
- Amphoric breath sounds in areas with large cavities
- Percussion: fluid accumulation suggested by flat, wooden sounds
- Grocco's sign: presence of paravertebral area of dullness on the opposite side
- May have no detectable abnormalities

INFECTIOUS DISEASE

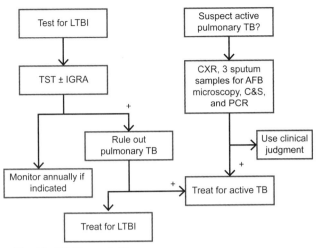

**Figure 2.** Flow Chart for TB Diagnosis [5,6]
AFB = acid fast bacilli, IGRA= IFN-γ release assay, LTBI = latent TB infection, PCR = polymerase chain reaction, TST = tuberculin skin test

### Investigation Notes
- Tuberculin skin test (TST) (used for latent infection, not for active TB infection; sensitivity = 90%, specificity >95% for 10 mm induration)[5,6]
    - False negatives common in immunosuppressed patients
    - False positives with nontuberculosis mycobacteria (NTM) and BCG vaccination
    - Induration NOT erythema should be measured (see **Table 4**)
- Interferon gamma release assays (IGRA)
    - Can be used in conjunction with TST
- CXR
    - Usually shows upper lobe infiltrates with cavities but in immunosuppressed patients, atypical pattern of lower lobe infiltration without cavities seen
- 3 specimens of AM sputum
    - Used to detect TB through microscopy for acid fast bacilli (AFB), C&S, and PCR (amplified *mycobacterium tuberculosis* direct test)
- CT and MRI can be used for imaging of extrapulmonary TB

**Table 4.** Tuberculin Skin Test Interpretation[5]

| Induration | Condition in which Size is Considered Positive |
|---|---|
| 0-4 mm | HIV infection with immune suppression AND the expected likelihood of TB infection is high |
| 5-9 mm | HIV infection, close contact of active contagious case, children suspected of having tuberculosis disease, abnormal chest X-ray with fibrotic disease, other immune suppression: TNF-α inhibitors |
| 10-15 mm | Recent immigrants from endemic countries, IV drug users, people working in high-risk settings (e.g. mycobacteriology laboratory personnel), children <4 yr or children exposed to adults in high-risk categories, people with clinical conditions that place them at high risk |
| >15 mm | Any person, even if no known risk factors for TB |

## Simplified Management Plan
- See **Table 5**
- Referral to Public Health is mandatory
- Completion of treatment is defined by total doses taken and not duration of treatment
- Drug resistance and poor rates of adherence:
  - Direct observation of treatment (DOT), especially during the initial phase, can be used to ensure adherence
  - Concurrently with treatment, monthly sputum examination is conducted until AFB and cultures become negative

**Table 5.** Treatment for Pulmonary TB[5]

| TB Status | Drug Regimens |
|---|---|
| Latent | INH for 9 mo OR<br>RMP for 4 mo* |
| Active | INH/RMP/PZA ± EMB for 2 mo, then INH/RMP for 4 mo OR<br>INH/RMP for 9 mo |
| MDR-TB† | Individualized therapy based on susceptibility/clinical situation, DOT should be carried out |

INH=isoniazid, RMP=rifampin, PZA=pyrazinamide, EMB=ethambutol, MDR-TB=multidrug resistant TB
*This regimen should only be used if INH cannot be used
†If you suspect multidrug resistant TB, referral to a specialized center is recommended

## 2.2 Extrapulmonary Tuberculosis

**Table 6.** Extrapulmonary Tuberculosis[5,7]

| Location | History | Physical Findings |
|---|---|---|
| Lymph Nodes | Accompanying HIV infection, immunosuppression | Painless swelling of lymph nodes, most commonly at cervical and supraclavicular sites |
| Upper Airways | Hoarseness, chronic productive cough | Ulcerations |
| Pleura | Asymptomatic, fever, pleuritic chest pain, dyspnea | Pleural effusion, dullness to percussion, absence of breath sounds |
| Pericardial | Subacute or acute with fever, dull retrosternal pain | Friction rub, cardiac tamponade, constrictive pericarditis |
| Peritoneal | No specific history | Abdominal/pelvic masses |
| Genitourinary | Asymptomatic, urinary frequency, dysuria, hematuria, flank pain | Females: infertility, pelvic pain, menstrual abnormalities<br>Males: epididymitis, prostatitis, orchiditis |
| Musculo-skeletal (spine) | Back pain, paraplegia, paraparesis | Kyphosis (gibbus deformity) |
| Sites Outside Spine | Monoarticular destructive arthritis | Hip, knee, ankle, or elbow pain |
| Miliary or Disseminated | Accompanying HIV infection, fever, night sweats, anorexia, weakness, weight loss | Hepatomegaly, splenomegaly, lymphadenopathy, choroidal tubercles in retina |
| CNS | Headache, mental lethargy, altered sensorium, neck rigidity | Obtundation, cranial nerve palsies |

INFECTIOUS DISEASE

## 3. HIV/AIDS

- Infection with the human immunodeficiency virus (HIV) (subtypes 1 or 2) causing immunodeficiency through the progressive depletion of CD4+ lymphocyte populations
- Acquired Immunodeficiency Syndrome (AIDS) is characterized by CD4+ cell counts below 200/mL or diagnosis of an AIDS-defining illness

### Epidemiology

- Approximately 37 million people infected worldwide
- Risk factors
  - Unprotected sexual activity, IV drug use
  - Men who have sex with men (MSM), sex workers, marginalized populations, immigrants from endemic countries

**Table 7.** Natural Progression of HIV/AIDS

| Stage | Characteristics |
|---|---|
| **Primary Infection/Acute HIV Syndrome** | • 50-70% experience this after primary infection<br>• Unexplained fatigue, sore throat, myalgias, malaise, fevers/night sweats, diarrhea, rash, weight loss, aseptic meningitis, lymphadenopathy, resolves spontaneously |
| **Asymptomatic Phase** | • Clinical latency, average 10 yrs for untreated patients<br>• May note generalized lymphadenopathy with minor opportunistic infections (e.g. herpes zoster, oral candidiasis), chronic diarrhea<br>• Progressive decline in CD4+ cells, but viral load can increase or remain stable |
| **Progression to AIDS** | • Persistent fever, fatigue, weight loss, diarrhea<br>• CD4+ count <200/mL or AIDS defining illness (e.g. *Pneumocystis jiroveci* [previously known as *P. carinii*] pneumonia [PJP], TB – pulmonary or extrapulmonary, recurrent bacterial pneumonia, cryptococcal meningitis, CNS toxoplasmosis, CMV retinitis), or neoplasms (Kaposi's sarcoma, lymphoma), clinical neurological disease – progressive multifocal leukoencephalopathy, HIV dementia |

CMV = cytomegalovirus

### Focused History

- Clinical presentation can vary widely depending on the stage of infection, underlying comorbid illness, and various aspects of patient history
- **HPI:**
  - Occurrence of opportunistic infections, malignancies, STIs, IV drug use associated conditions
    - STIs: hepatitis B and C, syphilis, genital warts, herpes simplex, gonorrhea, chlamydia
    - Other infections or malignancies (bacterial infections, fungal infections such as thrush, parasitic infections, mycobacterial infections)
- **Past Medical History**
  - Date and place of HIV testing and confirmation of test results
  - Any history of prior testing (e.g. for insurance, giving blood, pregnancy, other)
  - CD4+ count and viral load
  - TB skin test results
  - Syphilis test results
  - Date and results of last Pap smear (women)
- **Medications:**
  - Certain clinical manifestations are due to side effects of medication and antiretrovirals
  - Antiretroviral history (include adherence, response, CD4+, viral load), side effects/toxicity, any resistance testing and results
  - Participation in clinical trials
- It is very important to elicit a social history and thorough review of systems (see **General History and Physical Exam** chapter)

## Focused Physical Exam
- **General**
  - Vitals
  - Lipodystrophy and metabolic syndrome: central obesity and wasting of extremities and face
- **Head and Neck**
  - Fundoscopy (e.g. HIV retinopathy [cotton wool spots], cytomegalovirus retinitis)
  - Examine oral cavity
    - Candidiasis (thrush)
    - Kaposi's sarcoma lesions
    - Hairy leukoplakia on lateral tongue
    - Gingivitis
    - Bruises or bleeding from gums
    - Ulcers
  - Lymphadenopathy
- **Cardiovascular**
  - Signs of heart failure (edema, dyspnea)
  - Hypertension
- **Respiratory**
  - Focal chest findings associated with bacterial pneumonia
  - Chest findings may also be associated with TB
  - Absent chest findings compatible with *Pneumocystis jiroveci* pneumonia (PJP)
- **Abdominal**
  - Liver (hepatitis B and C, drug toxicity): stigmata of chronic liver disease, ascites, jaundice, hepatomegaly
  - Spleen: splenomegaly
  - Masses (lymphoma)
- **GU**
  - Ulcers or warts
  - Pelvic exam/Pap smear: cervical carcinoma
  - Rectal exam: anal/rectal carcinoma
- **Neurological**
  - Mental status: depression, memory loss, dementia, and psychosis
  - Sensory and motor exams
    - Focal neurological findings (e.g. weakness, photophobia) suggest CNS infection or tumor
    - Unsteady gait, poor balance, tremor
    - Loss of bladder or bowel control with myelopathy
    - Increased tone and deep tendon reflexes
    - Peripheral neuropathies
  - Meningeal irritation (see **Meningitis**, p.466)
- **MSK**
  - Arthritis in large joints: suggests HIV/AIDS-associated arthropathy
- **Dermatological**
  - Macular rash (seen with acute seroconversion syndrome)
  - Dermatitis, folliculitis, seborrhea
  - Herpes zoster
  - Karposi's sarcoma

## Investigations
- HIV antibody (1 and 2) + antigen (p24) test
  - If positive/inconclusive: Western blot
  - ELISA: >99% sensitivity, Western blot: >99% specificity[7,8]
- HIV viral load
- CD4+ T cell count
- HIV genotyping
- HLA-B*5701 allele testing prior to prescription of abacavir to check potential sensitivity
- Routine blood work (CBC-diff, electrolytes, Cr, LFTs, blood glucose, lipids, urinalysis, ACR)
- STI testing: HCV, HBV, VDRL, chlamydia/gonorrhea
- TB skin test
- Pap smear (once a year)

INFECTIOUS DISEASE

## Management
- Education and counseling
- Highly Active Anti-Retroviral Therapy (HAART)
- Prophylaxis of opportunistic infection if CD4 count < 200
- Immunizations (Pneumovax®, hepatitis A and B, influenza) if CD4 200+

## 4. SEXUALLY TRANSMITTED INFECTIONS
Bacterial, viral or parasitic organisms transmitted by any mode of sexual activity (oral, vaginal, anal).

### Focused History
- Please refer to the **General History** chapter for sexual history
- Both men and women can develop a reactive arthritis syndrome following *C. trachomatis* infection: conjunctivitis, urethritis or cervicitis, arthritis, and mucocutaneous lesions

### Focused Physical Exam
- **General Inspection**
  - ◆ Vitals
  - ◆ Examine conjunctiva, inspect mouth and tonsils, look for skin lesions
- **Adnexal Masses**
  - ◆ Tenderness and guarding in lower quadrants
  - ◆ Inspect perianal area and stool for mucopus
- **GU**
  - ◆ In men: inspect and palpate penis (especially meatus) and scrotum (especially epididymis), inspect for secretions
  - ◆ In women: inspection of vaginal orifice and Bartholin's gland for erythema and exudate, pelvic exam including inspection of cervix for redness, friability, discharge
  - ◆ Lymphadenopathy
- **MSK**
  - ◆ Arthritis
  - ◆ Polyarthralgias (especially wrists, knees, fingers, ankles)
  - ◆ Myalgias

**Table 8.** Signs/Symptoms and Diagnosis of Common STIs[8]

| Signs/Symptoms | Diagnosis | Treatment |
|---|---|---|
| **Chlamydia** (*Chlamydia trachomatis*) Asymptomatic (most); mucopurulent cervical discharge; erythematous cervix, often with infected erosion, urethral syndrome (dysuria, increased frequency, urgency, pyuria with no bacteria) | PCR | Azithromycin |
| **Gonorrhea** (*Neisseria gonorrhoeae*) Similar to chlamydia; offensive yellow-white discharge; tends to be thicker, more copious and painful than chlamydia | PCR (urine); Gram stain; culture of urethral or cervical discharge | Dual therapy with ceftriaxone/cefixime plus azithromycin or doxycycline (for MSM, ceftriaxone is recommended) |
| **Trichomoniasis** (*Trichomonas vaginalis*) Asymptomatic (up to 50%); profuse thin, frothy gray/yellow-green discharge, often foul-smelling; occasionally irritated, tender vulva; dysuria; petechiae on vagina and cervix (10%) | Saline wet mount culture on diamond medium | Metronidazole |

INFECTIOUS DISEASE

| Signs/Symptoms | Diagnosis | Treatment |
|---|---|---|
| **Condylomata Acuminata/Genital Warts** (HPV)<br>• Latent: no visible lesions, asymptomatic<br>• Subclinical: visible after acetic acid use<br>• Clinical: visible, wart-like hyperkeratotic, verrucous or flat, macular lesions; vulvar edema<br>• Lesions usually enlarge in pregnancy | Clinical, by visual inspection. Biopsy if uncertain or lesions worsen | Podophyllotoxin, imiquimod; trichloroacetic acid; excisional surgery or laser ablation |
| **Herpes Simplex** (HSV)<br>• May be asymptomatic<br>• Prodromal: tingling, burning, pruritus<br>• Multiple painful shallow ulcerations with small vesicles – may coalesce<br>• First infection: inguinal lymphadenopathy, malaise, fever<br>• If affect urethral mucosa: dysuria, urinary retention<br>• Recurrent: decreased duration, frequency, severity | Viral culture | Antiviral therapy (acyclovir, famciclovir, or valacyclovir) |
| **Syphilis** (*Treponema pallidum*)<br>• 1°: usually single, painless penile/vulval/vaginal/cervical chancre, inguinal lymphadenopathy 3 d to 4 wk after infection<br>• 2° (up to 3 mo later):<br>  • malaise, anorexia, headache, adenopathy; fever<br>  • generalized maculopapular rash; condylomata lata<br>• 3°: CNS/ascending aorta progressively destroyed; may involve other organs<br>• Congenital: possible fetal anomalies/stillbirth/neonatal death<br>• Latent: asymptomatic | Serology (non-treponemal screening test and confirmatory treponemal assay available) | Benzathine penicillin G dosed according to stage |

PCR = polymerase chain reaction

*Canadian Guidelines on Sexually Transmitted Infections.* Ottawa: Public Health Agency of Canada; 2010.

## 5. URINARY TRACT INFECTIONS
• See **Urological Exam** chapter

## 6. INFECTIOUS DIARRHEA
• Liquid or unformed stool passed at a higher frequency than usual >200 g/d
• 3 categories: acute (<2 wk), persistent (2-4 wk), chronic (>4 wk)

### Etiology
• Infectious (90% of cases), see Table 9

INFECTIOUS DISEASE

**Table 9.** Common Signs, Symptoms, and Epidemiology of Infectious Diarrhea[10]

| | Signs and Symptoms | Epidemiology |
|---|---|---|
| **Parasitic** | | |
| **Giardia, Cryptosporidia, Cyclospora, Isospora** | Persistent diarrhea (never blood), bloating, cramps, no fever; may have malabsorption | |
| **Amoebiasis** *(E. histolytica)* | Colitis with blood and mucus; absence of stool leukocytes | Rare, but serious |
| **Bacterial** | | |
| **Campylobacter, Salmonella, Shigella** | Watery diarrhea progressing to bloody diarrhea; severe lower abdominal cramps, vomiting, fever | Increasing incidence of *Campylobacter* in travelers; *Shigella* more common in children, MSM |
| **Listeria** | Diarrhea followed by muscle aches, fever, and nausea | Often foodborne (cold cuts, cheeses) |
| **ETEC** | Watery diarrhea, mild cramps, no fever | Traveler's diarrhea |
| **EHEC** (E. coli 0157:H7) | Bloody diarrhea; may cause hemolytic uremic syndrome (HUS) | Often foodborne |
| **Clostridium difficile** | Diarrhea with mucus ± blood | Associated with antibiotic use, often in long-term care homes and hospitals, but increasing community-acquired cases |
| **Viral** | | |
| **Hepatitis A** | Light-colored diarrhea | Often foodborne (raw seafood) |
| **Rotavirus, Norwalk-like Virus** (Norovirus) | Vomiting and diarrhea | Rotaviruses: children <2 yr Noroviruses: adults and children |

EHEC = enterohemorrhagic E. coli, ETEC = enterotoxigenic E. coli

## Focused History

- **HPI:** Appearance of stool: blood, mucus, fever, abdominal pain, tenesmus, vomiting. Refer to Table 9.
  - Features of diarrhea: frequency, duration
- **Past Medical History:** occupational history, recent stay in daycare center, hospital, ICU, recent antibiotic exposure
- **Medications:** recent use of antibiotics (broad-spectrum), laxatives, antacids, chemotherapy, colchicine, pelvic radiation therapy.
- **Social History:** travel and water exposure, sexual practice (including oral-anal and receptive anal contact)

## Focused Physical Exam
- Assess for intravascular volume depletion
  - Vitals
  - Postural lightheadedness and a reflex tachycardia >30 min indicates moderate to severe intravascular volume depletion
  - Urine output
  - Skin turgor, mucous membrane
  - Axillary moistness
  - Mental status changes

## Differential Diagnosis
- Pseudo-diarrhea (frequent passage of stool but total <200 g/d)
- Fecal incontinence
- Overflow diarrhea due to fecal impaction
- Post-infectious IBD
- Secondary lactose intolerance

## Investigations
- Fecal WBC count
- Stool microbiology
  - Gram stain
  - Culture
  - PCR (e.g. for noroviruses)
  - Electron microscopy (e.g. for noroviruses, rotaviruses)

## Management
- Fluid and electrolyte replacement
- In mild cases, observe
- In nonfebrile moderate cases without bloody stool or elevated WBC, antidiarrheal agents
- In febrile moderate to severe cases (significant volume depletion), consider empiric treatment with quinolone
- *Note:* antibiotic treatment of E. coli O157:H7 is contraindicated due to increased risk of progression to HUS and thrombotic thrombocytopenic purpura (TTP)[10]

# 7. VIRAL HEPATITIS
- 5 classes: hepatitis A-E (HAV, HBV, HCV, HDV, and HEV)
- Can be classified into two categories: fecal-oral (HAV, HEV) vs. parenteral/sexual (HBV, HCV, HDV)
- Of the 5 classes, HBV and HCV can cause chronic disease
- All RNA viruses except for HBV
- Wide range of symptoms from mild to severe

**Table 10:** Etiology and Management of five hepatitis classes

| Hepatitis Class | Etiology | Management |
|---|---|---|
| HAV | • Incubation period: ~4 wks<br>• From raw seafood or food prepared by an individual with active HAV<br>• Usually self-limiting, but occasionally fulminant, life-threatening disease | Infection is self-limited. Supportive care only. |
| HBV | • Incubation period: 8-12 wks<br>• Parenteral and sexual exposure<br>• Two peaks of exposure: infancy and adolescence<br>• Exposure in infancy usually leads to chronic infection, while exposure in adolescence can lead to acute infections that may become chronic<br>• Severe chronic and fulminant hepatitis can lead to cirrhosis and hepatocellular carcinoma | No intervention needed unless disease is chronic/persistent (HBeAg+) (adefovir or lamivudine) |

INFECTIOUS DISEASE

| Hepatitis Class | Etiology | Management |
|---|---|---|
| HCV | • Incubation period: ~7 wks<br>• Parenteral exposure (some sexual transmission)<br>• At risk groups: injection drug users, tattoo recipients, prison inmates, HIV patients, healthcare workers<br>• At least six different genotypes with different patterns of worldwide distribution<br>• Due to diversity, patients exposed to HCV will not have immunity against subsequent HCV infections<br>• Associated with cutaneous disorders such as porphyria cutanea tarda and lichen planus | Direct acting antivirals (i.e. simeprevir and sofosbuvir)<br><br>If pruritus present, give bile salt-sequestering resin cholestyramine |
| HDV | • Incubation period: ~ 8-12 weeks<br>• Absolute co-infection or superinfection with HBV (i.e. never alone)<br>• Cause of fulminant hepatic deterioration in individuals with active HBV | No intervention needed unless disease is chronic/persistent (HBeAg+) (adefovir or lamivudine) |
| HEV | • Incubation period: ~ 5-6 wks<br>• Enteric virus predominantly in India, Asia, Africa, and Central America<br>• Animal reservoir in pigs and other animals | Infection is self-limited. Supportive care only |

## Focused History
- **HPI:**
  - Constitutional symptoms: N/V, anorexia, fatigue, malaise, arthralgia, myalgia, headaches, photophobia, pharyngitis, cough, coryza
  - Fever: low grade (38-39°C) for HAV and HEV, others may have higher temperatures
  - Dark urine and clay-colored stool
  - Jaundice
- **PMHx**
- **Meds**
- **Social Hx:** IV drug use, incarceration, healthcare worker, travel, diet, alcohol use, sexual history, vaccination history

## Focused Physical Exam
- Focused abdominal exam
  - Palpation of enlarged masses (see **The Gastroinetestinal System** chapter)
  - Surface examination for signs of liver disease

## Investigations
- Most common investigation for patients suspected of viral hepatitis is a panel of serological tests: HBV surface antigen (HBsAg), anti-HBs IgM anti-HBc, IgM anti-HAV, and anti-HCV, plus viral load testing in patients with active HBV and HCV (see **Table 11** for diagnostic approach)
- Liver enzymes (AST, ALT)
- Liver function tests (albumin, INR, bilirubin, platelets)

INFECTIOUS DISEASE

**Table 11.** Simplified Approach to Diagnosis of Suspected Viral Hepatitis[10]

| HBsAg | IgM Anti-HAV | IgM Anti-HBc | Anti-HCV | Interpretation |
|:---:|:---:|:---:|:---:|:---|
| - | + | - | - | Acute hepatitis A |
| + | - | + | - | Acute hepatitis B |
| + | - | - | - | Chronic hepatitis B |
| - | - | + | - | Acute hepatitis B (HBsAg below detection threshold) |
| - | - | - | + | Acute hepatitis C |

## 8. MENINGITIS

Inflammation of the meninges that can be infectious or noninfectious in origin.

### Epidemiology
- Viral and bacterial meningitis are most common (fungal/parasitic causes less common)
- Pneumococcal and meningococcal infections are the most common causes of bacterial meningitis in adults

### Focused History
- **HPI**
  - ◆ Altered LOC: irritability/confusion/drowsiness/stupor/coma
  - ◆ Seizures
  - ◆ Neonates: signs of sepsis (fever, respiratory distress, apnea, jaundice)
  - ◆ Infants: fever, vomiting, irritability, convulsions, high-pitch cry, poor feeding, lethargy
  - ◆ Older children and adults:
    - ▪ Fever
    - ▪ Headache
    - ▪ Neck stiffness
    - ▪ Photophobia
- **PMHx**: STIs (HSV, syphilis, HIV), infection with *Mycobacterium tuberculosis*, parameningeal infections (e.g. otitis media, sinusitis), compromised immunity, persistent CSF leaks, head trauma, anatomical defects (including dermal sinuses), previous neurosurgical procedures
- **Meds:** Immunosuppressants
- **Social Hx:** Infectious contacts, travel to endemic regions

### Focused Physical Exam
- Vitals (fever, tachycardia/bradycardia, irregular respiration)
- Neonates and infants: inspect anterior fontanelle for bulging or tightness
- Nuchal rigidity (stiff neck) (see pg 557 for illustration)
  - ◆ **Brudzinski's Sign:** abrupt neck flexion with patient in supine position – involuntary flexion of hips and knees is positive sign
  - ◆ **Kernig's Sign:** strong passive resistance to attempts to extend knee from flexed thigh position
- Jolt accentuation
- Assess lethargy, level of consciousness (MMSE, Glasgow coma scale [GCS])
- Cranial nerves: typically IV, VI, VII affected by raised ICP or basilar inflammation
- Petechial or purpuric rash (typically in extremities)

### Investigations
- CBC and differential, electrolytes
- Blood cultures
- CT to exclude elevated ICP and mass lesion
- Lumbar puncture
- Opening pressure
- Protein, glucose, cell count and differential, Gram stain

## Management Principles
- Do not delay IV antibiotics
- The chosen antimicrobial agent should be bactericidal and penetrate the CSF
- Examples of empiric antibiotic treatment of bacterial meningitis include:
  - Ceftriaxone 2g IV q12h
  - Vancomycin 1.5g IV q12h
  - Ampicillin 2g IV q4h for individuals >50 yr or immunocompromised to cover *L. monocytogenes*
- Adjuvant dexamethasone treatment in adults with acute pneumococcal meningitis lowers mortality/risk of unfavorable outcome

### EBM: Adult Meningitis[11]

History alone is not useful in establishing a diagnosis of meningitis. Physical exam is useful for ruling out meningitis, and in determining which patients should proceed to more definitive testing (lumbar puncture).

| Physical Exam Finding | Sensitivity (%) |
|---|---|
| Fever | 77 |
| Neck Stiffness | 83 |
| Altered Mental Status (GCS <15) | 69 |

The absence of all three signs of the classic triad of fever, neck stiffness, and altered mental status virtually eliminates a diagnosis of meningitis (sensitivity of >1 sign present = 99%). 95% of patients will have at least 2/4 of headache, fever, neck stiffness, and altered mental status

## 9. SEPSIS

### Definitions: based on 2016 International Consensus[9]
- **Sepsis:** life-threatening organ dysfunction caused by a dysregulated host response to infection
- Clinical criteria:
  - Infection plus increase of 2 or more points in the Sequential (Sepsis-related) Organ Failure Assessment (SOFA) score (above baseline). SOFA score outlined in Consensus guidelines by Singer M *et. al.* (2016)
  - Outside the ICU, 2 or more of the quick-SOFA (qSOFA) score may be used as a screening tool to identify those who are likely septic
    - Respiratory rate >= 22/min
    - Altered mentation
    - SBP < 100mmHg
- **Septic Shock:** a subset of sepsis in which underlying circulatory, cellular and metabolic abnormalities are associated with a greater risk of mortality than sepsis alone
  - Clinical criteria: Hypotension requiring use of vasopressors to maintain MAP ≥65 mmHg and having a serum lactate >2 mmol/l persisting despite adequate fluid resuscitation

### Epidemiology/Etiology
- Approximately 2/3 of new cases are due to nosocomial infection
- See **Table 12** for common microorganisms that may generate sepsis response

**Table 12.** Common Microorganisms Generating Sepsis Response

| Microorganism | Common Examples |
|---|---|
| Gram-Negative Bacteria | *Enterobacteriaceae, P. aeruginosa* |
| Gram-Positive Bacteria | *S. aureus, enterococci, S. pneumoniae,* other *streptococci* |
| Classic Pathogens | *N. meningitidis, S. pneumoniae, H. influenzae, S. pyogenes* |

INFECTIOUS DISEASE

## Focused History
- **HPI:**Related to the site of origin of infection (skin and soft tissue, lungs, genitourinary tract, abdomen, CNS)
- **PMHx:** Previous medical or surgical interventions (chemotherapy, surgery, transplantation), history of immunosuppression (e.g. HIV/AIDS, chemotherapy, splenectomy, organ transplant), hypogammaglobulinemia, underlying chronic diseases affecting prognosis (DM, alcoholism, renal failure, resp disease, hematological malignanices and solid tumors), invasive procedures or indwelling devices, vascular catheterization, structural abnormalities in urogenital tract
- **Meds:** Antimicrobials, immunosuppressants (i.e. corticosteroid therapy, immunomodulatory biologic therapy (anti-TNF therapy))
- **Social Hx:** Diet, travel, infectious contacts

## Focused Physical Exam
- **Vitals**
- **Respiratory**
  - Cyanosis
  - Pulmonary infiltrates
- **CVS**
  - Signs of hypovolemia
- **Abdominal**
  - Jaundice
  - Hepatosplenomegaly
  - Murphy's sign
  - CVA/suprapubic tenderness
- **Dermatological**
  - Exanthems, i.e. erythema gangrenosum in *P. aeruginosa*
  - Contusions
  - Purpuric rash
  - signs of cellulitis
- **Neurological**
  - Altered mental status

## Investigations
- Culture and sensitivity of microorganisms:
  - Local site
  - Blood samples (2 x 10 mL samples from different venipuncture sites)
  - Midstream urine/catheter specimen if needed
- CBC with differential, comprehensive metabolic panel
- Chest X-ray

## Management
- IV antibiotics (following sample collection)
- Source management (e.g. abscess drainage)
- Oxygen saturation and fluid management
- Respiratory support

# 10. OSTEOMYELITIS

An infection of bone, characterized by progressive inflammatory destruction of bone, bone necrosis, and new bone formation.

## Epidemiology/Etiology
- Often community-acquired
- Commonly caused by staphylococci, streptococci, may be caused by *P. aeruginosa* and other gram negative rods (GNRs), anaerobic bacteria, and mycobacteria
- Microorganisms enter bone from a penetrating wound, or by spreading from a contiguous infectious focus or via hematogenous dissemination

INFECTIOUS DISEASE

## Focused History
- **HPI:** Pain history (onset, duration, severity, localized skeletal pain, similar pain previously), constitutional symptoms (fever, malaise, night sweats)
- **PMHx:** Previous trauma, sickle cell anemia, immunodeficiency, prosthetic joints, DM, vascular insufficiency, endocarditis, chronic skin ulcers
- **Meds:** Immunosuppressants
- **Social Hx:** IV drug use

## Focused Physical Exam
- Vitals
- Inspection:
    - Evidence of injury/trauma
    - Local source of infection (ingrown toenail, wound infection)
    - Cellulitis
- Peripheral vascular exam
- Probe-to-bone test

## Common Investigations
- CBC, ESR, CRP
- Blood cultures
- Bone biopsy: culture/sensitivity and histology
- X-ray, MRI

## Management
- **Medical**
    - Acute infection: IV antibiotics x 4-6 wk, can step-down to PO in selected cases
    - Chronic infection: as for acute followed by additional antibiotics using ESR/CRP, clinical signs and symptoms, and follow-up imaging as aids to determine antibiotic stop date
- **Surgical**
    - Acute infection: debridement of dead tissue
    - Chronic infection: debridement of all devitalized bone and soft tissue and removal of foreign bodies

# 11. SKIN, MUSCLE, AND SOFT TISSUE INFECTIONS
Tissue infection that involves the skin, subcutaneous fat, the fascia and/ or muscle.
## Epidemiology/Etiology
- Nosocomial vs. community-acquired
- Disruption of the epidermal layer by burns or bites, abrasions, foreign bodies, primary dermatologic disorders, surgery, or vascular/pressure ulcers allows penetration of bacteria to the deeper structures
- Hair follicles are a route of infection either for normal flora (e.g. staphylococci) or for extrinsic bacteria (e.g. *P. aeruginosa*)

## Focused History
- **HPI:** Fever, chills, sweats, pruritus, areas of erythema, warmth, and edema, areas of pain, tenderness, myalgia
- **PMHx:** Skin lesions, past infection (e.g. varicella zoster virus, herpes simplex virus), immune status, DM
- Meds
- **Social Hx:** Insect, tick, or animal/human bits, travel, IV drug use

## Focused Physical Exam
- **Lesion(s)**
    - Type of lesion (see **Dermatology** chapter and **Table 13**)
    - Exudates, hemorrhage
    - Arrangement (e.g. linear, clustered, annular, arciform, dermatomal) o Distribution and location (e.g. exposed surfaces, extremities, along skin folds)
    - Color (e.g. erythema in cellulitis)
    - Pain, tenderness, crepitus
    - Associated lymphangitis and regional lymph node involvement
    - Generalized lymph node enlargement
- **Fever**

**Table 13** Common Skin Lesions and Conditions[10]

| Lesion | Associated Conditions |
|---|---|
| Vesicles | Smallpox, chickenpox (primary varicella zoster virus infection), shingles (herpes zoster virus), "cold sores" (herpes simplex virus), genital ulcers (herpes simplex virus), hand, foot and mouth disease (coxsackievirus) |
| Bullae | Necrotizing fasciitis (group A streptococci, mixed Gram-negative, anaerobic infections, community-acquired methicillin-resistant *Staphylococcus aureus* [CA-MRSA]), staphylococcal scalded skin syndrome, gas gangrene (clostridial myonecrosis) |
| Crusted Lesions | Impetigo (streptococcal, staphylococcal), ringworm (dermatophytes), histoplasmosis, blastomycosis, sporotrichosis, cutaneous leishmaniasis |
| Papules and Nodules | Onchocerciasis nodule (Calabar swelling), lepromatous leprosy, secondary syphilis |
| Ulcers | Anthrax, leprosy, chancroid, primary syphilis (chancre) |
| Necrotizing Fasciitis | Staphylococcal necrotizing fasciitis (CA-MRSA), streptococcal gangrene (*S. pyogenes*), mixed aerobic and anaerobic bacteria, including Fournier's gangrene |
| Myositis and Myonecrosis | Pyomyositis (*S. aureus*), streptococcal necrotizing myositis (*S. pyogenes*), nonclostridial (crepitant) myositis (mixed infection), synergistic nonclostridial anaerobic myonecrosis (mixed infection), gas gangrene (*Clostridium* spp.) |

**Table 14.** Common Soft Tissue Infections

| Epidemiology/ Risk Factors | Location | Appearance of Lesions | Degree of Pain |
|---|---|---|---|
| **Impetigo** Common in children | Face, often perioral | Nonbullous honey-crust lesions, bullous-thin crust | Mild |
| **Erysipelas** Any age; may be spontaneous or post-traumatic; may complicate lymphedema | Face or extremities; involving the epidermis and dermis | Abrupt onset of fiery red swelling, well-defined indurated margins | Intense |
| **Cellulitis** As above | Epidermis, dermis, and subcutaneous fat | Swelling, erythema, warmth | Localized |
| **Necrotizing Fasciitis** Any age | Subcutaneous fascia | Swelling, edema, hemorrhagic bullae, cutaneous necrosis, patchy cutaneous anesthesia | Early reported pain may be out of proportion to the extent of skin findings |

INFECTIOUS DISEASE

## Common Investigations
- Aspiration or punch biopsy
- CT or MRI

## Management
- Appropriate empirical antibiotic treatment (dependent on site, route of infection, exposure history)
- Early/aggressive surgical management if necrotizing fasciitis, myositis or gangrene is suspected:
  - Visualization of deep structures
  - Removal of necrotic tissue
  - Reduction of compartment pressure
  - Obtain samples for Gram stain and culture

# 12. TRAVEL-RELATED ILLNESSES

- Fever from the tropics is:
  - A medical emergency and assumed to be malaria until proven otherwise (i.e. it is imperative to rule out malaria in any febrile traveler returning from the tropics or subtropics)
  - However, travel-related illnesses are often not tropical diseases

## Epidemiology
- The risk of acquiring tropical diseases is dependent on the travel environment, location, and duration
- Disease distribution varies with seasons (e.g. rainy seasons)
- For up-to-date information, visit a comprehensive website such as the Centers for Disease Control and Prevention (CDC)

## Focused History
- **HPI:** Fever hx (see Table 15 and 16), signs and symptoms (see Table 17)
- **PMHx**
- **Meds**
- **Social Hx**
  - Pre-Travel Preparation
    - Immunizations (e.g. hepatitis, meningitis, rabies, typhoid, yellow fever, etc.)
    - Malaria chemoprophylaxis (drug dose, adherence, duration)
    - Medications
  - Travel Itinerary
    - Countries visited, dates and duration
    - Accommodations (urban and/or rural, living conditions)
    - Purpose of travel
  - Exposure history
  - Ingestion of:
    - Raw, undercooked or "exotic" foods
    - Contaminated mild or unpasteurized dairy products
    - Contaminated water
  - Fresh water exposure
  - Walking barefoot
  - Sexual contact with local residents or fellow travelers
  - Transfusions, injections, receiving tattoos or body piercings
  - Insect bites (time of day, urban or rural)
  - Exposure to or bites from animals
  - Sick contacts
  - Accommodation (e.g. mud/thatched huts)

**Table 15.** Incubation Periods for Selected Tropical Diseases

| Incubation Period | Infection |
|---|---|
| **Short** (<10 d) | • Enteric bacterial infections<br>• Arboviral infections (dengue fever)<br>• Marburg viral disease |
| **Intermediate** (10-21 d) | • American trypanosomiasis (can include enteric fever)<br>• Leptospirosis<br>• Malaria (except *P. malariae*)<br>• Rickettsial infections (Rocky Mountain spotted fever, scrub typhus, Q fever, tick-bite fever, enteric fever) |
| **Long** (>21 d) | • Malaria (*P. malariae*)<br>• Schistosomiasis<br>• Tuberculosis<br>• Viral<br>• Hepatitis B virus<br>• Visceral leishmaniasis<br>• Filariasis (*W. bancrofti*) |

**Table 16.** Fever Pattern for Selected Tropical Diseases

| Pattern | Infection |
|---|---|
| **Continuous** | Enteric (typhoid or paratyphoid) fever, Lassa fever |
| **Remittent** | Tuberculosis |
| **Intermittent** | Malaria, tuberculosis |
| **Relapsing** | Relapsing fever, dengue fever, *P. malariae* |

## Focused Physical Exam
- **General**
  - Hydration, level of consciousness, malnourishment
  - Inspect the skin and sclera for jaundice, dermatological findings
- **Head and Neck**
  - Inspect the conjunctiva for infection
  - Assess for lymphadenopathy
- **Respiratory**
  - Signs of pneumonia
- **GU**
  - Hepatosplenomegaly, diarrhea
- **MSK**
  - Myalgia

**Table 17.** Basic Epidemiology and Symptoms of Major Tropical Diseases

| Illness | Vector or Exposure | Distribution | Symptoms |
|---|---|---|---|
| **African Sleeping Sickness** (African Trypanosomiasis) | Tsetse flies | Africa | Skin sore at the bite site, muscle and joint pain, swollen lymph nodes, fever |
| **Chagas Disease** (American Trypanosomiasis) | Night-biting reduviid bugs; mud, thatch or adobe houses | South and Central America | Pain and swelling in the area of an infected bug bite followed by a systemic illness including fever |

| Illness | Vector or Exposure | Distribution | Symptoms |
|---|---|---|---|
| **Dengue Fever** | Mosquitoes | Tropical regions of Africa, South and Central America, Caribbean, Asia, and Oceania | Fever, bone and joint pain, headache, swollen glands, hepatomegaly, fatigue, eschar, rash (hemorrhagic dengue fever) |
| **Filariasis** | Mosquitoes | South and Central America, Africa, Asia, India, Caribbean | Most asymptomatic or lymphedema of leg, scrotum, penis, arm, or breast |
| **Leishmaniasis** | Night-biting sandflies | Widespread | 1) Cutaneous: slow healing skin sores 2) Visceral: fever, weight loss, hepatosplenomegaly and anemia; months to years after exposure |
| **Malaria** | Mosquitoes | Widespread | Fever, chills, headache, myalgia, malaise, hepatosplenomegaly, jaundice |
| **Onchocerciasis** (River Blindness) | Day-biting black flies | Africa and South America | Dermatitis, subcutaneous nodules, lymphadenitis, ocular lesions (can lead to blindness); may occur months to years after exposure |
| **Schistosomiasis** (Bilharziasis) | Wading, swimming or bathing in fresh water | Sub-Saharan Africa, southern China, the Philippines, and Brazil | Most acute infections asymptomatic; acute syndrome: Katayama fever – fever, anorexia, weight loss, abdominal pain, hematuria, weakness, headaches, joint and muscle pain, diarrhea, nausea, and cough |
| **Yellow Fever** | Mosquitoes | Sub-Saharan Africa, Panama, Trinidad, South America | Sudden onset of fever, backache, headache, N/V, bradycardia, bleeding, jaundice |

**INFECTIOUS DISEASE**

## Diagnostic Investigations
- Blood films (thick and thin) × 3 (malaria) or rapid diagnostic test
- CBC, LFTs
- Blood, urine, stool cultures
- Serology (e.g. for dengue fever, schistosomiasis)
- Chest X-ray

## 13. IMMUNOCOMPROMISED POPULATION

**Table 18.** Important Opportunistic Infections and Common Associated Symptoms in HIV-Infected Individuals

| Infections | Common Signs and Symptoms |
|---|---|
| **Hepatitis C** | Jaundice, splenomegaly, stigmata of chronic liver disease |
| ***Pneumocystis jiroveci*** Pneumonia (previously *P. carinii*) | Fever, progressive dyspnea, nonproductive cough, fatigue; O/E: tachypnea, fever, inspiratory rales |
| **Tuberculosis** (pulmonary) | Fever, cough, sputum production, night sweats, weight loss, anorexia |
| ***Mycobacterium avium* Complex in HIV-Infected Individuals** | Nonspecific symptoms: high fever, night sweats, weight loss, anorexia, fatigue; hepatosplenomegaly, lymphadenopathy, diarrhea |
| **Cytomegalovirus** | Retinitis: floaters, visual field defects, scotoma; O/E: creamy white retinal exudates with hemorrhage, lesions obscure visualization of underlying vessels and other retinal structures; colitis: fever, diarrhea, weight loss, colon ulceration (± bleeding); esophagitis: fever, odynophagia, retrosternal pain |
| ***Candida* Species** | Thrush: white patches in oral cavity, scrape off with tongue depressor; esophagitis: fever, anorexia, dysphagia, retrosternal pain |
| **Toxoplasmic Encephalitis/ Cryptococcal Meningitis** | Insidious onset; fever, headache, mental status changes; focal neurologic signs, seizures |

## REFERENCES

1.  Rafei K, Lichenstein R. Airway infectious disease emergencies. *Pediatr Clin North Am.* 2006; 53(2):215-42.
2.  Mandell GL, Bennett JE, Dolin R (Editors). *Mandell, Douglas, and Bennett's Principles and Practice of Infectious Diseases,* 7th ed. New York: Churchill Livingstone/Elsevier; 2010.
3.  Choby BA. Diagnosis and treatment of streptococcal pharyngitis. *Am Fam Physician.* 2009; 79(5):383-390.
4.  Lim WS, Van der Eerden MM, Laing R, et al. Defining community acquired pneumonia severity on presentation to hospital: an international derivation and validation study. *Thorax.* 2003; 58(5):377-82.
5.  Long R, Ellis E (Editors). *Canadian Tuberculosis Standards,* 6th ed. Ottawa: Public Health Agency of Canada; 2007.
6.  Jensen PA, Lambert LA, Iademarco MF, et al. Guidelines for preventing the transmission of Mycobacterium tuberculosis in health-care settings, 2005. *MMWR Recomm Rep.* 2005; 30;54(RR-17):1-141.
7.  Heymann DL (Editor). *Control of Communicable Diseases Manual,* 19th ed. Washington: American Public Health Association; 2008.
8.  Public Health Agency of Canada. Canadian Guidelines on Sexually Transmitted Infections. Mar 2016. Accessed at: http://www.phac-aspc.gc.ca/std-mts/sti-its/cgsti-ldcits/index-eng.php#toc
9.  Singer M, Deutschman CS, Seymour CW, et al. The Third International Consensus Definitions for Sepsis and Septic Shock (Sepsis-3). *JAMA.* 2016; 315(8):801-810.
10. Fauci AS. *Harrison's Principles of Internal Medicine,* 17th ed. New York: McGraw-Hill; 2008.
11. Van de Beek D, De Gans J, Spanjaard L, et al. Clinical features and prognostic factors in adults with bacterial meningitis. *N Engl J Med.* 2004; 351(18):1849-59.

# CHAPTER 18:

# Medical Imaging

**Editors:**
Mohammed Firdouse, HBHSc
Kota Talla, BSc, BCom
Omid Shearkhani, HBSc

**Faculty Reviewers:**
Nasir Jaffer, MD, FRCPC
Eugene Yu, MD, RCPSC, ABR

## TABLE OF CONTENTS

MEDICAL IMAGING

# 1. ESSENTIALS OF IMAGING

### X-ray (Radiography)
- Denser structures are more opaque (metal > bone > fat > water > air)
- Poor delineation of soft tissues

### Computed Tomography Scan (CT)
- Multiplanar imaging using X-rays
- Bone is bright
- Delineates surrounding soft tissue better than a plain film
- Faster acquisition time than MRI has made it the modality of choice in many acute settings, such as cerebral hemorrhage

### Magnetic Resonance Imaging (MRI)
- No ionizing radiation but magnetic field exposure
- Safer for patients compared to CT and X-ray
- T1- vs. T2-weighted scans accentuate different tissues
- T1-weighted: fat is bright, water and CSF are dark
- T2-weighted: fat is dark, water is bright
- Many sequences available, including FLAIR and DWI
- FLAIR is a type of T2-weighted scan where CSF appears dark, and is used in assessment of several diseases of the central nervous system such as multiple sclerosis
- DWI assesses for fluid diffusion, where restricted diffusion (such as in ischemic stroke and cellular tumor) results in higher intensities
- Excellent delineation of soft tissues
- Costlier and higher acquisition time compared to CT and X-ray

### Ultrasound
- Image produced from reflected acoustic waves
- No ionizing radiation but can heat tissue

### Nuclear Imaging
- Radioactive nucleotides in patient show physiological functioning
- Location and amount of activity can be seen on scans

**Clinical Pearl: Importance of Clinical Context**
Medical images can be misleading if interpreted without clinical context or correlates. Always include relevant patient history when ordering medical imaging.

# 2. APPROACH TO THE CHEST X-RAY

### Types
Posterior-Anterior (PA) and left lateral
Portable: Anterior-Posterior (AP) – done supine or upright

**Clinical Pearl: Optimal Patient Positioning**
PA upright chest films are preferred because AP supine films obfuscate air-fluid levels and magnify mediastinal structures.

MEDICAL IMAGING

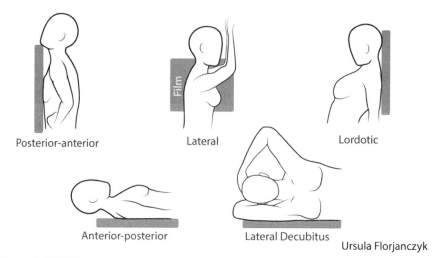

Posterior-anterior

Lateral

Lordotic

Anterior-posterior

Lateral Decubitus

Ursula Florjanczyk

**Figure 1.** CXR Views

### Interpretation
*Identifying Data*
- Exam date, name, sex, age, history number, position (supine, decubitus, upright), view (e.g. AP, PA), markers (R and L)

*Quality of Radiograph: RIP*
- **R**otation
  - ◆ Medial ends of the clavicle should be equidistant from the spinous process
  - ◆ Left and right ribcages, if not superimposed, should be within ~1-2 cm of each other on the lateral film (ideally <0.5 cm)
- **I**nspiration
  - ◆ Both the anterior segment of the 6th rib and the posterior segment of the 9th rib should be above the diaphragm (if inspiratory effort appropriate)
- **P**enetration
  - ◆ Vertebral bodies should be just visible through the cardiac shadow
  - ◆ Overexposed (vertebral bodies are very visible); underexposed (invisible)

*Looking for Pathologies: $A^2(BCDS)^2$ and Mediastinum*
- **A**irway
  - ◆ Follow trachea to carina and main bronchi (midline and patent)
- **A**orta
  - ◆ Follow arch to descending aorta on both frontal and lateral views
- **B**reathing (Lungs and Pleura)
  - ◆ Lung fields: upper, middle, and lower
    - ▪ Lung volumes, symmetry of markings (on frontal film)
    - ▪ Air space pathologies, interstitial pathologies, lobar collapse, and nodules
    - ▪ Lung periphery for pneumothorax and effusions
    - ▪ Examples of lung findings:
      - – Silhouette sign: loss of normally appearing interfaces implying opacification usually due to consolidation
      - – Air bronchogram: bronchi become visualized due to lung opacification, indicating air space disease, consolidation, etc.
      - – Kerley B lines: thickened connective tissue planes that commonly occur in pulmonary edema
      - – Net-like/reticular appearance: interstitial disease
      - – "Batwing" or "butterfly" appearance: alveolar edema
  - ◆ Pleura: costophrenic angles, entire perimeter of lung fields, position of fissures
    - ▪ Minor fissure from the right hilum to the 6th rib

- Major fissure laterally from T4-5 to the diaphragm
- Check for: blunting of costophrenic angles, focal or diffuse areas of pleural thickening, shifting of fissures, calcification, fluid collection

- **B**ones
  - Vertebrae, clavicles, ribs, sternum (best seen on lateral film)
  - Check for vertebrae and disc spaces, lytic or sclerotic lesions, rib fractures, osteoporosis (osteopenia, compression fracture, wedged)
- **C**irculation (including hila)
  - Central pulmonary arteries, veins, lymph nodes; mainstem and lobar bronchi
    - Deviation: left hilum should be 1-2 cm above the right (deviation may be due to lobar collapse or lobectomy)
    - Hilar enlargement
      - Smooth enlargement suggests arteries
      - Lobulated enlargement suggests lymphadenopathy
- **C**ardiac
  - Assess width of heart borders via the cardiothoracic ratio
    - Maximum heart width/greatest thoracic diameter should be <0.5
    - Right border = edge of right atrium
    - Left border = edge of left ventricle
  - Enlargement/distortion of cardiovascular shadow
    - Cardiomegaly, poor inspiration, supine position, obesity, pectus excavatum
    - Cardiomegaly suggests either myocardial hypertrophy, cardiac chamber dilatation or pericardial effusion
    - Cardiothoracic ratio <0.5 when cardiomegaly occurs alongside a hyperexpansive chest disorder (i.e. emphysema)
    - On expiration, heart size appears larger and mediastinum appears wider
- **D**iaphragm
  - Assess: position and costophrenic angles
    - Right hemidiaphragm may be up to 2 cm higher than the left
    - Check for: free air, calcifications, high or low diaphragm
      - Air underneath diaphragm: pneumoperitoneum (abnormal) or gastric bubble (normal)
      - Calcifications on diaphragm: asbestosis
      - Deviated diaphragm: either increased or decreased volume of peritoneal/thoracic structure
      - Elevated diaphragm: abdominal distention, lung collapse, pneumonectomy, pregnancy, pleural effusion
      - Depressed diaphragm: asthma, emphysema, pleural effusion, tumor
- **D**eformities
  - Assess: spine for deformity, asymmetry of pedicles/spinous processes
- **S**oft Tissues
  - Assess: neck, supraclavicular area, axillae, breast tissue, muscles
  - Check for: soft tissue masses, amount of soft tissue present
- **S**houlder
  - Look at bones and periphery
  - Continue in superior soft tissues/bones, up anterior chest wall, and down posterior ribs to the costophrenic angles
- **M**ediastinum
  - Mediastinal shift, abnormal widening and masses
  - Great vessels and mediastinal contours
  - Determine the mediastinal compartment where the abnormality is located (Table 1)

**Table 1.** Differential Diagnosis for a Mediastinal Mass

| | |
|---|---|
| **Anterior Mediastinal Mass** | **4 T**'s (thyroid lesions, thymic lesions, teratoma, terrible lymphoma), parathyroid lesions |
| **Middle Mediastinal Mass** | Bronchial carcinoma, bronchogenic cysts |
| **Posterior Mediastinal Mass** | Neurogenic tumors, esophageal lesions, hiatus hernia |
| **All Compartments** | Lymphoma, hematoma, abscess, aortic aneurysm |

MEDICAL IMAGING

# 3. CHEST PATHOLOGIES AND FINDINGS

## 3.1 Pneumothorax
- Air or gas in the pleural space

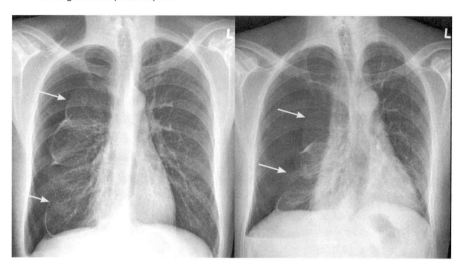

**Figure 2.** (A) CXR showing a right lung pneumothorax. With expiration, the tracheal and mediastinal shift becomes more pronounced

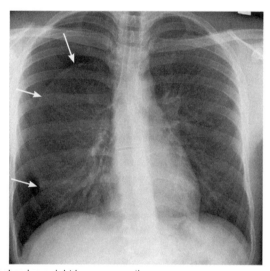

**Figure 2.** (B) CXR showing a right lung pneumothorax

| 1st Modality | 2nd Modality | 3rd Modality |
|---|---|---|
| **CXR:** decreased lung markings, partial or complete collapse of ipsilateral lung, contralateral mediastinal shift. | **CT:** the gold standard imaging investigation; lung markings will be absent in region of pneumothorax. | **CXR:** if a chest tube is inserted to re-expand the lung, repeat study after placement of chest tube. Look for proper placement. |
| **Tension pneumothorax:** severe contralateral mediastinal shift, inversion of hemidiaphragm. | **Indications:** an underlying pathology is suspected, for example: apical pleural blebs or bullae; pulmonary interstitial disease (lymphangiomyomatosis). Look for thin-walled cysts. | Then repeat CXR post chest tube removal |
| Sensitivity: 52% Specificity: 100% | | |

Ding W, et al. 2011. Chest 140(4):859-866.
Murphy FB, et al. 1990. AJR Am J Roentgenol 154(1):45-46.

### 3.2 Atelectasis (Loss of Volume)
- Collapse of a subsegment, segment, lobe or entire lung
- Atelectasis or loss of volume can be subsegmental, segmental, lobar, or involve the entire lung
- Atelectasis is often qualified by descriptors such as linear, discoid, or plate-like

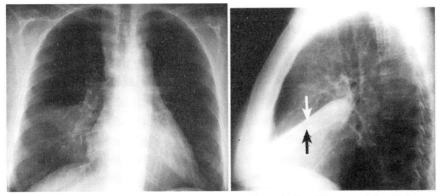

**Figure 3.** CXR showing complete right middle lobar atelectasis. Local increased density is seen in the region of the collapsed lung (see arrows)

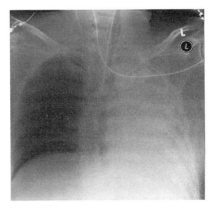

**Figure 4.** CXR showing complete atelectasis of left lung with air bronchogram and shift of the mediastinum to the left. The endotracheal tube is in the right lower bronchus resulting in the atelectasis

MEDICAL IMAGING

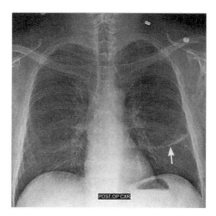

**Figure 5.** CXR showing subsegmental atelectasis on the left lower lobe (postoperative)

| 1st Modality | 2nd Modality |
|---|---|
| **CXR:** look for signs of loss of volume. Direct signs: Displacement of fissures Indirect signs: Local increased density, elevation of diaphragm, mediastinal displacement, compensatory hyperinflation, displacement of hila, absence of air bronchogram or increased opacity of the collapsed lung segment | **CT:** look for reduced volume and decreased attenuation in the affected part of the lung. Atelectasis is often associated with abnormal displacement of fissures, bronchi, vessels, diaphragm, heart, or mediastinal structures<br><br>**Indications:** only in cases where a malignant process is the suspected etiology, such as an endobronchial lesion (mucous plug, tumor or foreign body), intramural lesion (tumor or inflammatory lesion) or extrinsic lesions such as lymphadenopathy. CT is also used for staging the tumor |

### 3.3 Pneumonia
Inflammation and possible consolidation of the respiratory units of the lung

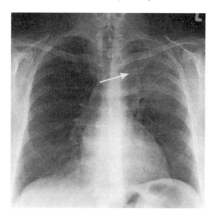

**Figure 6.** CXR showing L upper lobe pneumonia characterized by consolidation of affected segment

MEDICAL IMAGING

| 1st Modality | 2nd Modality |
|---|---|
| **CXR:** look for increased opacity of affected segment (consolidation) with air bronchogram, the hallmark for pneumonia. Other signs include silhouette sign of mediastinal structures and the spine sign on lateral CXR with increased opacity of lower lobes posterior. Some pneumonias may cause slight loss of volume (atelectasis) or increased volume (such as Klebseilla and Legionella bacteria) | **CT:** the gold standard imaging investigation. Consolidation appears as a homogeneous increase in pulmonary parenchymal attenuation that obscures the margins of vessels and airway walls. An air bronchogram may be present. The attenuation characteristics of consolidated lung rarely helpful in differential diagnosis (e.g. decreased attenuation in lipoid pneumonia and increased in amiodarone toxicity) |
| Sensitivity: 67%[1]<br>Specificity: 85% | **Indications:** atypical pneumonia on CXR or not resolving post treatment |

### 3.4 Obstructed Upper Airway
• Physical blockage of the upper respiratory tract

| 1st Modality | 2nd Modality |
|---|---|
| Depends on the patient's age group and the possible etiology and location of obstruction<br><br>**Cervical X Ray:** look for epiglottitis or foreign body. The classic radiographic findings of epiglottitis are a swollen epiglottis (i.e. a thumb sign; normal epiglottis is 3-5 mm thick), thickened aryepiglottic folds, and obliteration of the vallecula (vallecula sign) | **CXR:** look for air trapping on an exhalation phase film. Additionally, atelectasis may be present in the obstructed region<br><br>**Indications:** to assess for other causes of patient's dyspnea; the obstructed airway could affect any segments of the tracheobronchial tree<br><br>Sensitivity: 66%[2] |

### 3.5 Interstitial Lung Disease
• Disease of the nonconducting and nonrespiratory tissues of the lung

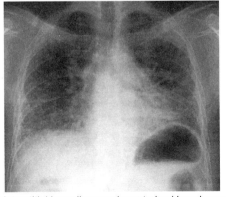

**Figure 7.** CXR showing interstitial lung disease characterized by a honeycomb appearance

MEDICAL IMAGING

| 1st Modality | 2nd Modality |
|---|---|
| **CXR:** interstitial lines fine, medium, and coarse (Kerley lines, septal) honeycomb with decreased or increased lung volume<br><br>Sensitivity: 59%<br>Specificity: 40%[3] | **High Resolution CT (HRCT):** the imaging modality of choice. Look for reticular opacities, honeycomb, ground glass opacities, and architectural distortion<br><br>**Indications:** to distinguish the different types of interstitial disease including: interstitial pulmonary fibrosis, sarcoidosis, interstitial pneumonia, and hypersensitivity pneumonitis<br><br>Sensitivity: 77-79%[3]<br>Specificity: 85-88% |

Hunninghake GW, et al. 2001. Am J Respir Crit Care Med 1 64(2):1 93-196.

### 3.6 Acute Bronchitis
- Inflammation of conducting bronchi (a clinical diagnosis)

| 1st Modality |
|---|
| **CXR:** bronchial wall thickening in more severe cases |

### 3.7 Chronic Obstructive Pulmonary Disease
- Irreversible obstruction of airways

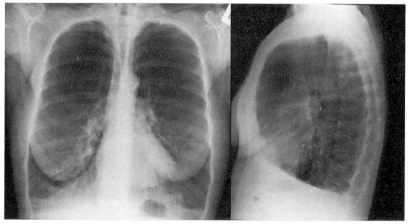

**Figure 8.** CXR showing hyperinflation and flattened diaphragms consistent with COPD

| 1st Modality | 2nd Modality |
|---|---|
| **CXR:** hyperinflation, decreased vascularity, flattened diaphragms, increased retrosternal air space. Basal emphysema suggestive of α-1 -antitrypsin deficiency | **CT:** imaging modality of choice. Similar findings as CXR but certain imaging findings suggestive of either panacinar or centrilobular emphysema<br><br>**Indications:** as an adjunct to find out the morphologic type of emphysema<br><br>Sensitivity: 63%[4]<br>Specificity: 88% |

MEDICAL IMAGING

## 3.8 Bronchiectasis
- Irreversible dilation of airways

| 1st Modality | 2nd Modality |
| --- | --- |
| **CXR:** the findings depend on the severity and type of bronchiectasis: 1) bronchial wall thickening: tram tracks (parallel line shadows) and 2) cystic type: cystic spaces, honeycombing, ring opacities. Other findings: finger-in-glove opacities result from mucous plugs within dilated bronchi<br><br>Sensitivity: 87%[5]<br>Specificity: 74% | **HRCT:** perform to distinguish types of bronchiectasis. Look for bronchial wall thickening and dilatation when bronchus is larger than the adjacent pulmonary artery (signet ring sign) or when bronchi are visible within 1 cm of the pleura; finger-in-glove mucous plugs in dilated bronchi. Three different forms of bronchiectasis will show different patterns: 1) cylindrical bronchiectasis, which shows smooth bronchial dilatation, 2) varicose bronchiectasis, which is characterized by beaded bronchial dilatation, and 3) cystic bronchiectasis, which is characterized by bronchial dilatation of greater 1 cm<br><br>**Indications:** to distinguish between the 3 different types of bronciectasis<br><br>Sensitivity: 84-95%[6]<br>Specificity: 93-100% |

Naidich DP, et al. 1982. J Comput Assist Tomogr 6(3):437-444
Hartman TE, et al. 1994. Radiographics 14(5):991-1 003

## 3.9 Pulmonary Embolism
Embolus blocking the arterial vessels in the lung

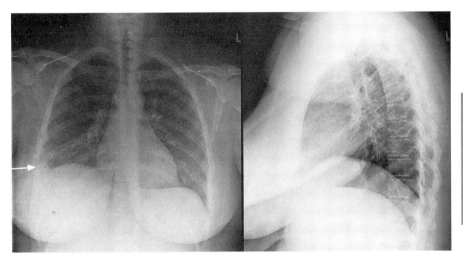

**Figure 9.** CXR of Hampton's hump at the right costophrenic sulcus shown in right lower lobe which is characteristic of a pulmonary embolism

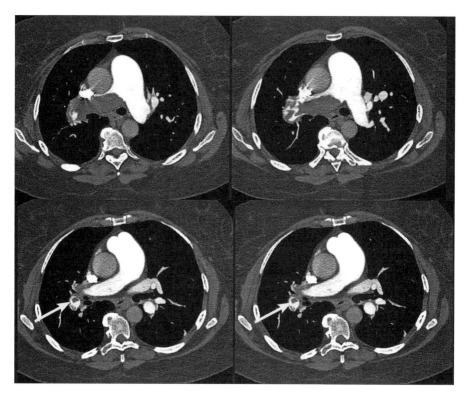

**Figure 10.** CT pulmonary angiogram showing a large embolus in the right main pulmonary trunk with smaller ones in left upper lobe pulmonary artery branch

| 1ˢᵗ Modality | 2ⁿᵈ Modality |
|---|---|
| **CXR:** most commonly normal (25%). Uncommon findings include: cardiomegaly (27%), pleural effusion (23%), elevated hemidiaphragm (20%), pulmonary artery enlargement (19%), atelectasis (18%), ill-defined opacity (17%), pulmonary edema (14%), oligemia (Westermark's sign) (8 %), overinflation (5%)[7]<br><br>Sensitivity: 33%[8]<br>Specificity: 59% | **CT Pulmonary Angiogram:** imaging of choice in moderate to high probability of pulmonary embolism. CT scan done with venous injection of contrast and imaging done at 20 s after<br><br>**Direct Findings:** railway track sign, rim sign, vessel cut-off, thrombus partially or completely occluding the artery with or without enlargement of artery<br><br>**Indirect Findings:** pulmonary hemorrhage or infarct, oligemia of affected segment, atelectasis, and small effusions<br><br>**Indications:** moderate or high probability of pulmonary embolism based on the Wells score<br><br>Sensitivity: 80%[9]<br>Specificity: 85.7% |

Greenspan RH, et al. 1982. Invest Radiol 17(6):539-543
Sood S, et al. 2006. IJIR 16(2):215-219

## 3.10 Pulmonary Edema

- Fluid accumulating in lung parenchyma or air spaces

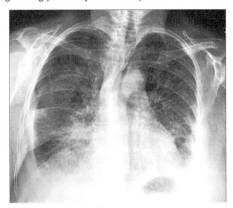

**Figure 11.** AP CXR showing a mixed interstitial and alveolar pulmonary edema with bilateral pleural effusions and cardiomegaly. Kerley B lines are seen at the bases

| 1ˢᵗ Modality | 2ⁿᵈ Modality |
|---|---|
| **CXR:** look for vascular redistribution, indistinct hilar vessels, interstitial edema (Kerley A and B lines), alveolar edema (consolidation), cardiomegaly, pleural effusions, and enlarged azygous vein | **CT:** look for extensive vascular markings and possible underlying lung pathologies |
| **Pulmonary Wedge Pressures (in mmHg):** normal CXR (4.5-1 2), cephalization of pulmonary veins (12- 17), Kerley lines (A, B, and C) (17-20), alveolar pulmonary edema (>25)<br><br>Sensitivity: 57%[10]<br>Specificity: 78% | **Indications:** acute respiratory distress syndrome is present in order to detect underlying lung pathology and complications |

Fonseca C, et al. 2004. Eur J Heart Fail 6(6):807-812

## 3.11 Lung Cancer

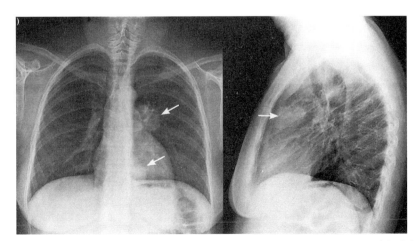

**Figure 12.** CXR of left lung cancer showing a 2.5 cm mass in the anterior segment of the left upper lobe. There is an additional lesion in the left lower lobe (behind the cardiac shadow).

MEDICAL IMAGING

| 1st Modality | 2nd Modality |
|---|---|

**CXR:**
**Malignant Characteristics:** pulmonary nodule or mass that: 1) doubles in volume within 1 to 18 mo, 2) irregular, speculated or lobulated edges, 3) noncalcified or calcification pattern that is not central nidus, laminated, popcorn or diffuse, 4) larger than 3 cm in diameter

**Adenocarcinoma:** solitary pulmonary nodule or mass usually in the upper lobe. Margins can be well- circumscribed, irregular, lobulated, or speculated. Can have a chronic airspace disease pattern

**Squamous Cell Carcinoma:** postobstructive pneumonia,
atelectasis, Golden S sign, apical mass with ill-defined borders and central lucency, asymmetrical pleural thickening

**Large Cell Carcinoma:** mass greater than 3 cm in diameter usually located in the lung periphery

**Small Cell Carcinoma:** hilar or perihilar mass, mediastinal widening, may be disseminated

**Nonbronchogenic Metastases:** multiple, noncalcified pulmonary nodules

Sensitivity: 78.3%[11]
Specificity: 97%

**CT:** preferred imaging because of better soft tissue delineation

**Adenocarcinoma:** solitary pulmonary nodule or mass usually in the upper lobe. Often have air bronchograms

**Squamous Cell Carcinoma:** subpleural mass with cavitation

**Large Cell Carcinoma:** mass greater than 3 cm in diameter

**Small Cell Carcinoma:** extensive lymph node involvement and soft tissue infiltration of the mediastinum

**Nonbronchogenic Metastases:**
multiple, noncalcified pulmonary nodules

**Indications:** require better characterization of the primary tumor, visualization of metastases and cancer staging

Sensitivity: 88.9%[11]
Specificity: 92.6%

### 3.12 Lung Abscess
Necrosis of lung tissue and cavitation

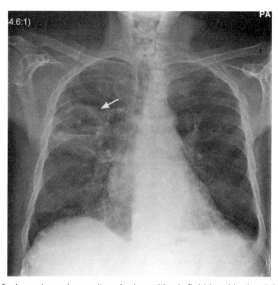

**Figure 13.** CXR of a large irregular cavitary lesion with air-fluid level in the right upper lobe

MEDICAL IMAGING

| 1st Modality | 2nd Modality |
| --- | --- |
| **CXR:** round, peripheral thoracic lesion. Has ill-defined margins (due to surrounding parenchymal inflammation) and may have cavitation with irregular margins and air-fluid levels. May be single or multiple (latter may be secondary to septicemia [e.g. from drug injection sites]) | **CT:** look for thick wall, nonuniform width, no pleural separation, no compression of uninvolved lung, acute chest wall angle, round shape, small size<br><br>**Indications:** CXR is inconclusive or not definitive |

Stark DD, et al. 1983. AJR Am J Roentgenol 141(1 ):163-1 67

### 3.13 Rib Fracture

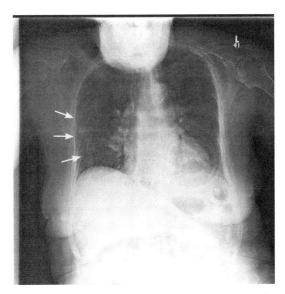

**Figure 14.** CXR of right rib fracture. Since more than two ribs are broken in two places, a flail chest is seen

| 1st Modality | 2nd Modality |
| --- | --- |
| **CXR:** displaced or nondisplaced rib fracture, can be associated with pneumothorax or hemothorax<br><br>Sensitivity: 40%[12] | CXR usually sufficient. Perform rib series if high suspicion of traumatic rib fracture without evidence on plain CXR. Perform a **bone scan** in the case of stress fractures<br><br>**Indications:** high suspicion of traumatic rib fracture without evidence on plain film or if suspecting stress fracture |

MEDICAL IMAGING

### 3.14 Mitral Valve Stenosis
- Narrowing of mitral valve opening

| 1st Modality | 2nd Modality |
|---|---|
| **CXR:** signs of left atrial hypertension (enlargement of the left atrium, right ventricle, and pulmonary trunk). Cephalization of pulmonary vasculature, septal (Kerley B lines), rarely calcification of mitral valve | **Transthoracic Echocardiogram and Doppler:** considered gold standard. Look for thickened mitral leaflets with reduced motion during diastole. Doming of the mitral valve. Enlarged left atrium and right ventricle with normal-sized left ventricle<br><br>**Indications:** need for visualization of abnormal leaflet motion and blood flow consistent with mitral valve stenosis |

Habib G. 2006. Heart 92(1 ):124-1 30

### 3.15 Angina with Nondiagnostic ECG and Negative Serum Markers

| 1st Modality | 2nd Modality |
|---|---|
| **Stress Radionuclide Myocardial Perfusion Imaging:** extensive reversible ischemia in multiple segments, left ventricular dilatation, increased lung uptake of radionuclide | **CT Coronary Angiogram:** gold standard imaging technique. Look for reduced coronary artery cross-sectional diameter<br><br>**Indications:** to determine the degree of arterial stenosis<br><br>Sensitivity: 99%[13]<br>Specificity: 96% |

### 3.16 Myocardial Infarction

| 1st Modality |
|---|
| **CXR:** may be normal or associated with nonspecific signs of CHF. Imaging is not usually recommended |

### 3.17 Aortic Dissection
- Separation of the walls of the aorta

| 1st Modality | 2nd Modality |
|---|---|
| **CXR:** widening of the aorta (ascending and descending) especially when compared to previous CXR, displaced intimal calcification from outer surface of the aorta (>10 mm), left apical pleural soft tissue cap (dissected left subclavian artery or apical pleural hemorrhage), widened mediastinum, left pleural effusion (hemothorax: rare)<br><br>Sensitivity: 67%[14]<br>Specificity: 86% | **CT Angiogram:** look for dilated aorta, intimal flap with two distinct lumens (false lumen and true lumen), beak sign, cobweb sign, intraluminal thrombus, pericardial effusion<br><br>**Indications:** to determine the type of aortic dissection in order to direct treatment<br><br>Sensitivity: 98%<br>Specificity: 100%[15] |

### 3.18 Esophageal Rupture

MEDICAL IMAGING

| 1st Modality | 2nd Modality | 3rd Modality |
|---|---|---|
| **CXR:** rupture common on left side of distal esophagus. Pneumomediastinum, air in the prevertebral space, widened lower thoracic mediastinum, left pleural effusion, subcutaneous emphysema. Pneumoperitoneum (if rupture extends toward gastric fundus) | **CT:** look for esophageal wall thickening and irregularity. Extra-esophageal air, mediastinal widening, air and fluid in left pleural space, abscess abutting the esophagus (in undiagnosed rupture)<br><br>**Indications:** to detect smaller esophageal ruptures | **Contrast Esophagography:** look for extravasation of contrast material, extraluminal gas<br><br>**Indications:** CXR and CT are inconclusive in making a diagnosis |
| Sensitivity: 86%[16] | Sensitivity: 95%[16] | |

### 3.19 Pericarditis
- Inflammation of pericardium

| 1st Modality | 2nd Modality |
|---|---|
| **CXR:** often normal. In severe cases, enlarged cardiac silhouette with clear lung fields, rapid cardiomegaly | **CT:** look for pericardial fluid, pericardial thickening/ enhancement, and pneumopericardium (rare)<br><br>**Indications:** for a definitive diagnosis |

### 3.20 Spontaneous Pneumomediastinum
- Air in the mediastinum

| 1st Modality | 2nd Modality |
|---|---|
| **CXR:** mediastinal lucencies that outline the aorta and pulmonary artery and distend the mediastinal pleura laterally or into the neck. Continuous diaphragm sign. Spinnaker sign. V sign of Naclerio (for esophageal rupture). Ring around the artery sign. Subcutaneous emphysema | **CT:** look for the same signs as on CXR<br><br>**Indications:** to improve sensitivity and provide a more definitive diagnosis |

## 4. ABDOMINAL PATHOLOGIES AND FINDINGS

### 4.1 Peritoneal Hemorrhage
- Bleeding within the peritoneum[17-21]

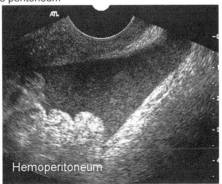

**Figure 15.** U/S of the pelvis showing hypoechoic fluid collection with small bowel (rounded structures) floating (not anechoic)

MEDICAL IMAGING

| 1st Modality | 2nd Modality |
|---|---|
| **U/S (FAST – Focused Assessment with Sonography in Trauma):** a hyperechoic fluid collection in the most dependent spaces (Morison's pouch, pouch of Douglas, and paracolic gutters) of the peritoneum<br><br>Sensitivity: 85%[20]<br>Specificity: 96% | **CT:** look for hyperdense fluid in the dependent spaces of the abdomen. Blood obscures, displaces or compresses the normal peritoneal structures. It can be distinguished from ascites since it has a higher attenuation than ascitic fluid<br><br>**Indications:** to determine cause of hemorrhage, better visualize surrounding structures, and plan therapeutic intervention. Patients must be hemodynamically stable to undergo CT scan<br><br>Sensitivity: 97.2%[20]<br>Specificity: 94.7% |

### 4.2 Intussusception

- Invagination of a bowel loop with its mesenteric fold (intussusceptum) into the lumen of a contiguous portion of bowel (intussuscipiens) as a result of peristalsis[22-27]

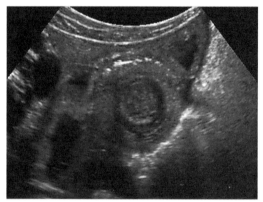

**Figure 16.** An U/S showing the target sign which is characteristic of intussusception. Intussusception of the jejunum is seen here

MEDICAL IMAGING

| 1st Modality | 2nd Modality | 3rd Modality |
|---|---|---|
| **Abdominal Plain Film:** look for distended bowel with absence of colonic gas. Crescent sign of air outlining the intussusceptum within the intussuscipiens (target sign). Signs better seen in children<br><br>Sensitivity: 80%<br>Specificity: 58%[22] | **U/S:** target sign or coiled spring lesion. Useful especially in pediatric age group<br><br>**Indications:** if you require a more sensitive and specific test for intussusception. This aids in determining the severity and complications of the pathology<br><br>Sensitivity: 97.9%[26]<br>Specificity: 97.8% | **CT Scan with Oral and IV Contrast:** useful in the adult population. Better visualization of surrounding structures allows for determination of cause of intussusception and assesses for complications such as bowel obstruction and strangulation<br><br>**Indications:** to determine etiology of intussusception<br><br>Sensitivity: 71.4-87.5%[26]<br>Specificity: 100% |

## 4.3 Ascites

- Pathologic fluid collection within the abdominal cavity (typically diagnosed based on clinical history and physical exam, imaging useful when suspect small volumes of ascitic fluid)[28-32]

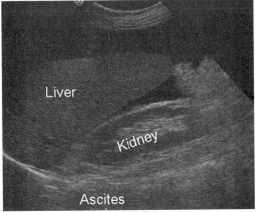

**Figure 17.** (A) U/S of ascitic fluid collection seen as the hypoechoic area between the liver and kidney in Morison's pouch

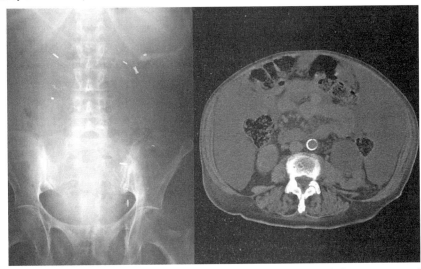

**Figure 17.** (B) The plain film of the abdomen (left image) shows a "ground glass appearance", and the corresponding axial CT image (right) shows large volume of clear fluid ascites

| 1st Modality | 2nd Modality |
|---|---|
| **Abdominal Plain Film**: look for loss of posterior liver edge (Morison's pouch), Mickey Mouse ear sign in pelvis (fluid in supravesicular peritoneal space), displacement of bowel loops, and increased haziness (large volume ascites) | **CT:** look for a hypodensity specifically in the perihepatic and subhepatic spaces. Can detect very small quantities of fluid |
| **U/S:** ascitic fluid is free-flowing and is typically found in the subhepatic recess, paracolic gutters, and in-between organs. If the fluid is transudative, the fluid is typically hypoechoic; whereas exudative fluids typically have multiple echoic foci | **Indications:** to determine cause of ascites, such as liver disease or malignancy |

### 4.4 Small Bowel Obstruction[53]
- Low grade or high grade blockage of the small intestine
- The small bowel is considered dilated when it exceeds 3 cm in diameter (3,6,9 rule)

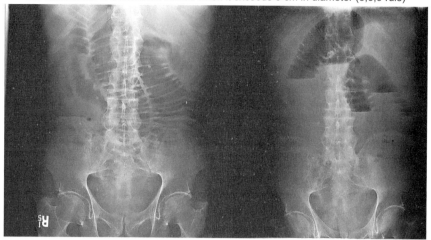

**Figure 18.** AXR of small bowel obstruction is characterized by dilated loops of bowel and "string of pearls" appearance. Plicae circulares are seen which confirms small bowel dilation with multiple air-fluid levels and minimal gas in the colon

| 1st Modality | 2nd Modality |
|---|---|
| **Abdominal Plain Film:** look for distended loops with multiple differential air-fluid levels, step ladder fluid levels, string of pearls sign, and minimal or no gas beyond point of obstruction | **CT Scan with Oral and IV Contrast:** look for a transition point of where the bowel abruptly changes. Absence of air or fluid in areas distal to this point. Proximal loops are distended and filled with fluid and gas |
| Sensitivity: 69%[33] | **Indications:** to determine etiology of bowel obstruction such as adhesions and strangulation |
| Specificity: 57% | Sensitivity: 81 -94%[33] |
| | Specificity: 96% |

### 4.5 Large Bowel Obstruction
- Partial or complete blockage of the colon or rectum

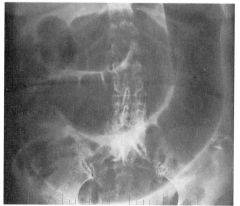 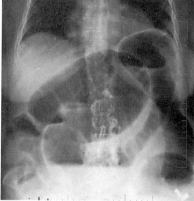

**Figure 19.** AXR of large bowel obstruction characterized by dilated loops of bowel as defined by the 3, 6, 9 rule. Haustra are seen on the portions of dilated bowel which confirms that it is large bowel

MEDICAL IMAGING

| --- | --- |
| **Abdominal Plain Film:** distended loops of bowel filled with gas and fluid proximal to point of obstruction. The colon is considered dilated when it exceeds 6 cm in diameter and the cecum is dilated when it exceeds 9 cm in diameter (3, 6, 9 rule)<br><br>Sensitivity: 77%[34]<br>Specificity: 50% | **CT Scan with IV, Oral, and Rectal Contrast:** look for dilated colon with an abrupt point of obstruction. Also can see associated complications such as ischemia and possible localized perforation (cecum)<br><br>**Indications:** to determine etiology (colon cancer, diverticulitis), severity and complications of obstruction<br><br>Sensitivity: 94%[34]<br>Specificity: 96% |

## 4.6 Perforated Bowel

- A hole penetrating through the wall of the intestines

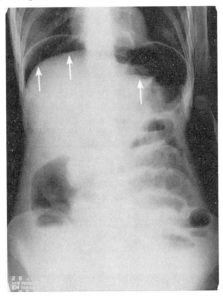

**Figure 20.** AXR of free air (arrows) under the diaphragm is seen and is characteristic of a bowel perforation

| --- | --- |
| **Abdominal Plain Films (Supine and Upright):** two types of free air – intraperitoneal and retroperitoneal air<br><br>**Intraperitoneal Air:**<br>· **Upright Film:** air under the diaphragm<br>· **Supine Film: signs include:** outlining of the falciform ligament, and Rigler's sign (bowel wall outlined on luminal and peritoneal sides)<br>**Retroperitoneal Air:** "streaky air"<br>· Look for air/gas outlining retroperitoneal organs: kidney, ascending/descending colon, and duodenum | **CT Scan with Oral and IV Contrast:** look for a collection of air or leakage of oral contrast locally around region of perforated bowel. There may be inflammatory changes shown in the pericolonic soft tissues and resultant focal abscess may be seen<br><br>**Indications:** suspect a small perforation since there is better visualization of small quantities of air/ gas<br><br>Sensitivity: 92%[35]<br>Specificity: 94% |

MEDICAL IMAGING

## 4.7 Peptic Ulcer Disease

- Mucosal erosions forming ulcers in the stomach or duodenum

| 1st Modality | 2nd Modality |
|---|---|
| **Single-Contrast or Double-Contrast Barium Studies:** poor mucosal coating of the barium and filling defects in the ulcerated regions are observed | **Esophagogastroduodenoscopy:** the imaging investigation of choice. Look for erosions and active bleeding sites in stomach lining. Additionally, can take a biopsy with this imaging method |
| | **Indications:** for confirmatory diagnosis and also to aid in determining cause of peptic ulcer disease |
| Sensitivity: 80-90%[36] | Sensitivity: >90% Specificity: >90%[36] |

## 4.8 Appendicitis[37]

- Inflammation of the appendix

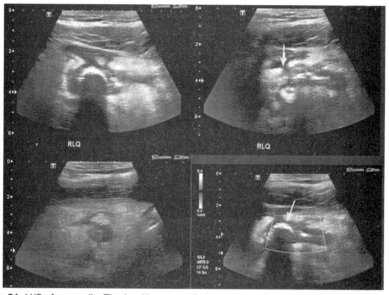

**Figure 21.** U/S of appendix. The healthy appendix is not normally seen on U/S. Here an inflamed appendix is seen surrounded by periappendiceal fluid. White semicircular area with shadowing in A and D display an appendicolith. Arrow points to a perforation in B

| 1st Modality | 2nd Modality |
|---|---|
| **U/S:** a healthy appendix is not normally seen on U/S. An inflamed appendix presents as a noncompressible structure >7 mm in diameter. The structure lacks peristalsis and typically has periappendiceal fluid surrounding it | **CT with IV Contrast Only:** look for an appendix with thickened walls which do not fill with contrast. May see appendicolith, mesoappendiceal inflammation, localized or diffuse perforation, and abscess. |
| | **Indications:** U/S is inconclusive and there is a high degree of suspicion. Also, can aid in developing a treatment plan since gives good visualization of surrounding structures. |
| Sensitivity: 66%[38] Specificity: 95% | Sensitivity: 98.5% Specificity: 98%[38] |

MEDICAL IMAGING

### 4.9 Diverticulitis

- Outpouching of the inner lining of the intestine which becomes infected or inflamed

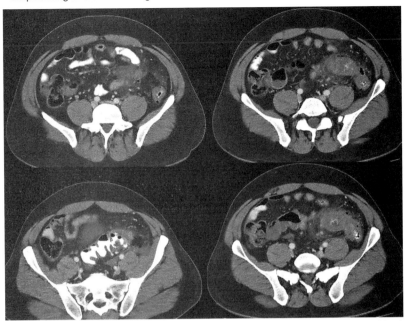

**Figure 22.** CT of pelvis with positive rectal contrast in sigmoid shows thickened sigmoid colon with few diverticula and inflamed mesentery

**1ˢᵗ Modality**

**CT with Oral, Rectal, and IV Contrast**: the gold standard in the diagnosis of diverticulitis. Look for pericolic fat infiltration, colonic diverticula, bowel wall thickening, phlegmon, abscesses, and localized perforation

Sensitivity: 97%[39]
Specificity: 97%

### 4.10 Cholecystitis

- Inflammation of the gallbladder

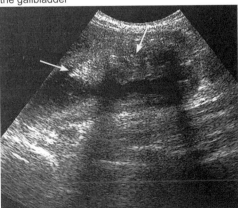

**Figure 23.** U/S of gallbladder. Thickened gallbladder walls visualized above are findings suggestive of cholecystitis

MEDICAL IMAGING

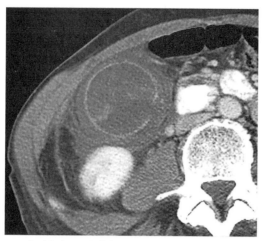

**Figure 24.** CT abdomen. Pericholecystic fluid and thickened gallbladder wall are seen on the CT suggestive of cholecystitis

| 1ˢᵗ Modality | 2ⁿᵈ Modality |
|---|---|
| **U/S:** look for pericholecystic fluid, gallbladder wall thickening (>4 mm), and gallstones | **CT:** look for gallbladder wall thickening (>4 mm), pericholecystic fluid, edema without the presence of ascites, and intramural gas |
| Sensitivity: 90-95%[39]<br>Specificity: 78-80% | **Indications:** require better visualization of the surrounding structures, which can aid in developing a treatment plan<br><br>Sensitivity: 95%[40] |

### 4.11 Pancreatitis

- Inflammation of the pancreas (typically a clinical diagnosis; however, imaging more useful to assess complications or pre-existing chronic pancreatitis)[41-45]

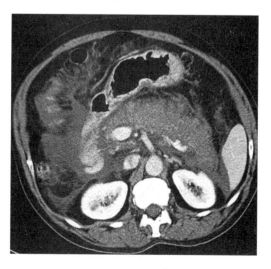

**Figure 25.** CT abdomen. Diffuse enlargement of the pancreas and blurring of the peripancreatic fat planes is seen, which is consistent with pancreatitis

MEDICAL IMAGING

| 1st Modality | 2nd Modality |
|---|---|
| **U/S:** look for pancreatic enlargement, peripancreatic fluid, hypoechoic foci suggestive of necrosis, and pancreatic pseudocysts | **CT with IV Contrast:** look for pancreatic enlargement, heterogeneous enhancement of the gland, irregular contour, blurring of peripancreatic fat borders, pseudocysts, abscesses, and necrosis |
| | **Indications:** to visualize complications of pancreatitis |
| Sensitivity: 60-70%[43] Specificity: 80-90% | Sensitivity: 70-90%[45] Specificity: 85% |

### 4.12 Peritonitis
- Inflammation of the peritoneum

**1st Modality**

**CT:** look for free intraperitoneal air, peritoneal thickening with enhancement, bowel wall and mesenteric thickening, and ascites. CT is only indicated if a clinical diagnosis of peritonitis is not definitive.

**Note:** plain film not useful

### 4.13 Renal Colic
- Acute abdominal pain due to kidney stones

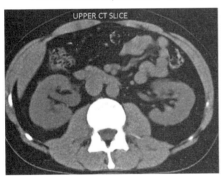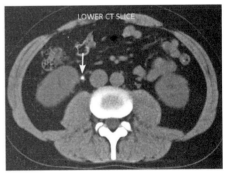

**Figure 26.** (A) CT abdomen. A small, calcified kidney stone (see arrow), seen as hyperdensity, is visualized in right ureter

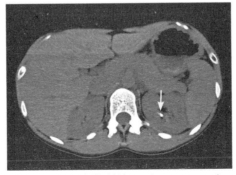

**Figure 26.** (B) CT Abdomen. A small, calcified kidney stone, seen as hyperdensity, is visualized in left pelvis

MEDICAL IMAGING

CT (No Contrast): often considered the gold standard. Look for renal pelvis and collecting system dilation, and obstructing kidney stones. Perinephric stranding or rarely urinoma may occur

Indications: for treatment planning since can visualize surrounding structures and can better determine characteristics of obstructing stone

Sensitivity: 91%[46]
Specificity: 91%

Abdominal Plain Film: used for prelithotripsy planning. Look for location, radiopacity of stone (calcium containing), and size of kidney stones

Sensitivity: 69%[46]
Specificity: 82%

### 4.14 Small Bowel Mesenteric Ischemia

- Insufficient blood flow from the mesenteric circulation resulting in ischemia and eventually necrosis of the small bowel wall

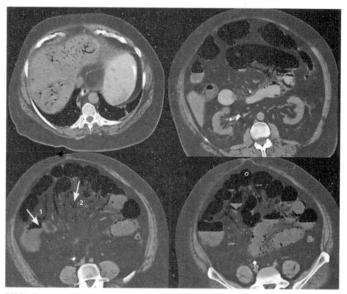

**Figure 27.** CT Abdomen. Small bowel ischemia visualized by bowel wall thickening and perienteric fat stranding (arrow 1). Additionally, portal venous gas and pneumatosis (arrow 2) are also shown

| 1st Modality | 2nd Modality |
|---|---|

Abdominal Plain Film: sometimes done as first-line imaging as clinical diagnosis often not apparent. Common findings: normal bowel gas pattern. Uncommon findings: ileus, wall thickening ("pinky printing"), pneumatosis, portal venous gas at periphery of liver edge (distinguishing portal versus biliary air)

CT Ischemic Protocol (Plain, Arterial, and Venous): look for bowel wall thickening, dilation, perienteric fat stranding, ascites, mesenteric arterial or venous thrombus, bowel infarction: pneumatosis and portal venous gas

Indications: to better characterize complications and severity of ischemia

Sensitivity: 96-100%[47]
Specificity: 89-94%

MEDICAL IMAGING

## 4.15 Ectopic Pregnancy
- Pregnancy that occurs outside the uterus

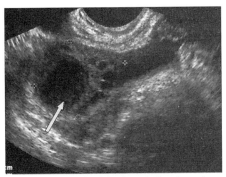 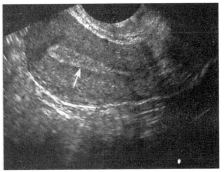

**Figure 28.** U/S of pelvis. A gestational sac is seen outside the uterus and there is no embryo present within the uterus. The uterine cavity has decidual reaction but no fetus

### 1ˢᵗ Modality

**US:** look for free intraperitoneal air, peritoneal thickening with enhancement, bowel wall and mesenteric thickening, and ascites. CT is only indicated if a clinical diagnosis of peritonitis is not definitive.

**Note:** plain film not useful

## 4.16 Gastritis
- Inflammation of the lining of the stomach

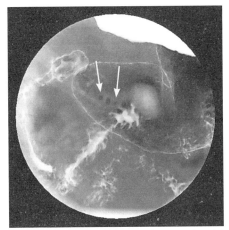

**Figure 29.** Upper GI Barium study. Gastric erosions and mucosal nodules seen, which is typical of gastritis

### 1ˢᵗ Modality

**Double-Contrast Upper GI Barium Studies:** look for thick gastric folds, gastric mucosal nodules, and gastric erosions

Sensitivity: 72%[49]
Specificity: 77%

MEDICAL IMAGING

## 4.17 Pyelonephritis
- Infection of the kidney

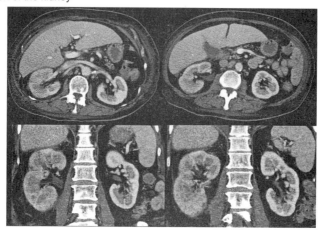

**Figure 30.** CT abdomen. Pyelonephritis of the right kidney seen characterized by kidney enlargement and decreased enhancement

| 1st Modality | 2nd Modality |
|---|---|
| **U/S:** often done as first-line imaging due to vague flank symptoms. Look for renal enlargement, loss of cortical medullar differentiation, mild hydronephrosis, and possible renal abscess | **CT:** the imaging investigation of choice. Contrast-enhancement typically indicated. Non-contrast used when stones are suspected. Look for enlargement of kidney, dilation of the collecting system, multi- focal abscess regions, and linear parenchymal striations <br><br>**Indications:** to better detect severity and complications of pyelonephritis <br><br>Sensitivity: 86.8%50 <br>Specificity: 87.5% |

## 4.18 Ischemic Colitis
- Insufficient blood supply to the colon resulting in ischemia and eventually necrosis

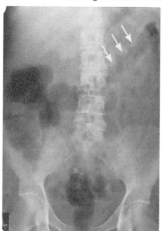

**Figure 31.** AXR. There is thumbprinting of the distal transverse colon (arrows) and narrowed descending colon: acute ischemic colitis in watershed area. The watershed area (branches from both the superior mesenteric artery [SMA] and inferior mesenteric artery [IMA]) is most vulnerable to ischemia since the SMA and the IMA do not have as many collaterals

| 1st Modality | 2nd Modality |
|---|---|
| **Abdominal Plain Film:** common radiographic findings include: normal gas pattern or ileus. Uncommon findings include: dilatation of a section of the colon (watershed area), mucosal edema (thumbprinting), pneumatosis | **CT Ischemic Protocol:** look for thromboembolism in the inferior mesenteric vessels, thickening of the bowel wall, absence of bowel wall enhancement with contrast-enhanced CT, narrowing of the bowel lumen due to mucosal edema, and bowel dilatation proximal to the ischemic segment of the bowel<br><br>**Indications:** the patient has abdominal pain and/or rectal bleeding or bloody diarrhea. The presence of any of the following risk factors elevates the pretest probability: age >60 yr, hemodialysis, HTN, DM, hypoalbuminemia, and constipation-inducing medications.<br><br>Sensitivity: 82%[51] |

### 4.19 Large Bowel Volvulus

- Twisting of the sigmoid or cecum on its respective mesentery leading to obstruction and ultimately ischemia

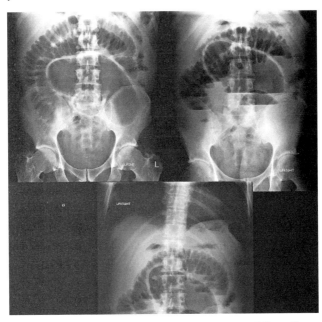

**Figure 32.** AXR. Abdominal plain films show dilated cecum in the midline with no air in the rest of the colon and dilated small bowel with air-fluid levels indicating a cecal volvulus

| 1st Modality | 2nd Modality |
|---|---|
| **Abdominal Plain Film:**<br>**Cecal Volvulus:** look for dilated cecum in left upper quadrant, small bowel obstruction, and no gas in the rest of colon (from hepatic flexure to rectum)<br><br>**Sigmoid Volvulus:** Look for dilated sigmoid colon extending from pelvis to epigastrium (coffee bean sign), and dilated and/or stool filled proximal colon | **CT:**<br>**Cecal Volvulus:** look for dilated edematous cecum, small bowl obstruction, whirl sign of twisted mesenteric and mesenteric vessel, ascites, rarely pneumatosis or free air<br><br>**Sigmoid Volvulus:** look for coffee bean sign of obstructed sigmoid and dilated colon proximally, whirl sign of twisted inferior mesenteric artery vessels and mesentery, and ascites |

MEDICAL IMAGING

## 4.20 Small Bowel Volvulus

- Obstruction and ischemia of the small bowel as a result of a loop of small bowel twisting

| 1st Modality | 2nd Modality |
| --- | --- |
| **Abdominal Plain Film:** look for bowel wall thickening and/or pneumatosis involving the affected segment of bowel. Poor sensitivity and specificity | **CT Abdomen and Pelvis with Oral, IV, and Rectal Contrast:** the imaging modality of choice. Look for single loop of dilated small bowel with two points of narrowing close to each other (bird beak), edema, delayed mucosal enhancement, and whirl sign of twisted vessels, and ascites<br><br>**Indications:** to allow for better visualization of surrounding structures, and for treatment planning<br><br>Sensitivity: 94%[52] |

## 4.21 Ileus

- Bowel obstruction in the absence of mechanical obstruction

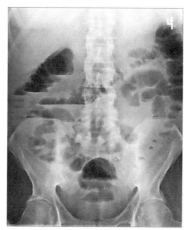

**Figure 33.** AXR. An upright view of the abdomen showing multiple air-fluid levels in nondilated small and large bowel including the rectum indicating ileus

| 1st Modality | 2nd Modality |
| --- | --- |
| **Abdominal Plain Film:** look for extensively gas-filled bowels without dilation | **CT:** may be required if symptoms getting worse and/or colon dilating despite treatment to rule out early perforation |
| There are several types of ileus depending on the etiologies and possible outcomes: | |
| **Localized Ileus (Sentinel Loop Sign):** secondary to underlying inflammatory process such as pancreatitis (C-Loop of duodenum); ileocecal ileus (appendicitis) or ileus affecting hepatic flexure (cholecystitis) | **Indications:** helpful in determining etiology and allow for treatment planning |
| **Diffuse Ileus:** usually either postoperative or infectious cause (C. difficile or garden variety gastroenteritis or electrolyte imbalance) | |
| **Ileus in ICU or Bedridden Orthopedic Patients:** colonic dilatation with competent ileocecal valve may lead to cecal dilatation and perforation – Ogilvey's syndrome | |

# 5. CENTRAL NERVOUS SYSTEM PATHOLOGIES AND FINDINGS

## 5.1 Epidural Hemorrhage
- Bleeding in between skull and dura mater from injury

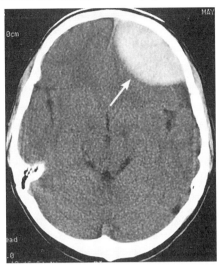

**Figure 34.** CT head. Epidural hematoma (see arrow) characterized by a biconvex hyperdensity between the skull and dura mater

| 1<sup>st</sup> Modality |
| --- |

**CT:** biconvex high density lesion between dura and skull

## 5.2 Subdural Hemorrhage
- Bleeding in between dura and arachnoid mater from ruptured veins

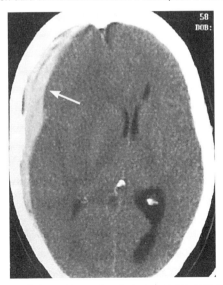

**Figure 35.** CT head. Crescent-shaped hyperdensity between the dura and arachnoid mater (see arrow) associated with the acute phase of a subdural hemorrhage. With time, the subdural collection becomes hypodense

MEDICAL IMAGING

| 1st Modality | 2nd Modality |
| --- | --- |
| **CT:**<br>**Acute Phase:** crescent-shaped area of high density between dura and arachnoid<br><br>**Chronic Phase:** crescent-shaped, low attenuation (fluid density). Sometimes there is an acute-on-chronic subdural bleed (hematocrit level) | **MRI:**<br>Better visualization of small collections of fluid and isodense hematomas55<br><br>**Indications:** in chronic presentations of subdural hemorrhage, since allows for better contrast |

### 5.3 Subarachnoid Hemorrhage (SAH)

- Bleeding underneath arachnoid mater from ruptured cerebral aneurysm or trauma

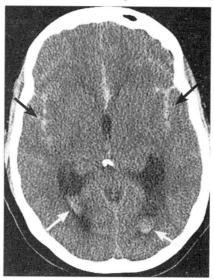

**Figure 36.** CT head. Interventricular hemorrhage is visualized by hyperdensities in the posterior horns of the lateral ventricles (white arrows). Subarachnoid hemorrhage is visualized by hyperdensity in the subarachnoid spaces (Sylvian fissure) (black arrows)

| 1st Modality | 2nd Modality | 3rd Modality | 4th Modality |
| --- | --- | --- | --- |
| **CT:** high density blood in CSF spaces around brainstem, Sylvian fissure, and sometimes the ventricles | **CT Angiogram:** useful to determine cause of SAH. Maximum intensity projection (MIP) reformats in the coronal and sagittal planes are helpful to visualize the intracranial vasculature<br><br>**Indications:** to determine cause of SAH<br><br>Sensitivity: 99%[57]<br>Specificity: 88%[57] | **Conventional Angiogram:** detection and coiling of aneurysm during interventional procedure<br><br>**Indications:** 1. CTA does not show a source and there is still urgent need to evaluate for a cause<br><br>2. CTA shows the source eg – aneurysm, vascular malformation and conventional angio is done as part of endovascular | **MRI:** may be used to detect an aneurysm. Increased signal intensity on fluid attenuated inversion recovery (FLAIR)<br><br>**Indications:** to determine cause of SAH if not well visualized on CT |

## 5.4 Hydrocephalus
- Accumulation of CSF in ventricles from obstruction

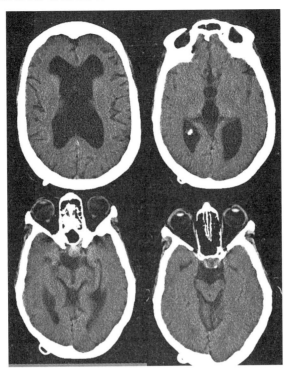

**Figure 37.** CT head. Markedly dilated ventricular system (lateral, third, and fourth ventricles) consistent with hydrocephalus

| 1st Modality | 2nd Modality |
|---|---|
| **Contrast CT:** enlargement of ventricles. Cause (e.g. colloid cyst) can be detected | **MRI:** more specific findings to determine underlying cause (communicating vs. non- communicating). Useful to visualize hyperintense white matter surrounding hydrocephalus demonstrating extent of edema from condition<br><br>**Indications:** the cause of hydrocephalus is unknown and needs to be determined for treatment. MRI has higher resolution images showing causes (e.g. blockages) better than CT |

## 5.5 Cerebral Abscess
- Accumulation of a pus-filled cavity due to an infectious process

| 1st Modality | 2nd Modality |
|---|---|
| **Contrast CT:** ring enhancement with a hypodense, necrotic core with contrast | **MRI:** T1-weighted image shows low intensity signal mass with isointense capsule. T2-weighted image demonstrates hyperintensity in mass and edema which frames abscess<br><br>**Indications:** patient has more specific clinical and imaging findings of abscess. Findings on MRI are more specific for cerebral abscess and can help distinguish from other pathologies (e.g. ring-enhancing gliomas)[56] |

MEDICAL IMAGING

## 5.6 Stroke (Ischemic Infarction)

- Loss of blood to brain region due to an emboli

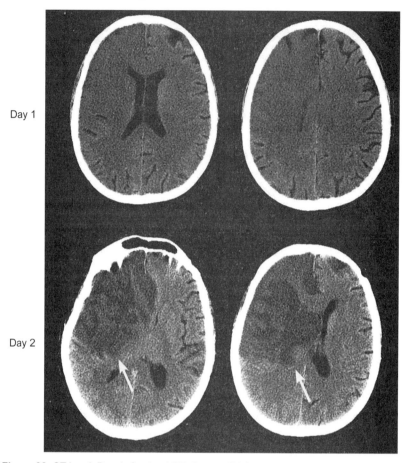

Day 1

Day 2

**Figure 38.** CT head. Day 1: Contrast CT shows mild decreased attenuation of right frontoparietal lobe with effacement of sulci. Day 2: A significant change with further decreased attenuation and mass effect compressing the ventricles (see arrows) and displacing the midline structure to the left. Hypodense area corresponding to area of ischemic stroke

| 1st Modality | 2nd Modality |
|---|---|
| **CT:** low density, wedge-shaped area corresponding to vascular distribution with little or no mass effect | **MRI:** used for patients who present within a couple of hours of onset. T2-weighted image shows hyperintense white matter with low differentiation between white/ gray matter[58] |
| Sensitivity: 61%[59] | **Indications:** completed for all patients within a couple hours of onset as the test has greater sensitivity |
| | Sensitivity: 91%[59] |

MEDICAL IMAGING

### 5.7 Multiple Sclerosis
- Demyelinating, autoimmune disease affecting the CNS

**1st Modality**

**MRI:** T2-weighted image shows round or ovoid white matter plaques often with periventricular or subcortical distribution. Plaques tend to be hyperintense, confluent and >6 mm in diameter

New lesions with active demyelination enhance with gadolinium while old lesions do not

Sensitivity: 57%[60]
Specificity: 95%[60]

### 5.8 Cord Compression
- Decreased space in the spinal canal causing deficits which follow affected nerve distribution

| **1st Modality** | **2nd Modality** |
|---|---|
| **MRI:** T1-weighted image shows narrowing of spinal cord in canal by disc herniation, fracture, tumors, etc<br><br>Sensitivity: 94%[61]<br>Specificity: 98%[61] | **CT:** better visualization of vertebrae involved around cord compression. Impingement of spinal cord at site of injury<br><br>**Indications:** to determine treatment plan, specifically surgical interventions, since able to visualize bony structures well |

## 6. MUSCULOSKELETAL PATHOLOGIES AND FINDINGS

### 6.1 Colles Fracture
- Fracture of the distal radius from a force causing posterior displacement: "dinner fork" deformity

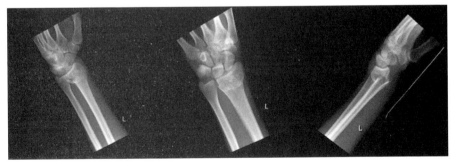

**Figure 39.** Xray of wrist. Fracture and posterior displacement of radius which is characteristic of a Colles fracture

**1st Modality**

**Plain Film (3 views):** radial displacement with dorsal displacement of distal fragment.

MEDICAL IMAGING

## 6.2 Dislocated Shoulder (Anterior)

- Complete separation of humerus from glenoid fossa: commonly from "falling on outstretched arm or direct blow"

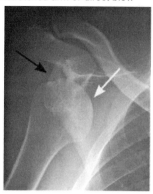 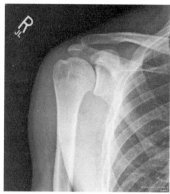

**Figure 40.** Xray of shoulder. (Left) Dislocation of the shoulder characterized by displacement of humeral head (white arrow) from glenoid fossa (black arrow). (Right) Normal shoulder

**1st Modality**

**Plain Film (3 views):** anterior displacement of humeral head on axillary view

## 6.3 Hip Fracture (Subcapital)

- Fracture of the proximal femur: femoral neck

**1st Modality**

**Plain Film (3 views):** anterior displacement of humeral head on axillary view

## 6.4 Dislocated Hip (Posterior)

- Complete separation of femoral head with acetabulum
- One leg will appear shorter in posterior dislocations

| **1st Modality** | **2nd Modality** | **3rd Modality** | **4th Modality** |
|---|---|---|---|
| **Plain Film (3 views):** adducted and internally rotated femur with superolateral displacement of femoral head | **MRI:** coronal T1-weighted image can detect early fractures if radiographs are inconclusive<br><br>**Indications:** suspicion of early fractures and this is not conclusive on plain film | **Bone Scan (Technetium 99m):** useful in equivocal cases if suspicion of avascular necrosis<br><br>**Indications:** suspicion of avascular necrosis[62] | **CT:** may be useful if more osseous details (e.g. degree of comminution and possible intraarticular bone fragments) are required<br><br>**Indications:** to allow for better visualization of bony structures and help direct treatment planning |

## 6.5 Torn Knee Ligaments

- Anterior cruciate ligament (ACL), posterior cruciate ligament (PCL), medial collateral ligament (MCL)

**1st Modality**

**MRI:** Poor visualization, an irregular contour or hyperintense signal in intrasubstance
Sensitivity (ACL): 76%[63]
Specificity (ACL): 52%[63]

## 6.6 Osteomyelitis

- Inflammation in the bone due to an infectious process

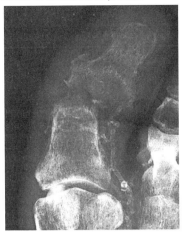

**Figure 41.** Xray of hand. Lytic bone lesions and osteoporosis seen in the distal phalanx which is characteristic of osteomyelitis

| 1st Modality | 2nd Modality | 3rd Modality | 4th Modality |
|---|---|---|---|
| **Plain Film (3 views):** soft tissue swelling, focal osteoporosis, with lytic bone destruction and periosteal reaction68 | **Bone Scan (Technetium 99m):** active phase: increased uptake in affected area (bone and soft tissues) | **Bone Scan (Technetium 99m):** useful in equivocal cases if suspicion of avascular necrosis | **CT:** may be useful if more osseous details (e.g. degree of comminution and possible intraarticular bone fragments) are required |
| Sensitivity: 43-75%[64] Specificity: 75-83%[64] | **Indications:** to allow for early detection of osteomyelitis Sensitivity: 65%[65] | **Indications:** suspicion of avascular necrosis[62] | **Indications:** to allow for better visualization of bony structures and help direct treatment planning |

## REFERENCES

1. Cortellaro F, Colombo S, Coen D, Duca PG. 2012. Lung ultrasound is an accurate diagnostic tool for the diagnosis of pneumonia in the emergency department. *Emerg Med J* 29(1):19-23.
2. Kwong JS, Adler BD, Padley SP, Müller NL. 1993. Diagnosis of diseases of the trachea and main bronchi: Chest radiography vs CT. *AJR Am J Roentgenol* 161 (3):519-522.
3. Raghu G, Mageto YN, Lockhart D, Schmidt RA, Wood DE, Godwin JD. 1999. The accuracy of the clinical diagnosis of new-onset idiopathic pulmonary fibrosis and other interstitial lung disease: A prospective study. *Chest* 116(5):1168-1174.
4. Mets OM, Buckens CF, Zanen P, Isgum I, van Ginneken B, Prokop M, et al. 2011. Identification of chronic obstructive pulmonary disease in lung cancer screening computed tomographic scans. *JAMA* 306(16):1 775-1781.
5. Van der Bruggen-Bogaarts BA, van der Bruggen HM, van Waes PF, Lammers JW. 1996. Screening for bronchiectasis. A comparative study between chest radiography and high-resolution CT. *Chest* 109(3):608-611.
6. Dodd JD, Souza CA, Müller NL. 2006. Conventional high-resolution CT versus helical high- resolution MDCT in the detection of bronchiectasis. *AMJ Am J Roentgenol* 187(2):414-420.
7. Hunninghake GW, Zimmerman MB, Schwartz DA, King TE Jr, Lynch J, Hegele R, et al. 2001. Utility of a lung biopsy for the diagnosis of idiopathic pulmonary fibrosis. *Am J Respir Crit Care Med* 164(2):193-196.
8. Elliott CG, Goldhaber SZ, Visani L, DeRosa M. 2000. Chest radiographs in acute pulmonary embolism. Results from the International Cooperative Pulmonary Embolism Registry. *Chest* 118(1):33-38.
9. Patel S, Kazerooni EA. 2005. Helical CT for the evaluation of acute pulmonary embolism. *AJR Am J Roentgenol* 185(1):135-149.
10. Gluecker T, Capasso P, Schnyder P, Gudinchet F, Schaller MD, Revelly JP, et al. 1999. Clinical and radiologic features of pulmonary edema. *Radiographics* 19(6):1507-1531.
11. Toyoda Y , Nakayama T, Kusunoki Y, Iso H, Suzuki T. 2008. Sensitivity and specificity of lung cancer screening using chest low-dose computed tomography. *Br J Cancer* 98(1 0):1602-1 607.
12. Crandall J, Kent R, Patrie J, Fertile J, Martin P. 2000. Rib fracture patterns and radiologic detection – A restraint-based comparison. *Annu Proc Assoc Adv Automot Med* 44:235-259.
13. Pugliese F, Mollet NR, Runza G, van Mieghem C, Meijboom WB, Malagutti P, et al. 2006. Diagnostic accuracy of non-invasive 64-slice CT coronary angiography in patients with stable angina pectoris. *Eur Radiol* 16(3):575-582.
14. Nienaber CA, von Kodolitsch Y, Nicolas V, Siglow V, Piepho A, Brockhoff C, et al. 1993. The diagnosis of thoracic aortic dissection by noninvasive imaging procedures. *N Engl J Med* 328(1):1- 9.
15. von Kodolitsch Y, Nienaber CA, Dieckmann C. 2004. Chest radiography for the diagnosis of acute aortic syndrome. *Am J Med* 116(2):73-77.
16. Hermansson M, Johansson J, Gudbjartsson T, Hambreus G, Jönsson P, Lillo-Gil R, et al. 2010. Esophageal perforation in South of

Sweden: Results of surgical treatment in 125 consecutive patients. *BMC Surg* 10:31.
17. Alexander ES, Clark RA. 1982. Computed tomography in the diagnosis of abdominal hemorrhage. *JAMA* 248(9):1104-1107.
18. Sagel SS, Siegel MJ, Stanley RJ, Jost RG. 1977. Detection of retroperitoneal hemorrhage by computed tomography. *AJR Am J Roentgenol* 129(3):403-407.
19. Lee BC, Ormsby EL, McGahan JP, Melendres GM, Richards JR. 2007. The utility of sonography for the triage of blunt abdominal trauma patients to exploratory laparotomy. *AJR Am J Roentgenol* 188(2):415-421.
20. Liu M, Lee CH, P'eng FK. 1993. Prospective comparison of diagnostic peritoneal lavage, computed tomographic scanning, and ultrasonography for the diagnosis of blunt abdominal trauma. *J Trauma* 35(2):267-270.
21. Lubner M, Menias C, Rucker C, Bhalla S, Peterson CM, Wang L, et al. 2007. Blood in the belly: CT findings of hemoperitoneum. *Radiographics* 27(1):109-125.
22. Smith DS, Bonadio WA, Losek JD, Walsh-Kelly CM, Hennes HM, Glaeser PW, et al. 1992. The role of abdominal x-rays in the diagnosis and management of intussusception. *Pediatr Emerg Care* 8(6):325-327.
23. Gayer G, Apter S, Hofmann C, Nass S, Amitai M, Zissin R, et al. 1998. Intussusception in adults: CT diagnosis. Clin Radiol 53(1):53-57.
24. Zubaidi A, Al-Saif F, Silverman R. 2006. Adult intussusception: A retrospective review. *Dis Colon Rectum* 49(10):1546-1551.
25. Barbiera F, Cusma S, Di Giacomo D, Finazzo M, Lo Casto A, Pardo S. 2001. Adult intestinal intussusception: Comparison between CT features and surgical findings. *Radiol Radiol* 102(1-2):37- 42.
26. HryhorczukAL, Strouse PJ. 2009. Validation of US as a first-line diagnostic test for assessment of pediatric ileocolic intussusception. *Pediatr Radiol* 39(10):1075-1079.
27. Kim YH, Blake MA, Harisinghani MG, Archer-Arroyo K, Hahn PF, Pitman MB, et al. 2006. Adult intestinal intussusception: CT appearances and identification of a causative lead point. *Radiographics* 26(3):733-744.
28. Testa AC, Ludovisi M, Mascilini F, Di Legge A, Malaggese M, Fagott A, et al. 2012. Ultrasound evaluation of intra-abdominal sites of disease to predict likelihood of suboptimal cytoreduction in advanced ovarian cancer: A prospective study. *Ultrasound Obstet Gynecol* 39(1 ):99-105.
29. Black M, Friedman AC. 1989. Ultrasound examination in the patient with ascites. *Ann Intern Med* 110(4):253-255.
30. Proto AV, Lane EJ, Marangola JP. 1976. A new concept of ascitic fluid distribution. *AJR Am J Roentgenol* 126(5):974-980.
31. Edell SL, Gefter WB. 1979. Ultrasonic differentiation of types of ascitic fluid. *AJR Am J Roentgenol* 133(1):111-114.
32. Gayer G, Hertz M, Manor H, Strauss S, Klinowski E, Zissin R. 2004. Dense ascites: CT manifestations and clinical implications. *Emerg Radiol* 10(5):262-267.
33. Maglinte DD, Reyes BL, Harmon BH, Kelvin FM, Turner WW Jr, Hage JE, et al. 1996. Reliability and role of plain film radiography and CT in the diagnosis of small-bowel obstruction. *AJR Am J Roentgenol* 167(6):1451-1455.
34. Suri S, Gupta S, Sudhakar PJ, Venkataramu NK, Sood B, Wig JD. 1999. Comparative evaluation of plain films, ultrasound and CT in the diagnosis of intestinal obstruction. *Acta Radiol* 40(4):422- 428.
35. Kim SH, Shin SS, Jeong YY, Heo SH, Kim JW, Kang HK. 2009. Gastrointestinal tract perforation: MDCT findings according to the perforation sites. *Korean J Radiol* 10(1):63-70.
36. Levine MS. Peptic ulcers. In: Gore RM, Levine MS. Textbook of Gastrointestinal Radiology, 2nd ed. New York: Saunders Elsevier; 2000.
37. Barloon, T.J., Brown, B.P., Abu-Yousef, M.M. et al. *Abdom Imaging* (1995) 20: 149
38. Doria AS, Moineddin R, Kellenberger CJ, Epelman M, Beyene J, Schuh S, et al. 2006. US or CT for diagnosis of appendicitis in children and adults? A meta-analysis. *Radiology* 241(1):83-94.
39. Sarma D, Longo WE. 2008. Diagnostic imaging for diverticulitis. *J Clin Gastroenterol* 42(10):1139- 1141.
40. Håkansson K, Leander P, Ekberg O, Håkansson HO. 2000. MR imaging in clinically suspected acute cholecystitis. A comparison with ultrasonography. *Acta Radiol* 41 (4):322-328.
41. Barakos JA, Ralls PW, Lapin SA, Johnson MD, Radin DR, Colletti PM, et al. 1987. Cholelithiasis: Evaluation with CT. *Radiology* 162(2):415-418.
42. Bastid C, Sahel J, Filho M, Sarles H. 1990. Diameter of the main pancreatic duct in chronic calcifying pancreatitis. Measurement by ultrasonography versus pancreatography. *Pancreas* 5(5):524-527.
43. Niederau C, Grendell JH. 1985. Diagnosis of chronic pancreatitis. *Gastroenterology* 88(6):1973- 1995.
44. Badea R. 2005. Ultrasonography of acute pancreatitis – An essay in images. *Rom J Gastroenterol* 14(1 ):83-89.
45. Luetmer PH, Stephens DH, Ward EM. 1989. Chronic pancreatitis: Reassessment with current CT. *Radiology* 171(2):353-357.
46. Balthazar EJ, Robinson DL, Megibow AJ, Ranson JH. 1990. Acute pancreatitis: Value of CT in establishing prognosis. *Radiology* 174(2):331-336.
47. Eray O, Cubuk MS, Oktay C, Yilmaz S, Cete Y, Ersoy FF. 2003. The efficacy of urinalysis, plain films, and spiral CT in ED patients with suspected renal colic. *Am J Emerg Med* 21 (2):152-154.
48. Wiesner W. 2003. Is multidetector computerized tomography currently the primary diagnostic method of choice in diagnostic imaging of acute intestinal ischemia? *Praxis* 92(31-32):1315-1317.
49. Kirk E. 2012. Ultrasound in the diagnosis of ectopic pregnancy. *Clin Obset Gynecol* 55(2):395- 401.
50. Dheer S, Levine MS, Redfern RO, Metz DC, Rubesin SE, Laufer I. 2002. Radiographically diagnosed antral gastritis: Findings in patients with and without Helicobacter pylori infection. *Br J Radiol* 75(898):805-811.
51. Craig WD, Wagner BJ, Travis MD. 2008. Pyelonephritis: Radiologic-pathologic review. *Radiographics* 28(1):255-277.
52. Taourel P, Aufort S, Merigeaud S, Doyon FC, Hoquet MD, Delabrousse E. 2008. Imaging of ischemic colitis. *Radiol Clin North Am* 46(5):909-924, vi.
53. Sandhu PS, Joe BN, Coakley FV, Qayyum A, Webb EM, Yeh BM. 2007. Bowel transition points: Multiplicity and posterior location at CT are associated with small-bowel volvulus. *Radiology* 245(1):160-167.
54. Frager D, Medwid SW, Baer JW, Mollinelli B, Friedman M. 1994. CT of small-bowel obstruction: Value in establishing the diagnosis and determining the degree and cause. *AJR Am J Roentgenol* 162(1) :37-4 1.
55. Senturk S, et al. 2010. Swiss Med Wkly 140(23-24):335-340.
56. Holmes TM, Petrella JR, Provenzale JM. 2004. *AJR Am J Roentgenol* 1 83(5):1247-1252.
57. Teksam M, McKinney A, Casey S, Asis M, Kieffer S, Truwit CL. 2004. Multi-section CT angiography for detection of cerebral aneurysms. *AJNR Am J Neuroradiol* 25(9):1485-1492.
58. Srinivasan A, et al. 2006. *Radiographics* 26(Suppl 1 ):S75-95.
59. Fiebach JB. 2002. CT and diffusion-weighted MR imaging in randomized order: Diffusion- weighted imaging results in higher accuracy and lower interrater variability in the diagnosis of hyperacute ischemic stroke. *Stroke* 33(9):2206-2210.
60. Barkhof F, Filippi M, Miller DH, Scheltens P, Campi A, Polman CH, et al. 1997. Comparison of MRI criteria at first presentation to predict conversion to clinically definite multiple sclerosis. *Brain* 120(Pt 11):2059-2069.
61. Parmar H, Park P, Brahma B, Gandhi D. 2008. Imaging of idiopathic spinal cord herniation. Radiographics 28(2):511-518.
62. Alavi A, McCloskey JR, Steinberg ME. 1977. *Clin Orthop Relat Res* 127:137-141.
63. Rayan F, Bhonsle S, Shukla DD. 2009. Clinical, MRI, and arthroscopic correlation in meniscal and anterior cruciate ligament injuries. *Int Orthop* 33(1):129-132.
64. El-Maghraby TA, Moustafa HM, Pauwels EK. 2006. Nuclear medicine methods for evaluation of skeletal infection among other diagnostic modalities. *Q J Nucl Med Mol Imaging* 50(3):167-192.
65. Williamson MR, Quenzer RW, Rosenberg RD, Meholic AJ, Eisenberg B, Espinosa MC, et al. 1991. Osteomyelitis: Sensitivity of 0.064 T MRI, three-phase bone scanning and indium scanning with biopsy proof. *Magn Reson Imaging* 9(6):945-948.
66. Naidich, D. P., Mccauley, D. I., Khouri, N. F., Stitik, F. P., & Siegelman, S. S. (1982). Computed Tomography of Bronchiectasis. *Journal of Computer Assisted Tomography*, 6(3), 437-444
67. Hartman, T. E., Primack, S. L., Lee, K. S., Swensen, S. J., & Müller, N. L. (1994). CT of bronchial and bronchiolar diseases. *RadioGraphics*, 14(5), 991-1003
68. Pineda C, Espinosa R, Pena A. 2009. *Semin Plast Surg* 23(2):80-89.

## ACKNOWLEDGEMENTS

We would like to thank Dr. Taebong Chung, Dr. Bob Bleakney, Dr. Nasir Jaffer, and Dr. Eugene Yu for their contribution of images in this chapter.

# CHAPTER 19:

# Oncology

**Editors:**
Angela Han, HBSc
Rebecca Stepita, BHSc
Armin Rahmani, BSc

**Faculty Reviewers:**
Raymond Jang, MD, FRCPC
Richard Tsang, MD, FRCPC

## TABLE OF CONTENTS

ONCOLOGY

# 1. SCREENING GUIDELINES

Primary prevention is essential in the management of cancer. **Figure 1** lists the rank estimates of cancer cases by incidence (excluding non- melanoma skin cancers) and mortality. **Table 1** lists the current Canadian Screening Guidelines for common cancer.

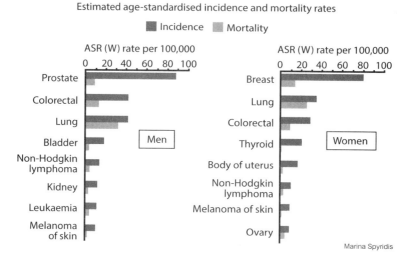

**Figure 1.** Canadian Cancer Statistics, 2012 [1]

**Table 1.** Canadian Cancer Screening Guidelines

| Cancer Type | Average Risk | High Risk |
|---|---|---|
| **Breast Cancer** [2,3,4]<br><br>Note: applies to women and trans women who have taken gender-affirming hormones for >5 years and trans men who have not had mastectomy | Age 40-49: mammography not recommended<br><br>Age 50-74: mammography every 2-3 years | High Risk: previous breast cancer, history of breast cancer in first degree relative, known BRCA1/BRCA2 mutation, received chest radiation, calculated as having >25% lifetime risk of breast cancer<br>• Age 30-69: annual mammography + MRI<br>• Age 70-74: annual mammography<br>• Age >74: patient preference with healthcare provider referral |
| **Colon Cancer** [5] | Age 50-74: FOBT every 2 years or flex sig every 10 years | High Risk: FAP, HNPCC, IBD, family history<br>• FAP: annual sigmoidoscopy or colonoscopy starting at age 10-12 [5]<br>• HNPCC: colonoscopy every 2 years starting at age 20-25, annual colonoscopy after age 40<br>• Previous colon cancer or polyps: colonoscopy every 3-5 years [5]<br>• IBD: colonoscopy every 1-2 years after 8 years of colitis [5]<br>• FHx that includes one or more first-degree relatives with the disease: colonoscopy at age 50, or 10 years earlier than age of diagnosis of youngest relative |

| Cancer Type | Average Risk | High Risk |
|---|---|---|
| **Cervical Cancer**[6,7,8]<br><br>Note: applies to all women (including trans women who have undergone surgery to create a neo-cervix) and trans men who have a cervix | **Pap test (cytology)**<br>• Age 21-70: Pap test if sexually active every 3 years<br>    ♦ If not sexually active, test when sexually active<br>    ♦ Stop at 70 years if unremarkable Pap smear for 10 previous years<br>**HPV DNA test**[12]<br>• HPV testing is not presently funded by the MOHLTC. As such, it is not used for screening purposes, though it may have a role in the workup of patients with abnormal Pap results | |
| **Prostate Cancer**[9] | Screening is not recommended with the PSA test | High risk: men of black race and men with a family history of prostate cancer<br>• Discuss the benefits and harms of screening with men at increased risk |

FAP = familial adenomatous polyposis, FOBT = fecal occult blood test, HNPCC = hereditary nonpolyposis colorectal cancer

## 2. PRINCIPLES OF ONCOLOGY

**HPI**
- Symptoms: what led to investigations
- Constitutional symptoms: fever, chills, fatigue, night sweats, weight loss, malaise
- Diagnostic results: imaging and pathology reports
- Treatment received to date (surgery, chemotherapy, radiation, interventional procedures such as stents and drains)
- Performance status: Eastern Cooperative Oncology Group (ECOG) scale (**Table 2**)
- Asymptomatic (detected by screening)

**PMHx**
- FHx of malignancies
- SHx: occupation, living situation, family, support system, activities of daily living, smoking, EtOH

**Patient's understanding of disease and prognosis**
**Other considerations for advanced disease:**
- Symptom burden assessment (e.g. the Edmonton Symptom Assessment Scale)
- End of life wishes (e.g. does the patient wish to die at home or hospital, Do Not Resuscitate [DNR] wishes)
- Power of Attorney (document)
- Advance directives indicating previously expressed wishes to guide end of life treatments and decision-making
- Spiritual or religious needs

**Table 2.** ECOG Performance Status[10]

| ECOG | Description |
|---|---|
| 0 | Fully active, able to carry on all pre-disease performance without restriction |
| 1 | Restricted in physically strenuous activity but ambulatory and able to carry out work of a light or sedentary nature, e.g., light house work, office work |
| 2 | Ambulatory and capable of all self-care but unable to carry out any work |
| 3 | Capable of only limited self-care, confined to bed or chair more than 50% of waking hours |
| 4 | Completely disabled. Cannot carry on self-care. Totally confined to bed or chair |
| 5 | Dead |

ONCOLOGY

## 3. FAMILIAL CANCERS AND CANCER SYNDROMES[11]

Clinical features that raise the suspicion of a familial form of cancer susceptibility in a patient diagnosed with any type of malignancy include:
- A cancer that occurs at an unusually young age compared with its usual presentation
- The development of multiple tumors in a single organ, or bilateral development of tumors in paired organs
- The development of more than one primary tumor of any type
- A family history of cancer of the same type or related type in one or more first-degree relatives
- A high rate of cancer occurrence in the family
- Cancer occurring in an individual or within a family with congenital anomalies or birth defects

### 3.1. BRCA1/2:
- Common cancers: breast cancer (including increased risk for men), ovarian cancer, prostate cancer
- Identifying patients at-risk: patients with relatives with breast cancer or ovarian cancer, particularly 1st degree relatives and/or relatives diagnosed at an early age; patients with breast and/or ovarian cancers and an Ashkenazi Jewish ethnicity
- Mitigating risk:
  - Genetic counselling
  - Screening beginning at a younger age, more frequently, consider mammography + MRI for breast screening
  - Consider role for chemoprevention and risk-reducing mastectomy and bilateral salpingo-oophorectomy

### 3.2. HNPCC / Lynch Syndrome:
- Common cancers: colorectal cancer, endometrial cancer, small bowel cancer, transitional cell carcinoma of the ureter or renal pelvis
- Identifying patients at-risk: Amsterdam Criteria
  - 3 or more relatives with HNPCC-associated cancers
    - 1 of whom is a 1st degree relative
    - 2 generations
    - 1 or more diagnosed before age 50

### 3.3. Familial Adenomatous Polyposis:
- Common cancers: early onset colorectal adenocarcinoma; extra-colonic malignancies including duodenal carcinoma, thyroid carcinoma, childhood hepatoblastoma, stomach adenocarcinoma, CNS tumors
- Identifying patients at-risk:
  - Genetic testing and counselling
    - In patients with a personal history of colorectal adenomas
    - In patients with a family history of FAP
- Mitigating risk:
  - Frequent flexible sigmoidoscopy or colonoscopy beginning at an early age
  - Consider role for prophylactic proctocolectomy

### 3.4. Li-Fraumeni Syndrome:
- Common cancers: breast cancer, sarcomas, central nervous system cancers, leukemias, and adrenocortical cancers
- Identifying patients at-risk:
  - Chompret diagnostic criteria (one of the following):
    1. A tumor belonging to the LFS tumor spectrum (soft tissue sarcoma, osteosarcoma, pre-menopausal breast cancer, brain tumor, adrenocortical carcinoma, leukemia, or lung bronchoalveolar cancer) before age 46 AND
    2. At least one first- or second-degree relative with an LFS tumor (except breast cancer if the proband has breast cancer) before age 56 or with multiple tumors;
    3. Multiple tumors (except multiple breast tumors), two of which belong to the LFS tumor spectrum and the first of which occurred before age 46
    4. Diagnosed with adrenocortical carcinoma or choroid plexus tumor, irrespective

ONCOLOGY

of family history
- ◆ Classic criteria (all of the following)
  - ▪ Sarcoma diagnosed before age 45
  - ▪ First-degree relative with any cancer before age 45
  - ▪ First- or second-degree relative with any cancer before age 45 or a sarcoma at any age

### 3.5. MEN1, MEN2A, MEN2B:
- Multiple endocrine neoplasia (MEN) includes several distinct syndromes, each with its own specific characteristics. There are three main types of MEN syndromes.
- Common cancers:
  - ◆ MEN 1: Parathyroid hyperplasia, pancreatic tumours (gastrinoma, insulinoma) and pituitary adenoma
  - ◆ MEN 2a: Medullary thyroid carcinoma (MTC), pheochromocytoma and parathyroid hyperplasia
  - ◆ MEN 2b: Medullary thyroid carcinoma, pheochromocytoma and mucosal neuroma
- Identifying patients at-risk:
  1. All first degree relatives of patients with MEN diagnosis
  2. MEN syndromes are inherited in an autosomal dominant fashion. If a person has MEN, each of their children has a 50% chance of inheriting their syndrome.
  3. Genetic causes for each type of MEN syndromes are very specific and families with one type of MEN do not have an increased risk of developing the other types.
  4. All patients with a MEN diagnosis, MEN mutation carriers and at risk family members with unknown carrier status are monitored for symptoms and signs of MEN associated tumours.

### 3.6. von Hippel Lindau:
- Common cancers: Hemangioblastomas of the brain (cerebellum) and spine, Retinal capillary hemangioblastomas (retinal angiomas), Clear cell renal cell carcinomas (RCCs), Pheochromocytomas, Endolymphatic sac tumors of the middle ear, Serous cystadenomas and neuroendocrine tumors of the pancreas, Papillary cystadenomas of the epididymis and broad ligament
  - ◆ Type 1: lower risk of developing pheochromocytomas
  - ◆ Type 2: high risk for developing pheochromocytoma
- Identifying patients at-risk:
  - ▪ Genetic testing for germline mutation of VHL gene
  1. Any blood relative of an individual diagnosed with VHL disease
  2. Any individual with TWO VHL-associated lesions: Hemangioblastoma, Clear cell renal carcinoma, Pheochromocytoma, Endolymphatic sac tumor, Epididymal or adnexal papillary cystadenoma, Pancreatic serous cystadenomas, Pancreatic neuroendocrine tumors)
  3. Any individual with ONE or more of the following: CNS hemangioblastoma, Pheochromocytoma or paraganglioma, Endolymphatic sac tumor, Epididymal papillary cystadenoma
  4. Any individual with: Clear cell renal carcinoma diagnosed at age <40 years, Bilateral and/or multiple clear cell RCCs, >1 Pancreatic serous cystadenoma, >1 Pancreatic neuroendocrine tumor, or Multiple pancreatic cysts + any VHL associated lesion

## 4. FUNDAMENTALS OF CANCER THERAPY
Most cancers involve a multidisciplinary approach to treatment and management. A thorough discussion of each cancer-specific strategy is beyond the scope of this handbook. Below we discuss the role of biopsy, and outline the fields of surgical, medical, and radiation oncology.

### 4.1. Biopsies
All cancers are diagnosed through a biopsy that is ultimately read by a pathologist. Biopsies may be done with (e.g. CT or U/S) or without image guidance. Biopsies may also be done as part of endoscopic procedures (e.g. bronchoscopy, OGD) (see **Table 3**).

**Table 3.** Biopsy Types*

| Biopsy Type | Description |
| --- | --- |
| Fine Needle Aspiration | Small needle, draw fluid out for cytology |
| Core Needle Biopsy | Large needle, preserves tissue architecture |
| Surgical (excisional) | Entire mass is removed |

*As the molecular profiling of cancers becomes more prevalent, it may be more important to collect larger tissue samples.

## 4.2. Surgical Oncology

For most solid tumor malignancies, surgery offers the best chance for cure. Palliative surgery can sometimes be used to relieve symptoms in a non-curative setting. Historically, surgery was the only effective form of treating cancer, but with developments in the fields of radiation and medical oncology, surgeons have to work with their colleagues in other disciplines to achieve the best results for patients.

**Principles of surgical oncology:**
- Curative surgery: Only performed when a total excision of the entire tumor size is possible. In many cases the associated lymph node drainage fields are also removed in continuity. The pathological findings from the surgical specimen will determine whether adequate tissue was removed during the operation.
- Palliative surgery: In this case the operation is performed to relieve symptoms caused by the tumor, either by resection or bypass. The surgeon tailors this type of surgery to the needs of patient to minimize morbidity and improve quality of life.
- Margins of surgical excision: The surgeon's goal is to remove all of the cancerous tumor with a rim of normal tissue around it. During or after the surgery, a pathologist examines the surgical specimen, determines whether the rim is clear of cancer cells, and measures the distance between the outer edge of the surrounding tissue and the edge of the cancer.

**Side effects of surgery:** Like other cancer treatments, surgery has its benefits, risks and side effects. The type and intensity of side effects vary from patient to patient and depend on several factors, such as:
- Type and stage of cancer
- Type of surgery
- The patient's overall health

**Some side effects of surgery include:**
- Pain
- Fatigue
- Appetite loss
- Swelling around the site of surgery
- Bleeding
- Infection
- Lymphedema: may occur after lymph nodes are removed
- Scarring and cosmetic concerns
- Stress and psychosocial implications

## 4.3. Medical Oncology

Medical oncology is involved in the systemic treatment of cancer, especially in the presence of metastatic dissemination. Medical oncology includes chemotherapy, hormonal therapy, targeted therapy, and immunotherapy.

**Principles of Chemotherapy:**
- Adjuvant Chemotherapy: for patients with successful initial treatment (no evidence of residual disease), but high risk for relapse (e.g. post- surgery)
- Neo-adjuvant Chemotherapy: for patients with bulky primary disease (not immediately amenable to initial therapy) with goal of reducing this bulk prior to initial treatment

("downstaging")
- ♦ Palliative Chemotherapy: to prolong life and improve symptoms
- ♦ without the intention of cure; not the same as palliative care

- **Acute Side Effects of Chemotherapy:**
  - ♦ Bone marrow – anemia, neutropenia, thrombocytopenia
  - ♦ GI tract – mucositis, nausea/vomiting, diarrhea
  - ♦ Fatigue
  - ♦ Hair thinning/loss

- **Chronic Side Effects of Chemotherapy:**
  - ♦ Cardiomyopathy
  - ♦ Secondary malignancies
  - ♦ Peripheral neuropathy

### 4.4. Radiation Oncology
Radiation oncology is involved in locoregional eradication of cancer with preservation of the normal structure and function of surrounding tissues.

Goals: treatment with curative vs. palliative intent

**Types of radiation therapy:**
- External beam radiation therapy
- Brachytherapy
- Unsealed radionuclide therapy (e.g. 131Iodine, free or tagged to MAb)

**Contraindications to radiation therapy:**
- Previous radiation therapy to normal tissue tolerance
- Pacemaker/defibrillator within the direct radiation field

**Side effects of radiation therapy:**
- Early radiation-induced reactions: acute, local (e.g. local skin reactions, alopecia, nausea, mucositis, esophagitis) or constitutional (e.g. fatigue), and myelosuppression for large volumes of bone marrow irradiation
- Late radiation-induced reactions: dose-dependent (particularly sensitive to high dose per fraction), occurring months to years after treatment, progressive (e.g. lung fibrosis, bone necrosis, myelopathy)
- Secondary malignancy: latency period generally >10 years, risk is higher in conjunction with chemotherapy

ONCOLOGY

# 5. APPROACH TO COMPLICATIONS IN ONCOLOGY

**Table 4.** DIMSH Approach to Complications in Oncology Patients

| Type of Complication | Example |
|---|---|
| Drug (consider both oncology and non-oncology drugs) | • Febrile neutropenia<br>• Chemotherapy-induced cardiomyopathy |
| Infectious | • Febrile neutropenia |
| Metabolic | • Electrolytes: hyponatremia, hypercalcemia, tumor lysis syndrome<br>• Organ failure: renal, liver failure |
| Structural (Think anatomically) | • CNS: brain metastases, spinal cord compression<br>• Organ obstruction: airway obstruction, biliary obstruction, bowel obstruction<br>• Blood vessels: superior vena cava obstruction syndrome, pulmonary embolus<br>• Excess fluid: pleural effusion, pericardial effusion, ascites |
| Hematologic | • Cytopenias: anemia, neutropenia, thrombocytopenia<br>• Thrombosis<br>• Disseminated intravascular coagulation (DIC) |

# 6. ONCOLOGIC EMERGENCIES

**Table 5.** Description, Risk Factors, and Management of Oncologic Emergencies

| Key Signs and Symptoms | Etiology | Risk Factors | Investigations |
|---|---|---|---|
| **Cancer Associated Thrombosis** | | | |
| • DVT: calf pain, leg swelling/erythema<br>• PE: dyspnea, cough, wheezing, chest pain, tachycardia, upper abdominal pain | • Activation of coagulation system → hypercoagulable state | • Malignancy increases risk of venous (DVT, PE) and arterial (stroke, MI) thrombo-embolic events<br>• Certain cancers: pancreas, stomach, lung, lymphoma<br>• Cancer chemo | • ECG<br>• CXR<br>• Venous leg Doppler<br>• CT angiography (if not, ventilation-perfusion [V/Q] scan) |
| **Hypercalcemia**<br>**(see Essentials of Fluids, Electrolytes, and Acid/Base Disturbances, p.463)** | | | |
| • Volume depletion<br>• Early: polyuria, polydipsia, nocturia, anorexia<br>• Late: apathy, irritability, muscle weakness, N/V | • May be from bony metastases or ectopic production | • Associated w/ cancers of: breast, lung, thyroid, kidney, prostate, and multiple myeloma | • Blood work including electrolytes, $Ca^{2+}$, $Mg^{2+}$, $PO_4^{3-}$, creatinine, and PTH<br>• ECG |

ONCOLOGY

| Key Signs and Symptoms | Etiology | Risk Factors | Investigations |
|---|---|---|---|

**Tumor Lysis Syndrome**

| | | | |
|---|---|---|---|
| • Electrolyte abnormalities: hypocalcemia, hyperphosphatemia, hyperkalemia, hyperuricemia<br>• Possible renal failure | • Massive release of uric acid, $K^+$, $PO4^{3-}$, tumor breakdown products from successful chemotherapy<br>• Occurs a few hours-days after treatment | • Associated with acute leukemia, Burkitt's lymphoma, and other hematologic malignancies | • Blood work including electrolytes, $Ca^{2+}$, uric acid, $K^+$, $PO4^{3-}$, and creatinine |

**Febrile Neutropenia**

| | | | |
|---|---|---|---|
| • Defined by: absolute neutrophil count <1.0 cell/mm$^3$ and temperature >38.0°C × 1 h or single temperature >38.3°C | • Susceptibility to infection due to immuno-suppressive state | • Granulocytopenia carries risk of bacterial infection (usually patient's own endogenous flora), and fungal infection if prolonged | • Blood work including CBC<br>• Blood cultures<br>• Urine culture<br>• CXR<br>• Other investigations guided by symptoms |

**Superior Vena Cava Obstruction Syndrome**

| | | | |
|---|---|---|---|
| • Tachypnea<br>• Collateral neck & chest vein engorgement<br>• Facial plethora<br>• Upper extremity edema<br>• Vocal cord paralysis<br>• Horner's syndrome (rare) | • Invasion /external compression of SVC by malignantstructures in right lung & mediastinum<br>• Thrombosis within SVC causing obstruction | • Associated with lung cancer (85%), advanced lymphoma (15%), metastatic disease | • CXR<br>• CT chest |

**Spinal Cord Compression**

| | | | |
|---|---|---|---|
| • Back pain<br>• Neurological deficits (muscle weakness, bladder and bowel dysfunction, and sensory deficit) | • Metastasis to the spine (thoracic spine most common) involving the vertebral body, paravertebral tissue, or epidural space* | | • X-ray (plain film)<br>• CT<br>• MRI (whole spine) |

*Note that residual neurological deficit is related to time from symptom onset to treatment; **spinal cord compression must be diagnosed and treated quickly**

ONCOLOGY

# REFERENCES

1. Globocan International Agency for Research on Cancer. Estimated Cancer Incidence, Mortality and Prevalence. France: IARC; 2012.
2. Canadian Task Force on Preventive Health Care, Tonelli M, Connor Gorber S, Joffres M, Dickinson J, Singh H, et al. Recommendations on screening for breast cancer in average- risk women aged 40-74 years. CMAJ. 2011; 183(17):1991-2001.
3. Cancer Care Ontario. OBSP Screening for Women at High Risk. Toronto: Cancer Care Ontario. 2016. Available from: https://www.cancercare.on.ca/pcs/screening/breastscreening/OBSP/highrisk/
4. Canadian Cancer Society. Breast cancer screening information for trans women. Toronto: Cancer Cancer Society. 2016. Available from: http://convio.cancer.ca/site/PageServer?pagename=SSL_ON_HCP_HCPTW_Breast
5. Cancer Care Ontario. Screening Guidelines - Colon Cancer. Toronto: Cancer Care Ontario. 2016. Available from: https://www.cancercare.on.ca/pcs/screening/coloscreening/cccstandardsguidelines/.
6. Canadian Cancer Society. Cervical cancer screening information for trans men. Toronto: Cancer Cancer Society. 2016. Available from: http://convio.cancer.ca/site/PageServer?pagename=SSL_ON_HCP_HCPTM_Cervical#.WC4I0eErLBJ
7. Cancer Care Ontario. Screening Guidelines - Cervical Cancer. Toronto: Cancer Care Ontario. 2016. Available from: https://www.cancercare.on.ca/pcs/screening/cervscreening/screening_guidelines/.
8. Murphy J, Kennedy EB, Dunn S, McLachlin CM, Fung Kee Fung M, Gzik D, et al. Cervical screening: A guideline for clinical practice in Ontario. J Obstet Gynaecol Can. 2012; 34(5):453-458.
9. Canadian Task Force on Preventive Health Care, Bell N, Connor Gorber S, Shane A, Joffres M, Singh H, Dickinson J, et al. Recommendations on screening for prostate cancer with the prostate-specific antigen test. CMAJ. 2014; 186(16):1225-34.
10. Eastern Cooperative Oncology Group-ACRIN Cancer Research Group. ECOG Performance Status. Philadelphia, Pennsylvania. 2016. Available from: http://ecog-acrin.org/resources/ecog-performance-status
11. UpToDate, Talley NJ, Lamont JT, Grover S. Familial adenomatous polyposis: screening and management of patients and families. Available from: https://www.uptodate.com/contents/familial-adenomatous-polyposis-screening-and-management-of-patients-and-families?source=search_result&search=fap&selectedTitle=2~116)
12. Cancer Care Ontario. Ontario Cervical Screening Guidelines Summary. Toronto: Cancer Care Ontario. 2016. Available from: https://www.cancercare.on.ca/common/pages/UserFile.aspx?fileId=13104

# CHAPTER 20:

# Ophthalmology

**Editors:**
Eli Kisilevsky, BSc (Hon.)
Fady Sedarous, BHSc

**Resident Reviewer:**
Manreet Alangh, MD, FRCSC

**Faculty Reviewers:**
Kathy Cao, MD, FRCSC
Daniel Weisbrod, MD, FRCSC

## TABLE OF CONTENTS

## GLOSSARY

**Common Abbreviations:**
- OD (oculus dexter) = right eye
- OS (oculus sinister) = left eye
- OU (oculus uterque) = both eyes

**Common Prefixes and Suffixes:**
- presby- = old
- core- = pupil
- blepharo- = eyelid
- kerato- = cornea
- dacryo- = tear
- -phakos/-phakic = lens
- -opsia = vision

## 1. ESSENTIAL ANATOMY

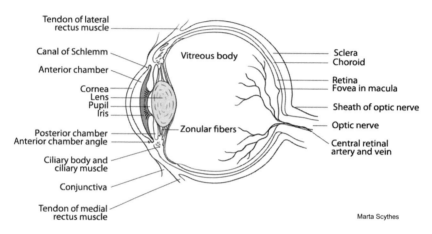

**Figure 1.** Anatomy of the Eye

Marta Scythes

## 2. DEFINITION OF REFRACTIVE ERROR
- Emmetropia: no refractive error
- Myopia: nearsightedness
  - ◆ focal point anterior to retina (nearsighted); correct with a minus lens
- Hyperopia: farsightedness
  - ◆ focal point posterior to retina; correct with a plus lens
- Presbyopia: decreased accommodation with aging
  - ◆ Correct with a positive lens for near vision
- Astigmatism: nonspherical cornea or lens; light rays not refracted uniformly
  - ◆ Correct with a cylindrical lens

## 3. APPROACH TO THE OPHTHALMOLOGICAL HISTORY AND PHYSICAL EXAM

### Overview of the History
In addition to general history taking, aspects of the ophthalmological history include:
- Ocular symptoms (see Table 1 and Table 4)
- Past ocular history (e.g. corrective lens use, prior trauma, surgery, infections, eye diseases)
- Past medical history (for ocular effects of systemic diseases)
- Family history of eye disease
- Ocular and systemic medications

## Overview of the Physical Exam
- Visual acuity (distance/near with correction)
- Visual fields (by confrontation)
- Extraocular muscle evaluation (motility, alignment)
- Pupillary examination (with hand-held light)
- External exam (orbit and 3 L's, see below)
- Fundoscopy (direct covered here, indirect more advanced)
- Slit lamp (front to back: sclera/conjunctiva to back of lens)
- Intraocular pressure (applanation or indentation)

# 4. FOCUSED HISTORY AND COMMON CHIEF COMPLAINTS

## Pain
Associated with:
- Blinking (e.g. corneal abrasions, foreign bodies, keratitis)
- Eye movement (e.g. optic neuritis)
- Headache and nausea (e.g. acute angle-closure glaucoma)
- Brow or temporal pain (e.g. temporal arteritis)
- Photophobia (e.g. iritis, corneal irritation)
- Irritation or "gritty sensation" (e.g. blepharitis, conjunctivitis, corneal abrasion)

**Table 1.** Common Differential Diagnoses for Pain and Possible Interpretation

|  | Acute Conjunctivitis | Acute Iritis | Acute Angle-Closure Glaucoma | Corneal Abrasion |
|---|---|---|---|---|
| **History** | Sudden onset | Fairly sudden onset, often recurrent | Rapid onset, possible previous attack | Trauma, pain |
| **Vision** | Normal, discharge may mildly obscure | Impaired if untreated | Impaired and permanently lost if untreated | Can be affected if central |
| **Associated Symptoms** | Gritty feeling | Photophobia, tenderness | Severe pain | Sharp pain |
| **Bilateral** | Frequent | Occasional | Rarely | Not usually |
| **Cornea** | Clear | Variable | Cloudy/ edematous | Irregular light reflex |
| **Pupil** | Normal, reactive | Sluggishly reactive, may be irregular shape, usually miotic | Mid-dilated, nonreactive, oval | Normal, reactive |
| **Discharge** | Watery and mucopurulent | None | None | Watery or mucopurulent |

## Red Eye[1]
Causes for a red eye can be divided into traumatic and nontraumatic:

**Table 2.** Traumatic vs. Nontraumatic Causes of Red Eye

|  | Causes |
|---|---|
| **Traumatic Red Eye** | Corneal abrasion*, corneal laceration, foreign body*, hyphema*, UV keratitis, chemical injury, globe rupture |
| **Non-traumatic Red Eye** | Blepharitis, conjunctivitis*, subconjunctival hemorrhage*, iritis*, orbital or periorbital cellulitis*, herpes simplex keratitis*, acute angle-closure glaucoma, episcleritis, scleritis |

*Common

OPHTHALMOLOGY

Further questions to ask:
- Associated eye pain or discharge?
- Contact with anyone with a red eye?

## Diplopia (Double Vision)[2]
- Due to misalignment of the eyes (compensatory head postures may be used)
- Can be with both eyes open (binocular) or noted only in one eye or with one eye open (monocular)
- Occurs in one or multiple fields of gaze when cranial nerves are affected

**Table 3.** Causes of Diplopia

| Classification | Example |
| --- | --- |
| **Ocular Motor Palsies** | Cranial nerves III, IV, VI |
| • **Inflammatory** | Multiple Sclerosis |
| • **Endocrine** | Diabetes Mellitus (pupil-sparing) |
| • **Intracranial Pathology** | Brainstem lesions, Circle of Willis aneurysms, neoplasm |
| **Autoimmune Disease** | Myasthenia gravis |
| **Thyroid Abnormalities** | Graves' disease |
| **Trauma** | Blowout fracture |

- Common causes of binocular diplopia are CN palsies, strabismus, and dysthyroid orbitopathy; common cause of monocular diplopia is a cataract

## Vision Loss

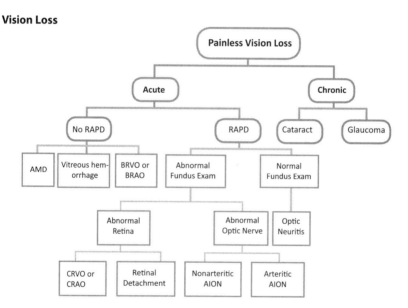

**Figure 2.** Common Causes of Painless Vision Loss
AION = anterior ischemic optic neuropathy, AMD = age-related macular degeneration, BRVO/BRAO = branch retinal vein/artery occlusion, CRVO/CRAO = central retinal vein/artery occlusion, RAPD = relative afferent pupillary defect

OPHTHALMOLOGY

**Table 4.** Other Common Visual Eye Symptoms and Disease States[3]

| Distinguishing Features | Differential Diagnosis |
| --- | --- |
| Colored Halos Around Light | Acute angle-closure glaucoma, opacities in lens or cornea |
| Color Vision Changes | Cataracts (rarely noticed by patient), drugs (e.g. digitalis increases yellow vision, Viagra® can cause a blue hue) |
| Difficulty Seeing in Dim Light | Myopia, vitamin A deficiency, retinal degeneration, cataract, diabetic retinopathy |
| Distortion of Vision | Wet age-related macular degeneration, macular pucker, central serous retinopathy, diabetic macular edema, macular hole |
| Flashes (photopsias) and Floaters | Migraine, retinal tear/detachment, posterior vitreous detachment, vitritis, vitreous hemorrhage, choroiditis |
| Glare, Photophobia | Iritis, cataracts |
| Loss of Visual Field or Presence of Shadow or Curtain | Retinal detachment or hemorrhage, branch retinal vein or arterial occlusion, NAION or AION, chronic glaucoma, stroke |
| Discharge | Watery: allergy/viral infection<br>Mucoid (yellow): allergy/viral infection<br>Purulent (creamy white/yellow): bacterial infection |
| Dryness | Decreased secretion due to aging, corneal abrasion, damage to lacrimal apparatus, dry-eye syndrome, Graves' disease, Bell's palsy, Sjögren's syndrome, anticholinergic drugs |
| Eyelid Swelling | Chalazion, hordeolum (stye), conjunctivitis, cellulitis, systemic edema, dacryocystitis |
| Protrusion of Eyes | Graves' proptosis, aging changes in the lid, retrobulbar tumor |
| Itching | Dry eyes, eye fatigue, allergies |
| Sandiness, Grittiness | Conjunctivitis, blepharitis |
| Tearing | Dry eyes (reflex tears), blocked nasolacrimal ducts, cholinergic drugs, ocular inflammation, entropion/ectropion, corneal abrasion/keratitis |

(N)AION = (non) anterior ischemic optic neuropathy

## Past Ocular History
- Use of eyeglasses and/or contact lenses: duration, frequency, cleaning practice
- Previous eye surgery, laser treatment, infections, trauma, foreign body presence (e.g. metal workers)
- Presence of chronic eye disease such as amblyopia, glaucoma, cataracts, macular degeneration, diabetic retinopathy

## Past Medical History
- Systemic diseases (may have ocular sequelae): DM, HTN, thyroid, autoimmune, systemic infections such as HIV, MS, connective tissue disorders
- Lung disease and kidney stones are possible contraindications for the prescription of topical β-blockers and carbonic anhydrase inhibitors, respectively
- Allergies: rhinoconjunctivitis (hay fever), preservatives in eye drops

## Family History
- Corneal disease, glaucoma, cataracts, retinal disease, strabismus, amblyopia
- Family history of systemic diseases that can affect eyes (see **Past Medical History**, above)

## Medications
- Ocular medications, current and prior use (e.g. anti-infectives, anti-inflammatories,

glaucoma medications)
- Many systemic medications have ocular side effects (e.g. corticosteroids can cause glaucoma, cataracts, and central serous retinopathy)

# 5. FOCUSED PHYSICAL EXAM[4]

## 5.1 Visual Acuity (VA)
- Tests the integrity of the entire visual system but only for central vision
- Test distance and near vision for best corrected visual acuity (BCVA, i.e. with glasses/contacts); one eye at a time (right eye first is standard practice) with the other eye occluded
- A pinhole occluder improves vision in an eye with uncorrected refractive error but NOT neural lesion or media opacity
- Legal blindness = 20/200 best corrected visual acuity (BCVA) in better eye or <20° of binocular visual field
- Canadian Ophthalmological Society recommends 20/50 BCVA OU, and a continuous visual field of 120° horizontally plus 15° both above and below fixation for driving in Canada

### Distance Visual Acuity Testing
- Snellen chart: test at 20 ft (6 m)
  - Recorded as a ratio: the numerator is the testing distance for the patient; the denominator is the distance at which a normal eye can read the line of letters.
  - e.g. 20/100 = the patient can read at 20 feet what a "normal" eye can read at 100 feet
- Ask patient to read smallest line of letters and record corresponding size (e.g. 20/30) if patient is able to read more than half the letters. Subtract for each incorrect letter in line (e.g. 20/30-2). If patient is able to read less than half the line record next largest line plus the number of letters correctly read in the smaller line (e.g. 20/40+1).
- Note whether patient is wearing corrective lenses (CC= cum correctione) or without (SC= sine correctione)
- If unable to read largest letters, then do the following from the longest distance the patient can see:
  1. **Count Fingers** (CF): e.g. CF @ 1 ft
  2. **Hand Motion** (HM): e.g. HM @ 2 ft
  3. **Light Perception** (LP) with a penlight: e.g. LP or NLP

### Near Visual Acuity Testing
- Test if near vision complaint or if distance testing is unavailable
- Use pocket vision chart with or without correction (e.g. Rosenbaum Pocket Vision Screener **found on the inside back cover**)
- Test at 14 in (30 cm) and record as Jaeger values (e.g. J2 at 14 in), which can be converted to distance equivalent (e.g. 20/30)

### Testing of Patients Who Cannot Read
- Use tumbling "E" chart or Landolt "C" chart with the patient describing/motioning the direction of the "E" or "C"
- Picture chart and the Sheridan-Gardiner matching test are often used for children between 2-4 yr and adults with expressive aphasia

## 5.2 Color Vision
- Ishihara pseudoisochromatic plates - present to patient with one eye occluded and ask them to identify the number as quickly as possible
  - Record how many were identified correctly and if there were delays in identification
- Assess macula/optic nerve function; often in pediatrics to screen for color blindness

## 5.3 Confrontation Visual Field Testing
- Approximates large field defects in the four quadrants of each eye
- Testing the patient's right eye:
  - ◆ Sit ~3 feet directly in front of the patient and close your right eye
  - ◆ Tell patient to cover left eye and focus right eye on your open left eye
  - ◆ Hold up 1 or 2 fingers in each quadrant (one quadrant at a time) and ask the patient to count fingers while looking at your open eye
- Repeat for the patient's left eye by covering the patient's right eye
- Note any areas of field loss and record as below:

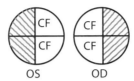

- Normal monocular visual field: 100° temporally, 60° nasally, 60° superiorly, and 75° inferiorly
- Amsler grid: tests central or paracentral scotomas
- Formal perimetry: Goldmann, Humphrey

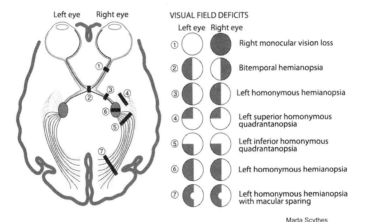

Marta Scythes

**Figure 3.** Brain Lesions and the Resulting Visual Field Defects

## 5.4 Extraocular Muscle Evaluation

### Motility
- Smooth pursuit: instruct patient to follow an object (e.g. tip of pen) in six cardinal positions of gaze; look for nystagmus (horizontal, vertical, or rotatory) and ask patient to report diplopia (double vision) in any position of gaze
- Saccadic movement: instruct patient to shift gaze rapidly from your index finger (positioned in the periphery) to your nose

### Alignment
- Strabismus: any type of ocular misalignment. Use the following tests:
  - ◆ **Hirschberg Corneal Reflex Test**: ask patient to fixate on a distant object. Shine penlight into both eyes from ~14 in (30 cm) away. Aligned eyes show symmetric light reflection near the center of both corneas. Misaligned eyes show displacement of corneal reflection in one eye
  - ◆ **Cover-Uncover Test**: ask patient to fixate on a distant object. Cover the patient's right eye and then uncover it. Repeat for the left eye. Positional shift during testing in the non-covered eye indicates presence of a tropia (a manifest or apparent deviation). A shift of the covered eye upon uncovering indicates the presence of a

OPHTHALMOLOGY

phoria (a latent deviation not apparent when both eyes are fixating).
- **Alternate Cover Test:** ask patient to fixate on a distant object. Cover the patient's right eye with a hand or an occluder, and observe for positional shift in the left eye. Rapidly change the cover to the patient's left eye, and observe for shift in the right eye. Positional shift in the non-covered eye reveals total deviation (phoria plus tropia)

**Table 5.** Possible Outcomes of Eye Alignment Tests

| | Eye Movement* | | | |
| --- | --- | --- | --- | --- |
| | Outward | Inward | Up | Down |
| **Tropia** | Esotropic | Exotropic | Hypotropic | Hypertropic |
| **Phoria** | Esophoric | Exophoric | Hypophoric | Hyperphoric |

*Tropia (constant misalignment) vs. phoria (latent deviation); eso/exo/hypo/hyper describe movement of eye during the application of the cover in each test

## Common Causes of Motility/Alignment Defects
- Congenital and late-onset strabismus, cranial nerve palsies, Graves' disease, myasthenia gravis, stroke, brain tumor, and orbital trauma

## 5.5 Pupil Examination
- Ask patient to fixate on distant target in dimly-lit room
- Shine a penlight obliquely to both pupils; assess pupil size, shape, and symmetry (measure using the pupil gauge found on the near vision card)

### Pupillary Light Reflex
- Shine penlight directly into the right eye and observe symmetric pupillary constriction in the right eye (direct response) and the left eye (consensual response)
- 3+ to 4+ = pupil constricts rapidly and completely; 1+ to 2+ = slowly and incompletely; 0 = does not constrict

**Table 6.** Differential Diagnosis of Constricted and Dilated Pupils

| Constricted Pupil | Dilated Pupil |
| --- | --- |
| Horner's syndrome | CN III palsy |
| Iritis | Acute glaucoma |
| Drug-induced* | Drug-induced†; Adie's pupil (mostly considered normal variant); post-trauma |

*Parasympathetic activation and/or sympathetic block; †Sympathetic activation and/or parasympathetic block

### Swinging Light Test
- Swing light from one pupil to the other to assess relative afferent pupillary defect (RAPD)/ Marcus Gunn pupil
- Pupil dilation in either eye as the light is shone on it indicates a RAPD, a sign of an optic nerve or retinal lesion
- Common causes of RAPD: optic neuritis, ischemic optic neuropathy, central retinal artery or vein occlusion, retinal detachment

### Accommodation Reflex
- Ask patient to look into the distance and then at an object (e.g. your finger) positioned 10 cm from the patient's nose
- Observe normal pupil constriction and eye convergence

**Clinical Pearl: Recording a Normal Pupil Exam**
Record normal pupil examination as "PERRLA": Pupils Equal, Round, Reactive to Light and Accommodation.

The Essentials of Clinical Examination Handbook, 8th ed.

## 5.6 External Ocular Examination
- Inspect the orbits looking for exophthalmos (protruding eye) and enophthalmos (sunken eye)
- Inspect the **4 L**'s (see **Figure 4**):
  - ◆ **Lymph Nodes**: preauricular, submandibular nodes
  - ◆ **Lids**:
    - Ptosis, swelling (allergy, inflammation: chalazion, hordeolum, blepharitis), crusting (blepharitis), xanthelasma (lipid deposits), smooth opening and closure, entropion/ectropion (inversion/eversion)
    - Chalazion: chronic inflammation of meibomian gland; localized painless swelling
    - Hordeolum/stye: acute inflammation of meibomian gland
    - Blepharitis: chronic inflammation of lid
  - ◆ **Lashes:**
    - Direction and condition
    - Trichiasis: inward turned lashes
  - ◆ **Lacrimal Apparatus:**
    - Tearing, obstruction, discharge, swelling
    - Dacryocystitis: infection of lacrimal sac
    - Keratoconjunctivitis sicca: dry eye syndrome
    - Epiphora: excessive tearing

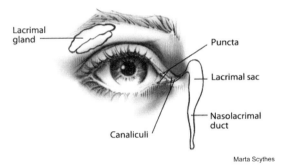

Marta Scythes

**Figure 4.** Lacrimal Apparatus

## 5.7 Upper Lid Eversion
- To look for foreign bodies or other conjunctival lesions
- May require topical anesthetic
- As patient looks down, grasp eyelashes and upper lid place cotton tip applicator gently on the skin at the lid fold (8 mm above lid margin), and press down as the lid margin is pulled up by the lashes

## 5.8 Direct Ophthalmoscopy/Fundoscopy
- Filters: red-free (visualize blood vessels and hemorrhages); polarizing (reduce corneal reflection); cobalt blue (to visualize fluorescein stain)
- Red numbers = minus lenses for myopic eye; green numbers = plus lenses for hyperopic eye

### Red Reflex
- Shine ophthalmoscope light into both pupils from ~30 cm away and look through the viewer
- Observe for evenness of color, presence of shadows/opacities
- An eye with clear ocular media (cornea, anterior chamber, lens, and vitreous) gives off bilaterally even red reflexes
- Common causes of abnormal red reflex (absent or dull): corneal scar, hyphema (blood in aqueous humor), cataract, vitreous hemorrhage, vitritis (infectious/noninfectious), large refractive error, ocular misalignment

## Fundoscopy technique
- Hold the ophthalmoscope in your R hand and use your R eye to examine the patient's R eye
- Use large aperture for dilated pupil, small aperture for undilated pupil. Use low light intensity!
- Set the focusing wheel at 0 and begin to look at the R eye at 1 foot away to detect the red reflex
- Slowly follow the red reflex moving closer to the patient until as close as possible without touching. Turn the focusing wheel until patient's retina comes into focus.
- Note: Visualizing the retina and optic disc may be obscured by corneal reflections and opacities in the medium. Focus on the most posterior image in the fundoscope to visualize the retina.
- Follow a retinal vessel from a bifurcation into the optic disc (nasally). Examine the following landmarks in order:
  - Optic disc: color, margin, cup (size and shape) symmetry, hemorrhages, elevation, cup-to-disc ratio (normal <0.5)
  - Retinal vessels: arteries are thinner and have a brighter reflex than veins. Follow arteries from the disc and veins back to the disc in each quadrant, noting arteriovenous (A/V) crossing patterns
  - Retinal background: color (normal red-orange), pigmentation, lesions (diffuse flecks, flame-shaped, cotton wool spots)
  - Macula: ask patient to look directly into the light; usually appears darker than surrounding retina and produces the foveolar reflex
- Repeat for the L eye (use L hand and L eye to examine patient's L eye)

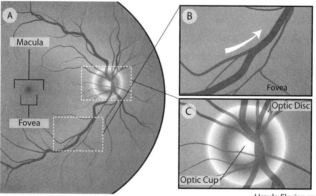

Ursula Florjanczyk

**Figure 5.** A represents the zoomed out view of the retina. B represents a typical fundoscopy examination view. Once a blood vessel is found in the view, follow the vessel in the opposite direction of the bifurcations to locate the optic disc (C).

**Table 7.** Findings on Ophthalmoscopy[5]

| Retinal Disease | Findings on Ophthalmoscopy |
| --- | --- |
| **Diabetic Retinopathy** | |
| Nonproliferative | Retinal hemorrhages, microaneurysms, cotton wool spots, exudates |
| Proliferative | Neovascularization, vitreous hemorrhage |
| **Central Retinal Artery Occlusion (CRAO)** | Whitened retina, cherry red spot in macula ± plaque |
| **Central Retinal Vein Occlusion (CRVO)** | Dilated, tortuous veins, flame-shaped hemorrhages, cotton wool spots, optic disc hyperemia/edema |
| **Hypertensive Retinopathy** | Arteriolar narrowing, and straightening with areas of silver-wire appearance, changes in arteriovenous crossings, cotton wool spots, flame-shaped hemorrhages, disc edema |

OPHTHALMOLOGY

| Retinal Disease | Findings on Ophthalmoscopy |
|---|---|
| Papilledema | Blurred elevated disc margins, ± flame-shaped hemorrhages |
| Glaucomatous Optic Neuropathy | Increased cup-to-disc ratio, asymmetric cup size between eyes, cup approaching disc margin, notching, optic nerve pallor, vessel displacement in disc |
| Retinal Detachment | Elevated retinal folds |
| Age-Related Macular Degeneration | Drusen (yellow deposits), retinal pigment epithelium atrophy (depigmentation in macula), subretinal fluid, subretinal hemorrhage or lipid |

### 5.9 Slit Lamp Examination[6]
- Provides stereoscopic and magnified views of all structures of the anterior segment of each eye
- Using a cobalt blue filter, corneal abrasions can be visualized upon staining with fluorescein dye
- Vertical fluorescein staining on the cornea may indicate a foreign body under the upper eyelid
- Stereoscopic view of the fundus and vitreous can be obtained with special lenses (78 or 90 diopter)

### Pupillary Dilation (Mydriasis)
- Mydriatics provide significantly better viewing of the lens, vitreous, and retina
- Contraindications: narrow angles, acute angle-closure glaucoma
- Usually with tropicamide 1% and phenylephrine hydrochloride 2.5%
- Wait 15-20 min after instilling mydriatic to allow dilation to occur
- To instill eye drop:
  - Seat patient, tilt head back, have patient look up, pull down on lower eyelid
  - Instill drop into sac made by lower eyelid and globe
  - Instruct patient to close eyes for a few seconds, provide a clean tissue

**Clinical Pearl: Eye Drops**
Mydriatic eye drops have red tops
Miotic eye drops have green tops

### Anterior Segment
- Examine the following structures of the anterior segment:
  - Lids and lashes (with lids everted if necessary)
  - Conjunctiva
    - Blood vessel dilatation, pigment, pallor, hemorrhage, redness (note pattern), swelling, nodules
    - Pinguecula: areas of benign elastotic degeneration of the conjunctiva near the nasal or temporal limbus
    - Pterygium: growth of fibrovascular tissue of the conjunctiva onto cornea
  - Sclera
    - Nodules, redness, discoloration (jaundice)
    - Episcleritis: self-limiting inflammation of the episclera, asymptomatic or with mild pain
    - Scleritis: bilateral, severely painful red eye with photophobia and decreased vision, vision threatening
  - Cornea
    - Abrasion, foreign body, clarity/opacity, scarring, ulceration
    - Keratitis: inflammation of cornea with pain, redness, and tearing with blinking
    - Corneal edema: cornea with irregular reflection and haze
    - Arcus senilis: white ring of lipid deposits in peripheral cornea related to atherosclerosis

OPHTHALMOLOGY

- Kayser-Fleischer ring: copper deposits in Wilson's disease
- AFTER examining corneal clarity, use fluorescein dye and cobalt blue filter to visualize corneal abrasions, ulcers, and foreign bodies; Rose Bengal dye for devitalized corneal epithelium

> **Clinical Pearl: Ulcers vs. Abrasions**
> To differentiate corneal ulcers from abrasions, view the cornea before staining with fluorescein. Ulcers have an opaque base, whereas abrasions have a clear base.

- ♦ Anterior chamber
  - Examine for blood (hyphema), pus (hypopyon), cells (graded 1+ to 4+)
  - Depth measurement (see Figure 7):
    - Slit lamp: direct narrow beam onto peripheral cornea at an angle of 60°; chamber is shallow if distance between cornea and iris reflexes is ≤1/4 of corneal reflex thickness
    - Penlight: shine light at an oblique angle from the temporal side of the head; chamber is shallow if ≥2/3 of nasal iris is covered by the shadow
- ♦ Iris
  - Cysts, nodules, color differences between eyes (congenital Horner's), neovascularization, synechiae (adhesions to cornea or lens)
- ♦ Lens
  - Opacities (cataracts), dislocation, intraocular lens implant

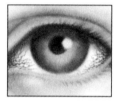
Conjunctival hyperemia

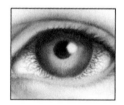
Ciliary flush

Marta Scythes 2010

**Figure 6.** Conjunctival Hyperemia vs. Ciliary Flush

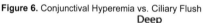

Deep                    Shallow

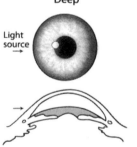
Light source →

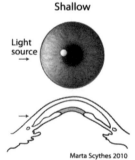
Light source →

Marta Scythes 2010

**Figure 7.** Anterior Chamber Depth Assessment

## Intraocular Pressure (IOP) Measurement
- Normal = 10-21 mmHg, mean = 16 mmHg
- Elevated IOP a risk factor for glaucoma
- Measured by:
  - Applanation: Goldmann applanation tonometry (GAT) using slit lamp, gold standard
  - Indentation: Tono-pen (widely used handheld instrument) or Schiotz; topical anesthetic with patient supine.
  - Noncontact applanation: air-puff tonometer

# 6. COMMON CLINICAL SCENARIOS

**Table 8.** Summary of Common Clinical Scenarios

| Etiology/Definition | Key Signs/ Symptoms | Risk Factors | Management |
|---|---|---|---|
| **Retinal Detachment** | | | |
| Detachment of neurosensory retina from the RPE<br><br>3 subtypes: rhegmatogenous, tractional and exudative (or serous) | Photopsia (light flashes in vision), floaters, and/or acute vision loss<br><br>Visual field loss ("black curtain") over hours to weeks | Aging, cataract surgery, myopia, family history, history of RD in the other eye, trauma, congenital, and diabetic retinopathy | Prevention is best achieved by treating retinal breaks by laser before they progress to retinal detachment Surgical correction usually required for repair (Pneumatic retinopexy, scleral buckling, vitrectomy) |
| **Primary Open-Angle Glaucoma (POAG)** | | | |
| Progressive damage to optic nerve without occlusion of outflow tract | Progressive peripheral visual field loss, elevated IOP >21, optic nerve cupping, visual field loss | IOP >22 mmHg, enlarged optic nerve cup (>0.5 cup-to-disc ratio), age >40 yr, black race, family history, myopia, vascular diseases | Directed at lowering IOP: medications, laser, trabeculoplasty/ trabeculectomy |
| **Acute Angle-Closure Glaucoma** | | | |
| Iris apposition or adhesion to the trabecular meshwork, leading to an increase in IOP and optic nerve damage | Corneal edema, conjunctival injection, mid-dilated, nonreactive, vertically oval pupil, IOP elevated, cells and flare in anterior chamber Headache and nausea | Family history, age >40 yr, female, family history of angle-closure symptoms, hyperopia, pseudoexfoliation race (Inuit > Asian > Caucasian = African) | Maximal medical therapy directed at lowering IOP: laser iridotomy |
| **Cataracts** | | | |
| Clouding and opacification of the crystalline lens of the eye | Blurred vision, decreased acuity and glare around lights at night; cloudiness and opacification of lens, and altered red reflex on physical exam | Age >40, family history, steroid use, diabetes, intraocular surgery, trauma, UV exposure, smoking | Surgery to remove the lens and replace with intraocular lens implant |

OPHTHALMOLOGY

## Dry Age-Related Macular Degeneration (Dry AMD)[7]

| | | | |
|---|---|---|---|
| Acquired retinal degeneration that causes significant central visual impairment | Blurred vision or distortion (metamorphopsia) often asymmetric | Female, family history, smoking, age, sunlight exposure, obesity, elevated cholesterol level, HTN | Vitamin C, E, lutein/zeaxanthin and zinc supplementation in patients with moderate to severe dry AMD decreases risk of progression to wet form |

## Neovascular (Wet) Age-Related Macular Degeneration (Wet AMD)

| | | | |
|---|---|---|---|
| AMD with choroidal neovascularization | Blurred vision or distortion (metamorphopsia) often asymmetric | Female, family history, smoking, age, sunlight exposure, obesity, elevated cholesterol level, HTN | Intravitreal injections of anti-VEGF; consider referral to a low vision specialist and low vision aids for those with legal blindness or low vision |

## Non-Proliferative Diabetic Retinopathy

| | | | |
|---|---|---|---|
| Progressive dysfunction of the retinal vasculature caused by chronic hyperglycemia | Microaneurysms, retinal hemorrhages, retinal lipid exudates, cotton wool spots, capillary nonperfusion, macular edema | Poorly controlled diabetes, duration of diabetes | Appropriate glucose control and regular ophthalmic follow-up, intravitreal injections of anti-VEGF or focal photocoagulation for macular edema |

## Proliferative Diabetic Retinopathy

| | | | |
|---|---|---|---|
| Diabetic Retinopathy with retinal neovascularization | Same signs as non-proliferative plus neovascularization | Poorly controlled diabetes, duration of diabetes | Appropriate glucose control. Vitrectomy and pan-retinal photocoagulation (PRP), intravitreal injections of anti-VEGF |

OPHTHALMOLOGY

# 7. SAMPLE OPHTHALMOLOGY NOTE[8]

**ID**: Mrs. A is a retired 50-yr-old African American female.

**CC**: Patient complains of sudden onset of right eye pain, severe headache, blurred vision, N/V.

**HPI**: These symptoms began 2 h ago without any inciting event. The patient was watching television when the symptoms began. The patient also reports seeing rainbow colored halos around lights. There is no history of trauma, flashing lights, curtains, metamorphopsia or diplopia.

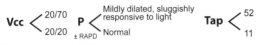

$$\text{Vcc} < \begin{matrix} 20/70 \\ 20/20 \end{matrix}_{\pm \text{RAPD}} \quad \text{P} < \begin{matrix} \text{Mildly dilated, sluggishly responsive to light} \\ \text{Normal} \end{matrix} \quad \text{Tap} < \begin{matrix} 52 \\ 11 \end{matrix}$$

Extraocular muscles intact

**SLE**:
*L/L*: Normal OU
*C/S*: Injected conjunctiva OD, normal OS
*K*: OD demonstrates corneal edema, normal OS
*A/C*: Shallow anterior chamber OD, normal depth OS
*Iris*: Appears pushed forward OD, normal OS
*Lens*: Normal OU
*Anterior Vit*: Normal OU
*Gonioscopy*: Closed-angle OD, demonstrating iris bombé; normal angle, but no apparent obstruction of trabecular meshwork OS

**DFE**:

Hazy view through edematous cornea
Macula: normal with no signs of retinal breaks or detachments
Vessels: no AV nicking
Periphery: normal
Disc: cup-to-disc ratio 0.3 OU

**Assessment Plan**:
- Acute angle-closure glaucoma
- Acetazolamide 500mg IV x 1 to reduce IOP
- Prednisolone acetate 1% to suppress inflammation
- Laser peripheral iridotomy for definitive treatment
- Follow-up with gonioscopy to assess the extent of peripheral anterior synechiae (PAS), and consider fundus exam as clinically indicated

**PMH**:
Osteoarthritis (knees)

**POH**:
Mild myopia
No surgeries, laser, injection or other treatment

**FH**:
Mother: Chronic primary angle-closure glaucoma
No history of macular degeneration, retinal detachment, blindness or autoimmune disorders

**Social History**:
20 pack yr smoking history
Drinks alcohol on occasion
No illicit drug use

**Meds**:
Daily Multivitamin
Tylenol 3 PM (uses it about 1 day/month when knee pain worsens

**Allergies**:
NKDA

**(From previous page)**
**ID** (identifying data), **CC** (chief complaint), **HPI** (history of present illness), **Vcc** (vision with glasses), **POH** (past ocular history), **FH** (family history), **SLE** (slit lamp exam), **Ext** (external), L/L (lids and lacrimation), **C/S** (conjunctiva and sclera), **K** (cornea), **A/C** (anterior chamber), **Vit** (vitreous chamber), **NKDA** (no known drug allergies), **DFE** (dilated fundus exam), **OD** (right eye), **OS** (left eye), **OU** (both eyes)

# REFERENCES

1. Leibowitz H. The Red Eye. N Engl J Med. 2000;343(5):345-351.
2. Gerstenblith A, Rabinowitz M. The Wills Eye Manual: office and emergency room diagnosis and treatment of eye disease. 6th ed. Philadelphia: Wolters Kluwer/Lippincott Williams & Wilkins; 2012:248-254.
3. Gerstenblith A, Rabinowitz M. The Wills Eye Manual: office and emergency room diagnosis and treatment of eye disease. 6th ed. Philadelphia: Wolters Kluwer/Lippincott Williams & Wilkins; 2012:1-6.
4. Bickley L, Szilagyi P, Bates B. Bates' Guide To Physical Examination And History-Taking. 11th ed. Philadelphia: Wolters Kluwer Health/Lippincott Williams & Wilkins; 2013:207-232.
5. Gerstenblith A, Rabinowitz M. The Wills Eye Manual: office and emergency room diagnosis and treatment of eye disease. 6th ed. Philadelphia: Wolters Kluwer/Lippincott Williams & Wilkins; 2012:293-348.
6. Nema H, Nema N. Diagnostic Procedures In Ophthalmology. 1st ed. Pangbourne, England: Alpha Science International; 2003:13-23.
7. Age-Related Eye Disease Study Research Group. A randomized, placebo-controlled, clinical trial of high-dose supplementation with vitamins C and E, beta carotene, and zinc for age-related macular degeneration and vision loss: AREDS report no. 8. Arch Ophthalmol. 2001;119(10):1417-1436.
8. Medical College of Wisconsin. Department of Ophthalmology Case Studies. Milwaukee: Medical College of Wisconsin. 2013. Available from: http://www.mcw.edu/ophthalmology/ education/ophthcstudies.htm

OPHTHALMOLOGY

CHAPTER 21:

# Pediatrics

**Editors:**
Zahra Sohani, PhD
Brandon Tang, BSc

**Resident Reviewers:**
Zenita Alidina, MD
Amy Rebecca Zipursky, BA, MD

**Faculty Reviewers:**
Hosanna Au, MD, DipMEd, FRCPC
Angela Punnett, MD, FRCPC

## TABLE OF CONTENTS

PEDIATRICS

# 1. APPROACH TO THE PEDIATRIC EXAM
- Overview
  - History often given by third party: identify their relationship with child
  - Observe parent-child interaction for nonverbal cues and family dynamics
  - Allow parent to discuss his/her feelings and acknowledge his/her concerns
  - Ask parents about specific concerns (this can be helpful in eliciting unexpressed fears or worries)

The following subsections outline important considerations for a history in the pediatric population, in addition to the concepts outlined in **The General History & Physical Exam** Chapter

## 1.1 Chief Complaint
- There may be multiple issues or concerns for why a child is seeking medical care. It is important to identify the patient's chief complaint amongst these

## 1.2 History of Presenting Illness
- Use the approach as presented in **The General History & Physical Exam** Chapter
- Risk Factors specific to HPI in the pediatric population:
  - Sick contacts (family members, daycare, school)
  - Recent travel
  - Family history of similar problems
  - Related medical problems (e.g. eczema and asthma)
- Medical care/interventions prior to this encounter

## 1.3 Past Medical History
The following are important considerations when taking a PMHx:
- Neonatal
  - Prenatal (see **Approach to the Neonate**)
  - Labor and Delivery (see **Approach to the Neonate**)
  - Feeding History (see **Approach to the Neonate**)
  - Common problems: jaundice, poor feeding, weight gain, sleeping, difficulty breathing, cyanosis (see **Approach to the Neonate**)
- Growth and Nutrition (including eating behaviours, typical diet, patterns of growth)
- Development (see **Table 30** in **Appendix**)
- Immunizations
  - Which and when?
  - Adverse reactions: local, systemic, or allergic
  - Are immunizations up to date? Refer to your local immunization schedule for details[1]
    - Example: Ministry of Health and Long-Term Care. Publicly Funded Immunization Schedules for Ontario – December 2016. Available from: http://www.health.gov.on.ca/en/pro/programs/immunization/docs/immunization_schedule.pdf
- Allergies
  - Environment, food, and medication: reaction experienced, action taken, time to resolution of symptoms, presence of a viral illness, exercise, heat, cold
  - Family history of atopy (allergic diseases such as eczema, allergies, asthma)
- Medications, including vitamins and supplements
  - Any recent changes to medications
  - Compliance
  - Recent antibiotic use
- "CASH"
  - Chronic illnesses
  - Accidents
  - Surgeries
  - Hospitalizations
- Other healthcare providers/services involved

### 1.4 Family History
- Genogram is helpful
- Ask about consanguinity
- Broader family as pertinent to the HPI: congenital abnormalities, allergies, recurrent illnesses, early deaths, frequent miscarriages

### 1.5 Social History
- Family
  - Extended/blended family, birth parents, custody and access
  - Household: space, pets, occupants, frequency of moves
  - Family dynamics: who cares for child?
  - Support systems, stress/discord/violence
    - Ask: "Do you feel safe at home?"
    - Recreation history: "What does the family do as a group?"
    - Major life events (deaths, accidents, separations, divorce)
- Parents
  - Occupational history (prolonged absences, exposures to toxins or infection)
  - Approach to discipline
  - Financial issues/problems (including any social assistance)
  - Substance abuse
- Neonatal
  - Inquire about the family's adaptation to the newborn, mother's emotional state (postpartum blues/depression), and supports for the parents
- Child
  - Interests and activities
  - School performance
  - Screen time

*ITHELLP Acronym for Social Screening*
- **I**ncome
- **T**ransportation
- **H**ousing
- **E**ducation
- **L**egal Status
- **L**iteracy
- **P**ersonal Safety

### 1.6 Review of Systems
- See age-appropriate sections (**Approach to the Neonate / Infant and Child / Adolescent**)

### 1.7 The Physical Exam
- A full physical exam should be done for every pediatric exam
- Knowledge of adult exam is assumed for pediatric exam. See the following "Approach to..." sections for more details on age-specific physical examinations

## Vital Signs
*Temperature*
- In children up to 2 yr:
  - For definitive temperature, take rectal temperature:
    - Use disposable slipcovers
    - Lubricate the thermometer prior to insertion. Spread the buttocks and insert a rectal thermometer slowly through the anal sphincter to 1-3 cm; read after 1 min

PEDIATRICS

**Clinical Pearl: Temperature[2]**

Normal rectal temperature > oral temperature > axillary temperature

| Method | Normal Temperature |
|--------|-------------------|
| Rectal | 36.6-38°C |
| Tympanic | 35.8-38°C |
| Oral | 35.5-37.5°C |
| Axillary | 34.7-37.3°C |

*Respiratory Rate (RR)*
- Count breaths for at least 30s
- Measure RR while baby/child is calm, prior to doing other physical exam maneuvers
- Place your hand just below the child's xiphoid process or listen to breath sounds through the stethoscope to get an accurate RR
- For each 1°C rise in temperature, the RR increases by ~3 breaths/min

*Pulse*
- Auscultate or palpate for 15-30s (sinus arrhythmia is normal)
- For each 1°C rise in temperature, the pulse increases by ~10 beats/min

*Blood Pressure*
- Measurement is not indicated for those under 3 yr, unless hospitalized or specific indication[3]
- Systolic is indicated in the table below; Diastolic BP = ~2/3 Systolic BP
- In the neonatal period, mean arterial pressure (MAP) should be at least the gestational age

*Oxygen Saturation*
- For pediatric patients in a hospital setting (or as an outpatient if available), the oxygen saturation is a valuable piece of information
- Measured by attaching an oxygen saturation probe to any well-perfused body part (e.g. finger, toe, or earlobe)
- Normal value is >92%, unless parameters are otherwise specified for a specific medical condition

**Table 1.** Average Ranges for Pediatric Vital Signs[4]

| Age | Respiratory Rate | Heart Rate | Systolic Blood Pressure | Weight (kg) |
|-----|------------------|------------|-------------------------|-------------|
| Infant | 30-50 | 120-160 | >60 | 3-4 |
| 6 mo-1 yr | 30-40 | 120-150 | 70-80 | 8-10 |
| 2-4 yr | 20-30 | 110-140 | 70-80 | 12-16 |
| 5-8 yr | 14-20 | 90-120 | 90-100 | 18-26 |
| 8-12 yr | 12-20 | 80-110 | 100-110 | 26-50 |
| >12 yr | 12-16 | 60-100 | 100-120 | >50 |

## 2. APPROACH TO THE NEONATE

### 2.1 Neonatal History
- Follow the outline in the **Approach to the Pediatric Exam**

PEDIATRICS

### Prenatal
- Mother's obstetrical history: previous pregnancies, miscarriages, abortions
- Pregnancy: planned or not, number of weeks, single or multiple pregnancies, complications
- Mother's health during pregnancy: age, hospitalizations, medications, bleeding, illnesses, accidents, vitamins, supplements, herbals, HTN, DM
- Tests: U/S, genetic screening such as First Trimester Screen, Amniocentesis/CVS (when and why), Group B Streptococcus (GBS), OGTT, serologies, STI testing, HIV testing
- Both parents: alcohol, smoking, drug exposure

### Labor and Delivery
- Spontaneous labour or induced? If induced, why?
- Premature or prolonged rupture of membranes?
- Labour duration and problems (maternal fever, non-reassuring fetal heart rate [FHR], meconium)
- Vaginal, forceps, vacuum or cesarean delivery
- Gestational age at birth, birth weight, Apgar scores
- Did the baby require admission to the neonatal intensive care unit (e.g. for ventilation) or antibiotics after birth? Was the baby kept in hospital for any reason?
- Postnatal period: jaundice, cyanosis, hypoglycemia, breathing or feeding problems, seizures

### Feeding
- Breastfeeding or formula?
  - Breastfed: frequency, duration
    - Vitamin D 400 IU/day
  - Formula: type, dilution, any formula changes, feeding frequency, and amount
  - Formula fed infants, if drinking less than 1L/day (neonates will not drink this amount), still need Vitamin D supplementation of 400IU
- Associated problems: difficulty latching on breast, vomiting
- Supplements: including vitamins and natural products
- Regurgitation: amount, frequency, bilious/non-bilious
- Outputs: urine/stool (number of diapers/day)
- Weight gain: neonates will regain birth weight by day 10-14 of life, and then gain 20-30g per day thereafter

### Review of Systems
- Head: any swelling of the head post-delivery, has it decreased?
- Eyes: conjunctivitis, scleral icterus
- Mouth/throat: cleft lip/palate, neck masses
- Cardiovascular: fatigue/sweating during feedings, cyanosis
- Respiratory: noisy breathing, work of breathing
- GI: appetite, weight gain, height, growth, vomiting
  - Bowel movements: timing of first meconium, frequency, consistency, color, blood, mucus, diarrhea or constipation, hernia
- GU: number of wet diapers
- Dermatological: jaundice (distribution, worsening or improving), birthmarks, rash
- Sleep: amount and quality

## 2.2 Neonatal Physical Exam
- Opportunistic exam, with baby undressed
- To optimize the exam, keep the baby quiet by placing the tip of your gloved finger in a crying baby's mouth, or ask parent to do so
- As much as possible, keep the baby warm

### General Survey and Vitals
- Appearance: Appears well? Any signs of respiratory distress (i.e. intercostal or sternal in-drawing, nasal flaring, stridor, etc.), color change, or abnormal vital signs?
  - Vital signs: RR, HR, temperature, BP, O2 saturation, and pre- and post-ductal O2 saturation

PEDIATRICS

♦ Assuming the patient is stable, note alertness, activity, facial features

*Assess Dehydration and Volume Depletion*
- Detailed signs of dehydration/volume status (see **Common Clinical Scenarios**, p.561)
- Weight loss (gold standard), capillary refill time, dry mucous membranes, decreased skin turgor, sunken fontanelles, decreased urine output, low blood pressure, increased heart rate, lethargy, sunken eyes
- Height: supine length
  - ♦ Average length 50cm
- Weight: loss of up to 10% of birth weight in first few days of life is normal (see **Table 2**)
  - ♦ Average weight 3.5 kg
- Classify birth weight on an intrauterine growth curve
- Small for gestational age (SGA) is <10th percentile
  - ♦ Asymmetric SGA: weight <10th percentile with head circumference and length >10th percentile
    - ▪ Implication: brain growth may be relatively spared
  - ♦ Symmetric SGA: weight, head circumference, and length all <10th percentile
    - ▪ Implication: growth overall restricted
- Appropriate for gestational age (AGA) is 10-90th percentile
- Large for gestational age (LGA) is >90th percentile
- See **Common Clinical Scenarios**, p.561 for associated disorders
- Head Circumference: measure the greatest circumference around the occipital, parietal, and frontal prominences above the brows and ears
  - ♦ Average circumference at term is ~35 cm
- To assess growth, plot height, weight, and head circumference on growth chart and determine percentiles. In the neonatal period, goal is 20-25 g/day of weight growth. Birth weight should be regained by 10-14 days of age

**Table 2.** Gestational Age and Birth Weight

| Birth Weight Classification | Weight |
|---|---|
| **Extremely Low Birth weight** | <1000 g |
| **Very Low Birth weight** | <1500 g |
| **Low Birth weight** | <2500 g |
| **Normal Birth Weight** | ≥2500 g |
| Gestational Age Classification | Gestational Age |
| **Preterm** | <37 wk |
| **Term** | 37-42 wk |
| **Postterm** | ≥42 wk |

## H.E.E.N.T.
*Head*
- Observe position, size, shape and symmetry of head
- After vaginal vertex delivery/prolonged labor:
  - ♦ Caput succedaneum: subcutaneous edema in occipito-parietal region that resolves 1-2 days postpartum; does not respect suture lines
- Cephalohematoma: subperiosteal hemorrhage that resolves in weeks to months; respects suture lines
- Subgaleal hemorrhage: bleeding below the periosteum; does not respect suture lines; risk of significant/occult bleeding
- Sutures and fontanelles
  - ♦ Sutures feel like ridges and usually flatten by 6 mo; persistent ridging suggests craniosynostosis
  - ♦ Fontanelles feel like soft concavities: anterior fontanelle is 2-5 cm and closes between 9-18 mo (median 14 mo), posterior fontanelle usually closes by 1-2 mo

## Eye
- Newborns respond best to human faces, so place your face directly in front of theirs
- Observe position of eyes, eyelids (ptosis), conjunctivae (for purulent conjunctivitis, hemorrhage), sclerae (for scleral icterus), irises, pupils
- Observe palpebral fissures: angle from line drawn from inner and outer canthus (e.g. up slanting may indicate Down syndrome, down slanting may indicate Noonan's syndrome, short may indicate fetal alcohol syndrome)
- Fundoscopy: observe red reflex (fundus) - absence due to opacification could be glaucoma, cataract, retinoblastoma

## Ear
- The tympanic membrane is obscured with accumulated vernix caseosa (white cheesy substance that covers baby's skin at time of birth) for the first few days of life
- Position, shape, and features of ears
- If an imaginary line is drawn from outer canthi of eyes, it should cross pinna or auricle. Low-set ears present if pinna is below this line; may indicate chromosomal anomaly (e.g. VACTERL, VATER)

## Nose
- Test for patency of nasal passages by gently occluding each nostril and checking for air passage (neonates or obligate nose breathers)

## Mouth
- Look at lips, gingival, and buccal mucosa for hydration and cyanosis
- Observe inside the mouth for any abnormalities with tongue depressor and light
  - Palpate the upper hard palate with your finger to make sure it is intact
- Notching of the posterior margin of the hard palate or a bifid uvula are clues of a submucosal cleft palate
- Epstein's pearls: tiny white or yellow rounded mucus retention cysts along the posterior midline of the hard palate
  - Disappear within a month of life
- A prominent protruding tongue may signal congenital hypothyroidism or Down syndrome

## Neck
- Webbing or extra neck folds may indicate Turner or Noonan Syndrome
- Midline or lateral congenital neck mass (e.g. thyroglossal duct cyst)
- Feel for enlarged nodes/glands, and the thyroid
- Palpable thyroid in newborns is always abnormal
- Congenital torticollis: "wry neck", bleeding during the stretching process of birth into the sternocleidomastoid, leaving a firm fibrous mass (fibromatosis coli); disappears over months
- Clavicles, to look for evidence of fracture (i.e. tenderness or a lump)

## Respiratory
- Use the bell of an adult stethoscope, or a pediatric stethoscope diaphragm; always compare both sides
- Signs of respiratory distress: tachypnea, tracheal tug, indrawing, retractions, nasal flaring, cyanosis, lethargy
  - Infants normally display more abdominal breathing
- Chest wall deformities (pectus excavatum)
- Respiration phases, depth, and rhythm
  - Rhythm irregularities may signify abnormalities such as apnea
  - Periodic breathing (up to 10s of apnea) can be normal, especially in premature infants

## Cardiovascular
- Cyanosis, pallor, perfusion (cap refill), respiratory distress, sweating with feeds
- Non-cardiac findings may indicate cardiac disease (e.g. poor feeding may be due to tachypnea)
- Heaves, thrills

PEDIATRICS

- Peripheral pulses: note strength/quality of femoral pulses
  - Normal pulse has sharp rise, is firm, and well localized
  - Patent ductus arteriosus is indicated by bounding pulses
  - Coarctation of the aorta is indicated by absence of femoral pulse, or lighter feel relative to the brachial pulse
- Note rate, rhythm, S1 and S2, murmurs (see **Common Clinical Scenarios**, p.561)
  - Soft precordial systolic murmur common in first few days after birth and is physiologic
  - If this murmur persists and is heard over the back, it may represent a patent ductus arteriosus
- If you hear a murmur, auscultate over the back, neck, and axillae to listen for radiation
- Sinus arrhythmia is a normal finding in children, with heart rate increasing on inspiration and decreasing on expiration

## Gastrointestinal
*Inspection*
- Protuberant abdomen expected in neonates; distended abdomen may indicate obstruction (see **Common Clinical Scenarios**, p.561)
- Scaphoid abdomen and respiratory distress may suggest congenital diaphragmatic hernia in a neonate
- Umbilicus
  - Check for umbilical hernia or signs of infection
  - Check for two arteries and one vein
- Abdominal wall
  - Rectus Diastasis (most common): gap between two sides of rectus abdominis muscle
  - Omphalocele: incomplete closure of anterior abdominal wall; herniated, overlying sac; typically associated with other anomalies
  - Gastroschisis: defect in anterior abdominal wall just lateral to umbilicus; herniated intestine with no covering sac; no associated anomalies
- Signs of jaundice, especially in neonates
- Anus: examine for redness, rash, imperforation and prolapse

*Auscultation*
- Bowel sounds normally present every 10-30s, but must listen for several minutes before determining that sounds are absent

*Palpation*
- Liver edge (normally <1-2 cm below costal margin) and kidneys are often palpable in the normal infant

*Genitourinary*
- Male
  - Ensure testes are descended, further work-up required if bilateral undescended testes
  - Check for hernia, hydrocele, hypospadias
- Female
  - Patent vagina, swollen labia, bloody or white vaginal discharge from maternal estrogen withdrawal (normal finding)
- In some newborns the genitalia may appear ambiguous, indicating either a chromosomal or endocrine abnormality
- Ambiguous genitalia should be considered a medical/social emergency

## Musculoskeletal
- With patient supine, test for developmental dysplasia of the hip with Barlow and Ortolani maneuvers; check each hip individually
- Barlow (mnemonic: back): flex knees, flex and slightly adduct hips, apply posterior pressure
  - POSITIVE if able to dislocate unstable hip
- Ortolani (mnemonic: out): flex knees and hips, abduct hips and apply anterior pressure

PEDIATRICS

- POSITIVE if audible and palpable clunk, able to reduce dislocated hip
- Club foot: plantar flexion of foot, heel inversion, medial forefoot deviation (this fixed deformity is pathological)
- Birth injury: clavicle fracture, brachial plexus injury (e.g. Erb's palsy)
  - Asymmetric Moro reflex with either of these injuries

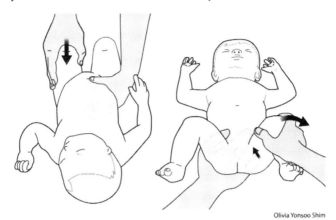

Olivia Yonsoo Shim

**Figure 1**. Barlow's and Ortolani's Tests for Hip Dislocation

## Neurological

Findings are greatly affected by internal factors: alertness, timing from last feeding, sleeping
- Moving all limbs symmetrically?
- Tone: increased, decreased, or normal?
- Positive Babinski is normal until 9 mo
- See **Table 3** below for primitive reflexes
- Neural tube defects
  - Spine/back: sacral dimple/hair tuft (spina bifida occulta), midline skin lesions

**Table 3.** Neonatal Primitive Reflexes

| Reflex | How to Elicit | Reaction | Age Observed |
|---|---|---|---|
| Galant | Stroke back about 1 cm from midline with baby held prone | Trunk curves toward stroked side | Birth to 4-6 mo |
| Placing | Baby upright, touch top of foot to table edge | Child mimics walking onto table | Birth to 4-6 mo |
| Rooting | Stroke cheek | Head turns to same side | Birth to 4 mo |
| Palmar/Plantar Grasp | Examiner places their finger into palm or sole of baby's foot | Fingers and toes grasp together | Birth to 4 mo |
| Moro | Startle baby with loud noise or suddenly lower supine baby | Arms extend, abduct with hands open; then arms come together | Birth to 4 mo |
| Asymmetric Tonic Neck Reflex (ATNR) | Turn head to one side | Arm/leg on same side extend, flex on opposite side (fencing position) | Birth to 6 mo |

## Dermatological
- Jaundice, pallor, mottling, diaper dermatitis, rashes, birthmarks, hemangiomas
- If lesions are present, describe their distribution, configuration, thickness, primary/secondary changes present, and color

# 3. APPROACH TO THE INFANT/CHILD

## 3.1 Infant/Child History
- If the infant/child is presenting for a regular "well-baby" check-up, document history, physical, immunizations, and patient education on the Rourke Baby Record
- Common problems: pharyngitis, earache, cough, asthma, dehydration, vomiting/diarrhea, urinary problems, limping/pain, headache, rashes, etc. (see **Common Clinical Scenarios**, p.561)
- Follow the outline in **Approach to the Pediatric Exam** p.540

## 3.2 Infant/Child Physical Exam
- For infants, do an opportunistic "head-to-toe" exam with child undressed and lying down
- Tips for examining children[5]:
    1. Use parent as a helper to soothe child: with younger children/infants, do most of exam with infant sitting/lying in the caregiver's lap
    2. Begin with observation: much of the exam can be done by observing the child play, move, and respond to outside stimuli
    3. Introduce yourself and your tools: let child see, and safely touch tools you will be using during the exam. You can also use toys as distractions
    4. Be flexible: perform distressing maneuvers toward the end of the exam. Give the child as much choice as possible (e.g. which body part to examine first?)
    5. Make a game out of the exam, for example:
        - **Respiratory**: to get the child to take a deep breath in and out, hold up your finger and tell them to practice blowing out the candle
        - **MSK/Neurological:** to test upper body strength, have the child "show you how strong they are". For the cranial nerve exam, "Simon Says" is a favorite

## General Survey and Vitals
- Assess appearance and degree of dehydration, refer to **Table 6**

## Growth and Development
- **Height:** supine length up to 2 yr, then standing >2 yr
- **Weight:** make sure diaper is off
- **Head Circumference:** measure the greatest circumference around the occipital, parietal, and frontal prominences above the brows and ears
- To assess growth, plot height, weight, and head circumference on growth chart and determine percentiles
    - WHO charts are now the Canadian standard
    - Focus on trend of growth longitudinally rather than individual values
    - Pay attention to crossing of percentile ranges
- **Failure to Thrive (FTT)**:
    - When a child's weight for height falls below the 3rd percentile
    - If weight drops two major percentile curves
- **BMI**: can be used in children aged ≥2 yr; growth chart available
- Calculate mid-parental height (MPH) to determine expected height of child when full-grown
- **Development**: always assess developmental milestones in infants/children, noting results on the Rourke Baby Record or chart
- If infant was born premature (<37 wk GA), use the "corrected age": the age based on the child's due date up to about 2 years old
    - E.g. if an 8 mo old baby was born 2 mo premature, use the 6 mo milestones

## H.E.E.N.T.
*Head*
- See **Approach to the Neonate**
- Asymmetry of the cranial vault (plagiocephaly) may result from consistently placing the child supine; ask about child's sleeping or playing positions
- Bulging, tense fontanelle when infant upright suggests increased intracranial pressure and is seen when baby cries, vomits, or has underlying pathology (CNS infection, neoplasm, hydrocephalus, injury)

**PEDIATRICS**

*Eye*

- Observe position of eyes, eyelids (ptosis), conjunctivae (for purulent conjunctivitis, hemorrhage), irises, pupils
- Observe palpebral fissures (see **Approach to the Neonate**)
- Assess fixation of eyes, refer to ophthalmology if any strabismus found
- **Cover-Uncover Test**: assess fixation by alternately covering one eye and observing for strabismus (present if covered eye moves toward object after being uncovered)
- **Corneal Light Reflex**: assess fixation by shining a bright light (e.g. penlight) in child's eyes. If the position of the reflected light on the child's pupil is different between the left and right eye, it may indicate a less-obvious strabismus (See **Table 4** for a list of differential diagnosis of findings)
- Pseudostrabismus: false appearance of eye misalignment. Commonly found in infants of East Asian and Aboriginal origin, where the medial epicanthal folds are especially apparent and the nasal bridge is widened. Unlike strabismus, the corneal light reflex will be normal in pseudostrabismus

**Table 4.** Differential Diagnosis of Findings on Observation of Eyes

| Finding | Differential Diagnosis |
|---|---|
| **Prominent sclera seen between upper lid and iris** | Hydrocephalus ("setting-sun" phenomenon), Graves' disease (proptosis) |
| **Drooping eyelid** | Paralysis of oculomotor cranial nerve |
| **Painful, red, swollen eyelid** | Stye, periorbital or orbital cellulitis, blepharitis |
| **Nodular, nontender area** | Cyst |
| **Sunken eye around eyelid** | Dehydrated |
| **Subconjunctival hemorrhages** | Normal in newborn; also seen with coughing or straining |
| **Red conjunctivae** | Bacterial or viral infection, allergy, irritation |
| **Pale conjunctivae** | Anemia |
| **Yellow sclerae** | Jaundice |
| **Bluish sclerae** | Osteogenesis imperfecta; can be normal in newborns |
| **Absence of color in iris** | Albinism |
| **Notch of outer edge of iris** | Visual field defect |
| **Constriction of pupils (miosis)** | Iritis, drug-induced (morphine) |
| **Fixed unilateral dilation of a pupil** | Local eye injury or head injury |
| **Dilation of pupils (mydriasis)** | Acute glaucoma, drug-induced, trauma, |
| **White pupils (leukocoria)** | Coloboma (failure of retinal development), intraocular tumor (retinoblastoma), cataract, |

- **Visual Acuity**
1. <3 yr old:
   - Use Tumbling E's or LEA Symbols eye chart
   - LEA Symbols eye chart: child holds chart with several shapes on it, points to matching shape held on a separate chart by the doctor
   - Visual acuity may not be possible if patient cannot identify pictures on eye chart
   - Optic blink reflex: for preverbal infants: blinking in response to bright light, or quick movement of object toward eyes
2. >3 yr old:
   - Use Snellen eye chart; average acuity is not 20/20 until 2-4 yr
- **Visual Fields**
  - Bring toy in from periphery; child's eyes should conjugately deviate toward object when it is seen

- **Fundoscopy**
    - Examine the red retinal (fundus) reflex and optic disc (lighter in color than adults, foveal light reflection may not be visible), looking for retinal hemorrhages, cataracts, corneal opacities (see **Common Clinical Scenarios**, p.561)

*Ear*
- Inspection
    - Position, shape, and features of ears
    - Assess for low-set ears
    - Look for discharge (rupture of tympanic membrane) and blood (foreign body irritation or scratching)
    1. Infant
        - Use smallest otoscope tip available to better visualize tympanic membrane, and steady hand against head
        - Pull auricle gently downward rather than upward for best view, since ear canal will be directed downward from the outside
        - Avoid insertion of otoscope too deeply; there is a risk of rupturing the tympanic membrane
        - Once tympanic membrane is visible, the light reflex may be diffuse and may not become cone-shaped for several months
    2. Child
        - Parents may need to help hold child in place for examination
        - Pull the auricle upward, outward, and backward for best view
- Hearing
    - Grossly test for hearing by whispering a command or question
    - An infant or child of any age can be referred for formal audiometric testing: if children fail screening maneuvers, you are doubtful in any way, parents have concerns, or if there is language delay, have the child tested!

*Nose*
- Nasolabial folds: asymmetry indicates facial nerve impairment or Bell's palsy
- With otoscope, inspect nasal mucous membranes, noting color and condition
- Look for nasal septal deviation and polyp

*Mouth and Pharynx*
- Inspection
    - First ensure the child is well positioned if using a tongue depressor for examination
    - Look at lips, gingival and buccal mucosa for hydration and cyanosis
    - Check hard and soft palate, uvula, and tonsils for exudates or enlargement
    - Assess breath
        - Odor may suggest metabolic conditions such as maple syrup urine disease or DKA
    - Teeth: examine for timing and sequence of eruption, number, character, condition and position; all of these characteristics are very variable between children
        - First teeth erupt at around 6 mo; permanent teeth erupt at 6 yr
        - Significant delay may be a sign of delayed skeletal development
        - Malformed teeth may indicate systemic insult
    - Tongue: common abnormalities include coated tongue from viral infection, and strawberry tongue found in scarlet fever, streptococcal pharyngitis, or Kawasaki disease
    - Tonsils: note size, position, symmetry, and appearance

*Neck*
- Inspection: look for enlarged nodes/glands and masses; note thyroid size
- Palpation
    - Infant: Best palpated while patient is supine since the neck is short
    - Child: Best examined while sitting
    - Neck mobility, either passive or active, depending on child's age
    - Ensure the neck is supple and mobile in all directions
    - Nuchal rigidity: for suspected meningitis, ask child to touch chin to chest and note

PEDIATRICS

pain/restriction
- ♦ Lymph nodes and presence of any additional masses (congenital cysts)
- ♦ The majority of enlarged lymph nodes in children are due to infection, not malignant disease
- ♦ Malignancy is more likely if node is >2 cm, hard, fixed, and accompanied by systemic signs such as weight loss

## Respiratory
- The pediatric respiratory exam should be completed using the same criteria as in the adult exam (see the **Respiratory System** Chapter)
- Infants and young children may have the respiratory exam done while sitting on a parent's lap: if they become agitated by the examiner's presence, they may need to be observed from a distance to better assess their respiratory status at rest

*Inspection*
- AP diameter: increased in cystic fibrosis, chronic asthma or chronic diffuse small airway obstruction
- Chest wall deformities
    - ♦ Pectus excavatum may be an isolated finding or may be associated with a chronic cardiorespiratory problem
    - ♦ Other chest wall deformities may be congenital or due to surgery
    - ♦ Spinal configuration
    - ♦ Kyphoscoliosis can affect shape of thoracic cage and pulmonary function
- Signs of respiratory distress
    - ♦ Retractions (suprasternal, intercostal, subcostal)
    - ♦ Nasal flaring
- Respiration phases, depth, and rhythm
    - ♦ Infants display more abdominal breathing, with a shift to chest excursion as they get older (thoracic breathing at ~6 yr)
- Rhythm irregularities beyond the neonatal period may signify abnormalities such as apnea
- Finger clubbing: may indicate chronic disease such as cystic fibrosis, respiratory, cardiac, and GI disorders
- Cyanosis: central cyanosis (indicates cardiorespiratory disease) vs. peripheral cyanosis
- Note level of consciousness

*Palpation*
- Use one or two fingers (based on size) to assess tracheal position
- Chest expansion and tactile fremitus have little use in young children

*Percussion*
- Diaphragmatic excursion is usually only performed on older children

*Auscultation*
- The bell of an adult stethoscope, or a pediatric stethoscope diaphragm, should be used in young children

## Cardiovascular
- See **Precordial Exam** Chapter

*Inspection*
- Failure to thrive and cyanosis are possible presentations of heart failure
- Clubbing may be associated with cyanotic congenital heart disease

*Palpation*
- Point of maximal apical impulse is found in the 4th intercostal space before age 7 then, 5th intercostal space

**PEDIATRICS**

*Auscultation*
- Murmurs are a common finding: up to 80% of children have murmurs, but only rarely have confirmed organic heart disease (see "Murmurs" under **Common Clinical Scenarios**, p.561)

## Gastrointestinal
- See the **Gastrointestinal System** Chapter
- Useful tips to relax child include flexing the child's knees, talking and playing with the child, and putting your hand flat on the abdomen

*Inspection*
- Protuberant abdomen
  - Expected in infants; feature disappears as early as 4 yr
  - Distended abdomen may indicate obstruction or abdominal mass
  - A large abdomen, with thin limbs and wasted buttocks, suggests severe malnutrition; seen in celiac disease or cystic fibrosis
- Umbilicus: check for umbilical hernia
- Abdominal wall
- Anus: redness and rash may indicate inadequate cleaning, diaper rash, or irritation from diarrhea

*Auscultation*
- See **Approach to the Neonate**

*Percussion*
- Should be tympanic except over the liver, fecal masses, or full bladder

*Palpation*
- Observe child's face carefully for pain while lightly palpating for tenderness and deeply palpating for abnormal masses
- Umbilical or inguinal hernia
- Palpate liver's lower margin; if margin indefinite, use percussion
- Pyloric stenosis: in later stages, described as a palpable "olive" just to the right of the midline in the epigastric area (usually in the first few months of life), associated with projectile vomiting
- Rectal exam should be done only if abdominal or pelvic disease suspected
- Prostate gland is not palpable in the young male

## Genitourinary: Male
*Inspection*
1. Infant
   - Penis
     - Foreskin completely covers the glans penis and is not retractable until months to years after birth
     - Shaft of penis: ensure penis appears straight, and note any ventral surface abnormalities. Fixed downward bowing of the penis is a chordee, and may accompany a hypospadias
     - Look for fibrous ring around meatus of foreskin (phimosis)
     - A small amount of white, cheesy material under the foreskin around the glans (smegma) is normal
   - Scrotum: poorly developed scrotum may indicate cryptorchidism (undescended testes)
   - Note rugae and presence or absence of testes in sac

2. Child
   - In precocious puberty, the penis and testes are enlarged due to conditions of excess androgens, including pituitary and adrenal tumors
   - As with adult men, swelling in the inguinal canal, especially after a Valsalva maneuver, may indicate inguinal hernia

## Palpation

1. Infant
   - ✦ Palpate the testes in the scrotum and then palpate up the spermatic cord to the external inguinal ring
   - ✦ If testis are palpated in the inguinal canal, gentle pressure can ease them down
   - ✦ Differentiate any swelling found in the scrotum from the testes
   - ✦ Hydroceles and inguinal hernias are two common scrotal masses, but only hydroceles transilluminate
   - ✦ Male infants with undescended testes should be referred to Urology by 1 year of age. The vast majority will descend spontaneously during this time
2. Child
   - ✦ Cremasteric reflex test: scratch the medial aspect of the thigh, ipsilateral testis moves upward
   - ✦ An extremely active cremasteric reflex may cause testis to retract upward and appear undescended
     - ▪ Absence of a cremasteric reflex is a sign of testicular torsion
   - ✦ To minimize retraction, examine when child is relaxed, use warm hands, and palpate from the lower abdomen along inguinal canal toward scrotum
   - ✦ Common causes of painful testicle are infection, trauma, torsion of the testicle, and torsion of the appendix testis

## Genitourinary: Female

*Inspection*
- Examine child in supine position; in younger children, child can sit in parent's lap with parent holding knees outstretched
- Inspect labia majora, labia minora, size of clitoris, presence of rashes, bruises or other lesions
- To examine more internal structures, separate the labia majora at midpoint to inspect urethral orifice and labia minora. Do not touch the hymen as it exquisitely sensitive
- Note condition of labia minora, urethra, hymen, and proximal vagina
- In children:
  - ✦ Labia majora and minora flatten out after infancy
  - ✦ Check for any rashes, bruises or external lesions
  - ✦ Examine labia minora, urethra, hymen, and proximal vagina by inspection only
  - ✦ Hymen is thin, translucent, and vascular, often with easily identifiable edges
  - ✦ Pubic hair before age 7 yr indicates premature adrenarche and potential precocious puberty
  - ✦ Labial adhesions (fusion of the labia minora) posteriorly may be noted in prepubertal girls

## Musculoskeletal
- Inspection, palpation, and range of motion
- Range of motion is greatest in the infant and then decreases with age

*Infant*
- Feet
  - ✦ Toeing-in:
    - ▪ 6-18 mo: commonly caused by internal tibial torsion
    - ▪ Rotate knees so patella faces forward, feet should face inward (usually disappears at 2 yr)
  - ✦ Flat feet are normal in children <2-3 yr
- Knee Alignment
  - ✦ Mild bow-legged (genu varum) pattern is normal until age 2 yr
  - ✦ Mild knock-knee (genu valgum) pattern is normal from 2-8 yr
- Hips
  - ✦ Barlow and Ortolani tests are recommended screening in infants up to 3 months of age; however, any persistent abnormality should have radiologic follow-up regardless of age
  - ✦ See **Approach to the Neonate**
  - ✦ Asymmetry of buttocks and thigh folds suggests congenital hip dysplasia

**PEDIATRICS**

- Spine
  - Look for vertebral deformities and pigmented spots, hairy patches, sacral dimple, or overlying skin in lumbosacral region (sign of spina bifida)

*Child*
- pGALS for MSK screening in school-aged children[6]
  - Contains a few additional maneuvers or alterations:
    - Foot and ankle – walk on heels then tiptoes
    - Wrists – palms together and then hands back to back
    - Temporomandibular joints – open mouth and insert three of child's own fingers
    - Elbow – reach up and touch the sky
    - Neck – look at the ceiling
- As child gets older, MSK exam is generally the same as an adult exam (see the **Musculoskeletal System** Chapter)
- Feet: In-toeing >12 yr: commonly caused by femoral anteversion
  - Rotate knees so patella faces forward, feet should now face forward
- Hips: check for hip pain or instability using Trendelenburg test
- Spine: check for scoliosis
  - Ask child to lean forward
  - Inspect curvature of spinous processes, rib humps (prominence of ribs due to convexity of spinal curvature), and look for asymmetry in hips and scapulae

## Neurological
- Findings are greatly affected by internal factors: alertness, timing from last feed, sleeping; and external factors: fear and anxiety, presence of parents
- Neurologic and developmental exams are often combined since neurologic abnormalities can present in young children as developmental abnormalities

*Infant*
- Mental status
  - Observe activities during alert periods
- Motor exam
  - Watch position at rest and as the infant moves spontaneously
  - Test resistance to passive movement noting any spasticity or flaccidity, increased or decreased tone
  - Specific maneuvers to assess tone:
    - Lift child by placing hands under arm pits. Axial tone is low if infant seems to "slip through" your hands
    - Hold infant prone, supporting them across the abdomen. Low tone if their head/neck flop over such that they are an "inverted U" shape
  - Can place infant on abdomen to observe movements, head position
- Deep tendon reflexes
  - Triceps, brachioradialis, and abdominal reflexes are hard to elicit before 6 mo
  - Anal reflex is present at birth and should be elicited if spinal cord lesion is suspected
  - Normal infants have an upgoing plantar (Babinski) response until approx 9 mo of age
  - Progressive increase in deep tendon reflexes in first year coupled with increased tone may indicate CNS disease such as cerebral palsy
- Sensory function
  - Pain sensation: touch or flick infant's palm or sole with your finger and observe for withdrawal, arousal, and change in facial expression

*Child*
- Motor exam
  - Observe child's gait while walking and running, noting any asymmetry, tripping, or clumsiness
  - Heel-to-toe walking, hopping, jumping (if developmentally appropriate)
  - Use toy to test for coordination, strength of upper extremities
  - If concerned about strength, test by having child sit on the floor and then stand up

- In children with weak hip and thigh strength, as seen in certain forms of muscular dystrophy, children get up by using their arms to "walk up" their legs to achieve an upright position (Gower's sign)
  - Hand preference in a child 1.5-2yr suggests weakness: must rule out hemiplegia
- Deep tendon reflexes: as assessed for adults (see **Neurological Exam**)
- Sensory exam
  - Test with cotton ball with child's eyes closed; do not use pinprick with young child
- Cerebellar exam
  - All cerebellar tests as done in adults, but make this into a game!
  - While developmental differences exist, significant asymmetry can suggest pathology
  - Look for nystagmus and gait disturbances and slurred speech

## Dermatological
- Done almost entirely on history and inspection, with a good source of light
- Inspection should begin with general observation of skin, hair, and nail color, pigmentation, and texture
- Skin temperature should be assessed as well
- If lesions are present, describe their distribution, configuration, thickness, primary/ secondary changes present, and color
- Be aware of lesions that raise concern for suspected child abuse, such as outlines of patterned objects
- Potential findings:
  - Contact dermatitis
    - Vesicular, erythematous, well-defined lesions
  - Atopic dermatitis (eczema)
    - Itchy, dry, slightly elevated papular lesions that form plaques
    - Face, neck, hands, and flexor surfaces of joints
  - Café-au-lait spots: consider neurofibromatosis type 1 if six or more café-au-lait spots greater than 5 mm in diameter before puberty, or greater than 15mm in diameter after puberty
  - Ash leaf spots (hypomelanic macules): consider tuberous sclerosis complex (Ash leaf spots may be the only visual sign in infancy)

# 4. APPROACH TO THE ADOLESCENT
- Adolescence is a time of tremendous physical and psychosocial change
- History and Physical Exam should focus on the following:
  - Puberty: signs of normal vs. abnormal maturation
  - Screening: for safety and risk-taking behaviors

## 4.1 Adolescent History
- With the adolescent's permission, at least part of the history should be obtained without parent in the room
  - Discuss confidentiality: inform adolescent that you will have to disclose to other people if they are suicidal, homicidal, or if they are being abused or have witnessed abuse of a minor
- ID: name, age, school grade, siblings, cohabitants in home
- CC: note that a teenager's initial CC may not represent his/her actual reason for seeking medical attention
- HPI (see **Approach to the Pediatric Exam**, p.540)
- PMHx: previous illnesses, surgeries, medications, allergies (medications and environmental), immunization history
- FHx: recurrent illnesses, early deaths, genetic diseases, cancer, psychiatric conditions, suicide, alcohol/substance abuse
- ROS: including menstrual patterns, urinary symptoms

## Psychosocial History
*The "HE²ADS³" Assessment*[7]
- Home
  - Living arrangements, relationship with parents and siblings, other occupants
  - Family issues, recent changes at home, feeling safe within the home

- Education and Employment
  - Name of school, current grade, academic performance, school attendance, behavior at school, plans for further education/vocation
  - Are you working? Where? How much?
- Eating
  - Diet: typical foods, types and frequency of skipped meals, vomiting, nutritional supplements, vitamin use, calcium/vitamin D intake
  - Eating Disorder Screen: "SCOFF"[8]
    - Do you make yourself **S**ick because you feel uncomfortably full?
    - Do you worry that you have lost **C**ontrol over how much you eat?
    - In 3 mo have you lost **O**ver 15 lbs?
    - Do you think you are **F**at when others think you are thin?
    - Does **F**ood dominate your life?
  - Body image and compensatory behaviours: recent weight gain or loss, dieting, use of weight loss drugs, vomiting, laxatives, exercise, diuretics, stimulants
- Activities
  - Online activities, screen time, exercise, sports, hobbies, parties/clubs
- Drugs
  - Do you have any friends who drink, smoke or use drugs?
  - Have you ever tried smoking or drinking alcohol (if yes, clarify frequency and amount)? What did you think? What about other drugs?
  - Have you ever gotten in trouble because of using these substances?
- Sex/Sexuality
  - Ask about the 5 P's, see **The General History & Physical Exam**
- Suicide/Mood
  - Screen for depression MSIGECAPS (see the **Psychiatry** Chapter)
  - Suicide assessment: past attempts, protective factors, current plan/means
  - Ask about bullying or stress
- Safety
  - From physical and sexual abuse at home, school, in relationships
  - Recent injuries: motor vehicle accidents, sports injuries, concussions
  - Risk-taking behavior (e.g. driving while intoxicated or being a passenger with an intoxicated driver)
  - Internet and social media safety, sexting

## 4.2 Adolescent Physical Exam
- As per adult exam, with particular emphasis on:
  - **Growth:** height, mass, BMI: should be plotted on curve to monitor growth
  - **H&N:** thyroid examination, screen for visual acuity and hearing
  - **GU** (Tanner staging):
    - Male: external genitalia; secondary sexual characteristics (body hair, pubic hair)
    - Female: external genitalia/breast/pubic hair; breast development
  - **MSK:** scoliosis
  - **Dermatological:** skin (acne, petechiae, pallor, pigmentation), hair (amount, distribution, hirsutism)

## General Survey and Vitals
- General Survey should consist of (1) General Inspection, (2) Growth Measurements
- 1. General Inspection: does this adolescent look "sick"?
  - Respiratory distress, level of alertness, general affect, nutritional status
- 2. Growth Measurements: measure height, weight, calculate BMI
  - Plot on growth chart and note trend and percentiles of growth
  - Height: growth spurt occurs during puberty, which accounts for 20-25% of final adult height; onset and duration of growth spurt is highly variable
    - Females: onset 7-13 yr
    - Males: onset 9-14 yr
  - Growth spurt lasts about 2 yr longer in males (into 3rd decade)
  - Weight: pubertal weight gain accounts for 50% of final adult body weight
    - Percentage body fat increases in females and decreases in males

PEDIATRICS

*Vital Signs*
- As per adults – note: teenage women often have lower BP than adults, but if otherwise well looking, this can be considered a variant of normal
- Ensure teenager is comfortable and not anxious before measuring vitals
- Hypertension in children is often due to a secondary cause whereas adolescent hypertension is usually essential hypertension

## H.E.E.N.T.
1. **Cranial Nerves** (see **The Nervous System** Chapter)
2. **Oral Cavity and Pharynx** (see **The Head, Neck, and Throat** Chapter)
   - Of particular note in adolescents:
     - Teeth: check for poor dental hygiene, enamel erosion from vomiting or tooth grinding (bruxism)
     - Tonsils
3. **Nose and Paranasal Sinuses** (see **The Head, Neck, and Throat** Chapter)
4. **Thyroid** (see **The Head, Neck, and Throat** Chapter)
   - In adolescence, Hashimoto's thyroiditis > asymptomatic goiter> Graves' disease
   - Hypothyroidism: mostly caused by Hashimoto's thyroiditis in adolescence
     - Growth and pubertal delay, menstrual dysfunction
     - Abnormally high weight gain, cold and dry skin
   - Hyperthyroidism: almost always caused by Graves' disease in adolescence
     - Emotional lability and sleep disturbance, change in school performance
     - Skin changes: eczema, erythema, excoriations, or smooth skin
5. **Neck** (see **The Head, Neck, and Throat** Chapter)
   - Lymph nodes
     - Infection (vast majority): red, <2 cm, mobile, location anterior (often strep throat) vs. posterior (mononucleosis)
     - Malignancy (rare): hard, fixed, >2 cm, with constitutional symptoms
       - Supraclavicular lymphadenopathy is malignancy until proven otherwise (prompt CXR needed to rule out mediastinal mass)
   - Neck stiffness: suggestive of meningitis, which can be assessed using Kernig and Brudnizki signs (described below)
     - A positive Kernig is pain on subsequent extension in the knee
     - A positive Brudnizki is indicated by involuntary lifting of the legs

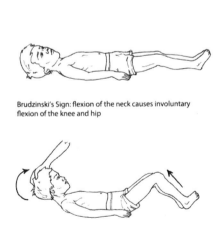
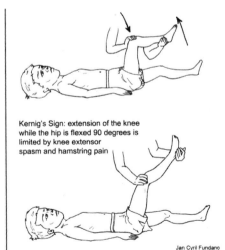

Brudzinski's Sign: flexion of the neck causes involuntary flexion of the knee and hip

Kernig's Sign: extension of the knee while the hip is flexed 90 degrees is limited by knee extensor spasm and hamstring pain

Jan Cyril Fundano

**Figure 2**. Kernig's and Brudzinski's Signs

6. **Eyes** (see **Ophthalmology** Chapter)
   - Adolescents should have visual acuity screened every 2-3 yr

- Use standard Snellen chart, with one eye covered

## Respiratory
- Similar to the adult exam (see **The Respiratory System** Chapter)

## Cardiovascular
- Similar to the adult exam (see **The Circulatory System** Chapter)
- Specific sign in adolescents:
  - Bradycardia, orthostatic vitals (hypotension and tachycardia with standing): associated with anorexia nervosa

## Gastrointestinal
- Similar to the adult exam (see **The Gastrointestinal System** Chapter)

*Inspection*
- Central adiposity vs. malnourishment/cachexia
- Lanugo (baby-like) hair: associated with anorexia nervosa

*Auscultation and Percussion*
- Bowel sounds
- Percuss all four quadrants, liver, and spleen
- Splenomegaly found in infectious mononucleosis, leukemia/lymphoma, hemolytic diseases

*Palpation*
- Light and deep palpation (tenderness, masses, peritoneal signs)
- Liver and spleen
- Kidney
- Special tests: appendicitis (see **The Gastrointestinal System** Chapter)
- Appendicitis is the most common indication for emergency abdominal surgery in childhood; its frequency peaks between ages 15-30 yr

## Genitourinary and Reproductive system
- Often the genitourinary/reproductive examination is left until the end, as teenagers can be embarrassed or sensitive about this area
- There should always be a chaperone for the GU and breast exams
- Onset of puberty is often variable; in general, onset is 8-13 yr in females, 9-14 yr in males
- Usual sequence of pubertal sexual maturation:
  - Females: thelarche (breast budding) → adrenarche (pubic hair) → growth spurt → menarche (onset of menstruation)
  - Males: testes enlargement → penile enlargement → adrenarche + axillary hair → growth spurt

PEDIATRICS

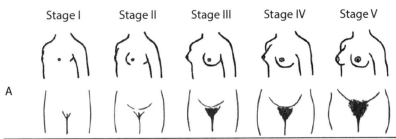

| I. | Breast: preadolescent, with elevated papilla<br>Pubic hair: prepubertal |
|---|---|
| II. | Breast: breast bud stage; small elevation of breast and papilla, areola diameter enlarges<br>Pubic hair: sparse hair at labia |
| III. | Breast: further enlargement of breast/areola, but their contours are not separated<br>Pubic hair: hair over pubis |
| IV. | Breast: projection of areola and papilla to form secondary mound<br>Pubic hair: coarse adult hair |
| V. | Breast: mature; areola recess to general contour of breast<br>Pubic hair: hair extends to medial thigh |

| I. | Testes: volume <1.5 mL<br>Pubic hair: prepubertal | Phallus: childlike |
|---|---|---|
| II. | Testes: volumes 1.6-6 mL<br>Scrotum: reddened, thinner, larger | Phallus: no change<br>Pubic hair: sparse hair at base of penis |
| III. | Testes: volume 6-12 mL<br>Scotum: greater enlargement | Phallus: increased length<br>Pubic hair: hair over pubis |
| IV. | Testes: volume 12-20 mL<br>Scrotum: further enlargement, darkening<br>Pubic hair: corse adult hair | Phallus: increased length, circumfrence |
| V. | Testes: volume >20 mL<br>Scrotum: adult | Phallus: adult<br>Pubic hair: hair extends to medial thigh |

Alison McFadden, Wendy Gu, Diana Kryski

**Figure 3**. Male and Female Tanner Staging

*Breast* (see the **Breast Exam** Chapter)
- Thelarche (budding of breast at onset of puberty) occurs at roughly 11 yr; is one of earliest signs of puberty
- Age of onset variable among different ethnicities; earlier in children of African descent
- Sexual maturation: can assign Tanner Stage (see **Figure 3**)
- In males: inspect for gynecomastia
  - Usually benign, self-limited; seen in up to 50-60% of adolescent boys
  - Etiology: idiopathic, 1° or 2° hypogonadism, obesity, marijuana use, hyperthyroidism, antiandrogen drugs, cancer chemotherapy

PEDIATRICS

- Typical appearance: 1-3 cm, round, freely mobile, often tender, firm mass beneath areola
- Further investigation if: large, hard, fixed enlargement or mass/ nodules
- Palpation (see the **Breast Exam** Chapter)

**Table 5.** Causes of Palpable Breast Masses in Children and Adolescents[9]

| Causes | |
| --- | --- |
| Classic or Juvenile Fibroadenoma | Intraductal Papilloma |
| Fibrocystic Changes | Fat Necrosis/Lipoma |
| Breast Cyst | Abscess/Mastitis |
| Neoplasm (carcinoma <1%) | Adenomatous Hyperplasia |

## Genitourinary
*Female*
- See the **Gynecological Exam** Chapter for detailed description
- Indications for pelvic examination (otherwise not necessary until 21 yr of age):
  - Abnormal vaginal discharge, pelvic pain, history of unprotected sexual intercourse, menstrual irregularities, suspicion of anatomic abnormalities, patient request
- **Inspection**
  - External genitalia
  - Pubic hair: assign Tanner staging (see **Figure 3**)
  - Internal genitalia (speculum examination)
  - Cervix, vagina
- **Palpation**
  - External genitalia (labia, clitoris, vagina), internal genitalia (cervix, uterus adnexae)

*Male*
- See the **Urological Exam** Chapter for detailed description
- Inspection
  - Assign Tanner stages of pubertal maturation (see **Figure 3**)
  - Not to be missed: red, tender, swollen testicle = torsion until proven otherwise (one of the few urological emergencies)
    - Differential Diagnosis: testicular torsion, torsion of appendix testes or epididymitis
- Palpation
  - Penis, scrotum, inguinal hernias, inguinal lymph nodes
  - Differential Diagnosis of painless scrotal mass in adolescent male: testicular cancer or other malignancy, hydrocele, spermatocele, varicocele, indirect inguinal hernia, abscess

## Common Investigations
- Gonorrheal and chlamydial swabs
- STI testing
- Pap smear (rarely performed on females <21 yr)
- See **Gynecological Exam** Chapter and **Infectious Disease** Chapter

## Musculoskeletal (see **The Musculoskeletal System** Chapter)

## Neurological (see **The Nervous System** Chapter)

## Dermatological
- Pubertal changes
- Acne (comedonal, papular or pustular inflammatory, nodulocystic); seen in 85% of adolescents
- Pigmentation of areolae, external genitalia
- Development of pubic and axillary hair
- Tinea pedis (athlete's foot): fungal infection

PEDIATRICS

- Scaling, fissuring, erythema at soles of feet and toe webs
- Psoriasis: 25% of cases have onset in adolescent years
  - Erythematous, circumscribed plaques with silvery scaly appearance
- Pitting and ridging nail changes: associated with anorexia nervosa

# 5. COMMON CLINICAL SCENARIOS

## 5.1 General
## Dehydration

**Table 6.** Clinical assessment of degree of dehydration[10]

| Mild (<5%) | Moderate (5-10%) | Severe (>10%) |
|---|---|---|
| Slightly decreased urine output | Decreased urine output | Markedly decreased or absent urine output |
| Slightly increased thirst | Moderately increased thirst | Greatly increased thirst |
| Slightly dry mucous membrane | Dry mucous membrane | Very dry mucous membrane |
| Slightly elevated heart rate | Elevated heart rate | Greatly elevated heart rate |
| | Decreased skin turgor | Decreased skin turgor |
| | Sunken eyes | Very sunken eyes |
| | Sunken anterior fontanelle | Very sunken anterior fontanelles |
| | | Lethargy |
| | | Cold extremities |
| | | Hypotension |
| | | Coma |

Canadian Paediatric Society, Nutrition and Gastroenterology Committee. Oral rehydration therapy and early refeeding in the management of childhood gastroenteritis, 2006. With permission

*Investigations*
- Electrolytes should be monitored daily for all children receiving >50% of their maintenance fluid volume via IV

*Management*
- The three basic principles of treating dehydration are: (1) Rehydration, (2) Replace ongoing losses, and (3) Provide maintenance fluid
- **Rehydrate** with oral rehydration therapy (ORT) such as Pedialyte for mild or moderate dehydration, and IV normal saline boluses (20mL/kg) for severe dehydration
- **Replace ongoing losses** 1:1 with fluid of similar tonicity to the fluid lost (e.g., ½ normal saline for gastroenteritis)
- **Provide maintenance fluid** according to the 4:2:1 rule (See **Fluids, Electrolytes, and Acid/Base Disturbances** Chapter)

## 5.2 H.E.E.N.T.

### 5.2.1 Ear

**Acute Otitis Media**
- Main causal organisms: *S. pneumoniae, H. influenzae, M. catarrhalis*
- Diagnosis of AOM requires all three of the following:
  - Acute onset of symptoms
  - Middle ear effusion (otorrhea, fixed tympanic membrane, visible air fluid levels)
  - Middle ear inflammation (discoloration of tympanic membrane: opaque, hemorrhagic, red/yellow)

PEDIATRICS

**Table 7.** Presentation and management of Acute Otitis Media

| KEY SYMPTOMS | PHYSICAL EXAM FINDINGS | INVESTIGATIONS | MANAGEMENT |
|---|---|---|---|
| Ear pain, fever, irritability, pulling at ears, persistent crying | Tympanic membrane appears cloudy, bulging, immobile and erythematous | Mainly clinical diagnosis. If complicated chronic infection, may consider CT/MRI head | <6 months old: Antibiotics (amoxicillin)<br><br>>6 months old, generally observe for 48-72 hours with antipyretics and without antibiotics<br><br>In any age group, always treat if patient is toxic, severe otalgia, temp >39°C, follow up cannot be assured |

### 6.2.2 Mouth

**Oral Candidal Thrush**
- Common up to 12 months; investigate for underlying condition/ immunodeficiency in older child
- Note: Milk can be scraped off with a tongue depressor, while thrush cannot

**Table 8.** Presentation and management of Oral Candidal Thrush

| KEY SYMPTOMS | PHYSICAL EXAM FINDINGS | INVESTIGATIONS | MANAGEMENT |
|---|---|---|---|
| Pain<br><br>Poor feeding | White plaques on buccal mucosa, lips, tongue, gums, and palate | Potassium hydroxide (KOH) slide preparation | Nystatin for mild to moderate; gentian violet in infants |
| Irritability | Scraping of the lesions may reveal erythema and bleeding at the base | | Fluconazole plus liposomal amphotericin B if severe (rare) |

PEDIATRICS

## Bacterial Pharyngitis/Tonsillitis

Table 9. Presentation and management of bacterial pharyngitis

| KEY SYMPTOMS | PHYSICAL EXAM FINDINGS | INVESTIGATIONS | MANAGEMENT |
|---|---|---|---|
| **Children <3yr:**<br>• Atypical presentations are common<br>• Scarlatiniform rash<br>• Vomiting<br>• Low-grade fever<br>• Nasal congestion<br>• Fatigue/irritability<br><br>**Children >3yr:**<br>• Fever<br>• Headache<br>• Abdominal pain<br>• Nausea<br>• Vomiting<br>• Sore throat<br>• Dysphagia<br>• Dyspnea | • Palatal petechiae<br>• Tonsillar enlargement +/- exudate<br>• Tender cervical nodes<br>• Stridor | RADT<br><br>Throat swab/ culture | Usually self-resolving course within 3-5 days<br><br>Antibiotic treatment such as Penicillin V often used to prevent complications<br><br>Tonsillectomy under special considerations (obstructive sleep apnea, recurrent throat infection, PFAPA syndrome, peritonsillar abscess)<br><br>Adenoidectomy under special circumstances (moderate/severe obstructive symptoms, adenoid facies, chronic sinusitis) |

## 5.3 Respiratory
### Asthma

- CC: Shortness of breath from: viral illnesses (most common trigger in younger children), physical activity, environmental allergens (animal dander, dust, house dust mites, pollen), food (eggs, seafood, peanuts), smoke, weather changes, exposure to cold, and stress[7]; Cough that is dry, tight, and occasionally wheezy (especially at night)
- Eczema in atopic child, especially in flexural surfaces
- Atopy in family members

Table 10. Presentation and management of asthma

| KEY SYMPTOMS | PHYSICAL EXAM FINDINGS | INVESTIGATIONS | MANAGEMENT |
|---|---|---|---|
| Wheezing<br><br>Cough<br><br>Dyspnea<br><br>Chest tightness<br><br>Sputum production | Vitals:<br>Tachypnea<br>Tachycardia<br><br>Accessory muscle use<br><br>Suprasternal retractions are commonly present<br><br>Loud biphasic (expiratory and inspiratory) wheezing<br><br>Expiratory phase longer than inspiratory phase, with high-pitched wheezes throughout most of expiration | Spirometry<br>Plethysmography<br><br>PFTs: reversible airway obstruction (children under age 6 cannot do PFTs so diagnosis based on clinical criteria*)<br><br>Consider CXR to rule out pneumonia | Controlling asthma triggers<br><br>Short-acting bronchodilators for quick-relief<br><br>Inhaled glucocorticoids, leukotriene modifiers, long acting bronchodilators for persistent asthma |

* For guidelines, refer to[11]: Ducharme FM, et al. Diagnosis and management of asthma in preschoolers: A Canadian Thoracic Society and Canadian Paediatric Society position paper. Can Respir J. 2015; 22(3): 135-43.

**Clinical Pearl: Asthma[12]**
Asthma is considered well-controlled if daytime symptoms are <4 d/wk, nighttime symptoms are <1 night/wk, there is normal physical activity, infrequent exacerbations, no absence from school, and the need for a β2-agonist is <4 doses/wk.

## 5.4 Cardiovascular

### Murmurs
- Soft precordial systolic murmur common in first few days after birth
- May indicate patent ductus arteriosus if it persists and is heard over the back

*Benign*
- Best heard best with bell of stethoscope and changes with patient position or respiration
- Could be physiologic (heard during fever, anemia)
- Could be specific type (see chart below)

**Table 11.** Benign Heart Murmurs in Children[13]

| Murmur | Age of Presentation | Location | Timing | Intensity, Quality, and Pitch |
|---|---|---|---|---|
| Carotid bruit | 2-10 years | Supraclavicular bilaterally (R>L) | Systolic ejection | Harsh or soft |
| Closing ductus | Neonate to 1 year | Upper left sternal border | Transient | Soft |
| Pulmonary flow murmur of newborn | Neonates, usually disappears by 3-6 months | Upper left sternal border, lung fields, axillae | Systole | Soft, slightly ejectile |
| Peripheral pulmonary branch stenosis | Neonates | Left upper sternal border | Systolic ejection | High pitch, radiates to axilla/back |
| Still's murmur | Preschool to early school age | Mid/lower left sternal border | Early and mid-systole | Grade I-II/VI, musical, vibratory, multiple overtones |
| Venous hum | Preschool to early school age | Under clavicle | Continuous | Soft, hollow, louder in diastole, can be eliminated by maneuvers that affect venous return or by contralateral neck rotation |

*Organic (non-innocent murmurs)*
- All diastolic murmurs (except venous hum), or systolic that are coarse, continuous, or ≥ Grade 3
- Consider both congenital and acquired causes

**Table 12.** Pathologic Heart Murmurs in Children[14]

| Defect | Location | Timing | Intensity | Pitch | Quality |
|---|---|---|---|---|---|
| Atrial septal defect (acyanotic) | Left second and third interspace | Wide and fixed split S2, peaks in mid-systole | Soft | Medium | Non-musical |

PEDIATRICS

| Defect | Location | Timing | Intensity | Pitch | Quality |
|---|---|---|---|---|---|
| Ventricular septal defect (acyanotic) | Left sternal border, third and fourth interspaces | Between S1 and S2 | Very loud | High | Blowing |
| Patent ductus arteriosus | Second left interspace, may radiate to left clavicle/sternum | Continuous; louder in late systole (just before S2); obscures S2; softer in diastole | Loud | Medium | Harsh |
| Tetralogy of Fallot | Second and third left interspaces | Between S1 and S2 | Not well transmitted | | No distinct characteristics |

- Adult murmurs such as aortic regurgitation and stenosis are less common, but still possible in children; refer to **Precordial Exam** Chapter
- Coarctation of the aorta may present with hypertension and a nonspecific systolic murmur in the left infraclavicular area
  - Clinical suspicion should prompt measurement of differential BP and O2 saturation (between upper extremities, or between upper and lower extremities) to confirm diagnosis

## Heart Failure
- Timing of HF is important
  - At Birth: rare (e.g. hemolysis, fetal-maternal transfusion, neonatal lupus)
  - First weeks of life: Obstructive lesion or persistent pulmonary hypertension (this can present later in cases of Trisomy 21, as their lungs are more compliant)
  - 4-6 weeks: Left-to-right shunting
  - After 3 months: Myocarditis, cardiomyopathy or supraventricular tachycardia

**Table 13.** Presentation and management of heart failure

| KEY SYMPTOMS | PHYSICAL EXAM FINDINGS | INVESTIGATIONS | MANAGEMENT |
|---|---|---|---|
| Shortness of breath, exercise intolerance<br><br>Pre-syncope or syncopal episodes<br><br>Diaphoresis and tiring with feeds in infants | Peripheral edema, failure to thrive, cyanosis, clubbing, heart murmur, hepatomegaly | CXR, ECG, 4 limb BPs, pre and post ductal saturations, consider echocardiogram | Treat underlying cause<br><br>Dietary measures<br><br>Refer to cardiology or consider pre-load reduction, inotropic therapy, afterload reduction, beta blockade |

## 5.5 Gastrointestinal
### Acute Gastroenteritis
- Classification of diarrhea
  - Definition: passage of ≥ 3 loose or watery stools per day
    - Acute diarrhea – Lasting several hours to days
    - Acute bloody diarrhea or dysentery
    - Persistent diarrhea – Lasting 14 days or longer
- Fecal-oral transmission
- Causes: Rotavirus and other viruses, Campylobacter, Salmonella, Shigella, Escherichia coli, C difficile, Giardia, and Cryptosporidium
- Differential Diagnosis: diet-related (e.g., milk protein intolerance, excess juice), ischemic intestinal damage (e.g., intussusception), malabsorption, lactase deficiency, cystic fibrosis, celiac disease, inflammatory bowel disease
- Caution in diagnosing acute gastroenteritis in patients with vomiting only!

**Table 14.** Presentation and management of acute gastroenteritis

| KEY SYMPTOMS | PHYSICAL EXAM FINDINGS | INVESTIGATIONS | MANAGEMENT |
|---|---|---|---|
| Diarrhea (frequent watery is suggestive of viral; blood or mucous in stool indicative of a bacterial pathogen; chronic may be a parasitic/non-infectious cause) | Vitals Fever Tachycardia Hypotension Increased malaise, lethargy, or irritability Signs of dehydration | Stool culture, EM, multiplex PCR, O&P If systemic infection suspected: CBC, blood cultures. Add urine cultures, chest radiography, and/or lumbar puncture if indicated | Assessment and management for dehydration Oral re-hydration, IV fluids, early re-feeding Antimicrobial, if indicated Early antiemetic, therapy can improve outcomes |
| Abdominal pain | Rash | | |

## Physiological Jaundice
- Second or third day of life
- Results from accumulation of unconjugated bilirubin

**Table 15.** Differential Diagnosis for Neonatal Jaundice Based on Age[15,16]

| Differential Diagnosis | Notes & Distinguishing Features |
|---|---|
| | **<24 h of Birth (\*\*\*Always pathologic\*\*\*)** |
| **Hemolysis: Rh/ABO incompatibility** | Positive Coomb's test, pallor, hepatosplenomegaly, +/- petechiae and dark urine |
| **Sepsis: GBS, TORCH, congenital** | Fever, labored breathing, decreased movements, vomiting/diarrhea, seizures |
| | **Typically 24-96 h of Birth** |
| **Physiologic** | R/O other causes, no other pathologic signs/symptoms |
| **Insufficient breastfeeding/dehydration** | Signs of dehydration, decreased urination, poor feeding |
| **Hemolysis: G6PD/PKU deficiency, thalassemia, spherocytosis** | Negative Coomb's test, anemia, splenomegaly, palor, fatigue; preceded by infection or medication use in G6PD |
| **Nonhemolytic: hematoma, polycythemia** | Ruddy complexion, hepatomegaly (polycythemia); Ecchymosis/hemorrhage (birthing trauma) |
| **Sepsis** | Same signs as above. Sepsis may present in first 24 of life or later |

PEDIATRICS

| Differential Diagnosis | Notes & Distinguishing Features |
|---|---|
| | **Typically >1 week** |
| **Breast milk jaundice** | Usually no other pathologic signs/symptoms |
| **Hypothyroidism** | Often asymptomatic clinically, but detected biochemically. May have: poor feeding, decreased activity, hypothermia, constipation |
| **Inborn errors of metabolism: galactosemia** | Poor weight gain, poor feeding, vomiting, seizures |
| **Neonatal hepatitis** | Appearance around 1-2 months of age, hepatosplenomegaly, poor growth, poor weight gain |
| **Biliary atresia** | Acholic stools are not noted at birth but develop over the first few weeks of life. Appetite, growth, and weight gain may be normal |

- Notable complications: kernicterus; presents as lethargy, slight hypotonia, poor sucking, high pitched cry, poor feeding

**Table 16.** Presentation and management of physiological jaundice

| KEY SYMPTOMS | PHYSICAL EXAM FINDINGS | INVESTIGATIONS | MANAGEMENT |
|---|---|---|---|
| Yellowed skin | Often unreliable | Heel prick | Phototherapy may be required depending on underlying risk and bilirubin levels as per nomogram (refer to Canadian Pediatric Society guideline) |
| Scleral icterus | | Serum bilirubin | |
| | | Transcutaneous bilirubinometry | |
| | | Depending on scenario: maternal and infant blood group, DAT, G6PD, CBC/ smear | Rarely, consider IVIG, exchange transfusion |

### Duodenal atresia
- Usually present in neonatal period

**Table 17.** Presentation and management of duodenal atresia

| KEY SYMPTOMS | PHYSICAL EXAM FINDINGS | INVESTIGATIONS | MANAGEMENT |
|---|---|---|---|
| Onset of vomiting within hours of birth | Scaphoid abdomen | Double bubble sign on X-ray | Adequate IV hydration, total parenteral nutrition until surgery |
| | Epigastric fullness | | |
| Bilious vomiting | | | Duodenoduodenostomy |
| Usually identified pre-natally | | | |

### Hirschsprung's Disease
- Many children diagnosed during first 2 years
- CC: abdominal distention, failure to pass meconium within the first 48 hours of life, and repeated vomiting
- 30% have family history
- Older infants and children typically present with chronic constipation
- Differential Diagnosis: Pediatric functional constipation

**Table 18.** Presentation and management of Hirschsprung's Disease

| KEY SYMPTOMS | PHYSICAL EXAM FINDINGS | INVESTIGATIONS | MANAGEMENT |
|---|---|---|---|
| **Newborn** | **Newborn** | Distended bowel | Swenson, Soave, |
| Delayed passage | Abdominal | loops with paucity of | Duhamel, and Boley |
| of meconium (>48 | distension | air in rectum on plain | procedures |
| hours of delivery) | | abdominal radiograph | |
| | Anal spasm | | Colostomy |
| Billious vomiting | | Narrowed distal colon | |
| | **Infant** | with proximal dilation | |
| Poor feeding | Palpable dilated | | |
| | loops of colon | Rectal biopsy (full | |
| Failure to thrive | | thickness/suction) | |
| | Forceful expulsion | demonstrating | |
| **Infant** | of fecal material | absence of ganglion | |
| Poor weight gain | upon completion | cells | |
| | of rectal exam | | |
| Chronic constipation | | | |

## 5.6 Genitourinary

### Nocturnal Enuresis
- Classification:
  - Primary: child has never achieved dryness; associated with family history of delayed bladder control; maturational
    - Usually spontaneously resolves over time: primary nocturnal enuresis occurs in 20% of 5 year olds, 7% of 7 year olds, and 5% of 10 year olds)
  - Secondary: child had achieved dryness for at least 6 months before new onset of "accidents"
- Differential Diagnosis: psychosocial stressors, behavioural, constipation, renal disease, UTI, DM, abuse, neurodevelopmental condition, cauda equina syndrome

**Table 19.** Presentation and management of nocturnal enuresis

| KEY SYMPTOMS | PHYSICAL EXAM FINDINGS | INVESTIGATIONS | MANAGEMENT |
|---|---|---|---|
| Involuntary urination at night | Look for evidence of underlying disease, such as: | Urinalysis (UTI, diabetes insipidus, diabetes mellitus) | Treat underlying cause |
| | | | If primary cause: |
| | | | · Education, motivational therapy |
| | · **General:** Poor growth, hypertension (renal dx) | Urologic imaging: Only if significant daytime complaints, suspicion for urological abnormality | · Active treatment only in older children around 9 years old (enuresis alarms, desmopressin) |
| | · **GI:** Palpable stool (constipation) | | |
| | · **GU:** Observed abnormal voiding such as slow stream or dribbling (urologic abnormality) | | |

### Urinary Tract Infection (UTI)
- CC: primarily age dependent, may present with fever, irritability, and smelly/cloudy urine at any age
- Main causal organisms: Staphylococci saprophyticus in adolescents, E. coli, Enterococcus, Klebsiella, Proteus, Pseudomonas (SEEK PP)

PEDIATRICS

**Table 20.** Presentation and management of urinary tract infection

| KEY SYMPTOMS | PHYSICAL EXAM FINDINGS | INVESTIGATIONS | MANAGEMENT |
|---|---|---|---|
| **Infant and young child (<2 yr):** Fever, Asymptomatic, GI symptoms (vomiting, poor feeding, etc.) <br><br> **Child (>2 yr):** *Cystitis* <br> • LUTS (frequency, urgency, dysuria) <br> • Hematuria <br> • Urinary retention or incontinence <br> • Suprapubic pain <br><br> *Pyelonephritis* <br> • N&V <br> • CVA pain | **General:** Fever, <br> **GI:** Suprapubic tenderness <br> **GU:** CVA tenderness | Urinalysis (positive leukocyte esterase, nitrites) <br><br> Urine culture (catheter or suprapubic aspiration for infant, clean catch for older child) | Usually outpatient antibiotics: 1st line = cefixime, cephalexin, amoxicillin-clavulanate, adjust according to sensitivities |

## 5.7 MSK
### Limp
- CC: painful or painless limp
- Differential Diagnosis:
    - Painless limp: weakness secondary to hip dysplasia, cerebral palsy, leg-length discrepancy
    - Painful limp (see **Table 21** for Differential Diagnosis)

**Table 21.** Differential Diagnosis of Painful Limp

| Differential Diagnosis | Notes & Distinguishing Features |
|---|---|
| **Septic arthritis (All ages)** | Fever, antalgic gait, refusal to weight bear, severely limited internal rotation, and adduction of hip. Typical presentation of limb: flexed, externally rotated, and abducted |
| **Osteomyelitis (All ages)** | Point tenderness, local edema, erythema, restricted movement/pseudoparalysis, ± fever |
| **Transient synovitis (3-10 years)** | Antalgic gait, hip fixed in flexion/external rotation, often recent viral infection <br> Note: TS is the most common cause of hip pain/limp in children |
| **Legg-Calve-Perthes (4-10 years)** | Mild, intermittent hip pain, referred to thigh/knee, limited internal rotation and abduction of hip |
| **Osgood-Schlatter (11-18 years)** | Pain with activity, relieved by rest, insidious onset over months, tenderness over tibial tuberosity ± erythema |
| **Slipped Capital Femoral Epiphysis (SCFE) (8-17 years)** | Obese child (especially boys), tenderness over hip joint capsule, restricted internal rotation and abduction; acute, painful limp |
| **Malignancy** <br> Leukemia <br> Neuroblastoma <br> Osteosarcoma | All: weight loss, constitutional symptoms <br> Night pain, pallor, petechiae, infections, bruising <br> Abdominal mass, night pain <br> Palpable mass, pathologic fracture |
| **Juvenile idiopathic arthritis (age varies)** | Persistent arthritis in children <16 yr; classified by affected joints; may have constitutional symptoms, fever, extra-articular signs, nail and eye abnormalities (sometimes) |

PEDIATRICS

| Differential Diagnosis | Notes & Distinguishing Features |
|---|---|
| Henoch-Schonlein Purpura (HSP) (3-7 years) | Following respiratory illness, purpuric rash over buttocks and legs, arthralgia, angioedema, abdominal pain |
| Growing pains (3-10 years) | Crampy night pain in calves and thighs, occasionally wakes child from sleep, bilateral; exam unremarkable, gone in the morning, no limitation of activity |

**Table 22.** Presentation and management of limp

| KEY SYMPTOMS | PHYSICAL EXAM FINDINGS | INVESTIGATIONS | MANAGEMENT |
|---|---|---|---|
| Limp<br><br>± Pain | • Gait exam<br>• MSK exam, proceed from areas of least to most concern<br>• Hip exam, especially rotation, Galeazzi test, Trendelenburg test, FABER test<br>• Skin exam<br>• Abdominal exam<br><br>Potential findings: antalgic gait, swelling/erythema of hip or knee joint, leg length discrepancy, unusual/fixed positioning of leg at rest, fever | Suspecting infection (CBC, ESR, CRP, blood culture; joint aspiration for septic arthritis)<br><br>Radiology:<br>• Plain XR<br>• Consider MRI, US | Treat underlying cause |

## Common MSK Injuries
### Knee
- Patellofemoral dysfunction: deep, aching anterior knee pain worsened by prolonged sitting, knee instability (common in female athletes)
- Anterior cruciate ligament (ACL) tear: after "cutting" movement in sports
- O'Donoghue's unhappy triad/skier's knee (ACL, medial collateral ligament, medial/lateral meniscus): after valgus knee injury

**Ankle**: most common acute injury in adolescent athletes
- Inversion: 85% acute ankle injuries
- Eversion: often more serious because higher risk of fracture or injury to tibio-fibular syndesmosis

### Uncommon, but not to be missed
- Legg-Calvé-Perthes disease: avascular necrosis of proximal femoral head which can disrupt the growth plate
  - Most common in boys 4-10 years
  - Common presentation: hip or groin pain, often minor; limp
- Slipped capital femoral epiphysis (SCFE): displacement of proximal femoral epiphysis (usually posteromedially) due to disruption of growth plate
  - Most common in obese adolescent male
  - Common presentation: acute, severe pain with limp
  - Key signs: limited internal rotation of hip and obligate external rotation on hip flexion (Whitman's sign)

## 5.8 Neurological

### Headaches

**Table 23.** Differential Diagnosis of Headaches

| Differential Diagnosis | Notes & Distinguishing Features |
|---|---|
| Meningitis | Fever, sensitivity to light, neck stiffness, nausea, vomiting, confusion, lethargy and/or irritability, positive Kernig and Brudzinski signs, bulging fontanelle, seizures |
| Other illness-related | Associated with focal signs of infection, fever, and may last for several days during the course of the illness |
| Trauma-related | Can occur at home, school or while playing sports; may be associated with nausea, vomiting, loss of consciousness, amnesia, seizure, discoordination |
| Tension-type headache | Described as tightness around both sides of the head; may rarely be associated with nausea, photo/phonophobia and lightheadedness, but not usually vomiting or throbbing |
| Migraine | Children: pounding and throbbing pain, lasting 1-2 hours, and may involve one or both sides of the head. Often associated with nausea, vomiting, and photo/phonophobia |
| | Adolescents: gradual onset and ending, often starts dull and steady and may progress to throbbing. May be worsened by motion, physical exertion, or head movement. Often identifiable triggers such as stress/sleep disturbance |
| | Some children/adolescents may experience aura (e.g. changes in vision preceding onset of headache) |
| Mass effect (e.g. brain neoplasm, hydrocephalus, hematoma) | Red flags: Worse headache of life, increasing severity and frequency, abnormal CNS exam, worse lying down, morning vomiting |

### Febrile Seizures
- Commonly in infants and young children 6 months to 5 year olds with febrile illness
- Associated with fever but without evidence of: 1) intracranial infection, 2) metabolic disturbance, or 3) history of previous afebrile seizures
- Differential Diagnosis: Rigors, CNS infection, genetic epilepsy with febrile seizures

**Table 24.** Presentation and management of febrile seizures

| KEY SYMPTOMS | PHYSICAL EXAM FINDINGS | INVESTIGATIONS | MANAGEMENT |
|---|---|---|---|
| Simple febrile seizures<br>• Short (<15 min), generalized seizure occurring once in 24h period<br>• No focal neurological findings before or after seizure<br><br>Complex febrile seizures<br>• Prolonged (>15 min), focal, multiple in a 24h period | Look for evidence of alternative etiology such as meningitis, structural abnormality in the brain (altered LOC, bulging fontanelle, focus of infection) | **Usually not required, done to rule out underlying cause:**<br><br>Bloodwork, neuroimaging, EEG<br><br>Lumbar puncture (if suspect meningitis) | Treat the underlying cause of the fever<br><br>Reassure and educate the parents<br><br>Usually spontaneously resolve<br><br>If persist >5 minutes: IV Benzodiazepines (diazepam, lorazepam) |

PEDIATRICS

## 5.9 Dermatological

### Diaper rash / dermatitis
- Consider nutritional deficiency (e.g. Zn) or Langerhans cell histiocytosis for diaper dermatitis that is unrelenting and severe despite proper treatment
- Treatment varies depending on etiology

**Table 25.** Differential Diagnosis of Diaper Dermatitis

| Disease | Primary Lesion | Secondary Lesion | Flexural Involvement | Other Sites |
|---------|----------------|------------------|---------------------|-------------|
| **Contact Irritant Dermatitis** | Shiny, red macules/ patches | Ulcerations, superficial erosions | Absent | None |
| **Seborrheic Dermatitis** | Yellow, greasy papules/ plaques on an erythematous base | Scales | Present | Scalp, Axillae, Trunk |
| **Candidal Dermatitis** | Bright red patches with peripheral scale, 'satellite lesions' | None | Present | Oral Thrush |

# 6. SPECIAL TOPICS

## 6.1 Genetic Disorders

**Table 26.** Common Genetic Disorders: Autosomal

| Condition | Cause | Signs |
|-----------|-------|-------|
| **Down's syndrome (Trisomy 21)**<br><br>1/650-1/1,000 live births | Chromosomal abnormality, extra chromosome 21 or Robertsonian translocation (less common); Associated with late' maternal age | • Hypotonia and microcephaly<br>• Epicanthal folds<br>• Upward slanting palpebral fissures<br>• Stenotic Eustachian tubes<br>• Single palmar creases<br>• Congenital heart and abdominal defects<br>• Mild to moderate cognitive impairment<br>• Frequent respiratory infections |
| **Edwards syndrome (Trisomy 18)**<br><br>1/5,000 births<br><br>Early mortality is most common but ~13% survive beyond 1 yr[17] | Chromosomal abnormality, extra chromosome 18; associated with late maternal age | • Growth retardation<br>• Simple, low-set ears<br>• Prominent occiput<br>• Micrognathia<br>• Overlapping fingers<br>• Rocker bottom feet<br>• Congenital heart, genital, and CNS defects<br>• Hypertonia |

**Table 27.** Common Genetic Disorders: Sex Chromosome

| Condition | Cause | Signs |
|-----------|-------|-------|
| **Klinefelter syndrome**<br><br>1/1,000 live male births | Aneuploidy of sex chromosomes, XXY in 80% of cases; associated with maternal age | • Long arms and legs, slim build<br>• Small testes 1-2 cm<br>• Gynecomastia<br>• Delays in language and emotional development<br>• Cognitive deficits variable; average IQ ~90<br>• Often not diagnosed until adolescence |
| **Turner syndrome**<br><br>1/2,000-1/5,000 live female births | Aneuploidy of sex chromosomes, usually XO | • Short stature<br>• Streak gonads<br>• Webbed neck<br>• Lymphedema<br>• Coarctation of aorta<br>• Hypoplastic nails<br>• Learning disabilities |

| Condition | Cause | Signs |
|-----------|-------|-------|
| **Fragile X syndrome**<br><br>1/5,000 male births (more severe presentation in male patients) | X-linked dominant, mutation of FMR1 gene | • Intellectual disability<br>• Associated with ADHD, autism<br>• Long narrow face, protruberant ears<br>• Joint hyperlaxity<br>• Macroorchidism |

## 6.2 Psychiatric and Behavioral Problems
- Some medical conditions may present with psychiatric/behavior problems, so a thorough history and physical exam is important in addition to a psychiatric assessment; see **Psychiatric** Chapter
- Refer to DSM-5 for specific diagnostic criteria

### Anxiety Disorders
- Note that transient development of age appropriate fears is common in childhood; therefore must evaluate degree of life disruption
- Watch for frequent repeat occurrences of anxiety related behaviors

### Attention Deficit/Hyperactivity Disorder
- Triad of inattentiveness, impulsivity, and hyperactivity such that behavior interferes with functional ability (social and academic)
- Hyperactivity can be associated with this disorder; not always present
- Signs: distractible, tendency to fidget, tendency to interrupt, low attention span

### Autism Spectrum Disorders
- Spectrum of developmental disorders characterized by[18]:
  - Deficits in social communication and interaction
    - Social initiation and response
    - Nonverbal communication
    - Social awareness and insight, ability to form relationships
  - Restricted or repetitive patterns of behaviour, interests, or activities
    - Atypical speech, movements, and play
    - Preoccupations with objects and topics
    - Rituals and resistance to change
    - Atypical sensory behaviours
- Checklist for Autism in Toddlers (CHAT screening tool) is available and has a good specificity, but a low sensitivity of 18%

### Depression
- Persistent depressed or irritable mood present for most of nearly every day, or anhedonia (markedly diminished interest/pleasurable activities)
- Signs and Symptoms:
  - Changes in sleeping patterns and appetite, inability to concentrate, feelings of worthlessness, fatigue, suicidal ideations and behaviors
  - Atypical presentations in adolescents include anger, oppositional behaviors, hypersomnia
- Highly associated with other psychiatric issues: anxiety, somatic complaints, relationship problems, academic concerns, drug usage
- Take suicide threats seriously; 80% of suicidal teens seek help beforehand

### Eating Disorders (Anorexia Nervosa and Bulimia Nervosa)
- Risk Factors: family history, low self-esteem, immaturity, poor family dynamics
- Expresses fears of obesity associated with alteration in perception of body image, and preoccupation with becoming or staying thin
- Disordered eating (especially anorexia) can be found as part of the "Female Athletic Triad": disordered eating, osteoporosis, and amenorrhea

**Table 28.** Anorexia Nervosa and Bulimia Nervosa

| | Anorexia Nervosa | Bulimia Nervosa |
|---|---|---|
| **Key Feature** | Intense fear of gaining weight. Persistent restriction of energy intake. Disturbance of body weight or shape perception | Recurrent binge eating with inappropriate compensatory behaviors (self-induced vomiting, laxatives, diuretics) |
| **Amenorrhea** | Yes | No |
| **Epidemiology** | 0.5% adolescent females 0.05% adolescent males Peak incidence 15-19 years old | 1-5% adolescent females Peak incidence early 20s |
| **Subtypes** | 1. Restricting (no compensatory behaviors) 2. Binge eating/purging | 1. Purging (vomiting, laxatives, diuretics) 2. Non-purging (compensatory behaviors: fasting, excessive exercise) |
| **Physical Signs** | Emaciation, muscle wasting, lanugo, hypothermia, starvation edema, bradycardia, arrhythmias | Muscle weakness, tooth decay, parotid gland enlargement, Russell's sign (knuckle calluses from self-induced vomiting), bloodshot eyes |
| **Body Weight** | BMI <18 kg/m$^2$ | Normal or higher than average |

## Aggressive Behaviors
- Oppositional Defiant Disorder
  - Negativistic, hostile, and defiant behavior
  - Features: losing temper, arguing with parents, refusal to comply with rules, blames others for mistakes, angry/resentful
  - Must cause clinically significant impairment in social, academic, or occupational functioning
  - May progress to conduct disorder; usually onset before 8 yr
- Conduct Disorder
  - Repetitive, persistent pattern of behavior in which basic rights of others and age-appropriate social norms/rules are violated
  - Features
    - Aggression: bullying, initiating fights, cruelty to animals or people
    - Property destruction: setting fires, destroying others' property
    - Deceitfulness or theft: lying to obtain goods, breaking and entering
    - Serious violation of rules: staying out, running away from home, truancy

## 6.3 Child Abuse
- Definition: Child maltreatment, sometimes referred to as child abuse and neglect, includes all forms of physical and emotional ill-treatment, sexual abuse, neglect, and exploitation that results in actual or potential harm to the child's health, development or dignity. Within this broad definition, five subtypes can be distinguished – physical abuse; sexual abuse; neglect and negligent treatment; emotional abuse; and exposure to intimate partner violence

## Physician's Role
- Mandatory Reporting Requirement: physicians are responsible for reporting any "reasonable grounds to suspect" child abuse; not reporting to Children's Aid Society is an offence (in Ontario)
- Physician's duty to report overrides provisions of confidentiality

## History
- Listen and believe reports with nonjudgmental and caring attitude
- Any statements made by a child about abuse should be recorded verbatim
- Using open-ended questions, obtain a thorough history of events leading up to injury, including the location and time of injury occurrence, who was present, and detailed events
- Red flags for non-accidental trauma include[19]:

PEDIATRICS

- Injury and history are not consistent
  - Mechanism, amount of force, developmental age of the child
- Inconsistent history
- Delay in seeking medical attention
- Multiple injuries
- Injuries of different ages
- Observe behaviors of child and caretaker
- Are caretaker responses appropriate and consistent?
- Does the child have exaggerated aggressiveness or passivity, or suggest sexualized overtones?

## Physical Exam

- Always do a complete physical exam (pictorializing on a diagram whenever possible), but especially noting the following:
  - **General:** height, weight, head circumference percentile
  - **H&N:** retina, behind the ears, eardrums, oral cavity for signs of occult trauma, frenula
  - **GU:** genitalia, rectum
  - **MSK:** bone and joint tenderness, fractures (new or healed), ROM
  - **Dermatological:** bruises, bites, cuts, scars, puncture wounds; unusual number, shape, and location warrant further investigation

## Common Disorders Related to Abuse

- Malnutrition; developmental delay
- Emotional difficulty: anxiety, depression, self-harm, suicide attempts, post traumatic stress disorder (PTSD)
- Head injury: leading cause of death from child abuse
- Physical and mental health problems as adults and high-risk lifestyle choices

**Table 29.** Indicators of Child Abuse[20]

| Type of Abuse | Signs and Symptoms | |
| | Behavioural Indicators | Physical Indicators |
| --- | --- | --- |
| **Physical Abuse**<br><br>Includes shaking, pushing, grabbing or throwing; hitting with hand; punching, kicking or biting; hitting with object; choking, poisoning or stabbing | · Cringe/flinch if touched unexpectedly<br>· Infants may have a vacant stare<br>· Delay in seeking medical attention<br>· Fear, anxiety, depression, low self-esteem, social withdrawal, poor school performance, self-harm | · Posterior rib fractures<br>· Distinct marks: cigarette burns, loop marks, belt buckles<br>· Untreated fractures<br>· Presence of several injuries over a period of time and/or in various stages of healing<br>· In abusive head trauma:<br>  • Minimal to no evidence of external trauma<br>  • Severe closed head injury, diffuse brain injury and swelling, subdural/subarachnoid and retinal hemorrhages<br>  • Fractures, especially posterior ribs |
| **Sexual Abuse**<br><br>Includes penetration; attempted penetration; oral sex; fondling; sex talk or images; voyeurism; exhibitionism; exploitation | · Age inappropriate play with toys, self or others displaying explicit sexual acts<br>· Age inappropriate sexually explicit drawing/description<br>· Bizarre, sophisticated or unusual sexual knowledge<br>· Prostitution and seductive behaviors | · Unusual or excessive itching in genital or anal area<br>· Torn, stained or bloody underwear<br>· Pregnancy; bruising, swelling or infection in genital or anal area, STIs |

**PEDIATRICS**

| Type of Abuse | Signs and Symptoms | |
| | Behavioural Indicators | Physical Indicators |
|---|---|---|
| **Neglect**<br><br>Includes failure to supervise leading to physical harm or sexual abuse; permitting criminal behavior; physical neglect; medical neglect; failure to provide psychiatric treatment; abandonment; educational neglect | • Frequent absence from school<br>• Delinquent acts, alcohol/drug abuse | • Pale, listless, unkempt<br>• Poor hygiene<br>• Failure to thrive without identifiable organic disease<br>• Indiscriminately seeks affection |
| **Emotional Maltreatment**<br><br>Includes threat of violence; verbal abuse; isolation or confinement; inadequate nurturing or affection; exploiting or corrupting | • Low self esteem<br>• Extremes in behavior, such as aggression, social withdrawal, desire to please others<br>• Psychiatric disorders like depression and anxiety; eating disorders; substance abuse | • May have increased physical health problems from chronic stress |
| **Exposure to Intimate Partner Violence**[21]<br><br>Includes direct witness to physical violence; indirect exposure to physical violence; exposure to emotional violence | • Poor academic performance<br>• Increased eating, sleeping, and pain complaints<br>• Increased use of health services for vague complaints such as headaches<br>• Behavioural disorders | • May have increased physical health problems from chronic stress |

# 7. APPENDIX

**Table 30.** Major Developmental Milestones

| GROSS MOTOR | FINE MOTOR | LANGUAGE (RECEPTIVE AND EXPRESSIVE) | SOCIAL/ BEHAVIOURAL |
|---|---|---|---|
| 1 month | | | |
| • Turns head side to side when supine | • Hands closed, thumb in fist | • Cries<br>• Startles to loud or sudden noises | • Calms down when comforted |
| 2 months | | | |
| • Briefly raises chin and chest when prone<br>• Briefly holds head erect when held upright | | • Has a variety of sounds (coos) | • Smiles<br>• Recognize and calm down to familiar gentle voice<br>• Follows movement with eyes |

PEDIATRICS

| GROSS MOTOR | FINE MOTOR | LANGUAGE (RECEPTIVE AND EXPRESSIVE) | SOCIAL/ BEHAVIOURAL |
|---|---|---|---|
| **4 months** | | | |
| • Head control (3 mths)<br>• Holds head steady when supported in sitting position<br>• Rolls prone to supine | • Hand regard (3 mths)<br>• Holds an object briefly when placed in hand<br>• Reach for objects if midline | • Turns head toward sound | • Laughs responsively<br>• Responds to people with excitement (leg movement /vocalizing) |
| **6 months** | | | |
| • Sits momentarily, tripod sitting | • Foot regard (5 mths)<br>• Transfers objects hand to hand<br>• Raking grasp | • Babbles | • Stranger anxiety begins |
| **9 months** | | | |
| • Sits well, no support<br>• Crawls or bum shuffles<br>• Pulls to stand<br>• Stands with support<br>• Starts cruising | • Pincer grasp | • Responds to 'NO' regardless of tone<br>• 'Mama' or 'Dada' nonspecific<br>• Non-verbal communication-starts pointing | • Makes sounds/ gestures to get attention or help<br>• Raises arms to be picked up/ held<br>• Develops object permanence<br>• Plays social games (peek-a-boo)<br>• Separation anxiety begins<br>• Seeks joint attention |
| **12 months** | | | |
| • Gets into sitting position without help<br>• Stands without support<br>• Walks while holding on | • Places cubes in cup with release<br>• Releases ball with throw<br>• Holds a cup to drink | • First word, up to 3 words (may not be clear)<br>• Follows simple commands (Don't touch, where's your toy?)<br>• Uses facial expressions, actions, and sounds to make needs known or to protest | • Responds to own name |
| **15 months** | | | |
| • Walks without support<br>• Crawls up stairs/ steps<br>• Attempts to squat to pick up toys | • Picks up and eats finger foods<br>• Imitates or scribbles<br>• Stacks 2 blocks | • Says 4-5 words (may not be clear)<br>• Looks at named object<br>• Imitates a few animal sounds<br>• Consistently points to needs/wants | • Looks at you to see how to react (e.g., after falling, when stranger enters room) |

PEDIATRICS

| GROSS MOTOR | FINE MOTOR | LANGUAGE (RECEPTIVE AND EXPRESSIVE) | SOCIAL/ BEHAVIOURAL |
|---|---|---|---|
| **18 months** | | | |
| • Walks forward pulling toys or carrying object<br>• Squats to pick up toy without falling<br>• Runs stiffly | • Stacks 3 blocks<br>• Eats with spoon | • Says >10 words (may not be clear)<br>• Points to a few body parts<br>• Uses familiar gestures and common expressions (i.e. waving, 'oh-oh')<br>• Follows directions when given without gestures, understands<br>• Identifies three body parts | • Shows affection towards people, pets or toys<br>• Points to show interest in something<br>• Makes eye contact when spoken to or playing together |
| **2 yrs** | | | |
| • Kicks a ball<br>• Plays in a squat position<br>• Runs well<br>• Jumps upstairs one at a time | • Puts objects into small container<br>• Turns pages one at a time<br>• Draws vertical or horizontal or circular strokes | • Combines 2 or more words<br>• 50% intelligible<br>• Understands 1 and 2 step directions<br>• Says >50 words | • Uses toys for pretend play (e.g., gives doll a drink)<br>• Copies actions (i.e., clapping hands)<br>• Parallel play<br>• Temper tantrums |
| **3 yrs** | | | |
| • Walks up stairs using handrail<br>• Stands on one foot briefly<br>• Rides tricycle | • Stacks 10 blocks<br>• Twists lids off jars or turns knobs<br>• Copies a circle | • Combines 3 or 4 words in sentence<br>• 75% intelligible<br>• Recognizes colors<br>• Understands 2 and 3 step directions | • Shares some of the time<br>• Plays make-believe games with actions and words, role-playing<br>• Plays alongside others comfortably, cooperative play<br>• Listens to music or stories for 5-10 minutes<br>• Toilet training |
| **4 yrs** | | | |
| • Walks up stairs alternating feet<br>• Hops on one foot | • Undoes buttons and zippers<br>• Dresses self with help<br>• Copies a cross | • Sings nursery rhymes<br>• 100% intelligible<br>• Understands 3-part directions | • Tries to comfort someone who is upset<br>• Fully toilet-trained by day |
| **5 yrs** | | | |
| • Stop, start and change direction when running<br>• Climb playground equipment easily<br>• Rides a bike | • Throws/ catches a ball<br>• Dresses and undresses with little help<br>• Copies a square and triangle | • Speaks clearly in adult-like sentences most of the time<br>• Counts to 10 and knows common colours/shapes<br>• Retells the sequence of a story | • Cooperates with adult requests most of the time<br>• Separates easily from parent/caregiver<br>• Group play |

# REFERENCES

1. Ministry of Health and Long-Term Care. Publicly funded immunization schedules for Ontario – December 2016. Available from: http://www.health.gov.on.ca/en/pro/programs/immunization/docs/immunization_schedule.pdf
2. Leduc D, Woods S. Temperature Measurement in Paediatrics. *Canadian Paediatric Society*. 2013.
3. U.S. Department of Health and Human Services. A pocket guide to blood pressure measurement in children. 2007; NIH Publication 07-5268.
4. Schafermeyer R. Pediatric trauma. *Emerg Med Clin North Am*. 1993; 11(1): 187-205.
5. Goldbloom RB. *Pediatric Clinical Skills*. Elsevier Health Sciences; 2010.
6. Jandial S, Foster HE. Examination of the musculoskeletal system in children: A simple approach. *Paediatr Child Health*. 2008; 18(2): 47-55.
7. Klein DA, Goldenring JM, Adelman WP. HEEADSSS 3.0: The psychosocial interview for adolescents updated for a new century fueled by media. 2014.
8. Anstine D, Grinenko D. Rapid screening for disordered eating in college-aged females in the primary care setting. *J Adolesc Health*. 2000; 26(5): 338-342.
9. Marcdante KJ, Kliegman RM, Jenson HB, Behrman RE. *Nelson Essentials of Pediatrics*, 6th ed. Philadelphia: Elsevier Saunders; 2011.
10. Leung A, Prince T. Oral rehydration therapy and early refeeding in the management of childhood gastroenteritis. Paediatr Child Health. 2006; 11(8): 527-31. Reaffirmed: 2016.
11. Ducharme FM, et al. Diagnosis and management of asthma in preschoolers: A Canadian Thoracic Society and Canadian Paediatric Society position paper. *Can Respir J*. 2015; 22(3): 135-43.
12. Becker A, et al. *CMAJ*. 2007; S12-S14.
13. Bickley LS, Szilagyi PG, Bates B. *Bates' Guide to Physical Examination and History Taking*, 10th ed. Philadelphia: Lippincott Williams & Wilkins; 2009.
14. Engel J. *Pocket Guide to Pediatric Assessment*. St. Louis: Mosby; 1989
15. Jaundice. Lecture for *CC3 Pediatric Seminar Series*. Toronto: University of Toronto; 2016.
16. Wong RJ, Bhutani VK. Pathogenesis and etiology of unconjugated hyperbilirubinemia in the newborn. Waltham, MA: UpToDate; 2017.
17. Nelson KE, Rosella LC, Mahant S, Guttmann A. Survival and surgical interventions for children with trisomy 13 and 18. *JAMA*. 2016; 316(4): 420-428.
18. Carpenter L. DSM¬5 Autism Spectrum Disorder. In: *Developmental & Behavioral Pediatrics, University of Washington Medical Center [Online]*. 2013.
19. Child Maltreatment. Lecture for *CC3 Pediatric Seminar Series*. Toronto: University of Toronto; 2016.
20. Trocmé N. Canadian incidence study of reported child abuse and neglect, 2008: Major findings. *Public Health Agency of Canada*; 2010.
21. Artz S, et al. A comprehensive review of the literature on the impact of exposure to intimate partner violence on children and youth. 2014.

PEDIATRICS

# CHAPTER 22:

# Pharmacology and Toxicology

**Editors:**
Waleed S. Ahmed, BHSc
Mark Shafarenko
Jane Wang, BSc

**Faculty Reviewers:**
Shinya Ito, MD, FRCPC
David Juurlink, BPhm, MD, PhD, FRCPC
Prateek Lala, MD, MSc

## TABLE OF CONTENTS

PHARM & TOXICOLOGY

# 1. DRUG PRESCRIBING PRACTICES

The following chapter provides a brief overview of common topics in practical drug prescribing and clinical pharmacology and toxicology. Please refer to the *Compendium of Pharmaceuticals and Specialties* (CPS), *United States Pharmacopeia Drug Information* (USP DI) or other pharmacology textbooks for more detailed information on the topics reviewed.

## 1.1 Common Abbreviations

Always consult the hospital formulary for approved abbreviations that are specific to each institution. To correct for common error-prone abbreviations, write out the order in full or use the correct abbreviation(s) (see **Table 1** and **Table 2**).

*For all error-prone abbreviations, it is best practice to write out the full order
Institute of Safe Medication Practices. List of Error-Prone Abbreviations, Symbols, and Dose Designations. 2013. http://www.ismp.org/tools/errorproneabbreviations.pdf

**Table 1.** Common Abbreviations for Medication Directions and Route of Administration

| Abbreviation | Interpretation |
| --- | --- |
| ac | Before meals |
| Amp | Ampule |
| BID | Twice a day |
| Cap | Capsule |
| cc | With meals |
| CVL | Central venous line |
| D5W | Dextrose 5% in water |
| GT | Gastrostomy tube |
| gtt | Drop |
| hs | At bedtime |
| IEN | In Each Nostril |
| IM | Intramuscular |
| IT | Intrathecal |
| IV | Intravenous |
| M or Mitte | Dispense this amount |
| mcg | microgram |
| mEq | milliequivalent |
| mg | milligram |
| mL | millilitre |
| NG tube | Nasogastric tube |
| NPO | Nothing by mouth (nil per os) |
| OTC | Over-the-counter |
| NS | Normal saline |
| pc | After meals (post cibum) |
| po | Oral route (per os) |
| pr | Rectal route (per rectum) |
| pv | Vaginal route (per vagina) |
| prn | When required (pro re nata) |
| q()h | Every () hour(s) |
| qAM | Every morning |

| Abbreviation | Interpretation |
|---|---|
| SC | Subcutaneous |
| SL | Sublingual |
| STAT | At once (statim) |
| Supp | Suppository |
| Susp | Suspension |
| TID | 3 times a day |
| TPN | Total parenteral nutrition |
| ud | As directed |
| v/v | Volume in volume |
| w/v | Weight in volume |
| w/w | Weight in weight |

Chabner D. The Language of Medicine. St. Louis; Saunders. 10th Ed. 2013.

**Table 2.** Common Error-Prone Abbreviations

| Full Order | Avoid Writing | Misinterpretations |
|---|---|---|
| Each ear | au | ou (each eye) |
| Each eye | ou | au (each ear) |
| Every other day | q.o.d. | QID (4 times a day) |
| Four times a day | QID | qd or q1d (once daily) |
| International units | IU | IV or number 10 |
| Intranasal | IN (instead, write IEN) | IM (intramuscular) |
| Left ear | as | os (left eye) |
| Left eye | os | as (left ear) |
| Microgram | μg (instead, write mcg) | mg (milligram) |
| Once daily | qd or q1d or OD | QID (4 times a day) OD (right eye) |
| Right ear | ad | od (right eye) |
| Right eye | od | ad (right ear) once daily |
| Units | U | number 0 |

## 1.2 Essentials of Writing a Prescription
- Name, address, and phone number of prescriber (and institution if applicable) - usually pre-printed on prescription pad
- Date of the written prescription
- Patient information: name and address
- Drug information and instructions: drug name, strength, route of administration (dosage form), frequency, and duration/timing
- Quantity to dispense (Mitte)
- Refill information (write 0 if no refills)
- Prescriber signature: write down the prescriber name if using an institution prescription pad
- May include allergies, date of birth/age, and weight of the patient where relevant (e.g. weight-based dosing)

Other points to consider when writing a prescription:
- Do not follow a decimal point with a zero (i.e. use 2 mg NOT 2.0 mg)

- Use zero before a decimal point when the dose is less than one whole unit (i.e. use 0.125 mg NOT .125 mg)
- Use commas for dosing units at or above 1,000 or or use full words
- Use complete drug names; do not abbreviate
- For narcotics and controlled substances
  - Write the total quantity (Mitte) to be prescribed OR ensure that it can be calculated based on the prescription (i.e. you cannot calculate total quantity for medications prescribed as PRN)
- Document or keep a copy of the prescriptions in the patient chart
- May include drug's indication for clarity (e.g. take 1 tab PRN back pain)

**Clinical Pearl: Narcotics and Controlled Substances[1]**
Since November 1, 2011, narcotics and controlled substances prescriptions in Ontario must include:
- The physician's College of Physicians and Surgeons of Ontario (CPSO) number
- The patient's government-issued ID number (same ID must be presented to pharmacist)

## 2. CLINICAL PHARMACOLOGY AND TOXICOLOGY

### 2.1 Factors Modifying Drug Actions and Localization
Individual factors may alter the effect of how the body absorbs, distributes, metabolizes, and eliminates a drug. The following are common modifying factors (see **Table 3**); for a complete list, a pharmacology text should be consulted.

**Table 3.** Factors Modifying Drug Actions and Localization

| Modifying Factor | Effect |
|---|---|
| Age | Children and the elderly may metabolize medications at different rates |
| Concurrent Illnesses | Renal disease, liver disease, cardiac failure, shock, and protein loss may alter pharmacokinetics |
| Concurrent Medications | May inhibit absorption, metabolism, and/or elimination<br>May produce additive, synergistic, or antagonistic pharmacodynamic effects |
| Food Intake | May alter the absorption of medications taken by mouth |
| Genetics | Genetic variations in drug metabolizing enzymes or target sites may increase toxicity or decrease effect |
| Pregnancy | Increased plasma volume, decreased protein binding, and changes in glomerular filtration rate may alter pharmacokinetics. Increased adiposity may alter volume of distribution and clearance of lipophilic drugs |
| Route of Administration | Each differs in rates or amounts of absorption and distribution:<br>• Oral (passive intestinal absorption, then first pass effect - this is the fraction of drug available to the systemic circulation after absorption)<br>• Rectal (local or systemic effects; hepatic portal circulation is bypassed, which minimizes first pass effect)<br>• SL (rapid diffusion into blood for direct systemic effects; no first pass effect)<br>• IV (no absorption barriers; no first pass effect; rapid effect; useful in continuous administration and in large volumes)<br>• IM (speed and duration of effect is dependent on formulation: aqueous [fast] or depot [sustained]) |

PHARM & TOXICOLOGY

| Modifying Factor | Effect |
|---|---|
| Route of Administration (continued) | • SC (slower than IV, similar to IM)<br>• Inhalation (rapid delivery across mucous membranes)<br>• Topical (local and direct effects) |
| Smoking | May affect drug absorption, distribution, metabolism and/or elimination |

Lew-Sang E. 1975. Aust Nurses J 4(10):21-22.
Brunton L., Chabner B., Knollman B. Goodman and Gilman's The Pharmacological Basis of Therapeutics. McGraw-Hill Education. 12th Ed. 2011. Section 1. Chapter 2.

## 2.2 Common Drug Interactions

Interacting agents can increase or decrease the actions of the following drugs (see **Table 4**). This list is not exhaustive (refer to drug monographs and other references for specific details and complete lists). Drug interactions may increase the risk for toxicity/overdose or may decrease the therapeutic response. Pharmacokinetic drug interactions commonly result from changes in absorption, distribution, metabolism, or elimination. Pharmacodynamic drug interactions may be additive, synergistic, or antagonistic. Genetic mutations in pharmacokinetic or dynamic pathways can alter efficacy and impact safety (pharmacogenetics). Changes in drug metabolism can often be predicted by consulting a table of known cytochrome P450 substrates (see **Online Resources** at the end of this chapter). Therapeutic drug monitoring may be required.

**Table 4.** Common Drug Interactions[2-5]

| Object Drug or Drug Class | Change in Drug Level or Effect | Precipitant Agent |
|---|---|---|
| **ACEIs and ARBs** | ↑ | Amiloride, cotrimoxazole, NSAIDs, spironolactone (additive hyperkalemia) |
| | ↓ | NSAIDs (antagonize hypotensive effect) |
| **Azole Antifungals** | ↓ | Antacids, H2-blockers, PPIs (increased gastric pH decreases absorption) |
| | ↓ | Barbiturates, rifampin (CYP3A4 induction) |
| **Benzodiazepines** | ↑ | Alcohol, opioids and other CNS depressants (additive CNS depression) |
| **β-blockers (CYP2D6 metabolism) (e.g. carvedilol, labetalol, metoprolol)** | ↑ | Fluoxetine, paroxetine (CYP2D6 inhibition) |
| **Calcium Channel Blockers** | ↑ | Azole antifungals, clarithromycin, erythromycin (CYP3A4 inhibition) |
| | ↓ | Barbiturates, carbamazepine, rifampin (CYP3A4 induction) |
| **Carbamazepine** | ↑ | Azole antifungals, cimetidine, clarithromycin, diltiazem, erythromycin, fluoxetine, fluvoxamine, isoniazid, verapamil (CYP3A4 inhibition leading to CBZ toxicity) |
| | ↓ | Rifampin, SJW (CYP3A4 induction) |
| **Codeine (prodrug of morphine)** | ↓ | Amiodarone, bupropion, fluoxetine, paroxetine (CYP2D6 inhibition leading to impaired morphine synthesis and reduced analgesia) |

| Object Drug or Drug Class | Change in Drug Level or Effect | Precipitant Agent |
|---|---|---|
| Cyclosporine | ↑ | Azole antifungals, clarithromycin, diltiazem, erythromycin, ritonavir, verapamil (CYP3A4 inhibition) |
| | ↓ | Barbiturates, carbamazepine, rifampin (CYP3A4 induction) |
| Dextromethorphan | ↑ | MAOIs (risk of serotonin syndrome): contraindicated |
| Digoxin | ↑ | Amiodarone, clarithromycin, diltiazem, erythromycin, verapamil (inhibition of PGP leading to increased absorption and reduced renal clearance) |
| | ↓ | Rifampin (induction of PGP clearance) |
| Diuretics | ↓ | NSAIDs (antagonistic) |
| HMG-CoA Reductase Inhibitors (CYP3A metabolism), does not include pravastatin and rosuvastatin | ↑ | Azole antifungals, clarithromycin, cyclosporine, erythromycin, grapefruit juice (CYP3A4 inhibition) |
| Lithium | ↑ | ACEIs, diuretics, NSAIDs (decreased renal clearance) |
| | ↓ | Theophylline (increased clearance: unknown mechanism) |
| MAOIs | ↑ | Anorexiants (e.g. amphetamines), other antidepressants (risk of serotonin syndrome): contraindicated |
| | ↑ | Sympathomimetics (risk of hypertensive crisis) |
| Nitrates | ↑ | Sildenafil, tadalafil, vardenafil (additive hypotensive effect): contraindicated |
| NSAIDs | ↑ | Anticoagulants, antiplatelets, ASA, SSRIs, warfarin (bleeding risk) |
| Phenytoin | ↑ | Amiodarone, co-trimoxazole, metronidazole (CYP2C9 inhibition) |
| | ↓ | Carbamazepine, rifampin (CYP2C9 induction) |
| Quinolones | ↑ | Drugs that can prolong QT interval (see p.385) |
| | ↓ | Antacids, calcium, iron, sucralfate: separate oral administration times by 2 hours |
| SSRIs | ↑ | MAOIs (risk of serotonin syndrome): contraindicated |
| | ↑ | NSAIDs (bleeding risk) |
| Sulfonylureas | ↑ | Amiodarone, co-trimoxazole, fluconazole, fluoxetine, fluvoxamine, metronidazole (CYP2C9 inhibition) |
| Sympathomimetics | ↓ | β-blockers (antagonistic) |
| | ↑ | MAOIs, TCAs (additive) |
| TCAs | ↑ | MAOIs (risk of serotonin syndrome): contraindicated |
| | ↑ | Amiodarone, cimetidine, haloperidol, SSRIs, terbinafine (CYP2D6 and 3A4 inhibition) |
| | ↓ | Barbiturates, rifampin (CYP3A4 induction) |
| Theophylline | ↑ | Cimetidine, ciprofloxacin, fluvoxamine (CYP1A2 inhibition) |

PHARM & TOXICOLOGY

| Object Drug or Drug Class | Change in Drug Level or Effect | Precipitant Agent |
|---|---|---|
| | ↓ | Rifampin, smoking (CYP1A2 induction) |
| Thiopurines | ↑ | Allopurinol (decreased metabolism) |
| Warfarin | ↑ | Acetaminophen, acute alcohol intake, allopurinol, amiodarone, azole antifungals, cimetidine, co-trimoxazole, fibrates, metronidazole (decreased metabolism) |
| | ↑ | Antibiotics (disrupts Vitamin K biosynthesis by gut flora) |
| | ↑ | ASA, antiplatelets, NSAIDs (bleeding risk) |
| | ↓ | Barbiturates, carbamazepine, phenytoin, rifampin (increased metabolism) |

ACEI = angiotensin conversion enzyme inhibitor, ARB = angiotensin receptor blocker, CBZ = carbamazepine, PGP = P-glycoprotein, PPI = proton pump inhibitor, SJW = St. John's wort

**Clinical Pearl: β-Blockers and Hypoglycemia**
β-blockers will mask symptoms of hypoglycemia except for sweating.

**Clinical Pearl: Histamine H2-Receptor Antagonists and Warfarin**
Less problematic alternatives to cimetidine from the same class are ranitidine and famotidine.

**Clinical Pearl: Penicillin Allergy[6]**
80% to 90% of patients who report a penicillin allergy are not truly allergic to the drug when assessed by skin testing. Patients who develop a rash while taking penicillins should not be labeled as penicillin allergic – the rash could, for example, be caused by an infection or other drugs – without considering other possibilities. For those patients who require penicillin and may have a history of allergic reaction, skin testing should be performed. However, many physicians will shy away from prescribing penicillins if the patient states an allergy.

**Clinical Pearl: Taking a Penicillin History[6]**
What to Ask:
• What was the patient's age at the time of the reaction?
• Does the patient recall the reaction? If not, who informed the patient of it?
• How long after beginning penicillin did the reaction begin?
• What were the characteristics of the reaction?
• What was the route of administration?
• Why was the patient taking penicillin?
• What other medications was the patient taking? Why and when were they prescribed?
• What happened when the penicillin was discontinued?
• Has the patient taken antibiotics similar to penicillin (e.g., amoxicillin, ampicillin, cephalosporins) before or after the reaction? If yes, what was the result?

## 2.3 Drugs That Can Prolong QT Interval

The following are selected medications that can prolong the QT interval with risk of inducing torsade de pointes arrhythmia when used according to labeling[6,7] (for more drugs, see **Online Resources** at the end of this chapter). Prior to prescribing these drugs, consideration should be given to duration of therapy, concurrent QT-prolonging drugs, and drug interactions. The patient should be assessed for risk factors including electrolyte abnormalities, congenital long QT

**PHARM & TOXICOLOGY**

interval, female gender, age, bradycardia, and myocardial injury. Consultation with a specialist or drug information service for use and monitoring guidelines is recommended

**Table 5.** Common drugs that can prolong QT interval

| Class | Examples |
|---|---|
| **Antiarrhythmics** | Amiodarone<br>Procainamide<br>Sotalol |
| **Antibiotics** | Macrolides (azithromycin)<br>Quinolones (moxifloxacin)<br>Pentamidine |
| **Antipsychotics** | Chlorpromazine<br>Pimozide<br>Thioridazine |
| **Others** | Chloroquine<br>Citalopram<br>Domperidone<br>Methadone |

## 2.4 Special Populations

### Important Variations to Consider when Deciding on Drug Therapy in the Pediatric, Adult, and Geriatic Populations

- Changes in body composition as a percentage of weight (e.g. fat, total body water)
- Changes in protein binding
- Physical size: body surface area
- Maturation and degeneration: hepatic metabolism, renal clearance
- Developmental changes in expression of drug target and ADME genes

These factors affect the absorption, distribution, metabolism, and elimination of drugs, as well as their localization. Refer to drug monograph or pediatric drug references for guidelines on pediatric dose adjustments[8].

### General Considerations for Geriatric Patients

- Assess for non-drug alternatives
- Define goal for drug therapy
- Take a detailed drug history including OTC and herbal products; rule out drug-induced symptoms
- Refer to the Beers Criteria that lists medications to avoid in the geriatric population, particularly those with certain diseases or syndromes[9] (see **Online Resources** at the end of this chapter)
- Simplify the number of drugs taken and number of administration times to increase compliance
- Ensure the drug is at steady state before changing dosing

### Pregnancy

Proper counseling should be provided to pregnant women who use medications. When considering therapeutics in pregnancy, the baseline risk for congenital abnormalities, the risks of the medication (teratogenic and perinatal), the risk of foregoing treatment, and the benefit of treatment must be weighed. Please consult a teratogen information service for more information, such as Motherisk (Canada) or the Organization of Teratology Information Specialists (USA).

A historically used drug cataloging system is the US Food and Drug Administration (FDA) risk classification system. This arrangement classifies medications into Category A, B, C, D, or X. In brief, drugs in Category A have failed to demonstrate fetal harm at certain doses, whereas drugs in Categories B to X are considered to be teratogenic in increasing levels. Category X is most likely to cause fetal harm[10]. See **Online Resources** at the end of the chapter for specific definitions for each category. Not all teratogenic medications are absolutely contraindicated in pregnancy. Pre-pregnancy planning is advised for all patients using these medications. The following are select medications in each category[11].

- **Category X**
  - Danazol, methyltestorenone, isoretinoin, etretinate, diethylstilbestrol
- **Category D**
  - Coumadin derivative (warfarin; under classification X as per manufacturer)
  - Oxytetracycline, tetracycline, phenytoin, valproic acid, clonazepam, carbamazepine
  - Azathioprine, cyclophosphamide, vincristine
  - ACE inhibitors in 2nd and 3rd trimesters
- **Category C**
  - Ethosuximide, lamotrigine, mephenytoin
  - ACE inhibitors in 1st trimester
- **Category B**
  - Acetaminophen, ranitidine
- **Category A**
  - Doxylamine/pyridoxine

*Note:* These classifications do not always distinguish between human versus animal data, doses, or differences in frequency, severity, and type of fetal developmental toxicities. Differences in these factors will pose different risks (see **Online Resources** at the end of this chapter for further details). Moreover, this letter category system is not a grading system, but often misinterpreted as such.

Therefore, the FDA has recently published a new rule for medication labelling to replace this risk classification system. The so-called "Pregnancy and Lactation Labelling Rule" (PLLR) or "final rule", requires each medication label to list a summary of risks for three subsections: "Pregnancy", "Lactation", and "Females and Males of Reproductive Potential". The PLLR removes pregnancy letter categories, and requires drug labels to be updated when information becomes outdated.

**In general, the following are considered safe at their recommended doses in pregnancy[12-15]:**
- Acetaminophen
- Antacids
- Antihistamines (e.g. diphenhydramine, hydroxyzine)
- Beta-lactams (penicillins)
- Doxylamine/pyridoxine
- Flu vaccine
- Ranitidine

## 2.5 Approach to the Toxic or Poisoned Patient

Drug toxicity can result from drug overdose; altered drug absorption, distribution, metabolism, and elimination; drug-drug interactions; and idiosyncratic hypersensitivity. Altered mental status, seizures, or cardiovascular changes are a few of the many symptoms that may lead to the suspicion of poisoning. Contact the local poison control center for consultation. The following includes an approach to a poisoned patient after airway, breathing, circulation, and glucose level have been assessed.

- Take the history from family/friends, police officers, paramedics about what substance(s) were taken; often the history is unreliable and if possible, ask for any bottles, syringes, or household products that were found around the patient
- To aid in the differential of possible poisons, assess the following and determine any characteristic toxic syndrome (see **Table 6**)
- Assess vital signs including pulse, RR, BP, and temperature:
  - Observe the eyes for miosis, mydriasis, nystagmus, or ptosis (not usually indicative of toxic ingestion unless botulism)
  - Assess the color, dryness, and temperature of the skin
  - Auscultate for bowel sounds to determine ileus or increased sounds
  - Perform a neurological exam
- Order a broad toxicology screen (blood and urine)

PHARM & TOXICOLOGY

- Decontamination procedures (including administration of activated charcoal, whole bowel irrigation, and thorough removal of any substances on the skin surface that may be absorbed transdermally e.g., nicotine patches on a child) should be individualized according to age, properties of substance(s) ingested, and the time elapsed since ingestion

**Table 6.** Common Toxic Syndromes and Treatments

| Agents | Signs and Symptoms | Treatment |
|---|---|---|
| **Acetaminophen** | GI upset, hepatotoxicity | N-acetylcysteine to prevent liver injury; consult Rumack-Matthew Nomogram for acetaminophen toxicity |
| **Amphetamines and Other Stimulants** | Agitation, acute psychosis, HTN, tachycardia, hyperthermia, seizures, serotonergic effects (see below) | Benzodiazepines for seizure; phentolamine for HTN if needed; manage serotonergic effects (see below) |
| **Anticholinergic Agents** | Blurred vision, dry skin and mucous membranes, confusion, hyperthermia, flushing, urinary retention **(see Essentials of Emergency Medicine)** | General support; physostigmine in selected patients: rule out tricyclic antidepressants before using (see below) |
| **Antipsychotics** | CNS depression, anticholinergic effects (see above), miosis (sometimes mydriasis), dystonia, akathisia, cardiac conduction delays with ventricular tachydysrhythmias | Sodium bicarbonate for ventricular tachydysrhythmias; magnesium for torsade de pointes |
| **Aspirin (salicylate)** | Initial hyperventilation and respiratory alkalosis, followed by AGMA | IV fluids; sodium bicarbonate; dialysis |
| **Benzodiaz-epines** | Amnestic effects, confusion, respiratory depression | General support |
| **β-blockers** | AV block, bradycardia, hypotension, hyperkalemia, hypoglycemia | Catecholamines; insulin with dextrose; dialysis for select β-blockers |
| **Calcium Channel Blockers** | AV block, bradycardia, hyperglycemia | Calcium; high dose insulin with dextrose |
| **Carbon Monoxide** | Confusion, headache, nausea, tachypnea | Oxygen |
| **Cholinesterase Inhibitors** | Muscarinic: Abdominal cramps, diaphoresis, diarrhea, lacrimation, salivation Nicotinic: Fasciculations, HTN, tachycardia, seizure | Atropine for muscarinic symptoms; pralidoxime can be considered for patients with organophosphate poisoning (not carbamate poisoning) |
| **Digoxin** | Hyperkalemia (with acute overdose), variety of cardiac rhythm disturbances, visual changes (yellow-green predominance), vomiting | Digoxin antibodies; avoid calcium except with severe hyperkalemia (usually chronic toxicity with renal failure) |
| **Ethylene Glycol and Methanol** | AGMA, osmolar gap, respiratory depression, visual disturbances | Sodium bicarbonate to correct acidemia; fomepizole or ethanol to prevent toxicity; dialysis |

PHARM & TOXICOLOGY

| Agents | Signs and Symptoms | Treatment |
|---|---|---|
| **Iron Salts** | Vomiting, diarrhea, abdominal pain, GI bleeding, hepatotoxicity, coagulopathy, AGMA, seizure; radio-opaque tablets on abdominal X-ray | Sodium bicarbonate to correct acidemia; deferoxamine for systemic toxicity |
| **Opioids** | N/V, constipation, respiratory depression, bradycardia, lethargy | Naloxone (start with small initial doses in patients with opioid-dependence) |
| **SSRIs** | Serotonin syndrome, agitation, confusion, hyperreflexia, rigidity, tremors, diarrhea, diaphoresis, HTN, tachycardia, hyperthermia | Aggressive cooling; benzodiazepines; consider cyproheptadine; discontinue offending agent |
| **Tricyclic Antidepressants** | Initial HTN, followed by hypotension in severe overdose, tachycardia, arrhythmia, anticholinergic effects (see above) | Sodium bicarbonate for arrhythmia; avoid physostigmine |

AGMA = anion gap metabolic acidosis, AV = atrioventricular , HTN = hypertension. Longo DL, et al. (Editors). Harrison's Online, 18th ed. 2012.

Micromedex Online: POISINDEX Database. Greenwood Village: Thomson Reuters (Healthcare) Inc.; 2013.

## 2.6 Common Recreational Drugs
It is not uncommon for patients to be using street drugs in addition to prescribed medications. Knowledge about the health effects produced
by these drugs along with some of the various street terms is useful (see **Table 7**).

**Table 7.** Common Recreational Drugs

| Drug | Alternative Street Names | Short-Term Health Effects |
|---|---|---|
| **Amphetamine family (e.g. amphetamines, methamphetamines, dextroamphetamine)** | Amphetamine family: speed, bennies, glass, crystal, crank, uppers, pep pills Methamphetamines: speed, crystal meth, meth, chalk, ice, crystal, jib | CNS stimulant drug; increased alertness, energy, restlessness; increased blood pressure, respiratory rate; paranoia, hallucinations |
| **Benzodiazepines** | Benzos, tranks, downers | CNS depressant; often used in conjunction with opioids or stimulants (to decrease their effect); produces calming and relaxing effect |
| **Cannabis: includes marijuana, hashish, and hash oil** | Marijuana: grass, weed, pot, dope, ganja Hashish: hash Hash oil: weed oil, honey oil | Perceptual distortions, drowsiness, spontaneous laughter, euphoria, relaxation or anxiety; increased appetite and heart rate; decreased blood pressure and balance; apathy |
| **Cocaine** | Blow, C, coke, flake, rock, snow, marching powder, nose candy | CNS stimulant drug; increased alertness and energy, awareness of senses; decreased sleep and hunger; increased heart rate, temperature, blood pressure, restlessness, anxiety; cardiac toxicity |

PHARM & TOXICOLOGY

| Drug | Alternative Street Names | Short-Term Health Effects |
|------|--------------------------|---------------------------|
| **Crack** | Freebase, rooster, tornado | Smoking form of cocaine; see cocaine (above) |
| **Ecstasy/ Methylenedioxymet- hamphetamine (MDMA)** | E, XTC, Adam, the love drug | Effects of both a stimulant and a hallucinogen; stimulant effects include increased blood pressure, heart rate, temperature, sense of euphoria; hallucinogen effects include hallucinations, distortion of perception |
| **Gamma Hydroxybutyrate (GHB)** | Goop, G, liquid ecstasy, liquid x | CNS depressant; at low doses, can allow user to feel euphoric, less inhibited, and more sociable; at higher doses, dizziness, memory loss, decreased consciousness, breathing, heart rate; loss of coordination; chronic use can lead to severe withdrawal syndrome |
| **Gravol® (Dimenhydrinate)** | | Antinausea medication available over-the-counter; can cause euphoria and hallucinations |
| **Jimson Weed** | Jamestown weed, angel's trumpet, devil's trumpet, devil's snare, devil's seed, mad hatter, zombie cucumber | Plant that contains atropine and scopolamine; may lead to confusion, euphoria, hallucinations, delirium, and an anticholinergic toxidrome |
| **Ketamine** | K, special K, ket, vitamin K, cat tranquilizers | Anesthetic drug and hallucinogen; produces intense hallucinations and sense that mind is detached from body (dissociation); also loss of coordination, confusion, memory loss, increased sleepiness |
| **Heroin** | Big H, China white, Mexican brown, smack, junk, dope | Opioid type of drug; sedative effect; euphoria; detachment from physical and emotional pain; respiratory depression, constipation, miosis |
| **Lysergic Acid Diethylamide (LSD)** | Acid, blotter, microdot, windowpane | Hallucinogen; can experience sense of joy, confusion, anxiety; vivid visual effects and altered sense of hearing, smelling, taste; GI upset, tremors, tachycardia |
| **Mescaline** | Cactus, cactus heads, cactus buttons, buttons, mesc, mese | Hallucinogen; abnormal visual perception, anxiety, paranoia; hyperreflexia |
| **Opioids (such as oxycodone, fentanyl)** | Hillbilly heroin, killers, OC, oxy, oxycotton, oxy80 | Opioid, sedative effect; respiratory depression (may be fatal); euphoria |
| **Phencyclidine (PCP)** | Angel dust, dust, crystal joint, tic tac, zoom, boat | Hallucinogen; hallucinations, anxiety, panic, increased heart rate, blood pressure, drowsiness, lack of coordination; agitation, hostility |

PHARM & TOXICOLOGY

| Drug | Alternative Street Names | Short-Term Health Effects |
|---|---|---|
| Psilocybin | Mushrooms, shrooms, magic mushrooms, musk, magic | Hallucinogen; hallucinations, calming effect, anxiety, panic, increased heart rate, blood pressure, drowsiness, lack of coordination |
| Rohypnol (Flunitrazepam) | Roofies, roachies, rope, rophies, ruffies, "date rape" drug | CNS depressant (part of the benzodiazepine family); calming effect, drowsiness, loss of consciousness at higher doses |
| Steroids | Juice, pumpers, weight trainers, roids | Increased muscle bulk, energy, irritability, anxiety, aggression; reduced fertility |

Longo DL, et al. (Editors). Harrison's Online, 18th ed. 2012.
Hindmarsh WK. Drugs: What your Kid Should Know. Gauteng: Pharmacy and Apotex Continuing Education; 2000.

## 2.7 Important Pharmacokinetic Formulae

### Clearance

$$Cl = \frac{\text{rate of drug elimination}}{\text{plasma drug concentration}}$$

### Creatinine Clearance (measured)

$$CrCl = \frac{U_{Cr} \times V}{P_{Cr}}$$

where CrCl = creatinine clearance, $U_{Cr}$ = creatinine concentration in collected urine sample, V = urine flow rate, $P_{Cr}$ = plasma creatinine concentration

### Single IV dose plasma concentration:

$$C = C_0 \, e^{-kt}$$

### Elimination rate constant:

$$k_e = \frac{Cl}{V_d} = \frac{(\ln C_1 - \ln C_2)}{(t_1 - t_2)}$$

### Estimated CrCl (Cockcroft Gault)

$$CrCl = \frac{1.23 \times Wt \times (140 - Age)}{Cr} \quad (\times 0.85 \text{ for females})$$

where CrCl = estimated creatinine clearance [mL/min], wt = weight in kg, age = years, Cr = serum creatinine [µM]

### Volume of Distribution

$$V_d = \frac{\text{amount of drug in body}}{\text{plasma drug concentration}}$$

PHARM & TOXICOLOGY

## Elimination Half-life

$$t_{1/2} = \frac{(0.693)(V_d)}{Cl} = \frac{(0.693)}{k_e}$$

## Ideal Body Weight (IBW)
- For Males:    IBW = 50.0kg + [2.3kg x (height in inches - 60)]
- For Females:   IBW = 45.5kg + [2.3kg x (height in inches - 60)]

Doses for certain drugs (e.g. acyclovir) should be calculated with IBW to avoid toxicity

## Steady State Drug Concentration (Css)

$$C_{ss} = \frac{(F)(\text{rate of drug administration})}{Cl}$$

where F = bioavailability fraction of dose, rate of drug administration = dose/time

### Loading Dose (LD)

$$LD = \frac{(C_p)(V_d)}{F}$$

where Cp = target plasma drug concentration, F=1 for IV drug and F<1 for oral drug

### Maintenance Dose (MD)

$$MD = \frac{C_p \text{ x } Cl \text{ x } \tau}{F}$$

where τ = dosing interval

- With Renal Impairment

$$MD = \frac{CrCl \text{ (patient)}}{CrCl \text{ (normal)}} \times \text{Standard Dose of Drug}$$

where CrCl = creatinine clearance (when drug is renally excreted)

## 2.8 Online Resources
- Cytochrome P450 Drug Interaction Table. Indiana University School of Medicine. www. drug-interactions.com
- QT Prolongation Drugs. Credible Meds. http://crediblemeds.org
- Beers Criteria. American Geriatrics Society. http://www. americangeriatrics.org/health_ care_professionals/clinical_practice/ clinical_guidelines_recommendations/2012
- FDA Pregnancy Categories. http://depts.washington.edu/druginfo/ Formulary/Pregnancy. pdf
- FDA Summary of Proposed Rule on Pregnancy and Lactation Labeling.http://www.fda. gov/Drugs/DevelopmentApprovalProcess/DevelopmentResources/Labeling/ucm093307. htm
- LactMed: for guidelines on medication usage during breastfeeding https://toxnet.nlm.nih. gov/newtoxnet/lactmed.htm
- For quick calculations, consider apps such as Calculate by QxMD, Epocrates, or RxCalc

PHARM & TOXICOLOGY

# REFERENCES

1. Ontario Ministry of Health and Long-Term Care. Ontario Public Drug Programs: Narcotics Monitoring System (NMS) Pharmacy Reference Manual. 2012. Available from: http://www.health.gov.on.ca/english/providers/program/drugs/resources/pharmacy_manual.pdf

2. Katzung B, Masters S, Trevor A. Basic and Clinical Pharmacology. New York: Lange Medical Books/McGraw-Hill, Medical Publications Division; 2012.

3. Regal R, Ong Vue C. Drug interactions between antibiotics and select maintenance medications: Seeing more clearly through the narrow therapeutic window of opportunity. Consult Pharm. 2004; 19(12):1119-1128.

4. Lesher BA. Clinically important drug interactions. Detail-Document #200601. Pharmacist's Letter. 2004; 20(6):200601.

5. Juurlink D. 2011. Drug Interactions for the Front-Line Clinician. Oral Presentation. Toronto, Ontario, Canada.

6. Arizona Center for Education and Research on Therapeutics (CERT). Drug Lists by Risk Groups: Drugs that Prolong the QT Interval and/or Induce Torsades de Pointes. 2013. Available from: http://www.azcert.org/medical-pros/drug-lists/drug-lists.cfm

7. Gowda RM, Khan JA, Wilbur SL, Vasavada BC, Sacchi TJ. Torsade de pointes: The clinical considerations. Int J Cardiol. 2004; 96(1):1-6.

8. Allegaert K, Verbesselt R, Naulaers G, van den Anker JN, Rayyan M, Debeer A, et al. Developmental pharmacology: Neonates are not just small adults... Acta Clin Belg. 2008; 63(1):16-24.

9. American Geriatrics Society Beers Criteria Update Expert Panel. American Geriatrics Society Updated Beers Criteria for potentially inappropriate medication use in older adults. J Am Geriatr Soc. 2012; 60(4):616-631.

10. Bánhidy F, Lowry B, Czeizel A. Risk and benefit of drug use during pregnancy. Int J Med Sci. 2005; 2(3):100-106.

11. Briggs GG, Freeman RK, Yaffe SJ. Drugs in Pregnancy and Lactation: A Reference Guide to Fetal and Neonatal Risk. London: Lippincott Williams & Wilkins; 2008.

12. Babb M, Koren G, Einarson A. Treating pain during pregnancy. Can Fam Physician. 2010; 56(1):25,27.

13. Schaefer C, Peters PWJ, Miller RK. Drugs During Pregnancy and Lactation. Amsterdam: Elsevier; 2007.

14. Einarson A, Maltepe C, Boskovic R, Koren G. 2007. Treatment of nausea and vomiting in pregnancy: An updated algorithm. Can Fam Physician. 2007; 53(12):2109-2111.

15. Law R, Maltepe C, Bozzo P, Einarson A. Treatment of heartburn and acid reflux associated with nausea and vomiting during pregnancy. Can Fam Physician. 2010; 56(2):143-144.

16. Madadi P, Koren G, Cairns J, Chitayat D, Gaedigk A, Leeder JS, et al. Safety of codeine during breastfeeding: Fatal morphine poisoning in the breastfed neonate of a mother prescribed codeine. Can Fam Physician. 2007; 53(1):33-35.

17. Kalant H, Grant DM, Eds MJ. Principles of Medical Pharmacology. Toronto: Elsevier; 2007.

18. Motherisk. Pregnancy and Breastfeeding Resources. 2013. Available from: http://www.motherisk.org/women/index.jsp

19. Garner J. The Rational Clinical Examination: Evidence-Based Clinical Diagnosis, edited by David L. Simel, MD, MHS, and Drummond Rennie, MD.Proceedings (Baylor University Medical Center). 2010; 23(1):0087.

# CHAPTER 23:

# Psychiatry

**Editors:**
Graham Mazereeuw, PhD
Jeremy Zung, MD

**Resident Reviewer:**
Zenita Alidina, MD

**Faculty Reviewers:**
Nathan Herrmann, MD, FRCPC
Ayal Schaffer, MD, FRCPC
Albert H.C. Wong, MD, PhD, FRCPC

## TABLE OF CONTENTS

# 1. APPROACH TO THE PSYCHIATRIC EXAMINATION

## Keys to a comfortable interview:
- Find a private room with a wall clock (avoid checking wristwatch)
- Have a box of facial tissues ready
- Avoid desks between the patient and physician, if possible
- Reiterate your commitment to confidentiality (exceptions include: harm to self/others/ children under 16, driving safety, and if required for court proceedings)
- Normalize answers to difficult questions, e.g. "Sometimes people in difficult situations like yours start to think life is not worth living. Does that describe you?"
- If the patient has a history of violence against others, review de-escalation techniques that have worked previously, notify staff when you enter the room, ensure your unrestricted access to the exit, clear the environment of potential weapons (loose objects, ties, scarves, furniture that is not readily movable, etc.), request security to be at hand

## Special Considerations
- Observation during history-taking provides the content of the dynamic mental status examination
- Introspection as to how examiner feels about the patient (counter-transference) is helpful for inferring how patient's friends/family feel
- Seek collateral for history: As some patients may lack insight (psychosis) or be hesitant to admit certain information (especially substance use, cognitive impairment), seeking information from collateral sources (relative, colleague, social worker, and health care professional) is almost always helpful. Consider the following:
  - What is this patient normally like at baseline?
  - What has been the major change in behaviour?
  - What specific encounter occurred and when?

## Different patient demeanours:

**Table 1.** Tailor your strategy to the patient's demeanour.

| Demeanour | Strategies |
|---|---|
| Agitated | • Focus on most relevant/important symptoms |
| | • Keep your voice calm |
| | • Avoid gestures that may suggest an imminent attack/ defense (e.g. hands behind back, hands raised in defense) |
| | • Avoid touching the patient to help calm him/her down |
| | • Allow patient plenty of personal space |
| Shutdown | • Try to engage patient in an area of conversation that is of interest to him/her (music, sports, politics, etc.) |
| | • Avoid sensitive topics |
| | • Avoid long pauses |
| | • Increase ratio of open-ended to closed-ended questions, often with several consecutive open-ended questions |
| Rationalizing | • Collateral sources of information may be extremely valuable |
| | • Be nonjudgmental |
| Unfocused | • Try to avoid gestures and sounds (note-taking included) that "feed the patient's lack of focus"[1] |
| | • Avoid structuring the patient too early: during the open-ended phase of the CC/HPI, let the patient explore his or her thoughts |
| | • Gradually increase the ratio of closed-ended to open-ended questions |
| | • Attempt to interject and focus the patient, gently at first, but more directly over time |
| | • Inform the patient that he or she is unfocused |

| Demeanour | Strategies |
|-----------|-----------|
| **Tearful** | • Allow patient some uninterrupted time to talk/cry |
|  | • Interject sensitively: patients may experience this as containing and organizing |
|  | • Monitor nonverbal cues, language, tone |
|  | • Say something comforting ("This must be very hard for you") |
|  | • The moment immediately after crying subsides is a good opportunity to learn more about the patient's pain |

Goldbloom DS (Editor). Psychiatric Clinical Skills. Philadelphia: Mosby Elsevier; 2006. Shea S. Psychiatric Interviewing: The Art of Understanding. Philadelphia: W.B. Saunders Company; 1988.

## 2. COMMON CHIEF COMPLAINTS AND DIFFERENTIALS

| Chief Complaint | Differential Diagnosis | Distinguishing Features |
|-----------------|------------------------|-------------------------|
| Sadness or euphoria (altered mood) | Major Depressive Episode | 2 weeks continuous depressed mood and anhedonia |
|  | Persistent depressive disorder (dysthymia) | 2 years continuous depressed mood and anhedonia |
|  | Bereavement | Response to a loss, waxing and waning, lasts <1 year |
|  | Bipolar I | Mania (1 week or hospitalized); functional in-between, unlike schizophrenia |
|  | Bipolar II | Hypomania (not psychotic, not hospitalized, ~4 days); greater depression, heritability |
| Hallucinations or delusions (Psychosis) | Schizophrenia | 6 months delusions, hallucinations, disorganized speech/behaviour, negative symptoms, dysfunctionality without substance use |
|  | Schizophreniform Disorder | 1-6 months psychosis |
|  | Brief Psychotic Disorder | 1 day-1 month psychosis |
|  | Major Depressive Disorder | Prominent depressed mood, often nihilistic delusions |
|  | Schizoaffective Disorder | Psychosis remains 2 weeks after altered mood abates |
|  | CNS injury (intoxication, temporal lobe epilepsy, tumour, stroke, brain trauma, neurosyphilis, lupus cerebritis, vitamin deficiency) | Past medical & ingestion history, localizing neurological deficits |

PSYCHIATRY

| Chief Complaint | Differential Diagnosis | Distinguishing Features |
|---|---|---|
| Anxiety | Generalized Anxiety Disorder | 6 months restless, fatigued, irritable, tense, disturbed sleep |
| | Panic Disorder | Recurrent panic attacks, transient 10-min palpitations, sweating, presyncope, trembling, dyspnea, chest pain, nausea, chills, paresthesias, fear of dying) |
| | Obsessive-Compulsive Disorder | Ego-dystonic thoughts, tension-relieving rituals, fear of contamination |
| | Post-Traumatic Stress Disorder | Exposure to actual or threatened death, intrusive memories, flashbacks, avoidance, irritability, and heightened startle |
| | Medical (Hyperthyroidism, Substance Use) | Associated syndrome/ toxidrome |
| Substance abuse | Alcohol | Breath odour, history, slurred speech, flushing |
| | Stimulants | Dilated pupils, hypertension, tachycardia, restlessness |
| | Sedatives | Orthostatic hypotension, lethargy, hypotonia |
| | Opiates | Pinpoint pupils, lethargy, hypotonia, flushing |
| | Hallucinogens | Hypertension, tachycardia, labile affect, delusional, hyperactive reflexes, flushing |
| Acute confusion/agitation | Delirium | Past medical history (drugs/intoxication, pain, infection, electrolyte disturbance, cardiac or brain ischemia); fluctuating course, night-time worsening ("sundowning") |
| | Dementia | Acute on chronic, gradual, or stepwise functional decline |
| | Psychosis | See above |
| | Borderline Personality Disorder | Long-term behavioural pattern: recurrent self-harm, fear of abandonment, extreme splitting, impulsivity, affective instability, sense of emptiness, intense rage, dissociation |

Black DW, Andreasen NC (Editors). Introductory Textbook of Psychiatry, 6th ed. Arlington: American Psychiatric Publishing; 2014.

## 3. FOCUSED HISTORIES
See **General History and Physical Exam** for a detailed approach to history taking. The following are elements of the history that are particularly relevant to the psychiatric exam:

### Past Psychiatric History
- Age of first symptoms and first contact with psychiatry
- Psychiatric hospitalizations: number of, diagnosis, treatment, outcome, date of last discharge (include psychiatric episodes for which patient did not see a mental health professional)
- Psychotropic medications (prescriber, indication, dose, adherence, and side effects), past psychotherapy or electroconvulsive therapy (ECT)

- Recent pregnancy (relevant to postpartum depression, mania, psychosis, etc.)
- Suicide attempts: lethality, medical attention, date of last attempt

## Collateral History
Note: Collateral history is key (especially in substance use, cognitive, or psychosis history), as patients may lack insight or minimize deficits out of shame
- What is this patient normally like at baseline?
- What has been the major change in behaviour?
- How much EtOH or recreational drug does he or she take?
- Ask for specific dates and accounts e.g. "She told me the same story three times in the last hour about how her neighbour was stealing her toothbrush." This is preferred to recording the interviewer's interpretation of the data, e.g., "She's just forgetting more things in her old age, and she's always been more suspicious."

## Past Personal/Developmental History
Summarize the patient's life from infancy to the present, with an emphasis on relationships with family and major life events (e.g. illness, divorce, deaths, etc.)
- Look for three themes[1]
  1. Recurring patterns of behavior
  2. Evolving sense of identity in "love, work, and play"
  3. Risk factors for illness (e.g. early childhood abuse, early loss of a parent, etc.)
- Can be divided into 5 phases[2]
  1. <u>Prenatal and perinatal</u>: maternal substance use; pregnancy/delivery complications
  2. <u>Early childhood (ages 0-3 yr)</u>: developmental milestones reached at usual age; temperament/childhood personality; attachment figures; separations; earliest memories
  3. <u>Middle/late childhood (ages 3-11 yr)</u>: development of gender identity; punishment; school performance; socialization, ability to make friends, etc. It is also very important to ask about neglect and abuse (verbal, physical, and/or sexual).
  4. <u>Puberty and adolescence</u>: early intimate relationships, sexual and nonsexual (if there are/were many, try to figure out why they usually ended, and what attracts the patient to others); school performance; extracurricular activities; friends; psychosexual development; experimentation with drugs and alcohol; onset of puberty and how it affected social relationships
  5. <u>Adulthood</u>: education; occupational history; marital and relationship history; sexual history; religion and spirituality; social activities; diet and exercise; current social support system; legal history; military history (if applicable); retirement (if applicable); bereavement (if applicable)
- Ask about the roles of parents during the patient's childhood[1]: "How would you describe your parents to someone who has never met them?"
- Ask about the patient's strengths, competencies, and interests as well. Patients who are not willing participants in psychiatric interviews may appreciate these questions[2,3]

## Family History of Psychiatric Illness
- Major psychiatric illness (symptoms, diagnosis, duration, treatment, response, hospitalization)
- Contact with a mental health professional
- Attempted or completed suicide
- Substance abuse
- Legal history

## History of Present Illness
- Invite patient to tell a bit about his or her story
- Consider precipitants from the three domains of "love, work, and play"[1]
  - Love: current familial and romantic relations, household environment, children, living arrangements
  - Work: occupation, source of income
  - Play: activities, habits, recreational drug use, OTCs

## Complaint-specific questions:

**Refer to Common Clinical Scenarios for greater detail on disorders (p. 607)**

Begin by normalizing answers to difficult questions, e.g. "Sometimes people in difficult situations like yours start to think life is not worth living. Does that describe you? [3]

Mood: Depressive symptoms, Anxiety, Manic symptoms
- Depressive symptoms:
  - "Have you been feeling down, depressed, hopeless, or blue?"
  - "How is it different from usual feelings of sadness for you?"
  - "Have you had little interest or pleasure in doing things that you usually enjoy doing?"
  - "Have you been feeling more tense, anxious, or irritable than usual?"
  - "Have you been thinking about death or about taking your own life?"
- Anxiety: including panic attacks, agoraphobia, obsessions, compulsions
  - "Do you ever feel overwhelming anxiety that is hard to control?"
  - "Do you find yourself worrying about a lot of different things?"
  - "Do you have worries or fears that you know are not rational but are unable to suppress?"
  - "Have you ever experienced a sudden uncomfortable attack of panic or fear?"
  - "Are you ever bothered by ideas that you can't remove from your head, such as being dirty? Do you have to perform certain actions over and over such as washing your hands or checking locks?"
- Manic symptoms:
  - "Have you had periods where you felt high and very different from your normal self?"
  - "Do you feel you are particularly important with special talents and abilities?"
  - "Have you had periods of racing thoughts and times when you can't sit still and need to finish a number of different projects?"
  - "Do you need less sleep than usual?"
  - "Have you done things that later caused you regret? Have you ever spent too much money or engaged in more sexual activity than is usual for you?"

Psychosis: Hallucinations, Delusions (see Mental Status Examination, p. 603)
  - "Have you ever heard voices talking to you or overheard conversations about you even when no one is visibly there?"
  - "Is anyone trying to find you and hurt you?"
  - "When watching TV or reading articles on the Internet, do you ever feel that there are special messages intended specifically for you?"

Substance Abuse
  - Phrase questions with an assumption of use[1] (e.g. "How much alcohol do you drink in a d/wk?" is better than "Do you drink?")
  - Alcohol (type of alcohol and weekly consumption)
  - Recreational drugs, tobacco, caffeine, marijuana
  - OTC medications, alternative medicines
  - Inquire about the reason for substance use

If alcohol abuse is suspected, the CAGE questions or the one-page AUDIT questionnaire are valid screening tools (average sensitivity = 0.71, specificity = 0.90 in psychiatric inpatients[4])
- C = "Have you ever felt the need to cut down on your drinking?"
- A = "Have people annoyed you by criticizing your drinking?"
- G = "Have you ever felt guilty about your drinking?"
- E = "Have you ever needed a drink in the morning to steady your nerves or get rid of a hangover (an 'eye opener')?"
  - $\geq 2$ affirmative responses suggests that formal investigation into alcoholism using DSM-V criteria is warranted[2]
  - Limitations of the CAGE questionnaire: does not perform as well in primary care settings, with women, or for detecting less severe forms of drinking
  - CAGE does not replace a full inquiry including symptoms of intoxication, withdrawal, dependence, and abuse (see Substance-Related Disorders, p. 611)

**PSYCHIATRY**

Disordered Eating & Body Dysmorphia
- ◆ "Are you happy with how your body looks and works?"
- ◆ "Do you find yourself constantly thinking about your weight? Food?"
- ◆ "Do you take any pills or supplements to lose weight?"
- ◆ "Do you ever cause yourself to vomit to lose weight?"

Cognitive Difficulties: memory, concentration, dementia
Collateral from family/friend is key
- ◆ "Does she need help now doing things that she could do just fine before? Finances? Driving? Cooking?"
- ◆ "Does the patient tend to repeat himself, have temper outbursts, be more demanding? Over what time period: stepwise or gradual? What specifically did you observe and when?"
- ◆ "Does the patient wake more at night, make accusations, engage in physical violence? Is he or she more suspicious of others lately?"

Somatic Symptoms
- ◆ Anorexia, weight loss/gain, insomnia/hypersomnia and pattern (trouble falling/staying asleep, early morning awakening), lethargy, agitation, decreased sexual energy or interest
- ◆ Neurological symptoms (e.g. seizures)
- ◆ Somatic problems with no known physical basis (psychosomatic)

## Suicide Risk Assessment
- • Risk factors for suicide: There are several sets of risk factors which may help you assess a patient's suicide risk. If possible, interview collateral sources (friends, family, etc.) about these risk factors and the presence of suicidal intent.
- • **SAD PERSONS** scale[5,6,7]
  - ◆ **S**ex: male
  - ◆ **A**ge >60 yr
    - ▪ In males, increased suicide risk also occurs in late adolescence[4]
  - ◆ **D**epression
  - ◆ **P**revious attempts (including aborted attempts and self-harm)
  - ◆ **E**thanol abuse
  - ◆ **R**ational thinking loss (psychosis, helplessness, hopelessness)
  - ◆ **S**uicide in family
  - ◆ **O**rganized plan
  - ◆ **N**o spouse/no support systems
  - ◆ **S**erious illness, intractable pain

**Clinical Pearl: SAD PERSONS Scale and Suicide Risk**
Do not rely solely on the SAD PERSONS scale to assess suicide risk, as it has been found to have low sensitivity and positive predictive value when predicting future suicide attempts.[8]

- • Shea's "Triad of Lethality"[11]
  1. Recent suicide attempt
  2. Acute psychosis suggesting lethality
  3. Elements from history that strongly suggest that the patient intends to harm him/herself

Psychotic processes: these should be actively and carefully explored if they arise during the interview[3].
- • Command Hallucinations: hearing voices that tell the patient to perform an act
- • Sense of Alien/Outside Control: the sensation that one's body is being controlled externally
- • Religious Preoccupation: performing suicidal (or homicidal) acts to please a higher power; preoccupation with certain verses from religious texts suggesting violence

Other considerations:

PSYCHIATRY

- Quality of the social environment: What will the patient return to if discharged? Are the family/friends supportive? Does the patient have unresolved interpersonal conflicts?
- Rapid change in medical condition: positive or negative, as this may indicate increased risk[3]
- Resilience factors: "What has kept you from committing suicide?" Determine if he/she has a "framework for meaning" (e.g. religion, cultural heritage, social obligations, children) that may deter him/her from suicide

## Suicidal Ideation (SI) and Lethality Assessment

### General approach
- Be aware of your own reactions/attitudes toward suicide and suicidal patients. Monitor these feelings when discussing SI with patients to ensure that they do not discourage disclosure
- Patients may give nonverbal cues of deception or anxiety when discussing SI; note-taking may hinder observation of such cues

### Chronological Assessment of Suicidal Events (CASE) approach[9]
1. Assess present SI or suicide event
2. Assess any SI over the preceding 2 months
3. Assess past SI
4. Assess any immediate SI

Note: When using this framework, inquire about all pertinent characteristics of SI noted above

### Inquiring about SI
General Advice:
- If a patient spontaneously mentions a particular method of suicide, he/she has likely considered that method
- If patient initially denies active SI, ask again later

Indirect:
- Ambiguous questions may spontaneously elicit SI: "Have you ever thought of a way of ending your pain?"
- Explore areas such as depression, psychosis, stressful life events, or abrupt social changes; disclosure of SI may naturally arise
  - May also inquire about passive ideation: "Have you ever thought life was not worth living?"

Direct:
- "Sometimes people who feel like you have been thinking about committing suicide. Do you ever feel that way?"
  - This approach helps normalize and reduce anxiety
- "Have you had thoughts of killing yourself/ taking your life/committing suicide?"

>
> **Clinical Pearl: Suicide**
> Discussing suicidal thoughts and plans does not put ideas into a patient's head. It is important to screen every patient for suicidal tendencies.

### SI Lethality Assessment
- Frequency
- Duration
- Pervasiveness (fleeting, sustained)
- Impulsivity of the patient
- Extent and details of any suicide plans: lethality of method; availability of method; likelihood of rescue; motive
- Extent and details of any action taken

### Management of SI
This is an emergency! Ensure that your patient goes to the emergency department to be referred for a psychiatric consultation.

PSYCHIATRY

If patient does not or cannot agree to this plan, he/she may be issued a Form 1 (see Mental Health Act Forms, p. 611); note that this form only applies in Ontario Hospitalization may be necessary (voluntary or involuntary)

**Note:** The utility of having a patient "contract for their safety" (no-suicide agreement) is highly controversial and should NEVER replace/supersede a clinical assessment

## 4. MENTAL STATUS EXAMINATION

The MSE, the psychiatrist's "physical examination", should be done with every patient at every visit.

Mnemonic: The MSE is **ASEPTIC**
- Appearance, behaviour, and motor activity
- Speech
- Emotions (mood and affect)
- Perception
- Thought content and process
- Insight and judgement
- Cognition

### 4.1 Appearance, Behaviour, and Motor Activity

**Appearance**
- Apparent vs. chronological age
- Dress appropriateness
- Grooming/hygiene
- Distinguishing physical features (including scars, tattoos)
- Facial expression
- Physical build
- Apparent physical health and presence of any physical limitations
- Get a sense of what the appearance says about the patient's self-esteem, interests, activities, attitudes, etc.

**Behavior**
- Does the patient exhibit acute distress?
- Patient's attitude toward examiner: cooperative, disinterested, agitated, guarded, seductive
- Appropriateness of attitude to context (e.g. whether patient sought help voluntarily or against his/her will)

**Motor Activity**
- Posture: slumped, stiffened
- Facial expression and eye contact: tearful, fearful/anxious
- Mannerisms
- Presence of nail biting, arms hugging the body, and echopraxia
- Agitated behavior (e.g. hair pulling, hand wringing)
- Presence of repetitive or involuntary movements (e.g. tics, chorea, tremor)
- Presence of tremor, jitteriness, lip-smacking, or tongue rolling that may indicate tardive dyskinesia (TD), akathisia, or medication-induced parkinsonism[3]
- *Note:* any abnormalities in motor activity should be further investigated with a neurological examination

### 4.2 Speech

Mnemonic: **FLAVouR**
- Fluency
  - Gross fluency of English language
  - Subtler issues such as stuttering, word finding difficulties, nonfluent aphasias, etc.
- Latency of response: there should normally be a short pause
- Amount: normal, increased, decreased
- Volume, tone: loud, soft, timid, angry, irritable, anxious, juvenile, insulting, etc.

- **R**ate: slowed, pressured/rapid

### 4.3 Emotions (Affect and Mood)
- Affect: patient's mood as observed by you (**OBJECTIVE**)
  - Quality: euthymic, depressed, elevated, anxious
  - Range: full, constricted, flat (an extreme form of constricted affect)
  - Intensity/Quantity: mild, moderate, severe
  - Stability: continuum from stable to labile
  - Appropriateness to thought content
- Mood: patient's mood as described by the patient (**SUBJECTIVE**)

### 4.4 Perception
Note the presence or absence of the following, as appropriate:
- Hallucinations: sensory perception in the absence of external stimuli[2]
  - Most frequently auditory, but can occur in all five modalities
  - Describe how patient feels and what he/she subjectively experiences during hallucinations, when they occur, and how often they occur
  - For auditory hallucinations, describe whether patient hears words, commands, or conversations
- Illusions: misperception of a real external stimulus[2]
- Depersonalization: a sense that one feels unreal, or has been detached from one's body[2]
- Derealization: a sense that one's surroundings have become unreal[3]

### 4.5 Thought Content
**Thought Content:** ideas/themes the patient communicates (**WHAT** the patient is thinking about)
- Obsessions: recurrent, often anxiety-provoking thoughts that the patient cannot suppress[2] (e.g. fear of contamination, obsession with order)
- Delusions: fixed, false beliefs that the patient maintains despite contradictory evidence, and which cannot be accounted for by the beliefs of a religious, cultural, or subcultural group.[2]
  - They can be classified into bizarre and non-bizarre delusions (see **Psychosis** for types of delusions)
    - Bizarre: content has no basis in reality (e.g. having a GPS tracking device inside one's body)
    - Non-bizarre: content is not true, but is within the realm of possibility (e.g. being followed/investigated by the government)
    - Determine the degree to which the patient challenges the delusion(s), how preoccupied the patient becomes, how consistent the delusion is, and the bizarreness of the delusion
- Preoccupations, phobias, somatic concerns
- Suicidal and homicidal ideation

Listed are some questions that can be useful when broaching the often sensitive issues of perceptual and thought content disturbances (see **Table 2**).

**Table 2.** Questions for Perceptual and Thought Content Disturbances

| MSE Subsection | Suggested Questions | Inquiring about... |
|---|---|---|
| **Perception** | "Have you ever felt as if the world around you suddenly changed or disappeared?" | Derealization |
| | "Have you ever felt as if you were outside your body and could watch yourself?" | Depersonalization |
| | "Have you ever heard/seen/felt/smelled/tasted anything that others could not?" | Hallucinations* |
| | "Have you noticed that you hear the voices of people speaking to you or about you when you are alone?" | Hallucinations (auditory) |

| MSE Subsection | Suggested Questions | Inquiring about... |
|---|---|---|
| **Thought Content** | "Do you have experiences that you think might be hard for others to understand?" | Delusions |
| | "Do you ever feel like you are being followed, watched, or spied on?" | Delusions (non-bizarre) |
| | "Do you ever feel like someone else is controlling your mind or body?" | Delusions (bizarre) |
| | "Do you ever feel like the television or radio was addressing you personally?" | Delusions of reference |
| | "Do you have thoughts that you can't seem to get out of your head, no matter what you do?" | Obsessions |

*Ask about only one modality at a time
Shader RI (Editor). Manual of Psychiatric Therapeutics, 3rd ed. Philadelphia: Lippin¬cott Williams & Wilkins; 2003.

**Thought Process**: the way that a patient comes to a conclusion (**HOW** the patient thinks)
- Components
  - Rate and flow of ideas
  - Coherence/logic
  - Presence/absence of goal-directed thinking
- Normal thought process is linear, organized, and goal-directed[2]
- Abnormalities of thought process
  - Blocking: patient cannot complete a thought, leading to cessation of speech
  - Perseveration: patient cannot seem to switch topics, and will continually return to the same topic despite attempts to change the subject
  - Circumstantiality: patient is indirect and includes irrelevant details, but eventually answers the question
  - Tangentiality: patient digresses from initial topic, and never returns to original point
  - Flight of ideas: patient rapidly "jumps" from one topic to another, but all topics are logically connected
  - Loosening of associations: patient moves between topics that are not logically connected
  - Word salad: jumble of words/phrases that is often repetitious and has no coherent meaning
  - Neologism: a fabricated/made-up word that is often incomprehensible
  - Clang association: a sequence of thoughts that is driven by the sounds of preceding words, often leading to rhyming or punning

## 4.6 Insight and Judgment
- Insight: the patient's degree of awareness and understanding of his/her illness and the potential causes. It can be good, partial, or poor.
  - "What do you think is going on with you now?"
- Judgment: the patient's ability to make sound decisions and to act accordingly.
  - Better determined by examining the decisions that the patient has made during the course of his/her illness rather than using hypothetical situations[2,6]

## 4.7 Cognition
- Asking patient to state age and date of birth as part of ID at the beginning of the assessment can be used as a quick cognitive screen
- Many cognitive screening tools are available, each with advantages and disadvantages (see **Cognitive Screening Tools**, p. 606)
- Levels of consciousness/alertness: hyperalert, alert, drowsy, confused, stuporous, unconscious
- Orientation: to time, person (others), place, and self
  - If patient has arrived on time to the appointment (by him/herself), orientation may not have to be assessed formally

- For time and place, ask questions from easiest to hardest: "What year is it? Month? Day of the week? Date?" or "What country are we in? Province? City? Road? Address?"
- Attention and concentration
  - Months of the year (forward and backward)
  - Digit span test (forward and backward)
  - Serial 7's subtraction test (or serial 3's)
  - Observing how the patient interacts in the interview will also indicate his/her attention and concentration
- Memory[5,6]
  - Immediate recall: name 3-5 unrelated objects, and have patient repeat them back
  - Delayed recall: ask patient to repeat the same 3-5 objects after roughly 5 min
    - If the patient has trouble, offer a hint (category hint first, then multiple choice)
  - Long-delayed recall: ask patient to repeat the same 3-5 objects after roughly 30 min
    - More commonly tested by neuropsychologists, less commonly by physicians
  - Recall of remote personal memory
    - Names and dates from patient's past, birthdays and anniversaries (spouse, parents, etc.)
  - Recall of general cultural knowledge
    - "Who was Christopher Columbus?"
- Abstraction
  - Take into consideration patient's education, IQ, native language, and culture
  - Proverb interpretation: "How would you explain the meaning of 'Don't judge a book by its cover'?"
  - Similarities test: "What is similar about apple and an orange" (Abstract answer: they are both fruit. The answer "they are both round" is the concrete response).

## Cognitive Screening Tools

**Table 3.** Common Cognitive Screening Tools

| Comparison of Cognitive Screening Tools | | |
|---|---|---|
| MMSE | Advantages | • Fast and easy to administer<br>• Long history of clinical use<br>• Focuses on short-term memory loss and recognition problems |
| | Limitations | • Not sensitive to early/mild changes in cognition<br>• Does not test executive functioning<br>• Emphasis on verbal ability<br>• Fee for usage (copyrighted)<br>• Affected by education levels<br>• Developed for English speaking patients but has been translated into dozens of languages |
| MoCA | Advantages | • Free<br>• More sensitive to mild or early cognitive changes (MMSE ≥24-26)<br>• Useful when patients have cognitive complaints but no functional impairment<br>• Better measures of apraxia, visuospatial function, and executive function vs. MMSE |
| | Limitations | • Slightly longer than MMSE (but not by much)<br>• Affected by education levels |

| | | |
|---|---|---|
| **Mini-Cog** | Advantages | • Not limited by education levels or language<br>• Similar sensitivity and specificity for dementia compared to MMSE<br>• Short testing time and easy to administer (three-item recall and clock drawing)[10] |
| | Limitations | • Limited cognitive dimensions are tested |
| **Clock-Drawing** | Advantages | • Score correlates with MMSE (high sensitivity, specificity, and inter-rater reliability)<br>• Fast and easy to administer (less than 1 min to conduct and score)[11]<br>• Widely used in clinical settings<br>• Tests visuospatial and executive functioning<br>• May be less affected by language and education |
| | Limitations | • Not a sensitive test for mild dementia<br>• Not a direct test of memory<br>• Multiple scoring schemes |

MMSE = Mini-Mental State Examination, MoCA= Montreal Cognitive Assessment

**Clinical Pearl: Caregiver Beliefs**
When caregiver believes that something is wrong, he/she is often correct.[1]

## 5. COMMON INVESTIGATIONS

**Laboratory Tests**: TSH, vitamin B12, folate, ferritin, CBC, electrolytes, calcium profile, blood glucose, blood culture, serum and urine toxicology screen, BUN, creatinine, liver enzymes and liver function tests, serum medication levels

**Imaging**: CT head (e.g. first episode psychosis), MRI head
CT imaging guidelines (according to 2006 CCCD recommendations)[12]:   A cranial CT scan is recommended in the context of the psychiatric examination if one of the following is present:
- ◆ Rapid (e.g. over 1-2 mo) unexplained decline in cognition or function or "short" duration of dementia (less than 2 years) and age <60
- ◆ Recent and significant head trauma
- ◆ Use of anticoagulants or history of bleeding disorder
- ◆ Unusual or atypical cognitive symptoms or presentation (e.g. progressive aphasia)
- ◆ Neurologic symptoms: new severe headache, seizures, localizing signs
- ◆ Early urinary incontinence and gait disorder

**MRI indication**: to monitor structural intracerebral disease, usually preferable to CT.

**Weight and BMI**: to monitor side effects of psychotropic drugs; health pertaining to psychiatric disorders

**ECG**: to monitor side effects of psychotropic drugs (e.g. QTc)

**Cognitive assessments** (see **Table 3**)

## 6. COMMON CLINICAL SCENARIOS

*Note:* The following sections are meant to assist in optimizing the interview process and setting for patients who present with psychiatric symptoms. For specific diagnostic criteria, classification, epidemiology, and differential diagnosis of psychiatric disorders, please refer to the DSM-IV or an equivalent manual. Clinical practice guidelines from the American Psychiatric Association (APA) are also available at http://psychiatryonline.org/guidelines.aspx.

PSYCHIATRY

| Key Symptoms | Physical Exam Findings | Investigations | Management |
|---|---|---|---|

**Anorexia nervosa**

| | | | |
|---|---|---|---|
| • Discrepancy between weight and perceived body image<br>• Fear of gaining weight<br>• Binging, purging, laxative, diuretic use | Psychiatric exam:<br>• Intense fear of gaining weight/prevention of weight gain<br>• Distorted perception of body shape/weight<br>• ↓ energy intake<br>Physical exam:<br>• BMI <16 (severe)<br>• Check vitals for hypotension, bradycardia, hypothermia<br>• Dry skin, lanugo hair, dependent edema, acrocyanosis | • CBC, lytes, Cr, glucose, beta hCG<br>• ECG | Non-pharmacologic:<br>Refeeding and positive reinforcement<br><br>CBT, IPT |

**Anxiety disorders**

| | | | |
|---|---|---|---|
| Panic attacks present with:<br><br>Students Fear the 3 Cs:<br>Sweating<br>Trembling or shaking<br>Unsteadiness or dizziness<br>Derealization or depersonalization<br>Excessive heart rate, palpitations<br>Nausea or abdominal distress<br>Tingling and numbness (paresthesia)<br>Shortness of breath or smothering sensation<br>Fear of loss of control, going crazy, or dying<br>Chest pain or discomfort<br>Choking sensation<br>Chills or hot flushes | Psychiatric exam:<br>• Worries or fears that patients knows are irrational but has difficulty suppressing, more days than not<br><br>Physical exam:<br>• None specific. | • Clinical diagnosis<br>• Rule out organic causes: CBC, lytes, TSH, hCG, urine toxicology | Non-pharmacologic:<br>CBT<br><br>Pharmacologic:<br>SSRIs (fluoxetine, fluvoxamine, paroxetine, sertaline), SNRIs (venlafaxine), buspirone, benzodiazepines |

PSYCHIATRY

| Key Symptoms | Physical Exam Findings | Investigations | Management |
|---|---|---|---|

**Bipolar disorder**

| Key Symptoms | Physical Exam Findings | Investigations | Management |
|---|---|---|---|
| • Extreme, atypical fluctuations in mood<br><br>• Mania/hypomania: elevated mood<br><br>• Depression: decreased mood | Psychiatric exam:<br>**GST PAIID**<br>**Grandiosity**<br>inflated self-esteem<br>**Sleep**<br>decreased need<br>» Highly "useful and reliable criterion for mania"[1]<br>**Talkative**<br>more than usual or feels pressured to talk<br>**Pleasurable activities**<br>performed to excess (e.g. spending, sex, substance abuse) with potentially harmful consequences<br>**Activity**<br>increase in impulsive or disinhibited behavior<br>**Ideas**<br>flight of (racing thoughts)<br>**Increased mood**<br>**Distractible**<br>by irrelevant environmental stimuli | • Clinical diagnosis | Pharmacologic:<br>Lithium, valproic acid, olanzapine, risperidone, quetiapine, aripiprazole, ziprasidone, carbamazepine, asenapine, paliperidone +/- SSRIs for depressive symptoms (if present) |

**Borderline personality disorder**

| Key Symptoms | Physical Exam Findings | Investigations | Management |
|---|---|---|---|
| • Impulsivity<br>• Unstable and intense interpersonal relationships<br>• Recurrent self-harm and self-mutilation | Physical exam:<br>• Wrist/arm scars<br>• Labile mood | • Clinical diagnosis | Non-pharmacologic:<br>DBT<br><br>Pharmacologic:<br>SSRIs, antipsychotics |

**Bulimia nervosa**

| Key Symptoms | Physical Exam Findings | Investigations | Management |
|---|---|---|---|
| • Binge eating<br>• Lack of control over eating during episode<br>• Compensatory behaviours to prevent weight gain (induced vomiting, excessive exercise, laxatives, diuretics) | Physical exam:<br>• Callus on dorsal hands<br>• Dental erosions, caries<br>• Parotid enlargement | • Lytes, Cr, liver enzymes<br>• ECG | Non-pharmacologic:<br>CBT, IPT, psychodynamic psychotherapy<br><br>Pharmacologic:<br>Fluoxetine, other SSRIs |

**PSYCHIATRY**

| Key Symptoms | Physical Exam Findings | Investigations | Management |
|---|---|---|---|

### Cognitive impairment

| Key Symptoms | Physical Exam Findings | Investigations | Management |
|---|---|---|---|
| • Family note significant decline in cognitive function e.g. memory<br>• Labile emotions, subtle personality changes, restricted activities<br>• Rapid onset<br>• Night awakening | • Mental status exam<br>• Focal neurologic deficits<br>• Ability to use tools or feed self | • Neuropsycho-logical and cognitive testing<br>• Neuroimaging, LP<br>• CBC, lytes, Cr glucose, B12, folate, TSH, syphilis, HIV serology, U/A | • Address treatable causes<br><br>Pharmacologic: Donepezil, rivastigmine, galantamine, memantine |

### Delirium

| Key Symptoms | Physical Exam Findings | Investigations | Management |
|---|---|---|---|
| • Acute inattention<br>• Fluctuating course<br>• Disorientation and perceptual disturbances<br>• Toxic/medication ingestion | • Mental status exam<br>• Focal neurologic deficits | • CBC, lytes, Cr, glucose, calcium<br>• Neuroimaging<br>• Toxin screen, CXR, urinalysis, ABG, LP | Non-pharmacologic: Reorientation<br><br>Pharmacologic: Treat the underlying cause Review all medications Haloperidol, risperidone, olanzapine, quetiapine for controlling aggression |

### Depression

| Key Symptoms | Physical Exam Findings | Investigations | Management |
|---|---|---|---|
| • Depressed mood<br><br>and/or<br><br>• Reduced ability to experience pleasure | Psychiatric exam:<br><br>Mood↓<br>Sleep ↑/↓<br>Interest or pleasure ↓<br>Guilt or worthlessness<br>Energy ↓<br>Concentration ↓<br>Appetite or weight ↑/↓<br>Psychomotor activity: agitation or retardation)<br>Suicidal Ideation/ intent | Rule out organic causes: CBC, lytes, TSH, hCG, urine toxicology | Non-pharmacologic: CBT, IPT, Mindfulness-based cognitive therapy<br><br>Pharmacologic:<br>1st line: SSRIs (e.g. sertraline), SNRIs (e.g. venlafaxine), bupropion, escitalopram, mirtazapine, moclobemide, mianserin, reboxetine, tianeptine<br><br>2nd line: tricyclics, quetiapine, trazadonem selegline transdermal<br><br>3rd line: MAO inhibitors |

PSYCHIATRY

| Key Symptoms | Physical Exam Findings | Investigations | Management |
|---|---|---|---|
| **Psychosis** | | | |
| • Loss of contact with reality, manifesting as delusions and/or hallucinations | Psychiatric exam, mental status exam: <br>• Delusion of grandeur <br>• Persecutory or paranoid delusion <br>• Delusion of reference <br>• Thought broadcasting <br>• Thought insertion or withdrawal <br>• Mind reading <br>• Delusion of control <br>• Delusion of guilt <br>• Somatic delusion | Rule out organic causes: <br>• TSH, T3/T4, glucose, vit B12, HIV, TB, ceruloplasmin, cortisol, autoimmune, etc <br><br>Set baseline before starting antipsychotics: <br>• CBC, liver enzymes, Cr, prolactin, fasting glucose, lipids, weight, ECG | Atypical antipsychotics: olanzapine, risperidone, quetiapine, clozapine, aripiprazole, etc. <br><br>Typical antipsychotics: haloperidol, chlorpromazine, perphenazine, flupenthixol |
| **Substance – related disorders** | | | |
| • Aberrant pattern of use <br>• Non-medical use of prescription substance for physiological effects <br>• Use of illicit substance for physiological effects | Psychiatric exam: <br>• Depression, anxiety, agitation, sleep disturbance, psychosis, fatigue, anorexia <br><br>Physical exam: <br>• Needle track marks <br>• Nasal-septal perforation <br>• Conjunctival injury <br>• Tobacco-stained fingers or teeth <br>• Alcoholic breath odour <br>• Weight loss | • Liver enzymes <br>• Hep B/C serology <br>• Drug testing in urine, blood, hair, sweat, saliva, breath | Non-pharmacologic: Assess motivation for use and barriers to behavior change <br><br>Harm reduction strategies <br><br>Pharmacologic: Consult treatment guidelines for substance-specific therapy (http://psy-chiatryonline.org/guidelines.aspx) |

## 7. MENTAL HEALTH ACT FORMS

Ontario Mental Health Act Forms enable physicians to be decision makers about their patients' care (**Table 4**).

Basic Criteria for Certification:
1. Serious bodily harm to the person; or
2. Serious bodily harm to another person; or
3. Imminent and serious physical impairment of the person

**Table 4.** Ontario Mental Health Act Forms

| Form | Form Name/Function | Purpose |
|---|---|---|
| FORM 1 (FORM 42 to patient) | Application by Physician for Psychiatric Assessment | Duration: 72 h from admission <br>Reason: meets criteria for certification and for psychiatric assessment <br>Issued: by examining physician within 7 d |

| Form | Form Name/Function | Purpose |
| --- | --- | --- |
| FORM 2 | Order for Examination under Section 16 | Duration: 7 d to get patient to hospital<br>Reason: hospitalization and psychiatric assessment<br>Issued: by Justice of the Peace |
| FORM 3 (FORM 30 to patient) | Certificate of Involuntary Admission | Duration: Lasts 2 wk from date signed<br>Reason: meets criteria for certification<br>Issued: by attending physician different from Form 1 physician |
| FORM 5 | Change to Informal or Voluntary Status | Reason: when physician feels that patient does not require involuntary admission, but does not necessarily mean that patient is ready for discharge |
| FORM 33 | Notice to Patient that Patient is Incompetent | Reason: patient not mentally capable to consent to collection, use or disclosure of personal health information; patient not mentally capable to manage property; patient is not mentally capable to consent to treatment of mental disorder |

## REFERENCES

1. Shea SC. Psychiatric Interviewing: The Art of Understanding. Philadelphia: W.B. Saunders Company; 1988.
2. Sadock BJ, Sadock VA, Ruiz P (Editors). Kaplan & Sadock's Comprehensive Textbook of Psychiatry, 9th ed. Philadelphia: Lippincott Williams & Wilkins; 2009.
3. Goldbloom DS (Editor). Psychiatric Clinical Skills. Philadelphia: Mosby Elsevier; 2006.
4. Dhalla S, Kopec JA. The CAGE questionnaire for alcohol misuse: A review of reliability and validity studies. Clin Invest Med. 2007; 30(1):33-41.
5. Carlat DJ. The Psychiatric Interview: A Practical Guide, 2nd ed. London: Lippincott Williams & Wilkins; 2005.
6. Shader RI (Editor). Manual of Psychiatric Therapeutics, 3rd ed. Philadelphia: Lippincott Williams & Wilkins; 2003.
7. Patterson WM, Dohn HH, Bird J, Patterson GA.. Evaluation of suicidal patients: The SAD PERSONS scale. Psychosomatics. 1993; 24(4):343-349.
8. Bolton JM, Spiwak R, Sareen J. Predicting suicide attempts with the SAD PERSONS scale: A longitudinal analysis. J Clin Psychiatry. 2012; 73(6):e735-e741
9. Shea SC. The Practical Art of Suicide Assessment: A Guide for Mental Health Professionals and Substance Abuse Counselors. New York: John Wiley; 1999.
10. Borson S. The mini-cog: A cognitive "vital signs" measure for dementia screening in multi¬lingual elderly. Int J Geriatr Psychiatry. 2000; 15(11):1021-1027.
11. Shulman KI, Gold DP, Cohen CA, Zucchero CA. Clock-drawing and dementia in the community: A longitudinal study. Int J Geriatr Psychiatry. 1993; 8(6):487-496.
12. Patterson CJ, Gauthier S, Bergman H, Cohen CA, Feightner JW, Feldman H, et al. The recognition, assessment and management of dementing disorders: Conclusions from the Canadian Consensus Conference on Dementia. CMAJ. 1999; 160(12 Suppl):S1-S20.

# CHAPTER 24:

# Primer on Evidence Based Medicine

**Editors:**
Zahra Sohani, PhD

**Faculty Reviewers:**
Lawrence Mbuagbaw, MD, MPH, PhD, FRSPH
Fahad Razak, MD, MSc, FRCPC

## TABLE OF CONTENTS

**EBCP**

EBCP

# 1. BACKGROUND AND INTRODUCTION

## 1.1 What is evidence-based medicine?

The philosophical principles of evidence based medicine (EBM) find its origins in mid-19th century Paris and describes the 'conscientious, explicit, and judicious use of current best evidence in making decisions about the care of individual patients'[1]. Currently, we understand evidence-based medicine as a paradigm predicated on integrating clinical expertise with evidence from well-designed and conducted systematic research. In addition to expert judgment and research, decisions should integrate patient values and preferences to maximize clinical outcomes[2–4].

## 1.2 Sources of evidence

The 6S pyramid is arranged as a hierarchy in which resources should be used to guide clinical decisions. When answering a clinical question, clinicians should search for evidence based resources at the highest possible tier. Whereas for some questions, the highest resource may be a computerized decision support system, for others it may be a systematic review.

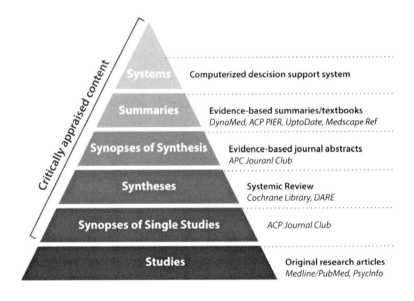

**Figure 1.** The Information Pyramid[5]

## 1.3 Validity of clinical research

The utility of studies in making clinical decisions is determined in large part by its internal and external validity
- **Internal Validity:** the extent to which the design and conduct of the study minimizes bias (described further below)
- **External Validity:** the extent to which the results of a study can be generalized to the target population

Bias in epidemiology is understood as systematic error that results in incorrect assumption of the true effect of an exposure on the outcome of interest. Bias in design, implementation, analysis, and interpretation can affect the conclusions drawn from the research findings and ultimately impact patient care.

EBCP

Below we outline types of biases that can be present in primary studies[6]

1. **Selection Biases** result when the groups being compared differ in baseline prognostic factors relevant to the outcome; common types of selection bias include:
   - **Volunteer Bias:** individuals who volunteer to participate in the study are different from non-volunteers
   - **Non-Respondent Bias:** responders and non-responders differ

2. **Measurement Biases** result when systematic errors occur during the collection of data. Several types of measurement biases exist, including:
   - **Instrument Bias:** calibration errors lead to inaccurate measurements
   - **Differential misclassification bias:** the probability of misclassification of exposure or outcome is different across groups (e.g. unreliable instrument incorrectly misclassifies exposure among cases but not controls)
   - **Non-differential misclassification bias:** the probability of misclassification of exposure or outcome is the same across groups (e.g. unreliable instrument incorrectly misclassifies exposure among both cases and controls)
   - **Insensitive Measure Bias:** lack of tool sensitivity precludes measurement of differences in variables of interest
   - **Expectation Bias:** prior expectations of those assessing the results influences their judgment
   - **Recall Bias:** individuals' responses to questions are dependent on memory and may be affected by the outcome (e.g. sick patients are more likely to remember an exposure vs. less sick/non-sick patients)
   - **Spectrum Bias:** differing case-mixes in various clinical settings affects the performance of diagnostic and screening tests

3. **Intervention Biases** commonly affect research studies that compare groups, and include:
   - **Contamination Bias:** members of one group receive the intervention of the other group, therefore minimizing the difference between groups
   - **Compliance Bias:** subject adherence to interventions affects study outcomes
   - **Attrition Bias:** subjects who drop out of the study differ from those who remain

4. **Confounder:** an extraneous variable (separate from the independent variable) that is related to the outcome of interest, potentially confusing the results

## 1.4 Study designs, their strengths and limitations

Numerous study designs can be used to answer clinical questions. The choice of design is dependent on the type of question, resources (including funding) available, prevalence of exposure and/or outcome, as well as previously published literature on the topic. Below we outline study designs common to clinical epidemiology[3,6]

**Table 1.** Study designs in clinical research[3,6]

| Study design | Description | Strengths | Limitations |
|---|---|---|---|
| **Randomized controlled trial** | Individuals from the population of interest are randomly allocated to either the group receiving the treatment under investigation or to a standard treatment (or placebo treatment) as the control | · Minimizes selection bias<br>· Prognostic balance of groups<br>· Treating physicians and patients are usually blinded to group assignment<br>· Allocation concealment<br>· "Gold standard" for establishing cause-effect relationships | · Noncompliance with group assignment<br>· Attrition bias<br>· Possible poor generalizability (external validity) as a result of specific inclusion criteria<br>· Clinical equipoise – trial can only be ethically permissible if treatment is not known to be better than placebo or control<br>· Possible long length of follow-up |

EBCP

| Study design | Description | Strengths | Limitations |
|---|---|---|---|
| **Prospective cohort studies** | Two groups: exposed vs. not exposed to factor of interest are followed forward in time until development of outcome | • Able to establish temporality<br>• Those with and without outcomes in both groups are derived from same population<br>• Allows calculation of incidence<br>• Facilitate study of rare exposures | • Expensive<br>• Bias in assessment of outcome as a result of no blinding to exposure<br>• Information bias – varied information quality between exposed and non-exposed<br>• Differential attrition in exposed and non-exposed<br>• Long length of follow-up |
| **Retrospective cohort studies** | Two groups: exposed vs. not exposed to factor of interest are followed forward in time until development of outcome based on <u>historic data</u> | • Less expensive<br>• Short or no follow-up needed<br>• Those with and without outcomes in both groups are derived from same population<br>• Facilitate study of rare exposures | • Selection of a comparable non-exposed control group<br>• Bias in assessment of both exposure and outcome<br>• Unable to establish temporality<br>• Absence of data on potential confounding factors if the data was recorded in the past<br>• Differential attrition in exposed and non-exposed |
| **Case-control studies** | Two groups: cases (with outcome) vs. controls (without outcome) are assessed retrospectively for exposure to harmful agent (exposure of interest) | • Relatively inexpensive<br>• No follow-up needed<br>• Facilitate study of rare diseases<br>• Facilitate study of diseases with long latency | • Selection bias: selection of cases (e.g. very sick cases) and controls (e.g. hospitalized controls)<br>• Lack of matching<br>• Recall bias<br>• Unable to establish temporality |
| **Cross sectional** | Exposure and outcome of interest are measured at the same time-point | • Cheap, flexible<br>• No follow-up<br>• Cases and non-cases drawn from the same population | • Unable to establish temporality<br>• Non-response bias<br>• Cannot infer incidence<br>• Sample chosen may not be representative<br>• Not suitable for studying rare diseases or diseases with a short duration |
| **Case reports** | One (report) or multiple (series) cases with observed association between exposure and outcome | • Highlights potential unknown relationships | • Does not involve hypothesis testing |
| **Interviews** | • Structured: set, rigid interview questions/ prompts<br>• Semi-Structured: interview questions/ prompts can be personalized<br>• Unstructured: conversational | • Allow for full exploration of each patient's experience and perspective<br>• Study questions can evolve between interviews<br>• Permit discussion of sensitive topics | • Time-consuming<br>• Interviewer-patient relationship can affect responses to questions<br>• Current views may impact interpretations of past events |

EBCP

| Study design | Description | Strengths | Limitations |
|---|---|---|---|
| **Focus Groups** | • Structured; semi- structured; unstructured | • Allow pilot- testing of novel study questions <br> • Participants can benefit from/build on the responses of others <br> • Efficient use of time in obtaining multiple perspectives | • Interviewer- group relationship can affect responses <br> • Responses can be affected by the group dynamic and contrived setting |

The effect of an intervention or an exposure on the outcome of interest can be expressed in a multitude of ways, such as odds ratio and number needed to treat, among others. **Appendix 1** outlines commonly reported outcome measures.

## 2. TOOLS TO CRITICALLY APPRAISE INDIVIDUAL STUDIES AND SYSTEMATIC REVIEWS

When appraising medical literature, it can be challenging to consolidate considerations of study design, associated strengths and weaknesses, and common biases to answer "is this study valid?" and consequently "are the results true and applicable to my patients?". To facilitate this process, several tools have been developed. We outline some of these tools below:

### 2.1 Randomized controlled trials (RCTs)

The Cochrane Collaboration's tool for assessing risk of bias overviews domains in RCTs that can introduce bias[7]. This tool can be used to evaluate individual studies or quantify risk of bias in systematic reviews of trials. Bias is assessed as a judgment (high, low, or unclear) for elements from five domains: selection, performance, attrition, reporting, and other. It is important to note that this tool only assess the risk of bias, and therefore internal validity of studies; the generalizability, or external validity, should be separately appraised.

**Table 2.** Cochrane risk of bias tool for randomized studies

| Domain | Assessment | Support for judgement |
|---|---|---|
| **Selection bias** | | |
| Random sequence generation | + High <br> - Low <br> ? Unclear | Describe the method used to generate the allocation sequence in sufficient detail to allow an assessment of whether it should produce comparable groups |
| Allocation concealment | + High <br> - Low <br> ? Unclear | Describe the method used to conceal the allocation sequence in sufficient detail to determine whether intervention allocations could have been foreseen in advance of, or during, enrolment |
| **Performance bias** | | |
| Blinding of participants and personnel Assessments should be made for each main outcome (or class of outcomes) | + High <br> - Low <br> ? Unclear | Describe all measures used, if any, to blind study participants and personnel from knowledge of which intervention a participant received. Provide any information relating to whether the intended blinding was effective |

EBCP

| Domain | Assessment | Support for judgement |
|---|---|---|
| **Detection bias** | | |
| Blinding of outcome assessment Assessments should be made for each main outcome (or class of outcomes) | + High<br>- Low<br>? Unclear | Describe all measures used, if any, to blind outcome assessors from knowledge of which intervention a participant received. Provide any information relating to whether the intended blinding was effective |
| **Attrition bias** | | |
| Incomplete outcome data Assessments should be made for each main outcome (or class of outcomes) | + High<br>- Low<br>? Unclear | Describe the completeness of outcome data for each main outcome, including attrition and exclusions from the analysis. State whether attrition and exclusions were reported, the numbers in each intervention group (compared with total randomized participants), reasons for attrition/exclusions where reported, and any re-inclusions in analyses performed by the review authors |
| **Reporting bias** | | |
| Selective reporting | + High<br>- Low<br>? Unclear | State how the possibility of selective outcome reporting was examined by the review authors, and what was found |
| **Other bias** | | |
| Other sources of bias | + High<br>- Low<br>? Unclear | State any important concerns about bias not addressed in the other domains in the tool. If particular questions/entries were pre-specified in the review's protocol, responses should be provided for each question/entry |

Based on the above domains, an overall risk of bias for individual studies or for a review of studies can be determined:

1. Summary assessment for the individual study:
   - **Low**: low risk of bias for all key domains
   - **Unclear**: Unclear risk of bias for one or more key domains
   - **High**: High risk of bias for one or more key domains.

2. Summary assessment across studies (for example in a systematic review):
   - **Low**: Most information is from studies at low risk of bias
   - **Unclear**: Most information is from studies at low or unclear risk of bias
   - **High**: The proportion of information from studies at high risk of bias is sufficient to affect the interpretation of results.

### 2.2 Observational Studies

The Newcastle-Ottawa scale has been modified to assess both cohort and case-control studies[8]. As with RCTs, this tool can be used to quantify risk of bias in individual studies. Assessments are based on the domains described below and take in to account both internal and external validity of studies.

EBCP

**Table 3.** Risk of bias assessment for case-control studies

| Domain | Component |
|---|---|
| **Selection** | Is the case definition adequate?<br>a) yes, with independent validation *<br>b) yes, e.g. record linkage or based on self-reports<br>c) no description |
| | Representativeness of the cases<br>a) consecutive or obviously representative series of cases *<br>b) potential for selection biases or not stated |
| | Selection of Controls<br>a) community controls *<br>b) hospital controls<br>c) no description |
| | Definition of Controls<br>a) no history of disease (the outcome of interest) *<br>b) no description of source |
| **Comparability** | Comparability of cases and controls on the basis of the design or analysis<br>a) study controls for _____ (Select the most important factor.) *<br>b) study controls for any additional factor * (This criterion could be modified to indicate specific control for a second important factor.) |
| **Exposure** | Ascertainment of exposure<br>a) secure record (e.g. surgical records) *<br>b) structured interview where blind to case/control status *<br>c) interview not blinded to case/control status<br>d) written self-report or medical record only<br>e) no description |
| | Same method of ascertainment for cases and controls<br>a) yes *<br>b) no |
| | Non-Response rate<br>a) same rate for both groups *<br>b) non-respondents described<br>c) rate different and no designation |

**Table 4.** Risk of bias assessment for cohort studies

| Domain | Component |
|---|---|
| **Selection** | Representativeness of the exposed cohort<br>a) truly representative of the average _____ (describe) in the community *<br>b) somewhat representative of the average _____ in the community *<br>c) selected group of users e.g. nurses, volunteers<br>d) no description of the derivation of the cohort |
| | Selection of the non-exposed cohort<br>a) drawn from the same community as the exposed cohort *<br>b) drawn from a different source<br>c) no description of the derivation of the non-exposed cohort |
| | Ascertainment of exposure<br>a) secure record (e.g. surgical records) *<br>b) structured interview *<br>c) written self-report<br>d) no description |

EBCP

ESSENTIALS OF CLINICAL EXAMINATION HANDBOOK, 8TH ED.

| Domain | Component |
|---|---|
| | 4) Demonstration that outcome of interest was not present at start of study<br>a) yes *<br>b) no |
| **Comparability** | Comparability of cohorts on the basis of the design or analysis<br>a) study controls for _____ (select the most important factor) *<br>b) study controls for any additional factor * (This criterion could be modified to indicate specific control for a second important factor.) |
| **Outcome** | Assessment of outcome<br>a) independent blind assessment *<br>b) record linkage *<br>c) self-report<br>d) no description |
| | Was follow-up long enough for outcomes to occur<br>a) yes (select an adequate follow up period for outcome of interest) *<br>b) no |
| | Adequacy of follow up of cohorts<br>a) complete follow up - all subjects accounted for *<br>b) subjects lost to follow up unlikely to introduce bias - small number lost<br>- > ____ % (select an adequate %) follow up, or description provided of those lost) *<br>c) follow up rate < ____% (select an adequate %) and no description of those lost<br>d) no statement |

Tools are available to assess risk of bias, internal validity, and external validity of studies across various study designs, such as genetic association studies and non-randomized studies[9-11].

### 2.3 The Grades of Recommendation, Assessment, Development, and Evaluation (GRADE)

- The GRADE Framework rates the quality of a body of evidence, of which one is a systematic review, relevant to a particular question[12]
- The domains described below can be used to upgrade or downgrade the evidence
- GRADE Pro (https://gradepro.org) can be used to rate evidence based on the dimensions below and create summary of findings tables

Downgrade evidence based on
1. Inconsistency: widely varying differences in estimates among studies
2. Indirectness: study population or intervention differs in relevant ways from patients, the intervention in practice, surrogate outcomes measured or interventions not compared head-to-head
3. Imprecision: wide confidence intervals around the effect estimate or small sample population studied
4. Publication Bias: not all relevant studies were considered
5. Bias: systematic error in study design or execution

Upgrade evidence based on
1. Large and consistent effects
2. Dose-response gradient
3. All plausible confounders would reduce the size of the effect

Worked Example # 1 – A body of evidence is rated using dimensions described above. These ratings are then translated into an overall assessment of the evidence for that outcome and presented using summary of findings tables. Below, we provide an example of one such table based on a systematic review of studies comparing antibiotics versus placebo for otitis media infections in children[13].

EBCP

EBCP

**Table 5.** Summary of finding: antibiotics for acute otitis media in children

## Antibiotics compared with placebo for acute otitis media in children

Patient or population: Children with acute otitis media
Setting: High- and middle-income countries
Intervention: Antibiotics
Comparison: Placebo

| Outcomes | Estimated risks (95% CI) | | Relative effect (95% CI) | No. of Participants (studies) | Quality of the evidence (GRADE) | Comments |
| --- | --- | --- | --- | --- | --- | --- |
| | Control risk[a] Placebo | Intervention risk Antibiotics | | | | |
| Pain at 24h | 367 per 1,000 | 330 per 1,000 (286 - 382) | RR 0.9 (0.78 - 1.04) | 1229 (5) | ⊕⊕⊕⊕ High | |
| Pain at 2 - 7 d | 257 per 1,000 | 185 per 1,000 (159 - 213) | RR 0.72 (0.62 - 0.83) | 2791 (10) | ⊕⊕⊕⊕ High | |
| Hearing, inferred from the surrogate outcome abnormal tympanometry - 1 mo | 350 per 1,000 | 311 per 1,000 (262 - 375) | RR 0.89 (0.75 - 1.07) | 927 (4) | ⊕⊕⊕◯ Moderate[b] | |
| Hearing, inferred from the surrogate outcome abnormal tympanometry - 3 mo | 234 per 1,000 | 227 per 1,000 (178 - 290) | RR 0.97 (0.76 - 1.24) | 808 (3) | ⊕⊕⊕◯ Moderate[b] | |
| Vomiting, diarrhea, or rash | 113 per 1,000 | 156 per 1,000 (123 - 199) | RR 1.38 (1.09 - 1.76) | 1,401 (5) | ⊕⊕⊕◯ Moderate[c] | Ideally, evidence from nonotitis trials with similar ages and doses (not obtained) might improve the quality of the evidence |

Abbreviations: CI, confidence interval; RR, risk ratio; GRADE, Grading of Recommendations Assessment, Development, and Evaluation
[a] The basis for the control risk is the median control group risk across studies. The intervention risk (and its 95% CI) is based on the control risk in the comparison group and the relative effect of the intervention (and its 95% CI)
[b] Because of indirectness of outcome
[c] Generally, GRADE rates down for inconsistency in relative effects (which are not inconsistent in this case). Inconsistency here is in absolute effects, which range from 1% to 56%. Contributing factors to the decision to rate down in quality include the likely variation between antibiotics and the fact that most of the adverse events come from a single study. Consideration of indirect evidence from other trials of antibiotics in children (not undertaken) would likely further inform this issue.

## 2.4 Qualitative Studies

- Critically appraising a qualitative study means evaluating its quality and its applicability in clinical practice
- Quality reflects the appropriateness of choices made by the researchers and the transparency of the study, while applicability is concerned with the similarity between the study context and the context of clinical practice, or alternatively, the extent to which the study results inform clinically-applicable theory
- Six questions below can be considered when appraising a qualitative research study:
    1. Was the sample used in the study appropriate to the research question? Did the sample have appropriate breadth and depth, and was the sociocultural context acknowledged?
    2. Was the data collected appropriately? Were methods chosen that were appropriate to the research question?
    3. Was the data analyzed appropriately? Is the study explicit about what was done, how, and by whom? Was the analysis conducted in a way that is congruent with the study's theoretical framework?
    4. Does the study adequately address potential ethical issues? Does the study address reflexivity or the researcher's influence on the research process?
    5. Can I transfer the results of this study to my own setting? Does the study advance our understanding of a particular situation? Careful attention should be paid to the influence of context on the applicability of the results for practice
    6. In conclusion: is what the researchers did clear?
- Similar to quantitative studies, tools can be used to appraise internal and external validity of qualitative studies; these can be found in the quoted references[14–16]

# 3. SCREENING AND DIAGNOSTIC TESTS

Clinical tests are used to screen for illness or diagnose the presence of a disease, such as the use of fecal occult blood test to screen for colon cancer and serum ferritin for the diagnosis of iron deficiency anemia. Ideally such tests would identify all patients with the disease as 'positive' and identify all patients who are disease free as 'negative'. Furthermore, no patient without a disease would be identified as 'positive' and similarly no patient with a disease would be identified as 'negative' by the test. Most clinical tests, however, do not meet this ideal. Measures of sensitivity, specificity, positive predictive values, negative predictive values, and likelihood ratios are used to understand the utility of a clinical test. We will review these below.

## 3.1 Sensitivity and Specificity

In the context of medical tests, sensitivity of the test will **reflect the extent to which true positives are not missed** and specificity will define **the extent to which a positive test means the condition is actually present**. Neither sensitivity nor specificity are dependent on the prevalence of disease in the population of interest. Sensitivity can be used to rule out a disease (**SNout**; **S**ensitive test, if **N**egative, rules **out**), such that if a negative result is achieved on a test that is highly sensitive, the patient most likely does not have the disease. Specificity, on the other hand, can be used to rule in a disease (**SPpin**; **Sp**ecific test, if **P**ositive, rules **in**); a positive result on a specific test is suggestive of the disorder[17,18].

EBCP

$$Sensitivity = \frac{True\ positive}{True\ positive + False\ negative}$$

$$Specificity = \frac{True\ negative}{True\ negative + False\ positive}$$

## 3.2 Positive and negative predictive values

Unlike sensitivity and specificity, the positive predictive value (PPV) and negative predictive value (NPV) are dependent on the prevalence of disease in the population. They are defined as below:

$$PPV = \frac{True\ positive}{True\ positive + False\ positive}$$

$$NPV = \frac{True\ negative}{True\ negative + False\ negative}$$

Since PPV and NPV are dependent on prevalence of the disease, the same diagnostic test will have a different predictive accuracy according to the clinical setting in which it is applied. This concept is illustrated in the example below.

Worked Example # 2 – Let's consider a test for diabetes with a sensitivity of 99% and a specificity of 95% in two populations: 1) a sample of 30 year olds with a prevalence of 1% and 2) a sample of 70 year olds with a prevalence of 20%[18].

| | Young (age = 30) | Old (age = 70) |
| --- | --- | --- |
| Prevalence in the population | 1% | 20% |
| Number in population (A) | 1000 | 1000 |
| Number diseased (B) | 10 | 200 |
| Number not diseased (C) | 990 | 800 |
| True positives (B x 0.99) | 9.9 | 198 |
| False positives (C x (1-0.95)) | 49.5 | 40 |
| Total number positive on test | 59.4 | 238 |
| PPV | 16.7% | 83.2% |

Therefore, with the same test (sensitivity of 99% and specificity of 95%), we see a different positive predictive value since the number of true positives and false positives is contingent on the total population and proportion diseased. In other words, a positive test result is much more likely to be a true positive (i.e., the patient has diabetes) in an older population (in which diabetes is more prevalent).

### 3.3 Likelihood ratios

Likelihood ratios (LRs) reflect how much more likely a patient is who tests positive to have a disease than one who tests negative. They are divided into negative and positive LRs as described below:

$$LR+ = \frac{sensitivity}{1 - sepcificity}$$

Positive LRs indicate how much more likely a patient is to test positive with the disease than to test positive without the disease.

$$LR- = \frac{1 - sensitivity}{specificity}$$

Negative LRs indicate how much more likely a patient is to test negative with the disease than to test negative without the disease.

### 3.4 Receiver operating characteristic (ROC) curves

A test's sensitivity, specificity, PPV, and NPV is dependent on the cut-off point used (e.g. a serum ferritin of 45 µg/L to diagnose anemia[19] in **Figure 2**) to declare a positive test.

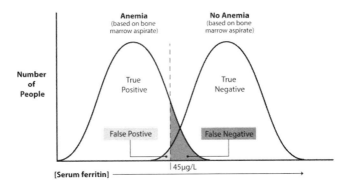

**Figure 2.** Overlap of normal distributions describing an anemic and non-anemic population, based on a bone marrow aspirate (gold standard), with 'true positive', 'true negative', 'false positive' and 'false negative' values

If this threshold is increased (e.g. 50µg instead of 45µg), there will be fewer false negatives but an increased number of false positives results. With the new threshold, the test will be more sensitive, but less specific. The converse is also true; a lower threshold will give a more specific and less sensitive test.

Sensitivity and specificity of a test can be plotted with varying thresholds (**Figure 3**). This curve can be used to identify an optimal threshold based on the requirements of the test.

EBCP

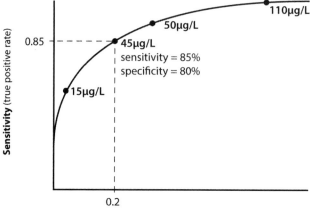

0.85 - - - - - - 45µg/L
sensitivity = 85%
specificity = 80%

50µg/L

110µg/L

15µg/L

Sensitivity (true positive rate)

0.2

1-Specificity (false positive rate)

\* the numbers used in this figure are hypothetical and
do not reflect a study of serum ferritin and anemia

**Figure 3.** Receiver operating characteristic curve demonstrating how varying thresholds for
serum ferritin to designate 'anemia' will change sensitivity and specificity of a test

## 4. APPENDIX 1 – SUMMARY OF OUTCOME MEASURES USED IN CLINICAL RESEARCH

**Table 6.** Outcomes measures reported in clinical research, their definitions, and formulas

| Concept | Definition | Formula |
|---|---|---|
| **Odds ratio** | Ratio of the odds of event A among the exposed population compared to the odds of event A among the unexposed population | $OR = \dfrac{Exposed\ in\ disease \div Exposed\ in\ healthy}{Not\ exposed\ in\ disease \div Not\ exposed\ in\ healthy}$ |
| **Absolute risk** | the proportion of individuals in a particular population who experience event A | $AR = \dfrac{Number\ with\ outcome}{Total\ population}$ |
| **Relative risk** | the absolute risk of event A in a population exposed to X, divided by the absolute risk of event A in a population not exposed to X. One needs to have sampled the population prior to exposure. Thus, the relative risk can be calculated from cohort studies, randomized trials, and controlled clinical trials, but cannot be calculated from case control studies or cross-sectional studies | $RR = \dfrac{AR_{exposed}}{AR_{unexposed}}$ |

EBCP

| Concept | Definition | Formula |
|---------|-----------|---------|
| **Absolute risk reduction** | the absolute risk of adverse event A in a population exposed to the protective effects of X, compared to the absolute risk of adverse event A in a population not exposed to X | $ARR = AR_{unexposed} - AR_{exposed}$ |
| **Absolute risk increase** | the absolute risk of adverse event A in a population exposed to the deleterious effects of X, compared to the absolute risk of adverse event A in a population not exposed to X | $ARI = AR_{exposed} - AR_{unexposed}$ |
| **Relative risk reduction** | the reduction in rate of harmful outcomes in the exposed group compared to the non-exposed group, expressed as a proportion of the non-exposed group rate | $RRR = \dfrac{ARR}{AR_{unexposed}}$ |
| **Relative risk increase** | the increase in rate of harmful outcomes in the exposed group compared to the non-exposed group, expressed as a proportion of the non-exposed group rate | $RRI = \dfrac{ARI}{AR_{unexposed}}$ |
| **Number needed to treat** | the number of patients that would have to be treated with X in order for one patient to benefit by avoiding one harmful outcome | $NNT = \dfrac{1}{ARR}$ |
| **Number needed to harm** | the number of patients that would have to be treated with X in order for one patient to experience one harmful outcome | $NNH = \dfrac{1}{ARI}$ |

EBCP

# REFERENCES

1. Sackett DL. Evidence-based medicine. *Semin Perinatol.* 1997;21(1):3-5. doi:10.1016/S0146-0005(97)80013-4.
2. Miles A, Loughlin M. Models in the balance: evidence-based medicine *versus* evidence-informed individualized care. *J Eval Clin Pract.* 2011;17(4):531-536. doi:10.1111/j.1365-2753.2011.01713.x.
3. Guyatt G, Rennie D, Meade MO, Cook. DJ. *Users' Guides to the Medical Literature: Essentials of Evidence-Based Clinical Practice.* 2nd ed. New York: McGraw-Hill Medical; 2008.
4. Straus S, Glasziou P, Richardson W, Haynes RB. E*vidence-Based Medicine: How to Practice and Teach It. New York:* Churchill-Linvingstone; 2011.
5. DiCenso A, Bayley L, Haynes RB. Accessing preappraised evidence: fine-tuning the 5S model into a 6S model. *Ann Intern Med.* 2009;151(6):JC3. doi:10.7326/0003-4819-151-6-200909150-02002.
6. Gordis L. *Epidemiology.* 5th editio. Elsevier; 2014. https://elsevier.ca/product.jsp?isbn=9781455737338. Accessed May 11, 2015.
7. Higgins JPT, Altman DG, Gøtzsche PC, et al. The Cochrane Collaboration's tool for assessing risk of bias in randomised trials. *BMJ.* 2011;343(oct18_2):d5928. doi:10.1136/bmj.d5928.
8. Wells G, Shea B, O'Connell D, et al. The Newcastle-Ottawa Scale (NOS) for assessing the quality of nonrandomised studies in meta-analyses. Ottawa Hospital Research Institute. http://www.ohri.ca/programs/clinical_epidemiology/oxford.asp. Published 2014. Accessed September 3, 2014.
9. Sohani ZN, Sarma S, Alyass A, et al. Empirical evaluation of the Q-Genie tool: a protocol for assessment of effectiveness. *BMJ Open.* 2016;6(e010403).
10. Sohani ZN, Meyre D, de Souza RJ, et al. Assessing the quality of published genetic association studies in meta-analyses: the quality of genetic studies (Q-Genie) tool. *BMC Genet.* 2015;16(1):50. doi:10.1186/s12863-015- 0211-2.
11. Sterne JA, Hernán MA, Reeves BC, et al. ROBINS-I: a tool for assessing risk of bias in non-randomised studies of interventions. *BMJ.* 2016;355. http://www.bmj.com/content/355/bmj.i4919. Accessed May 23, 2017.
12. Guyatt GH, Oxman AD, Schünemann HJ, Tugwell P, Knottnerus A. GRADE guidelines: a new series of articles in the Journal of Clinical Epidemiology. *J Clin Epidemiol.* 2011;64(4):380-382. doi:10.1016/j.jclinepi.2010.09.011.
13. Guyatt G, Oxman AD, Akl EA, et al. GRADE guidelines: 1. Introduction—GRADE evidence profiles and summary of findings tables. *J Clin Epidemiol.* 2011;64(4):383-394. doi:10.1016/j.jclinepi.2010.04.026.
14. Popay J, Rogers A, Williams G. Rationale and Standards for the Systematic Review of Qualitative Literature in Health Services Research. *Qual Health Res.* 1998;8(3):341-351. doi:10.1177/104973239800800305.
15. Dixon-Woods M, Shaw RL, Agarwal S, Smith JA. The problem of appraising qualitative research. *Qual Saf Heal Care.* 2004;13(3):223-225. doi:10.1136/qhc.13.3.223.
16. Walsh D, Downe S. Appraising the quality of qualitative research. *Midwifery.* 2006;22(2):108-119. doi:10.1016/j.midw.2005.05.004.
17. Lalkhen AG, McCluskey A. Clinical tests: sensitivity and specificity. *Contin Educ Anaesthesia, Crit Care Pain.* 2008;8(6):221-223. doi:10.1093/bjaceaccp/mkn041.
18. University of Ottawa. Sensitivity, Prevalence and Predictive Values. https://www.med.uottawa.ca/sim/data/Sensitivity_and_Prevalence_e.htm. Accessed April 8, 2017.
19. Guyatt GH, Patterson C, Ali M, et al. Diagnosis of iron-deficiency anemia in the elderly. *Am J Med.* 1990;88(3):205-209. http://www.ncbi.nlm.nih.gov/pubmed/2178409. Accessed April 8, 2017.

EBCP

# APPENDIX 1:

# Commonly Used Medications

**Editors:**
Florentina Teoderascu, MD, HBHSc

---

## TABLE OF CONTENTS

APPENDIX 1

# 1. COMMONLY-USED THERAPEUTICS IN CLINICAL MEDICINE

| Clinical Application | Examples |
| --- | --- |
| **Analgesia** | |
| **NSAIDs** | Acetylsalicylic acid (Aspirin®) <br> Diclofenac (Voltaren®, Pennsaid Solution®) <br> Ibuprofen (Motrin®, Advil®) <br> Indomethacin <br> Ketorolac (Toradol®) <br> Meloxicam (Mobicox®) <br> Naproxen (Naprosyn®) |
| **NSAIDs-COX-2 Selective Inhibitors** | Celecoxib (Celebrex®) |
| **Analgesia** | |
| **Opioid Analgesics** (narcotics) | Codeine <br> Fentanyl <br> Hydromorphone (Dilaudid®) <br> Hydrocodone (Hycodan®) <br> Methadone (Metadol®) <br> Morphine (Statex®) |
| **Opioid Antagonists** | Naloxone (Naloxone HCl Injection®) <br> Naltrexone (ReVia®) |
| **Other Analgesics** | Acetaminophen (Tylenol®) <br> Acetaminophen with codeine <br> (Tylenol #2®, Tylenol #3®) |
| **Anesthesia/Sedation** | |
| **General Anesthetics: IV** | Propofol (Diprivan®) <br> Ketamine injection (Ketalar®) <br> Thiopental |
| **General Anesthetics: Inhaled** | Isoflurane <br> Desflurane (Suprane®) <br> Nitrous oxide <br> Sevoflurane (Sevorane AF®) |
| **Muscle Relaxants** | Atracurium besylate <br> Neostigmine (Prostigmin®) <br> Rocuronium (Zemuron®) <br> Succinylcholine (Anectine®) |
| **Sedatives: Benzodiazepines** | Diazepam (Diastat®, Valium®) <br> Lorazepam (Ativan®) <br> Midazolam (Midazolam Injection®)* <br> Oxazepam (Serax®) <br> Temazepam (Restoril®; primarily for insomnia) <br> Triazolam (Halcion®; primarily for insomnia) <br><br> *most common adjunct for anesthesia |
| **Sedatives: Other** | Chloral hydrate (Chloral Hydrate Odan®) <br> Zopiclone (Imovane®) |

APPENDIX 1

ESSENTIALS OF CLINICAL EXAMINATION HANDBOOK, 8TH ED.

| Clinical Application | Examples |
|---|---|
| **Cardiology** | |
| **ACE Inhibitors** | Captopril (Capoten®)<br>Enalapril (Vasotec®)<br>Fosinopril (Monopril®)<br>Lisinopril (Zestril®)<br>Perindopril (Aceon®)<br>Ramipril (Altace®) |
| **Angiotensin II Receptor Blockers (ARBs)** | Candesartan cilexetil (Atacand®)<br>Irbesartan (Avalide®, Avapro®)<br>Losartan (Cozaar®)<br>Telmisartan (Micardis®)<br>Valsartan (Diovan®) |
| **Antiadrenergics** (central acting) | Clonidine (Catapres®; both central/peripheral)<br>Methyldopa (Aldomet®, Supres®)<br>Prazosin (both central/peripheral) |
| **Antiadrenergic** (peripheral acting) | Reserpine |
| **Anticoagulant** | **Vitamin K Antagonist:**<br>Warfarin (Coumadin®)<br>**Low Molecular Weight Heparins (LMWH):**<br>Dalteparin (Fragmin®)<br>Enoxaparin (Lovenox®)<br>Tinzaparin (Innohep®)<br>**Direct Thrombin Inhibitors:**<br>Bivalirudin (Angiomax®)<br>Dabigatran (Pradax®) |
| **Antiplatelet Agents** | Acetylsalicylic acid (Aspirin®)<br>Dipyridamole (Persantine®)<br>Dipyridamole/ASA (Aggrenox®)<br>**Adenosine Diphosphate Receptor Inhibitors:**<br>Clopidogrel (Plavix®)<br>Prasugrel (Effient®)<br>Ticagrelor (Brilinta®)<br>Ticlopidine (Ticlid®)<br>**GP IIb/IIIa Inhibitors:**<br>Abciximab (ReoPro®)<br>Tirofiban (Aggrastat®) |
| **β-Blockers** | Atenolol (Tenormin®; β1 selective)<br>Acebutolol HCl (Monitan®; β1 selective)<br>Metoprolol (Lopressor®; β1 selective)<br>Nadolol (nonselective)<br>Propranolol (Inderal-LA®; nonselective)<br>Timolol (Azarga®, Blocadren®; nonselective) |
| **Calcium Channel Blockers** | **Non-dihydropyridine:**<br>Diltiazem (Cardizem®)<br>Verapamil (Chronovera®)<br>**Dihydropyridine:**<br>Amlodipine besylate (Norvasc®)<br>Nifedipine (Adalat®) |

APPENDIX 1

| Clinical Application | Examples |
|---|---|
| **Inotropes (increase contractility)** | **Cardiac Glycosides:**<br>Digoxin (Lanoxin®)<br>**Phosphodiesterase Inhibitors:**<br>Milrinone lactate (Primacor®)<br>**Sympathomimetic Amines:**<br>Dopamine (Intropin®)<br>Dobutamine HCl<br>Epinephrine (Alveda®)<br>Norepinephrine bitartrate (Levophed®) |
| **Nitrates** | Isosorbide dinitrate (Isordil®)<br>Isosorbide mononitrate<br>Nitroglycerin (Minitran®) |
| **Thrombolytics (lytics)** | Alteplase (Activase®; tPA)<br>Reteplase (Retavase®)<br>Streptokinase (Streptase®)<br>Tenecteplase (TNkase®) |
| ***Agents for Dyslipidemia*** | |
| **Bile Acid Sequestrants** | Cholestyramine (Olestyr®)<br>Colestipol (Colestid®)<br>Colesevelam (Lodalis®) |
| **HMG-CoA Reductase Inhibitors** (statins) | Atorvastatin (Lipitor®)<br>Fluvastatin (Lescol®)<br>Lovastatin (Advicor®, Mevacor®)<br>Pravastatin (Pravachol®)<br>Rosuvastatin (Crestor®)<br>Simvastatin (Zocor®) |
| **Cholesterol Absorption Inhibitor** | Ezetimibe (Ezetrol®) |
| **Fibrates** | Fenofibrate (Fenomax®)<br>Gemfibrozil (Lopid®) |
| **Nicotinic Acid** | Niacin |
| ***Diuretics*** | |
| **Carbonic Anhydrase Inhibitor** | Acetazolamide (Diamox Sequels®) |
| **Loop Diuretics** | Bumetanide (Burinex®)<br>Ethacrynic acid (Edecrin®)<br>Furosemide (Lasix®) |
| **Osmotic Diuretics** | Mannitol (Osmitrol®)<br>Glycerol<br>Urea (Hydrophil®, Uremol®) |
| **K⁺ Sparing Diuretics** | Amiloride (Midamor®)<br>Spironolactone (Aldactone®) |
| **Thiazide and Related Diuretics** | Hydrochlorothiazide (Accuretic®, Altace HCT®)<br>Chlorthalidone |
| ***Other Clinical Scenarios*** | |
| **Acute MI** | ACE inhibitors<br>Acetylsalicylic acid (Aspirin®)<br>β-blockers<br>Clopidogrel<br>Heparin<br>Morphine<br>Nitroglycerin<br>Thrombolytics |

APPENDIX 1

| Clinical Application | Examples |
|---|---|
| **Angina Pectoris** | Acetylsalicylic acid (Aspirin®)<br>β-blockers<br>Calcium channel blockers<br>Nitrates |
| **CHF** | ACE inhibitors<br>Angiotensin receptor antagonists<br>β-blockers<br>Digoxin<br>Diuretics |
| **HTN** | ACE inhibitors<br>Angiotensin receptor antagonists<br>β-blockers<br>Calcium channel blockers<br>Diuretics |

## Endocrinology

| | |
|---|---|
| **Addison's Disease** | Fludrocortisone (Florinef®)<br>Hydrocortisone |
| **DM Type 1** | **Intermediate-Acting Insulin:**<br>NPH<br>**Long-Acting Insulin:**<br>Glargine<br>**Rapid-Acting Insulin:**<br>Aspart<br>Lispro<br>**Short-Acting Insulin:**<br>Insulin |
| **DM Type 2** | **α-Glucosidase Inhibitor:**<br>Acarbose (Glucobay®)<br>**Biguanides:**<br>Metformin (Sandoz®)<br>**Gliptins (DPP-IV Inhibitors):**<br>Sitagliptin (Januvia®)<br>Sitagliptin + Metformin (Janumet®)<br>**Insulin:**<br>Rapid, short, intermediate, long<br>**Meglitinides:**<br>Nateglinide (Starlix®)<br>Repaglinide (GlucoNorm®)<br>**Sulfonylureas:**<br>Chlorpropamide<br>Glyburide (DiaBeta®)<br>Gliclazide (Diamicron®)<br>Glimepiride (Amaryl®)<br>**Thiazolidinediones:**<br>Pioglitazone (Actos®)<br>Rosiglitazone (Avandia®)* |

APPENDIX 1

| Clinical Application | Examples |
|---|---|
| Hypercalcemia | **Bisphosphonate:**<br>    Pamidronate disodium (Aredia®)<br>**Bone Reabsorption Inhibitor:**<br>    Calcitonin (Calcimar®, Miacalcin®)<br>**Calcimimetic Agent:**<br>    Cinacalcet (Sensipar®)<br>**Precipitating Agent:**<br>    Potassium phosphate*<br><br>*poses significant risks |
| Hyperkalemia | **β-Agonist:**<br>    Salbutamol (Ventolin®)<br>**Electrolyte Supplements:**<br>    Calcium chloride<br>    Calcium gluconate<br>    Furosemide (Lasix®)<br>    Insulin with Dextrose<br>**Potassium Binding Resins:**<br>    Sodium polystyrene sulfonate (Kayexalate®)<br>    Sodium bicarbonate |
| Hyperthyroidism | β-blocker (alleviates symptoms)<br>Iodine-131<br>Methimazole (Tapazole®)<br>Propylthiouracil |
| Hypothyroidism | Levothyroxine (Levotec®, Eltroxin®; T4)<br>Liothyronine (Cytomel®; T3)*<br><br>*can be used in conjunction with levothyroxine |
| **Gastroenterology** | |
| Antacids | Aluminum hydroxide (Amphojel®)<br>Calcium carbonate (Caltrate®)<br>Magnesium hydroxide/carbonate<br>**OTC Preparations:**<br>    Alka-Seltzer®<br>    Gaviscon®<br>    Maalox®<br>    Rolaids® |
| Antiemetics | **Anticholinergic Agent:**<br>    Scopolamine (Buscopan®)<br>**Antihistamine:**<br>    Dimenhydrinate (Gravol®)<br>**Dopamine Receptor Antagonists:**<br>    Metoclopramide (Maxeran®)<br>    Prochlorperazine<br>**Serotonin Receptor Antagonists:**<br>    Dolasetron mesylate (Anzemet®)<br>    Ondansetron (Zofran ODT®)<br>    Granisetron (Kytril®) |
| H2-Receptor Antagonists | Cimetidine (Tagamet®)<br>Famotidine (Pepcid®)<br>Nizatidine (Axid®)<br>Ranitidine (Zantac®) |

APPENDIX 1

| Clinical Application | Examples |
|---|---|
| **Proton Pump Inhibitors (PPIs)** | Esomeprazole (Nexium®) |
| | Lansoprazole (Prevacid®) |
| | Omeprazole (Losec®) |
| | Pantoprazole (Pantoloc®) |
| | Rabeprazole (Pariet®) |
| **Agents for Constipation** | **Bulk-Forming Laxative:** |
| | Psyllium (Metamucil®) |
| | **Decompaction:** |
| | Mineral oil |
| | **Osmotic Agents:** |
| | Magnesium hydroxide |
| | Lactulose |
| | Magnesium citrate |
| | Magnesium |
| | Polyethylene glycol |
| | **Stimulant Laxatives:** |
| | Bisacodyl (Bi-PegLyte®, Correctol®) |
| | Senna (Senokot S®) |
| | **Surfactant:** |
| | Docusate (Colace®) |
| **Agents for Diarrhea** | Attapulgite (Kaopectate®) |
| | Bismuth subsalicylate (Pepto-Bismol®) |
| | Diphenoxylate (Lomotil®) |
| | Loperamide (Imodium®, Loperacap®) |
| | Oral rehydration therapy |
| **Agents for GI Bleed** | Pantoprazole (Pantoloc®) |
| | Octreotide |
| **Agents for Irritable Bowel Syndrome** | **Antidepressant:** |
| | TCA (for pain) |
| | **Bile Acid Sequestrant:** |
| | Cholestyramine (Questran®) |
| | **Bulk-Forming Laxative:** |
| | Psyllium (Metamucil®) |
| | **Opioid:** |
| | Loperamide (Imodium®, Loperacap®) |
| **Agents for Inflammatory Bowel Disease** | **Steroids:** |
| | Budesonide |
| | Hydrocortisone |
| | Prednisone |
| | **Other:** |
| | 5-Aminosalicylic acid (Salofalk®, Pentasa®) |
| | Azathioprine (Imuran®) |
| | Cyclosporine (Restasis®, Sandimmune®) |
| | Infliximab (Remicade®) |
| | Mercaptopurine (Purinethol®) |
| | Methotrexate |
| | Sulfasalazine (Salazopyrin®) |
| **Head and Neck** | |
| **Bell's Palsy** | Artificial tears |
| | Corticosteroids |
| | Ocular ointment |
| | **Oral Antivirals:** |
| | Acyclovir |
| | Prednisolone |

APPENDIX 1

| Clinical Application | Examples |
|---|---|
| Acute Otitis Externa | Analgesics<br>**Otic Drops:**<br>Betamethasone + Gentamicin (Garasone®)<br>Ciprofloxacin (Cipro®)<br>Ofloxacin (Floxin®, Ocuflox®)<br>Moxifloxacin (Vigamox®) |
| Sudden Sensorineural Hearing Loss | Corticosteroids |
| Otitis Media | **1st line Antibiotics:**<br>Amoxicillin<br>Sulphamethoxazole-Trimethoprim (Septra®)<br>Macrolides<br>**2nd line Antibiotics (When Amoxicillin Fails):**<br>Amoxicillin/Clavulanic acid (Clavulin®)<br>Cephalosporins<br>**For Symptoms:**<br>Analgesics<br>Antipyretics |
| Vertigo | **Anticholinergic Agent:**<br>Transdermal scopolamine<br>**Antihistamine:**<br>Diphenhydramine (Benadryl®)<br>**Benzodiazepine:**<br>Diazepam (Valium®)<br>**Ménière's Disease:**<br>Betahistine (Serc®)<br>**Phenothiazine Antiemetics:**<br>Prochlorperazine maleate (Nu-Prochlor®) |
| Rhinorrhea | **Antihistamines:**<br>Desloratadine (Aerius®)<br>Diphenhydramine (Benadryl®)<br>Fexofenadine (Allegra®)<br>Loratadine (Claritin®)<br>**Topical/Systemic Decongestants:**<br>Phenylephrine (Neo-Synephrine®)<br>Pseudoephedrine (Promatussin®)<br>**Topical Glucocorticoids:**<br>Budesonide (Rhinocort®)<br>Fluticasone proprionate (Advair®) |
| Anterior Epistaxis | **Topical Vasoconstrictors:**<br>Cocaine<br>Oxymetazoline (Dristan®, Vicks Sinex®) |
| **Infectious Diseases - Anti-bacterial** | |
| Cell Wall Synthesis Inhibitors | Cephalosporins<br>Carbapenems<br>Glycopeptides (Vancomycin)<br>Penicillin |
| DNA Complex Agent | Metronidazole (Flagyl®)*<br><br>*The major mechanism of action involves cross-linking with, and inactivation of, cysteine-containing bacterial and protozoal enzymes |
| DNA-Directed RNA Polymerase Inhibitor | Rifampin (Rifadin®) |

APPENDIX 1

ESSENTIALS OF CLINICAL EXAMINATION HANDBOOK, 8TH ED.

| Clinical Application | Examples |
|---|---|
| **DNA Gyrase Inhibitor** | Fluoroquinolones |
| **Folic Acid Metabolism Inhibitors** | Sulfamethoxazole (Bactrim®)<br>Trimethoprim (Polytrim®) |
| **Protein Synthesis Inhibitors** (50S ribosomes) | Clindamycin (Dalacin®)<br>Macrolides |
| **Protein Synthesis Inhibitors** (30S ribosomes) | **Aminoglycosides:**<br>Gentamicin<br>Tobramycin<br>Tetracyclines |

*Clinical Scenarios*

| | |
|---|---|
| **Community-Acquired Pneumonia** | Amoxicillin/Clavulanic acid<br>Cephalosporins<br>Doxycycline (Doxycin®)<br>Macrolides<br>**Quinolones:**<br>Gatifloxacin (Zymar®)<br>Levofloxacin (Levaquin®)<br>Moxifloxacin (Avelox®) |
| **Otitis Media** | Amoxicillin<br>Amoxicillin/Clavulanic acid<br>Cefixime (Suprax®)<br>Cefuroxime axetil (Ceftin®)<br>Sulfamethoxazole/Trimethoprim (Septra®) |
| **TB** | **1st Line:**<br>Ethambutol (Etibi®)<br>Isoniazid (INH)<br>Vitamin B6<br>Pyrazinamide<br>Rifampin (Rifadin®)<br>Streptomycin (SteriMax®)<br>**2nd Line:**<br>Fluoroquinolones (Levofloxacin) |
| **UTI** | Amoxicillin<br>Amoxicillin/Clavulanic acid<br>Cephalexin (Keflex®)<br>Nitrofurantoin<br>**Quinolones:**<br>Ciprofloxacin (Cipro®)<br>Norfloxacin (Noroxin®)<br>Trimethoprim/Sulfamethoxazole (Septra®) |

**Infectious Diseases - Antifungal**

| | |
|---|---|
| **Echinocandin** | Capsofungin (Cancidas®; intravenous) |
| **Polyenes** | Amphotericin B (Fungizone®; systemic)<br>Nystatin (Nyaderm®; topical) |
| **Imidazoles** | Clotrimazole (Lotriderm®)<br>Ketoconazole (Ketoderm®)<br>Miconazole (Desenex®) |
| **Triazoles** | Fluconazole (Diflucan®)<br>Itraconazole (Sporanox®)<br>Voriconazole (Vfend®) |

APPENDIX 1

| Clinical Application | Examples |
|---|---|
| **Infectious Diseases - Antifungal** | |
| **HIV** | Fusion inhibitors<br>Protease inhibitors<br>NNRTIs (non-nucleoside reverse transcriptase inhibitors)<br>NRTIs (nucleoside reverse transcriptase inhibitors) |
| **Nucleoside Reverse Transcriptase Inhibitors (NRTIs)** | Abacavir sulfate (Ziagen®)<br>Lamivudine (Epivir®)<br>Stavudine (Zerit®)<br>Zidovudine (Retrovir®) |
| **Non-Nucleoside Reverse Transcriptase Inhibitors (NNRTIs)** | Delavirdine mesylate (Rescriptor®)<br>Efavirenz (Sustiva®; also known as EFV)<br>Nevirapine (Viramune®) |
| **Protease Inhibitors** | Amprenavir<br>Atazanavir<br>Indinavir<br>Lopinavir<br>Nelfinavir<br>Ritonavir<br>Saquinavir |
| **Integrase Inhibitor** | Raltegravir potassium (Isentress®) |
| **Combination Antiretrovirals** | Abacavir + Zidovudine + Lamivudine (Trizivir®)<br>Zidovudine + Lamivudine (Combivir®) |
| **Fusion Inhibitors** | Enfuvirtide (Fuzeon®)<br>Maraviroc (Celsentri®) |
| **Other Antivirals** | Oseltamivir (Tamiflu®; against influenza virus)<br>Ribavirin (Virazole®; inhibits wide range of viruses) |
| **Nucleoside Polymerase Inhibitors** | Acyclovir (Zovirax®)<br>Ganciclovir (Cytovene®) |
| **Musculoskeletal** | |
| **Osteoarthritis** | Acetaminophen (Tylenol®)<br>Capsaicin topical (Rub A535®)<br>Intra-articular glucocorticoid injection<br>Intra-articular hyaluronan injection<br>NSAIDs<br>Opioids<br>Selective COX-2 inhibitors |
| **Osteoporosis** | Alendronate (Fosamax®)<br>Etidronate (Didrocal®)<br>Risedronate (Actonel®)<br>Calcium and Vitamin D supplementation<br>Calcitonin (Calcimar®, Caltine®)<br>Estrogen (Premplus®, Premarin®)<br>Parathyroid hormone<br>Raloxifene (Evista®) |

APPENDIX 1

| Clinical Application | Examples |
|---|---|
| Rheumatoid Arthritis | **Disease Modifying Therapy (DMARDs):**<br>Hydroxychloroquine sulfate (Plaquenil®)<br>Sulfasalazine (Salazopyrin®)<br>Methotrexate<br>**Immunosuppressive Therapy:**<br>Azathioprine (Imuran®)<br>Cyclosporine (Restasis®)<br>Cyclophosphamide (Procytox®)<br>Leflunomide (Arava®)<br>**NSAIDs** |

### Neurology

| | |
|---|---|
| Alzheimer's Disease | **Cholinesterase Inhibitors:**<br>Donepezil (Aricept®)<br>Galantamine (Reminyl ER®)<br>Rivastigmine (Exelon®)<br>Memantine (Ebixa®) |
| CVA/TIA | Alteplase (Activase®; tPA)<br>Acetylsalicylic acid (Aspirin®)<br>Clopidogrel (Plavix®)<br>Dipyridamole + Aspirin® (Aggrenox®)<br>Warfarin (Coumadin®) |
| Epilepsy | **Atypical Absence/Myoclonic/Atonic:**<br>Lamotrigine (Lamictal®)<br>Topiramate (Topamax®)<br>**Focal:**<br>Carbamazepine (Tegretol®)<br>Phenytoin (Dilantin®)<br>**Generalized-Onset Tonic Clonic:**<br>Lamotrigine (Lamictal®)<br>Topiramate (Topamax®, Topiragen®)<br>Valproic acid (Depakene®)<br>**Partial Seizures (Narrow-Spectrum AEDs):**<br>Gabapentin (Neurontin®)<br>Vigabatrin (Sabril®)<br>**Typical Absence:**<br>Ethosuximide (Zarontin®)<br>Valproic acid (Depakene®)<br>**Other (Acute Therapy):**<br>Diazepam (Valium®)<br>Lorazepam (Ativan®) |
| MS | Glatiramer acetate (Copaxone®)<br>Glucocorticoids<br>Interferon-$\beta$1a (Avonex®) or 1b (Betaseron®) |
| Parkinson's Disease | **Dopamine Agonists:**<br>Pramipexole (Mirapex®)<br>Ropinirole (ReQuip®)<br>Levodopa/Carbidopa (Sinemet®)<br>**Other:**<br>Anticholinergics (Benztropine)<br>COMT inhibitors (Entacepone)<br>MAO-B inhibitors (Selegiline)<br>NMDA antagonists |

APPENDIX 1

| Clinical Application | Examples |
|---|---|
| **Obstetrics and Gynecology** | |
| **Nutritional Supplementation** | Folic acid |
| | Multivitamins (Materna®, Pregvit®) |
| **Antinausea** | Benzamides (serotonin antagonists) |
| | Dimenhydrinate (Gravol®) |
| | Doxylamine + Pyridoxine (Diclectin®) |
| **Hypertension** | **Severe HTN (>160mmHg systolic or >90mmHg diastolic):** |
| | Hydralazine |
| | Labetalol (Trandate®) |
| | Nifedipine (Adalat®) |
| | **Non-Severe HTN:** |
| | Methyldopa (Aldomet®) |
| | Labetalol (Trandate®) |
| | Other β-blockers |
| **Inducing Agents** | Oxytocin |
| | Prostaglandin E2 |
| **Medical Abortion** | Methotrexate + Misoprostol |
| **Rh- Mother and Rh+ (or Unknown) Fetus; uterine bleeding; ectopic pregnancy; procedures (eg. amniocentesis, chorionic villus sampling)** | RHO immune globulin (RhoGAM®) |
| **Ophthalmology** | |
| **Anesthetics** | **Na+ channel blocker (drops)** |
| | Tetracaine (0.5%, 1%) |
| | Proparacaine |
| **Antibiotics** | **Fluoroquinolone (drops)** |
| | Moxifloxacin drops (0.5%) |
| | Ciprofloxacin |
| | Gatifloxacin |
| | **Aminoglycoside (drops)** |
| | Tobramycin (0.3%) |
| | **Others (drops)** |
| | Vancomycin |
| | Polymyxin B (0.1%, 0.25%) |
| **Anti-inflammatory** | **NSAIDs (drops)** |
| | Diclofenac (0.1%) |
| | Ketorolac |
| | Nepafenac |
| | **Corticosteroids (drops)** |
| | Prednisolone acetate |
| | Dexamethasone |
| | Fluoromet.halone |
| **Anti-virals** | Acyclovir (ointment) |
| | Trifluridine (drops) |
| **Dilating Agents** | **Anticholinergic (drops)** |
| | Atropine |
| | Cyclopentolate |
| | Tropicamide |
| | **Alpha-adrenergic agonist (drops)** |
| | Phenylephrine |

APPENDIX 1

| Clinical Application | Examples |
|---|---|
| Glaucoma | **Alpha-2 agonist (drops)**<br>Brimonidine<br>**Carbonic anhydrase inhibitor (drops)**<br>Acetazolamide<br>Dorzolamide<br>Brinzolamide<br>**Prostaglandin analogue (drops)**<br>Latanoprost<br>Bimatroprost<br>Travoprost<br>**Cholinomimetics (drops, gel)**<br>Pilocarpine<br>**Non-selective beta-blocker (drops)**<br>Timolol<br>Betaxolol<br>Levobunolol<br>**Combination therapies (drops)**<br>Timolol & brimonidine<br>Timolol & brinzolamide<br>Timolol & dorzolamide<br>Timolol & travoprost |

## Psychiatry

### Antidepressants

| | |
|---|---|
| **Selective Serotonin Reuptake Inhibitors** | **SSRIs:**<br>Citalopram (Celexa®)<br>Escitalopram (Cipralex®)<br>Fluoxetine (Prozac®)<br>Paroxetine (Paxil®)<br>Sertraline (Zoloft®) |
| **Tricyclic Antidepressants** | **TCAs:**<br>Amitriptyline (Elavil®)<br>Clomipramine (Anafranil®)<br>Doxepin (Sinequan®)<br>Imipramine (Tofranil®)<br>Nortriptyline (Aventyl®) |
| **Serotonin-Norepinephrine Reuptake Inhibitors** | **SNRIs:**<br>Duloxetine (Cymbalta®)<br>Venlafaxine (Effexor®) |
| **Monoamine Oxidase Inhibitors (MAOIs)** | Phenelzine sulfate (Nardil®)<br>Tranylcypromine sulfate (Parnate®) |
| **Other** | Bupropion (Wellbutrin®)<br>Mirtazapine (Remeron®)<br>Tryptophan (Tryptan®) |

### Antipsychotics

| | |
|---|---|
| **Typical** | Chlorpromazine (Largactil®)<br>Flupenthixol (Fluanxol®)<br>Haloperidol (Haldol®)<br>Perphenazine (Trilafon®) |
| **Atypical** | Clozapine (Clozaril®)<br>Olanzapine (Zyprexa®)<br>Quetiapine (Seroquel®)<br>Risperidone (Risperdal®)<br>Ziprasidone (Zeldox®) |

APPENDIX 1

| Clinical Application | Examples |
|---|---|
| *Other* | |

**Antianxiety Agents**

SSRIs, TCAs, MAOIs
**Benzodiazepines:**
  Alprazolam (Xanax®)
  Clonazepam (Rivotril®)
  Lorazepam (Ativan®)
  Oxazepam (Serax®)
  Temazepam (Restoril®)
  Diazepam (Valium®)
**β-Blockers:**
  Atenolol (Tenormin®)
  Oxprenolol (Trasicor®; non-selective)
  Pindolol (Visken®)
  Propranolol
**Other:**
  Buspirone (BuSpar®)
  Hydroxyzine (Atarax®)
  Pregabalin (Lyrica®)
  Venlafaxine (Effexor®)

**Mood Stabilizers** (for bipolar disorder)

**Anticonvulsants:**
  Carbamazepine (Tegretol®)
  Lamotrigine (Lamictal®)
  Lithium (Lithane®, Carbolith®)
  Valproic Acid (Depakene®)

**Opioid Agonists**

Buprenorphine + Naloxone (Suboxone®; for opioid addiction)
Methadone (Metadol®)

**Notes for Psychiatry**
- Cognitive behavioral therapy (CBT) is an effective first-line treatment for mild to moderate depression and anxiety disorders
- Electroconvulsive therapy (ECT) is indicated and effective for severe and medically refractory depression

## Respirology

**Asthma**
(relief medication)

**Anticholinergic:**
  Ipratropium bromide (Atrovent®)
**β-Agonists:**
  Epinephrine
  Isoprenaline
  Salbutamol
  Terbutaline
**Methylxanthine:**
  Theophylline (Uniphyl®)

**Asthma**
(long-term control medication)

**Inhaled Glucocorticoids:**
  Beclomethasone (Qvar®)
  Budesonide (Pulmicort®)
  Fluticasone (Flovent®)
**Leukotriene Inhibitor:**
  Montelukast (Singulair®)
**Mast Cell-Stabilizing Agents:**
  Cromolyn (Nascrom®)
  Nedocromil (Alocril®)

APPENDIX 1

| --- | --- |
| **COPD** | **Anticholinergics:**<br>Ipratropium bromide (Atrovent®)<br>Tiotropium (Spiriva®)<br>**β-Agonists:**<br>Salmeterol (can also be used for asthma)<br>Salbutamol<br>**Inhaled Glucocorticoids:**<br>Beclomethasone (Qvar®)<br>Budesonide (Pulmicort®)<br>Fluticasone (Flovent®)<br>**Methylxanthine:**<br>Theophylline (Uniphyl®) |
| **Urology** | |
| **Benign Prostatic Hyperplasia** | **5α-Reductase Inhibitor:**<br>Finasteride (Proscar®)<br>**α-Adrenergic Blockers:**<br>Terazosin (Hytrin®)<br>Doxazosin (Cardura®)<br>Tamsulosin (Flomax®) |
| **Chronic Renal Failure** | ACE inhibitors<br>Angiotensin receptor blockers<br>Protein restriction |
| **Erectile Dysfunction** | Sildenafil (Viagra®)<br>Tadalafil (Cialis®)<br>Vardenafil (Levitra®) |
| **Agents for Urinary Incontinence**<br>(hyperactive bladder) | **Anticholinergic Drugs:**<br>Propantheline bromide<br>**Antispasmodics:**<br>Oxybutynin (Ditropan®)<br>Tolterodine (Detrol®)<br>Trospium (Trosec®)<br>**TCAs** |
| **Agents for Urinary Incontinence**<br>(stress incontinence) | Estrogen<br>Pseudoephedrine hydrochloride<br>**TCAs:**<br>Imipramine<br>Desipramine<br>Amitriptyline |
| **Vascular** | |
| **DVT/PE** | Heparin<br>Warfarin (Coumadin®)<br>**LMWH:**<br>Dalteparin (Fragmin®)<br>Enoxaparin (Lovenox®)<br>Tinzaparin (Innohep®) |
| **Temporal Arteritis (GCA)** | Prednisone (high dose, starting at 60 mg/d PO for approximately 1 month) |

APPENDIX 1

## 2. DRUG CATEGORY NAMING SHORTCUTS

Although there are several exceptions, drugs in the same therapeutic/ mechanistic category often have similar endings/beginnings. It is also worth noting that there may be other drugs that also belong to the classes described below that have different endings

| Prefixes/Suffices | Therapeutic Class | Examples |
|---|---|---|
| -afil | PDE-5 inhibitors | sildenafil, tadalafil, vardenafil |
| -ane | Inhaled general anesthetics | halothane, enflurane, isoflurane |
| -ase | Thrombolytics | streptokinase, alteplase, tenecteplase |
| -azine | Phenothiazine antipsychotics and Antihistamines | chlorpromazine, fluphenazine, perphenazine, promethazine |
| -azole | Antifungals | ketoconazole, itraconazole, fluconazole |
| -barbital | Barbiturates | phenobarbital, pentobarbital, secobarbital |
| Ceph-/Cef- | Cephalosporins | ceftriaxone, cefuroxime, cefazolin, cephalexin, cefprozil |
| -cillin | Penicillin antibiotics | penicillin, amoxicillin, cloxacillin |
| -curonium | Non-depolarizing neuromuscular blockers | pancuronium, rocuronium, vecuronium |
| -cycline | Tetracycline antibiotics | tetracycline, doxycycline, minocycline |
| -dipine | Dihydropyridine calcium channel blockers | nifedipine, felodipine, amlodipine |
| -dronate | Bisphosphonates | alendronate, etidronate, risedronate |
| -floxacin | Fluoroquinolones | moxifloxacin, levofloxacin, ciprofloxacin |
| Gli-/Gly- | Second generation sulfonylureas | gliclazide, glimepiride, glibenclamide/ glyburide |
| -ipramine | Tricyclic antidepressants | clomipramine, imipramine, desipramine |
| -lol | β-blockers | propranolol, metoprolol, labetalol |
| -mab | Monoclonal antibodies | rituximab, trastuzumab, bevacizumab |
| -micin/ -mycin | Aminoglycoside antibiotics | gentamicin, neomycin, tobramycin |
| -navir | Antiretroviral protease inhibitors | ritonavir, indinavir, saquinavir |
| -(pa)rin | Anticoagulants | heparin, warfarin, enoxaparin |
| -penem | Carbapenems | ertapenem, meropenem, imipenem |
| -platin | Platinating antineoplastics | cisplatin, carboplatin, oxaliplatin |
| -prazole | Proton pump inhibitors | omeprazole, pantoprazole, lansoprazole |
| -pressin | Antidiuretic hormones | desmopressin, vasopressin |
| -pril | ACE inhibitors | captopril, enalapril, lisinopril |
| -rubicin | Anthracycline antineoplastics | doxorubicin, daunorubicin, epirubicin |
| -sartan | Angiotensin II receptor blockers | losartan, irbesartan, valsartan |
| -(s)one | Corticosteroids | cortisone, prednisone, prednisolone |
| -statin | HMG-CoA reductase inhibitors | atorvastatin, lovastatin, pravastatin |

APPENDIX 1

| Prefixes/Suffices | Therapeutic Class | Examples |
| --- | --- | --- |
| -terol | β2-agonist bronchodilators | salmeterol, formoterol, albuterol |
| -thromycin | Macrolide antibiotics | erythromycin, clarithromycin, azithromycin |
| -tidine | H2-receptor antagonists | cimetidine, ranitidine, famotidine |
| -tilide | Class III antiarrhythmics | dofetilide, ibutilide |
| -triptan | Serotonin (5-HT) agonists | sumatriptan |
| -zepam/ -zolam | Benzodiazepines | midazolam, diazepam, lorazepam |
| -zosin | α-adrenergic blockers | prazosin, terazosin, doxazosin |

## REFERENCES

1. Browne A, Dugani S, Hutson J, McSheffrey G, Stefater M. *Pharmacology You See: A High-Yield Pharmacology Review for Health Professionals*, 1st ed. Toronto: McGraw-Hill; 2011.
2. Compendium of Pharmaceuticals and Specialties. Ottawa: Canadian Pharmacists Association. 2012. Available from http://www.e-therapeutics.ca.
3. Harvey R, Clark M, Finkel R, Rey J. *Lippincott's Illustrated Reviews: Pharmacology*, 5th ed. Baltimore: Lippincott Williams & Wilkins; 2011.
4. Micromedex Online. Greenwood Village: Thomson Reuters (Healthcare) Inc.; 2013.
5. Wells PS. Venous Thromboembolism. In Repchinsky C (Editor). *Therapeutic Choices*, 6th ed. Ottawa: Canadian Pharmacists Association; 2011.

APPENDIX 1

# APPENDIX 2:

# Common Laboratory Values

**Editors:**
Yuhao Shi, BSc

## TABLE OF CONTENTS

# 1. HEMATOLOGY

| Test | Conventional Units | SI Units / Notes |
|---|---|---|
| **Complete Blood Count (CBC)** | | |
| **Hemoglobin (Hb)** | M: 13.3-16.2 g/dL<br>F: 12.0-15.8 g/dL | M: 133-162 g/L<br>F: 120-158 g/L |
| **Hematocrit (Hct)** | M: 38.8-46.4%<br>F: 35.4-44.4% | M: 0.388-0.464<br>F: 0.354-0.444 |
| **Erythrocyte Count (RBC)** | M: 4.3-5.6 x $10^6$/mm$^3$<br>F: 4.0-5.2 x $10^6$/mm$^3$ | M: 4.3-5.6 x$10^{12}$/L<br>F: 4.0-5.2 x$10^{12}$/L |
| **Mean Corpuscular Volume**<br>(MCV=Hct/Hb) | 79.0-93.3 fL | 79.0-93.3 µm$^3$ |
| **Mean Corpuscular Hb**<br>(MCH=Hb/RBC) | 26.7-31.9 pg/cell | 26.7-31.9 pg/cell |
| **MCH Concentration**<br>(MCHC=MCH/MCV) | 32.3-35.9 g/dL | 323-359 g/L |
| **Leukocyte Count (WBC)** | 4.5-11.0 x $10^3$/mm$^3$ | 4.5-11.0 x $10^9$/L |
| **Differential Count**<br>Neutrophils<br>Bands<br>Lymphocytes<br>Monocytes<br>Eosinophils<br>Basophils | Percent (%)<br>40-70<br>0-5<br>20-50<br>4-8<br>0-6<br>0-2 | Cells x $10^9$/L<br>1.42-6.34<br>0-0.45<br>0.71-4.53<br>0.14-0.72<br>0-0.54<br>0-0.18 |
| **Platelet Count** | 1.65-4.15 x $10^5$/mm$^3$ | 165-415 x $10^9$/L |
| **Miscellaneous Hematology Values** | | |
| **Erythrocyte Sedimentation Rate (ESR)** | M: 0-15 mm/h<br>F: 0-20 mm/h | M: 0-15 mm/h<br>F: 0-20 mm/h |
| **Reticulocyte Count** | M: 0.8-2.3% of RBC's<br>F: 0.8-2.0% of RBC's | M: 0.008-0.023<br>F: 0.008-0.020 |

# 2. COAGULATION

| Test | Conventional Units | SI Units / Notes |
|---|---|---|
| **International Normalized Ratio (INR)** | 0.8-1.1 | 0.8-1.1 |
| **Prothrombin Time (PT)** | 12.7-15.4 s | 12.7-15.4 s |
| **Partial Thromboplastin Time** | 60-70 s | 1.5-2.5x greater<br>w/ anticoagulants |
| **Activated Partial Thromboplastin Time (aPTT)** | 25-35 s | |
| **Bleeding Time** | <7.1 min | <7.1 min |
| **D-dimer** | 220-740 ng/mL FEU | Low: not thrombosis |
| **Fibrinogen** | 233–496 mg/dL | Low: clotting |

# 3. SERUM CHEMISTRY

| Test | Conventional Units | SI Units / Notes |
|---|---|---|
| **Electrolytes** | | |
| **Sodium** | 136-146 mEq/L | Critical: <120, >160 |
| **Potassium** | 3.5-5.0 mEq/L | Critical: <2.5, >6.5 |

| Test | Conventional Units | SI Units / Notes |
|------|--------------------|--------------------|
| Chloride | 102-109 mEq/L | Critical: <80, >115 |
| Bicarbonate (HCO$_3$) | 22-30 mEq/L | Critical: <15, >40 |
| Anion Gap [Na-(Cl+HCO$_3$)] | 7-16 mEq/L | 12-20 mEq/L w/ K$^+$ |
| **Calcium**<br>Total<br>Ionized | 8.7-10.2 mg/dL<br>4.5-5.3 mg/dL | 2.2-2.6 mmol/L<br>1.12-1.32 mmol/L |
| Magnesium | 1.5-2.3 mg/dL | Critical: <0.5, >3 |
| Phosphorus | 2.5-4.3 mg/dL | 0.81-1.4 mmol/L |
| Lactate | Arterial: 4.5-14.4 mg/dL | Venous: 4.5-19.8 mg/dL |
| **Non-electrolytes** | | |
| Blood Urea Nitrogen (BUN) | 7-18 mg/dL | 2.5-6.4 mmol/L |
| Creatinine | M: 0.6-1.2 mg/dL<br>F: 0.5-0.9 mg/dL | M: 53-106 µmol/L<br>F: 44-80 µmol/L |
| Uric Acid | M: 3.1-7.0 mg/dL<br>F: 2.5-5.6 mg/dL | M: 180-410 µmol/L<br>F: 150-330 µmol/L |
| Glucose (fasting) | 75-100 mg/dL | 4.2-5.6 mmol/L |
| **Non-electrolytes** | | |
| Osmolality | 280-325 mOsm | Critical: <265, >320 |
| Osmolal Gap | <10 mOsm/kg | <10 mOsm/kg |
| **Liver / Pancreas Tests** | | |
| Alanine Aminotransferase (ALT) | 8-20 U/L | Viral hepatitis:<br>ALT/AST >1 |
| Aspartate Aminotransferase (AST) | 12-38 U/L | Liver disease: ALT/AST <1 |
| γ-Glutamyltransferase (GGT) | M: 9-50 U/L<br>F: 8-40 U/L | Marker of hepatobiliary disease and chronic alcohol use |
| Alkaline Phosphatase (ALP) | 30-120 U/L | Liver disease if elevated w/ 5'-nucleotidase, otherwise bone |
| 5'-Nucleotidase | 0-11 U/L | |
| **Bilurubin**<br>Total<br>Conjugated (direct)<br>Unconjugated (indirect) | 0.3-1.3 mg/dL<br>0.1-0.4 mg/dL<br>0.2-0.9 mg/dL | 5.1-22 µmol/L<br>1.7-6.8 µmol/L<br>3.4-15.2 µmol/L |
| Amylase | 20-96 U/L | Acute pancreatitis: rise in amylase paralleled w/ later rise in lipase |
| Lipase | 3-43 U/L | |
| Albumin | 4.0-5.9 g/dL | 40-50 g/L |
| **Lipids** | | |
| **Total Cholesterol**<br>Recommended<br>Moderate risk<br>High risk | <200 mg/dL<br>200-239 mg/dL<br>≥240 mg/dL | <5.2 mmol/L<br>5.2-6.2 mmol/L<br>≥6.2 mmol/L |

APPENDIX 2

| Test | Conventional Units | SI Units / Notes |
|------|--------------------|--------------------|
| **HDL-Cholesterol** | M: >29 mg/dL<br>F: >35 mg/dL | M: >0.75 mmol/L<br>F: >0.91 mmol/L |
| **LDL-Cholesterol**<br>  Recommended<br>  Moderate risk<br>  High risk | <br><130 mg/dL<br>130-159 mg/dL<br>≥160 mg/dL | <br><3.37 mmol/L<br>3.37-4.12 mmol/L<br>≥4.12 mmol/L |
| **Free Fatty Acids (FFAs)** | 8-25 mg/dL | 0.28-0.89 mmol/L |
| **Triglycerides (TG)** | M: 40-160 mg/dL<br>F: 35-135 mg/dL | M: 0.45-1.81 mmol/L<br>F: 0.40-1.52 mmol/L |
| **Apolipoprotein A-1** | 119-240 mg/dL | Component: HDL |
| **Apolipoprotein B** | 52-163 mg/dL | Component: LDL, VLDL |
| **Serum Proteins** | | |
| **Albumin** | 35-50 g/dL | High: dehydration; half-life of 12-18 days |
| **Serum Proteins** | | |
| **Immunoglobulins (Ig)** | IgA: 70-350 mg/dL<br>IgD: 0-14 mg/dL<br>IgE: 0-212 mg/dL<br>IgG: 700-1700 mg/dL<br>IgM: 50-300 mg/dL | 15% of Ig<br>rarely detected<br>allergic response<br>75% of Ig<br>ABO blood types and rheumatoid factor (RF); doesn't cross placenta |
| **Protein**<br>  Total<br>  Electrophoresis of globulins | <br>6.7-8.6 g/dL<br>$\alpha_1$: 0.2-0.4 g/dL<br>$\alpha_2$: 0.5-0.9 g/dL<br>$\beta$: 0.6-1.1 g/dL<br>$\gamma$: 0.7-1.7 g/dL | <br>67-86 g/L<br>$\alpha_1$: 2-4 g/L<br>$\alpha_2$: 5-9 g/L<br>$\beta$: 6-11 g/L<br>$\gamma$: 7-17 g/L |
| **C-Reactive Protein (CRP)** | <1.0 mg/dL | Cardiac risk indicator |
| **Markers for Neoplasia** | | |
| **α-Fetoprotein (αFP)** | <8.5 ng/mL | Detects fetal defects |
| **Carcinoembryonic Antigen (CEA)** | Non-smokers:<br><2.5 ng/mL | Smokers:<br><5.0 ng/mL |
| **Prostate Specific Antigen (PSA)** | <4.0 ng/mL | Cancerous: <10% free PSA |
| **CA-125** | 0-35 U/mL | Detects ovarian cancer |
| **Markers for Cardiac / Skeletal Muscle Injury** | | |
| **Lactate Dehydrogenase (LDH)** | 115–221 U/L | Peak: 2-3 d w/ MI |
| **Isoenzymes** | Fraction 1: 18-33%<br>Fraction 2: 28-40%<br>Fraction 3: 18-30%<br>Fraction 4: 6-16%<br>Fraction 5: 2-13% | Origin: heart, RBC<br>Origin: heart, lung<br>Origin: lung<br>Origin: kidney, pancreas<br>Origin: muscle, liver |
| **Creatine Kinase** | M: 0.87-5.0 µkat/L<br>F: 0.66-4.0 µkat/L | M: 51-294 U/L<br>F: 39-238 U/L |
| **CK-MB Isoenzyme** | 0-5.5 ng/mL | Myocardial cell specific |
| **Myoglobin** | M: 20-71 µg/L<br>F: 25-58 µg/L | Elevated within 3 h of MI |

| Test | Conventional Units | SI Units / Notes |
|---|---|---|
| **Cardiac Troponin I** | 0-0.04 ng/mL | Elevated until 7-10 d after MI |
| **Cardiac Troponin T** | 0-0.1 ng/mL | Elevated until 10-14 d after MI |
| **Nutrition** | | |
| **Folate** | | |
| Serum | 5.4-18 ng/mL | 12.2-40.8 nmol/L |
| Eyrthrocytes | 150-450 ng/mL | 340-1020 nmol/L |
| **Iron** | 41-141 µg/dL | 7-25 µmol/L |
| **Ferritin** | M: 15-200 ng/mL<br>F: 12-150 ng/mL | M: 15-200 µg/L<br>F: 12-150 µg/L |
| **Nutrition** | | |
| **Transferrin** | 200-400 mg/dL | Low: Fe deficiency anemia |
| **Total Iron Binding Capacity (TIBC)** | 300-360 µg/dL | Indirectly measures transferrin |

## 4. SERUM ENDOCRINE TESTS

| Tests | Conventional Units | SI Units / Notes |
|---|---|---|
| **Adrenocorticotropin Hormone (ACTH)** | | |
| 0800 hours | 10-60 pg/mL | 2.2-13.3 pmol/L |
| 1600 hours | <20 pg/mL | <4.5 pmol/L |
| **Aldosterone** | | |
| Supine | <16 ng/dL | <443 pmol/L |
| Upright | 4-31 ng/dL | 111-858 pmol/L |
| **β-human Chorionic Gonadotrophin (β-hCG)** | <5.0 mIU/mL | <5.0 IU/L |
| **Cortisol** | | |
| 0800 h | 8-20 µg/dL | 251-552 nmol/L |
| 1700 h | 3-13 µg/dL | 83-359 nmol/L |
| **C-Peptide** | 0.8-3.5 ng/mL | 0.27-1.19 nmol/L |
| **Dehydroepiandrosterone Sulfate (DHEAS)** | | |
| M: | 10-619 µg/dL | 0.9-17 µmol/L |
| F: Premenopausal | 12-535 µg/dL | 0.9-9.9 µmol/L |
| F: Postmenopausal | 30-260 µg/dL | <4.8 µmol/L |
| **Estradiol** | | |
| M: | <20 pg/mL | <184 pmol/L |
| F: Follicular phase | 20-145 pg/mL | 184-532 pmol/L |
| F: Ovulatory peak | 112-443 pg/mL | 411-1626 pmol/L |
| F: Luteal phase | 20-241 pg/mL | 184-885 pmol/L |
| F: Postmenopausal | <59 pg/mL | <217 pmol/L |
| **Follicle Stimulating Hormone (FSH)** | | |
| M: | 1.0-12.0 mIU/mL | 1.0-12.0 IU/L |
| F: Follicular phase | 3.0-20.0 mIU/mL | 3.0-20.0 IU/L |
| F: Ovulatory peak | 9.0-26.0 mIU/mL | 9.0-26.0 IU/L |
| F: Luteal phase | 1.0-12.0 mIU/mL | 1.0-12.0 IU/L |
| F: Postmenopausal | 18.0-153.0 mIU/mL | 18.0-153.0 IU/L |

APPENDIX 2

| Tests | Conventional Units | SI Units / Notes |
|---|---|---|
| **Growth Hormone (GH)** | M: <5 ng/mL<br>F: <10 ng/mL | M:<5 µg/L<br>F: <10 µg/L |
| **Hemoglobin A1C (Hb-A1C)** | <6% | Poor diabetic control >9% |
| **Luteinizing Hormone (LH)** | | |
| M: | 2.0-12.0 mIU/mL | 2.0-12.0 IU/L |
| F: Follicular phase | 2.0-15.0 mIU/mL | 2.0-15.0 IU/L |
| F: Ovulatory peak | 22.0-105.0 mIU/mL | 22.0-105.0 IU/L |
| F: Luteal phase | 0.6-19.0 mIU/mL | 0.6-19.0 IU/L |
| F: Postmenopausal | 16.0-64.0 mIU/mL | 16.0-64.0 IU/L |
| **Progesterone** | | |
| M: | <1.0 ng/mL | <3.18 nmol/L |
| F: Follicular phase | <1.0 ng/mL | <3.18 nmol/L |
| F: Luteal phase | 3-20 ng/mL | 9.54-63.6 nmol/L |
| **Prolactin** | | |
| M: | 2-18 ng/mL | 2-18 µg/L |
| F: Non-pregnant | 3-30 ng/mL | 3-30 µg/L |
| F: Pregnant | 10-209 ng/mL | 10-209 µg/L |
| F: Postmenopausal | 2-20 ng/mL | 2-20 µg/L |
| **Parathyroid Hormone (PTH)** | 8-51 pg/mL | Shows diurnal variation |
| **Serotonin (5-HT)** | 50-200 ng/mL | 0.28-1.14 umol/L |
| **Testosterone** | | |
| Free | M: 90-300 pg/mL<br>F: 3-19 pg/mL | M: 312-1041 pmol/L<br>F: 10.4-65.9 pmol/L |
| Total | M: 270-1070 ng/dL<br>F: 6-86 ng/dL | M: 9.36-37.10 nmol/L<br>F: 0.21-2.98 nmol/L |
| **Thyroid Stimulating Hormone (TSH)** | 0.5-5 µU/mL | Shows diurnal variation |
| **Thyroxine ($T_4$)** | | |
| Free | 0.7-1.24 ng/dL | 9-16 pmol/L |
| Total | 5-12 µg/dL | 65-155 nmol/L |
| **Triiodothyronine ($T_3$)** | | |
| Free | 2.4-4.2 pg/mL | 3.7-6.5 pmol/L |
| Total | 77-135 ng/dL | 1.2-2.1 nmol/L |
| **Vasoactive Intestinal Polypeptide (VIP)** | <60 pg/mL | <60 ng/L |

## 5. URINALYSIS

| Tests | Conventional Units | SI Units / Notes |
|---|---|---|
| **pH** | 5.0-9.0 | 5.0-9.0 |
| **Specific Gravity** | 1.001-1.035 | Easy to obtain |
| **Osmolality** | 50-1200 mOsm/kg | More exact results |
| **Creatinine** | 1.0-1.6 g/day | 8.8-14 mmol/d |
| **Creatinine Clearance** | M: 82-125 mL/min<br>F: 75-115 mL/min | M: 1.37-2.08 mL/s<br>F: 1.25-1.92 mL/s |
| **Urea Nitrogen** | 6-17 g/day | 214-607 mmol/d |
| **Sodium** | 100-260 mEq/d | 100-260 mmol/d |
| **Potassium** | 25-100 mEq/d | 25-100 mmol/d |
| **Calcium** | <300 mg/d | >7.5 mmol/d |

| Tests | Conventional Units | SI Units / Notes |
|---|---|---|
| Phosphate | 400-1300 mg/d | 12.9-42.0 mmol/d |
| Uric Acid | 250-800 mg/d | 1.49-4.76 mmol/d |
| Glucose | 50-300 mg/d | 0.3-1.7 mmol/d |
| Albumin | 10-100 mg/d | 0.01-0.1 g/d |
| Protein | <150 mg/d | <0.15 g/d |
| Urine Sediment<br>    Leukocytes<br>    Erythrocytes | <br>0-2/high power field<br>0-2/high power field | <br>0-2/high power field<br>0-2/high power field |
| Urinary Catecholamines | <100 µg/d | <5.91 nmol/d |
| Dopamine | 60-440 µg/d | 392-2876 nmol/d |
| Epinephrine | 0-20 µg/d | 0-109 nmol/d |
| Norepinephrine | 15-80 µg/d | 89-473 nmol/d |

## 6. CEREBROSPINAL FLUID (CSF)

| Tests | Conventional Units | SI Units / Notes |
|---|---|---|
| Cell Count | 0-5 cells/mm$^3$ | Presence of white blood cells is considered abnormal |
| Chloride | 116-130 mEq/L | Decreased with meningeal infections, tubercular meningitis, and low blood chloride levels; increased levels correlated with blood levels |
| Glucose | 40-70 mg/dL | 2.2-3.9 mmol/L; a level <60% of blood glucose level may indicate meningitis or neoplasm |
| Opening Pressure | 50-180 mmH$_2$O | If blockage in CSF circulation is suspected in the subarachnoid space, perform a Queckenstedt-Stookey test |
| Protein<br>    Albumin | <br>6.6-44.2 mg/dL | <br>Increased levels indicate a breakdown in the blood-brain barrier |
|     IgG | 0.9-5.7 mg/dL | Increased levels may be suggestive of inflammatory and autoimmune diseases of the CNS (e.g. MS) |
|     Lumbar | 15-50 mg/dL | Most common method; needle placed in the subarachnoid space of the spinal column |
|     Cisternal | 15-25 mg/dL | Needle placed below the occipital bone; done with fluoroscopy |
|     Ventricular | 6-15 mg/dL | Rarely done; recommended in people with possible brain herniation |

## 7. ARTERIAL BLOOD GASES

| Test | Conventional Units | SI Units/Notes |
|---|---|---|
| pH | 7.35-7.45 | Critical: <7.25, >7.55 |
| HCO$_3$ | 22–30 meq/L | Critical: <15, >40 |
| pCO$_2$ | 35–45 mmHg | Critical: <20, >60 |
| pO$_2$ | 80-100 mmHg | Critical: <40 |
| SaO$_2$ | 95-100% | Critical: ≤ 75% |

     ESSENTIALS OF CLINICAL EXAMINATION HANDBOOK, 8TH ED.

# 8. ASCITIC FLUID

| Condition | Gross Appearance | Protein, g/L | Cell Count | | Other Tests/ Notes |
|---|---|---|---|---|---|
| | | | Red Blood Cells, 10,000/µL | White Blood Cells /µL | |
| **Transudates** | Serum albumin: ascites albumin difference >11 g/L | | | | |
| **Cirrhosis** | Straw-colored or bile-stained | <25 (95%) | 1% | <250 (90%); predominantly mesothelial | Hepatic sinusoids have been damaged |
| **Congestive Heart Failure** | Straw-colored | Variable, 15-53 | 10% | <1000 (90%); usually mesothelial, mononuclear | Hepatic sinusoids are normal and allows passage of protein into the ascites |
| **Exudates** | Serum albumin: ascites albumin difference <11 g/L | | | | |
| **Neoplasm** | Straw-colored, hemorrhagic, mucinous, or chylous* | >25 (75%) | 20% | >1000 (50%); variable cell types | Cytology, cell block, peritoneal biopsy |
| **Tuberculous Peritonitis** | Clear, turbid, hemorrhagic, chylous | >25 (50%) | 7% | >1000 (70%); usually >70% lymphocytes | Peritoneal biopsy, stain and culture for acid-fast bacilli |
| **Pyogenic Peritonitis** | Turbid or purulent | If purulent, >25 | Unusual | Predominantly neutrophils | Positive Gram stain, culture |
| **Nephrosis** | Straw-colored or chylous | <25 (100%) | Unusual | <250; mesothelial, mononuclear | If chylous, ether extraction, Sudan staining |
| **Pancreatic Ascites (pancreatitis, pseudocyst)** | Turbid, hemorrhagic, or chylous | Variable, often >25 | Variable, may be blood-stained | Variable | Increased amylase in ascitic fluid and serum |

APPENDIX 2

# 9. PLEURAL FLUID

| Condition | Gross Appearance | pH | Glucose mmol/L | Amylase PF: Serum | Cell Count | |
|---|---|---|---|---|---|---|
| | | | | | Red Blood Cells (1000/mm³) | White Blood Cells (1000/mm³) |
| **Transudates** | Light's criteria: pleural fluid/serum protein <0.5 AND pleural fluid/serum LDH <0.6 AND pleural fluid LDH <2/3 upper normal serum limit | | | | | |
| **Congestive Heart Failure** | Clear, straw | >7.4 | >3.3 | ≤1 | 0-1 | <1 predominantly mononuclear |
| **Cirrhosis** | Clear, straw | >7.4 | >3.3 | ≤1 | <1 | <0.5 predominantly mononuclear |
| **Pulmonary Embolus: Atelectasis** | Clear, straw | >7.3 | >3.3 | ≤1 | <5 | 5-15 predominantly mononuclear |
| **Exudates** | Light's criteria: pleural fluid/serum protein >0.5 OR pleural fluid/serum LDH >0.6 OR pleural fluid LDH >2/3 upper normal serum limit | | | | | |
| **Pulmonary Embolus: Infarction** | Turbid to hemorrhagic, small volume | >7.3 | >3.3 | ≤1 | Bloody in 1/3 to 2/3 of patients | 5-15 predominantly neutrophils; may show many mesothelial cells |
| **Pneumonia** | Turbid | ≥7.3 | >3.3 | ≤1 | <5 | 5-40 predominantly neutrophils |
| **Empyema** | Turbid or purulent | 5.50-7.29 | <3.3 | ≤1 | <5 | 25-100 predominantly neutrophils |
| **TB** | Straw; serosanguineous in 15% | <7.3 (20%) | 1.7-3.3 (20%) | ≤1 | >10 | 5-10 predominantly mononuclear |
| **Malignancy** | Straw to turbid to bloody | <7.3 (30%) | <3.3 (30%) | ≤1 | 1 to >100 | <10 predominantly neutrophils |
| **RA Effusion** | Turbid or green or yellow | <7.3; usually ~7.0 | <1.7 (95%) | ≤1 | <1 | 1-20 neutrophils in acute; mononuclear in chronic |
| **SLE** | Straw to turbid | <7.3 (30% | <3.3 (30%) | ≤1 | <1 | Neutrophils in acute; mononuclear in chronic |
| **Rupture of Esophagus** | Purulent | 6.0 | N or D | >2 Salivary type | Can be bloody | Predominantly neutrophils |
| **Pancreatitis** | Serous to turbid to serosanguineous | >7.3 | >3.3 | >2 | 1-10 | 5-20 predominantly neutrophils |

## REFERENCES

1. Longo DL, et al. (Editors). *Harrison's Online*, 18th ed. 2012. Available from: http://accessmedicine.ca.
2. Porter RS, Kaplan JL. *The Merck Manual*, 19th ed. Appendix II, Table 1. 2011. Available from: http://www.merckmanuals.com.
3. Pagana KD, Pagana TJ. *Mosby's Manual of Diagnostic and Laboratory* Tests, 4th ed. St. Louis: Mosby; 2010.

APPENDIX 2

APPENDIX 3:

# Basics of Suturing and Needles

**Authors:**
Maya Deeb, HBSc
Mark Shafarenko

**Faculty Reviewers:**
Kyle Wanzel, MD, MEd, FRCSC

## SUTURE CHOICE[1]

### I. Suture Type

#### Absorable vs. Nonabsorbable (Permanent)
- **Absorbable:** Degrade and lose strength over time. Synthetic sutures degrade in a hydrolytic manner whereas natural sutures degrade in a proteolytic manner
- **Nonabsorbable:** Elicit a milder cell-mediated reaction to the suture. When removed, there is less inflammation and minimal scarring

*Indications:*
- Closure under slight tension: rapidly absorbing sutures are a good option
- Closures under short-term tension: absorbable sutures that can maintain strength for a longer period of time (4-6 weeks)
- Maintenance of long-term tension: permanent sutures

#### Monofilament vs. Multifilament (twisted or braided)
- **Monofilament:** single filament, easier gliding through tissue, less prone to infection, but knots are more difficult to tie and require more throws (lower knot security)
- **Multifilament:** multiple filaments twisted or braided together, stronger (higher knot security), more pliable, but may be more prone to weak spots

#### Barbed vs. Nonbarbed (twisted or braided)
- Barbed are useful in knotless closure, help to maintain tension
- Barbed are also faster to deploy
- Harder to backtrack with barbed sutures

**Table 1.** Suture Materials: Absorbable vs. Non-Absorbable and Monofilament vs. Multifilament[2]

| Suture Materials | Examples |
|---|---|
| **Non-absorbable, monofilament** | Nylon, polypropylene (Prolene®), stainless steel |
| **Non-absorbable, multifilament** | Silk, Ti-Cron®, Mersiline®, Ethibond® |
| **Absorbable, monofilament** | Monocryl®, Biosyn®, Caprosyn®, gut, chromic gut, fast absorbing gut |
| **Absorbable, multifilament** | Vicryl®, Polysorb® |

### II. Suture Caliber:

- Choose the smallest caliber that provides the strength required
- General guidelines[2]:
  - Face: 5-0 or 6-0
  - Body: 4-0 or 5-0
  - Tendon: 3-0 or 4-0

### III. Suture Needle:

#### Needle Point Configuration (Figure 1)[1]:
- Cutting needles:
  - Sharp edge along the full length of the needle tip
  - Permanent and absorbable sutures on cutting needles are used for subcutaneous, dermis, and skin closures
  - **Conventional cutting vs. reverse cutting needles:**
    - Conventional: sharp edge on the interior of the curve; may cut through skin edge and compromise closure
    - Reverse: sharp edge on the exterior of the curve; better for skin closure

- Taper needles:
  - Sharp tip, no sharp edges; less likely that the suture material would cut through tissue
  - Permanent sutures on taper needles are used for fascia, muscle, tendon, or cartilage under tension

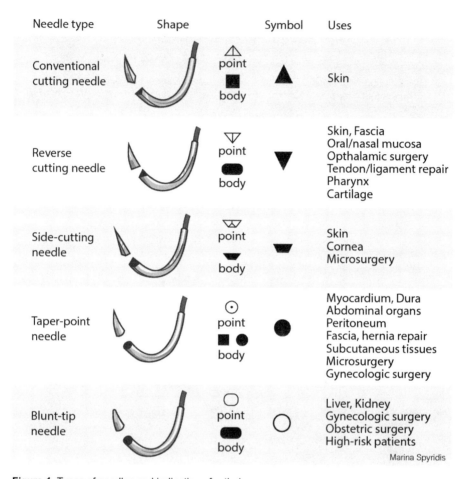

| Needle type | Shape | Symbol | Uses |
|---|---|---|---|
| Conventional cutting needle | | point △ ▲ body ■ | Skin |
| Reverse cutting needle | | point ▽ ▼ body ⬭ | Skin, Fascia Oral/nasal mucosa Opthalamic surgery Tendon/ligament repair Pharynx Cartilage |
| Side-cutting needle | | point ▽̱ ▼̱ body ▽̱ | Skin Cornea Microsurgery |
| Taper-point needle | | point ⊙ ● body ■ ● | Myocardium, Dura Abdominal organs Peritoneum Fascia, hernia repair Subcutaneous tissues Microsurgery Gynecologic surgery |
| Blunt-tip needle | | point ◯ ◯ body ⬭ | Liver, Kidney Gynecologic surgery Obstetric surgery High-risk patients |

Marina Spyridis

**Figure 1**. Types of needles and indications for their use

## SUTURING TECHNIQUES[2-3]

### A. Simple Interrupted Suture:
- Most commonly used suture
- Everts the skin edges. The edges will overlap if the suture is not placed at the same depth on both sides of the incision or wound
- Guidelines: place sutures roughly 5-7 mm apart and 1-2 mm from the skin edge

### B. Simple Running Suture (Continuous Over-and-Over Suture):
- Wound edges need to be approximated beforehand
- Not as precise as simple interrupted sutures
- Can provide hemostasis if placed in a locking fashion
- Useful in scalp closures

APPENDIX 3

### C. Vertical Mattress Suture:
- Used when skin eversion is difficult with simple sutures alone

### D. Horizontal Mattress Suture:
- Reliable skin edge approximation and eversion
- Good for thick skin (e.g. hands, feet) closure

### E. Subcuticular (Intradermal) Suture:
- Continuous fashion
- Needle passed horizontally through the superficial dermis, parallel to the skin surface
- Sutures must be placed at the same level
- Eliminates the need for external skin sutures
- Leaves no suture marks on the skin
- Cannot be used in trauma

### F. Half-Buried Horizontal Mattress Suture:
- Leaves suture marks on only one side of the suture line
- Used in cosmetically important areas

### G. Buried Deep Dermal Suture:
- Placed completely under the skin

Note: the most important techniques for clerks to know are simple interrupted, simple continuous, and subcuticular

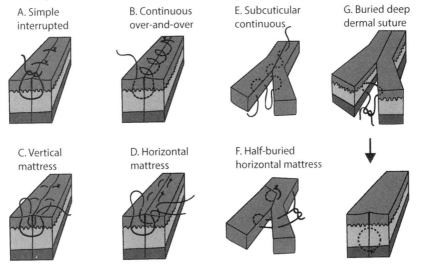

Alison McFadden

**Figure 2**. Suturing techniques. A. Simple interrupted, B. Continuous over-and-over, C. Vertical mattress, D. Horizontal mattress, E. Subcuticular continuous, F. Half-buried horizontal mattress, G. Buried deep dermal suture

## SUTURE REMOVAL[4]:

### Timing of Suture Removal
- Face (including lips): 5-7 d
- Eyelids: 3-5 d
- Hands/feet: 10-14 d
- Trunk: 7-10 d
- Breast: 7-10 d Note: if staples were used as opposed to sutures, remove as early as day 3 (regardless of site) and replace with Steri-strips

# REFERENCES

1. Janis, J. E. (2014). Essentials of plastic surgery (2nd ed.). Boca Raton, FL: CRC Press.
2. Merali, Z., & Woodfine, J. D. (2016). Toronto Notes 2016 (32nd ed.). Toronto, ON: Toronto Notes for Medical Students.
3. Thorne, C. H. (2014). Grabb and Smith's Plastic Surgery (7th ed.). Philadelphia, PA: Lippincott Wiliams & Wilkins.
4. Ashley SW (Editor). ACS Surgery: Principles and Practice. Hamilton: BC Decker; 2012.s

# INDEX

**Note:** Page numbers followed by *f* and *t* indicate figures and tables, respectively. Boxed materials are indicated by *b*.

INDEX

Apraxia, 216*t*
Arachnoid cyst, 78
Arboviral infections, 472*t*
Arcus cornealis, 89
Arcus senilis, 533
Areflexia, 227*t*
Arrhythmia(s), 23*t*, 44*t*, 45*f*, 217*t*, 441
    hypocalcemia and, 88
Arterial blood gases, 337
    laboratory values, 652
    normal values, 419, 419*t*
    pregnancy-related changes in, 283*t*
Arterial insufficiency, 52, 56, 59–62
Arterial occlusion
    acute, 57*t*, 59–61, 60*b*
    chronic, 58*t*, 61–62
Arterial palpation/auscultation, 53–55
Arthritis, 364*t*, 461. *See also* Gout;
    Osteoarthritis; Psoriatic arthritis;
    Rheumatoid arthritis (RA)
    Chlamydia trachomatis and, 461
    in HIV-infected (AIDS) patients, 460
    inflammatory vs. non-inflammatory, 213*t*
    juvenile idiopathic, 569*t*
    midfoot, 210
    septic, 197, 205, 569*t*
Arthropod bite, 357*t*
Articulation, testing/exam, 226
Ascending colon, 92*f*, 92*t*
Ascites
    in HIV-infected (AIDS) patients, 460
    imaging, 493, 493*f*
    and jugular venous pressure (JVP),
    101*b*
    malignant, 653
    pancreatic, 653
    tests for, 103, 103*f*
Ascitic fluid, 653
Asherman's syndrome, 265*t*
Ash leaf spots, 555
Aspiration, 330*t*
Aspirin
    adverse effects of, 382
    and gastrointestinal bleeding, 98
    ototoxicity, 119*t*
    overdose, 420
    toxicity/toxidrome, 403*t*, 589*t*
Asterixis, 228*t*
Asthma, 329*t*, 330*t*, 339, 339*t*, 342, 563,
563*t*, 564*b*, 642
    occupational, 333*t*
    testing for, 338
Astigmatism, 524
Astrocytoma, 243*t*
Asymmetric tonic neck reflex, 547*t*
Ataxia, 227*t*, 242*t*
    cerebellar, 239*t*
    cerebellar appendicular, 229*t*
Atelectasis, 481
    imaging, 481*f*–482*f*, 482
    pleural fluid with, 654

Atherosclerosis, 61
    risk factors for, 51
Athetosis, 228*t*
Athlete's foot. *See* Tinea pedis
Atopy, 563
Atrial fibrillation, 32*t*, 37*t*, 39–40
    on ECG, 44*t*
Atrial flutter, on ECG, 44*t*
Atrial septal defect, 33*t*, 564*t*
Atrioventricular (AV) block, 32*t*
    on ECG, 44*t*
Atrioventricular (AV) dissociation, 32*t*
Atrioventricular (AV) node, 19*f*, 20
Atrophy, 227*t*, 228*t*
Attention, assessment of, 606
Attention-deficit/hyperactivity disorder, 573
Auditory acuity testing, 121*t*
AUDIT questionnaire, 600
Auscultatory gap, 12
Autism spectrum disorders, 573
Autoimmune disorders
    neck pain caused by, 137*t*
    oral involvement in, 130*t*
Autoimmune polyglandular syndrome, 81,
    88
Automatisms, 229*t*
Avascular necrosis, of hip, 197
Axillae, palpation, in breast exam, 255
Axillary nerve, 232*f*
    mononeuropathy, 166
Axis (C2), 185*f*

## B
Babinski's sign, 235, 554
Backache, pregnancy-related, 284*t*
Back pain, 186, 227*t*
    acute, 50*t*
    common patterns of, 186*t*
    referred, 186
Bacterial vaginosis, 274*t*
Baker's cyst, ruptured, 203
Band keratopathy, 87*t*
Barbiturates
    adverse effects of, 382, 419
    nomenclature, 644
    toxidrome, 403*t*
Bariatric surgery, hypocalcemia due to, 88
Barium studies
    in gastritis, 501, 501*f*
    in peptic ulcer disease, 496
Barlow's test, 546–547, 547*f*, 553
Barrel chest, 188, 331, 333
Barrier protection, 9
Basal cell carcinoma (BCC), 376
    pigmented, 357*t*
    precursors, 378*t*
Basal ganglia, 227*t*, 228*t*
Basal skull fracture, 387, 388*f*
Battle's sign, 387
Beau's lines, 362, 363*t*, 364*f*

INDEX

INDEX

INDEX

INDEX

INDEX

INDEX

INDEX

Frontal lobe dysfunction, 241t
Frontal lobe tumor, 124t
Frontal sinus, 123f
Frozen shoulder. See Adhesive capsulitis
Functional residual capacity (FRC), 337f,
    338, 339t
Fundoscopy, 531–532, 532f
    in HIV-infected (AIDS) patients, 460
    in infant/child, 550
    in neonate, 545
Fungal infection
    cutaneous, 371–372, 371t
    systemic, 81
Funnel chest. See Pectus excavatum
Fusion inhibitors, 638

## G

Gag reflex, 134, 223t, 226
Gait
    antalgic, 164, 195, 200
    assessment, 164, 205, 445, 554
    in child, 554, 555
    in elderly, 445
    examination, 195, 239
    hemiplegic, 239t
    knee and, 200
    parkinsonian, 239t, 445
    pathologic patterns, 239, 239t
    scissor, 239t
    spastic, 215t, 239t
    Trendelenburg, 164, 195
    wide-based, 227t
Gait apraxia, 241t
Gait disorders, 215t
Galactosemia, 567t
Galant reflex, 547t
Gallbladder, 92f, 92t, 101–103
Gallbladder disease, abdominal pain
    caused by, 95t
Gallstones, 97, 110t
Gamma glutamyltransferase, laboratory
    values, 648
Ganglion cyst, 373t
    of hand, 182
    of wrist, 179
Gangrene, 52, 53, 471
    Fournier's, 470t
    streptococcal, 470t
Gas gangrene, 470t
Gastric cancer, 95t, 97
Gastric outlet obstruction, 93t, 101
Gastrinoma, 98t, 517
Gastritis, barium studies of, 501, 501f
Gastrocnemius muscle, testing/exam, 230t
Gastroenteritis, 93t, 96t
    acute, 565, 566t
    in children, 565, 566t
Gastroenterology, commonly used drugs in,
    634–635
Gastroesophageal reflux disease (GERD),

22t, 95t, 97, 108t, 329t
    and hoarseness, 141t
    nausea and vomiting in, 93t
Gastrointestinal (GI) bleeding, 98, 98t, 635
    drug-induced, in elderly, 448b
Gastrointestinal (GI) system
    anatomical regions of, 92f
    in children, 565–568
    exam
        in adolescent, 558
        in elderly, 445
        in neonate, 546
    malignancy, 93t
    obstruction, 93t, 96t, 98
    symptoms to ask about, 5t
Gastroparesis, 93t
Gastroschisis, 546
Gender history, 6–7
General anesthesia, 353
General anesthetics, 630
    nomenclature, 644
Generalized anxiety disorder, 598
Genetic disorders
    autosomal, 572t
    sex chromosome, 572t–573t
Genetics, and pharmacokinetics/
    pharmacodynamics, 583t
Genitalia. See also Female genitalia; Male
    genitalia
    ambiguous, 546
Genitourinary system. See also Female
    genitalia; Male genitalia
    common investigations, in adolescent,
        560
    exam, 316–319
        in adolescent, 556, 558
        in elderly, 445
        female-specific maneuvers, 319
        male-specific maneuvers, 317–318
        in neonate, 546
    female, in infant/child, 553
    male
        anatomy of, 310f
        in infant/child, 552–553
    pediatric male-specific disorders, 326
    in pediatric patient, 568–569
    symptoms to ask about, 5t, 6
Genogram, 3, 3f
Genohyoid muscle, 123f
Genu recurvatum, 200
Genu valgum, 10f, 200
    in child, 553
Genu varum, 10f, 200
    in infant, 553
Gerber lift-off test, 169t, 171, 171f, 172
Geriatric giants, 444t
Geriatric patient(s)
    activities of daily living, assessment,
        443
    adverse effects of medications in, 448b
    anxiety in, 441

INDEX

Growth hormone–releasing hormone (GHRH), 79f
Guarding, voluntary vs. involuntary, 106
Guillain-Barré syndrome, 218t, 419
    neonatal, 566t
Gum hypertrophy, 134t
Guyon's ulnar nerve entrapment, 177
Gynecology
    adnexal exam, 271, 272
    benign neoplasms in, 275t–276t
    common chief complaints, 265t–266t
    common investigations, 272t
    drugs commonly used in, 640
    general screening exam, 16t
    history-taking in, 266–268
    malignant neoplasms in, 276t–277t
    rectovaginal exam, 272
    speculum examination, 269–270, 269f
Gynecomastia, 71t, 101, 559

# H

Haemophilus influenzae
    otitis media, 561
    pneumonia, 341t
    sepsis, 467t
Hair
    examination, 362
    general screening exam, 15t
    hypocalcemia and, 88
    hypothyroidism and, 84, 85t
HAIR-AN syndrome, 86t
Hair loss, 362. See also Alopecia
    history-taking for, 358
    metabolic reproductive syndrome and, 85
    telogen, 373b
Hair pull test, 373
Hairy leukoplakia, 460
Hallucinations, 597, 604, 604t, 611
    command, 601
    history-taking about, 600
Hallucinogens, abuse, 598
Hallux valgus, 210
Hamstrings
    distal, tendinopathy, 203
    strain/tear, 199
    testing/exam, 230t
Hand(s)
    abnormalities, 364t
    deformities of, 182t–183t, 183f
    FOOSH-related injury, 185
    foot and mouth disease, 470t
    history-taking for, 182
    ligamentous injury, 184
    liver disease and, 101
    nerves of, 181–182
    pain in, 182
    physical exam, 11, 182–184
    range of motion, 183, 184t
    swelling of, 182

Hand hygiene, 9
Hand preference, in very young child, 555
Hard palate, 123f
Hashimoto's thyroiditis, 71t, 84, 557
Hashish/hash oil, abuse/recreational use, 590t
Hawkins-Kennedy test, 169t, 171
Headache, 215t, 242t–243t. See also Migraine
    causes, 402t
    cluster, 215t, 242t
    differential diagnosis, 571t
    history-taking for, 402
    in hyperthermia, 391t
    illness-related, 571t
    investigations, 246t
    management, 246t
    onset, 402
    in pediatric patient, 571
    physical exam for, 246t, 402
    quality, 402
    tension, 215t, 242t, 402, 571t
    thunderclap, 215t, 242t
    timing, 402
    trauma-related, 571t
Head and neck
    general screening exam, 15t
    inspection, 138
    lymph node groups of, 135f, 136t
    palpation, 138
    physical exam, 9, 9t–11t
        in adolescent, 556
        in infant/child, 548
        neonatal, 544–545
        in trauma, 387
    symptoms to ask about, 4t
Head circumference
    of infant/child, 548
    neonatal, 544
Head injury, in children, 575
HE2ADS3 assessment, for adolescent, 555–556
Head trauma, anosmia after, 124t
Hearing, assessment, in infant/child, 550
Hearing loss, 227t
    autoimmune, 118t
    conductive, 118t, 225, 225t, 226b
    in elderly, 444
    medication-induced, 118t
    noise-induced, 118t
    sensorineural, 118t, 225, 225t, 636
Heart. See also entries under Cardiac
    anatomy of, 19f
    blood supply to, 19
    on chest X-ray, 479
    electrical conduction system, 19f, 20
    innervation of, 20
    physiology, 19–20
    valvular dysfunction, 23t, 24t
    venous drainage of, 20
Heart block, 26t, 32t

INDEX

INDEX

INDEX

physical exam and investigations in, 296–299
postterm, 295
preterm, 285t, 295, 299
speculum exam in, 299
stages of, 300–302
term, 295
true, 295, 296t
Labral tear, 165, 198
Lachman test, for anterior cruciate ligament tear, 201
Lacrimal apparatus, 531, 531f
Lactate, serum, laboratory values, 648
Lactate dehydrogenase (LDH), serum, 649
Lactic acidosis, 420
Lactose intolerance, diarrhea caused by, 94t
Langerhans cell histiocytosis, 572
Language exam, 219t
Lanugo, 558
Large bowel obstruction, imaging, 494f, 495
Large for gestational age (LGA) infant, 544
Laryngitis, 131t
Laryngocele, 137t
Larynx, 123f, 133t
Lasègue test. See Straight leg raise test
Lassa fever, 472t
Lateral collateral ligament, special test for, 202
Lateral epicondylitis, 173t, 176
Lavender oil, adverse effects of, 71t
Laxatives, 635
diarrhea caused by, 94t, 98
Lead, ototoxicity, 119t
Lead-pipe rigidity, 229, 229t
LEA Symbols chart, 549
Left atrium, 19, 19f
enlargement, 45, 45f
Left ventricle, 19, 19f
Left ventricular failure, 32t
Left ventricular hypertrophy, 33t
on ECG, 45
Leg(s), rubor on dependency, 56
Legg-Calvé-Perthes disease, 569t, 570
Legionella, pneumonia, 341t
Leg length
discrepancy, acceptable, 195
measurement of, 195
Leg pain, 52
acute onset nontraumatic, 50t
constant, 50t
intermittent, 50t
musculoskeletal, 50t
referred, 162
Leiomyomata. See Fibroids, uterine
Leishmaniasis, 473t
cutaneous, 470t, 473t
visceral, 472t, 473t
Lentigines, 378
Lentigo maligna melanoma, 357t
Leopold's maneuvers, 290, 292t

Leprosy, 470t
Leptospirosis, 472t
Leriche's syndrome, 61
Leukemia(s), 516–517, 558, 569t
Leukocoria, 549t
Leukocyte count, 647
Leukonychia, 363t
Leukoplakia, 134t
Leukorrhea, pregnancy-related, 284t
Leukotriene inhibitor, for asthma, 642
Lichenification, 362
Lichen planopilaris, 374
Lichen planus, 357t, 361t, 381t
Lichen sclerosus, 275t
Li-Fraumeni syndrome, 516–517
Light's criteria, for pleural fluid, 654
Likelihood ratios (LRs), 625
Limb ischemia
acute, 50t, 51–52
chronic, 50t
critical, 50t, 52, 61
Limp. See also Gait
in children, 569
painful, differential diagnosis, 569t–570t
Lindsay's nails, 363t, 364f
Lingual tonsil, 123f, 147t
Lingula, 329f
Lipase, pancreatic, laboratory values, 648
Lipemia retinalis, 89
Lipids, serum, laboratory values, 648–649
Lipoma, 359t
neck swelling caused by, 137t
Lipoprotein lipase (LPL), deficiency, 88
Lisfranc injury, 210
Listeria, 463t, 467
Lithotomy position, 268, 268f
Livedo reticularis, 53
Liver, 92f, 92t
abscess, 94t
exam, 101–103
laboratory tests, 648
palpation, 102, 102f
in neonate, 546
percussion, 102, 102f
Liver disease, 97
abdominal pain caused by, 94t
cholestatic, 88, 98
dermatological manifestations, 381, 381t
and gastrointestinal bleeding, 98
and jugular venous pressure (JVP), 101b
Liver failure, 71t, 72t, 75, 420
color abnormalities in, 9t
Liver span, 102
Load and shift test (shoulder), 167t
Lobule (ear), 116f
Local anesthesia, 352t
Local anesthetic systemic toxicity (LAST), 352
Lochia, 303

INDEX

INDEX

INDEX

in mental status exam, 604
Mood stabilizers, 642
Moon facies, 10t, 381t
Moraxella catarrhalis, otitis media, 561
Morning sickness, 94t
Moro reflex, 547t
    asymmetric, 547
Morton's neuroma, 210
Motility disorder, 93t
    diarrhea caused by, 94t
Motor activity, in mental status exam, 603
Motor exam, in infant/child, 554–555
Mouth, exam
    in infant/child, 550
    in neonate, 545
Movement(s)
    abnormal, 228t–229t
    involuntary, 227t
MRCP. See Magnetic resonance
    cholangiopancreatography (MRCP)
Mucosa, vasculitis and, 53
Multiple endocrine neoplasia, 81, 87, 517
Multiple myeloma (MM), 71t
Multiple sclerosis (MS), 215t–218t,
    238t–240t, 247t, 311, 639
    and diplopia, 526t
    imaging, 509
    RAPD in, 223b
    signs and symptoms, 245t
Multivitamins, for pregnant patient, 640
Murphy's sign, 106t
Muscle(s)
    examination, 228
    lesions, 227t
    myotomal distribution, 230t
    strength
    wasting/weakness, distribution, and
        cause, 228t
    weakness, 164, 227t
Muscle pain, 215t
Muscle relaxants, 630
Muscle tension dysphonia, 131t
Muscle tone, 229
    abnormal, causes, 229t
    assessment, in infant, 554
Musculocutaneous nerve, 232f
Musculoskeletal exam, 162–164
    in elderly, 445
    general screening, 16t
    in infant/child, 553–554
    neonatal, 546–547
    screening, in child, 554
    in trauma, 388
Musculoskeletal injury(ies), in children, 570
Musculoskeletal system
    drugs commonly used in, 638–639
    history-taking for, 162
    imaging, 509–511
    power assessments/isometric
        movements, 164
    symptoms to ask about, 5t

Myalgia, 227t, 461
    in hyperthermia, 391t
Myasthenia gravis (MG), 131t, 216t, 218t,
    530
    and diplopia, 526t
Mycobacteria, osteomyelitis, 468–469
Mycobacterium avium complex, in HIV-
    infected (AIDS) patients, 474t
Mycobacterium tuberculosis. See
    Tuberculosis
Mycophenolate mofetil, diarrhea caused by,
    94t, 98
Mycoplasma pneumoniae, pneumonia, 341t
Mycosis fungoides, 357t
Mydriasis, 223t, 533, 549t
Myocardial infarct/infarction, 20t, 95t, 97.
    See also Non-ST-segment elevation
    myocardial infarction (NSTEMI); ST-
    segment elevation myocardial infarction
    (STEMI)
    acute, 38, 46, 47f, 632
    acute Q-wave, 46, 47f
    chest X-ray and, 490
    investigations for, 35t
    localization, 47t
    non-Q wave, 47
    silent, 38
    transmural, on ECG, 46
Myocardial ischemia, 46
Myocardial perfusion imaging, in angina
    with nondiagnostic ECG, 490
Myoclonus, 228t
Myoglobin, serum, laboratory values, 649
Myokimia, 215t
Myonecrosis, 26t, 470t
    clostridial, 470t
Myopathy, 215t, 229t
Myopia, 524, 527t
Myositis, 215t, 470t, 471
Myotome(s)
    of upper and lower limbs, 230t, 231f
Myringitis, 117t
Myxedema, 218t
Myxedema coma, 84

# N

Naegele's rule, 288
Nail(s). See also Clubbing, of nails
    anorexia nervosa and, 561
    atrophy, 381t
    brittle, 381t
    changes, history-taking for, 358
    disease and, 363t, 364f
    examination, 362
    general screening exam, 15t
    hypocalcemia and, 88
    hypothyroidism and, 85t
    liver disease and, 101
    palpation, 363t
    physical exam, 11

INDEX

INDEX

INDEX

INDEX

INDEX

INDEX

of external ear, 117t
head, 215t
history-taking in, 387
of middle ear, 117t
neck pain caused by, 137t
physical exam in, 387–388
in pregnancy, 285t
rapid primary survey (RPS) of, 385–387
secondary survey in, 387–388
and sensory loss, 238t
vaginal, 265t
Traumatic brain injury, 245t, 247t
Travel-related illness, 471–473
Tremor, 216t, 227t, 229t
classification of, 240t
drug-induced, 216t
essential, 229t, 240t
functional, 240t
in hand, 364t
intention, 227t, 229t, 240t
physiological, 216t, 229t, 240t
postural/action, 240t
resting, 240t
Trendelenburg test, 195
Triangular fibrocartilaginous complex
(TFCC) injury, 179
Triazoles, 637
Triceps muscle, testing/exam, 230t
Triceps tendon reflex, 234
Trichiasis, 531
Trichomoniasis, 461t
Tricuspid regurgitation, 33t, 34t
Tricuspid valve, 19f
Tricyclic antidepressants, 610, 635, 641,
642
adverse effects of, 419
drug–drug interactions with, 585t
for neuropathic pain, 350, 351f
nomenclature, 644
toxicity/toxidrome, 403t, 590t
for urinary incontinence, 643
Trigeminal neuralgia, 124t, 402
Trigger finger, 182, 183f, 184
Triglycerides, serum
increased, 88–89
laboratory values, 649
Triiodothyronine (T3), 79f, 82
overproduction, 82
serum, laboratory values, 651
Tripoding, 333
Trisomy 13, prenatal diagnosis, 294t
Trisomy 18. See Edwards syndrome
Trisomy 21. See Down's syndrome
Trochanteric bursa, 194f
Troponins, cardiac, 35t, 400t
laboratory values, 650
Trousseau's sign, 88, 415, 415f
Tryptophan, 641
Tubal tonsils, 147t
Tuberculin skin test, 457, 457f, 457t
Tuberculosis, 78, 81, 87, 228t, 330t, 339,

340t, 453t, 456–458, 472t, 637
diagnosis, 158, 456–457, 457f
extrapulmonary, 458t
history-taking for, 456
in HIV-infected (AIDS) patients, 459t,
474t
lymph node involvement in, 149t, 150t,
158
management of, 158
miliary, 158, 458t
multidrug resistant, 458, 458t
neck swelling/mass in, 137t
physical exam in, 456
pleural fluid in, 654
pulmonary, 456–458, 458t
Tuberous sclerosis, 555
Tubo-ovarian abscess, 265t
Tumescent anesthesia, 352t
Tumor(s). See also Neoplasms/neoplasia
and abnormal vaginal bleeding, 265t
cerebral, 238t
CNS, 516
of external ear, 118t
intracranial, 216t
of middle ear, 118t
nasal, 125t
neck pain caused by, 137t
nervous system, 215t
neurological, 243t
neurologic disorders caused by, 218t
oropharyngeal, 130t
respiratory symptoms with, 330t
retrobulbar, 527t
skin, 359t
testicular, 316t
Tumor lysis syndrome, 521t
Turf toe, 210
Turner syndrome, 545, 572t
Two-point discrimination test, 238
Tympanic membrane
anatomy of, 116f
otoscopic exam of, 121, 122t
perforation, 118t
Tympanometry, 122t
Typhoid, 472t

## U

Uhthoff effect, 216*t*
Ulcer(s)
aphthous, 130*t*, 134*t*
arterial, 50*t*
corneal, 534, 534*b*
diabetic, 50*t*, 74
gastric, 97
in HIV-infected (AIDS) patients, 460
malignant, 50*t*
nasal, 53
oral, 53, 130*t*, 132
skin, 50*t*, 52, 53, 360*f*, 362, 470*t*
traumatic, 50*t*

INDEX

INDEX

INDEX

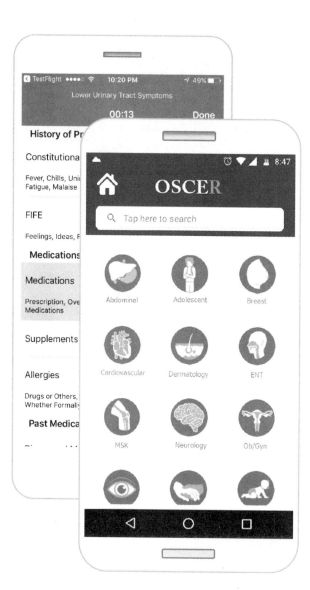

# OSCE**R**

Available in September, 2017!

Use the new companion mobile app to the Essentials of Clinical Examination Handbook, 8th ed. to prepare for your next Objective Structured Clinical Exam (OSCE)!

Visit:
http://www.thieme.com for more details.

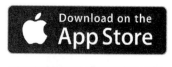

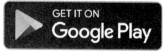